PEDIATRIC NEUROPSYCHOLOGY

Also Available

Developmental Social Neuroscience
and Childhood Brain Insult: Theory and Practice
Edited by Vicki Anderson and Miriam H. Beauchamp

Diagnosing Learning Disorders,
Third Edition: From Science to Practice
Bruce F. Pennington, Lauren M. McGrath, and Robin L. Peterson

Mild Traumatic Brain Injury
in Children and Adolescents
Edited by Michael W. Kirkwood and Keith Owen Yeates

Pediatric Neuropsychology

Research, Theory, and Practice

THIRD EDITION

Edited by
Miriam H. Beauchamp
Robin L. Peterson
M. Douglas Ris
H. Gerry Taylor
Keith Owen Yeates

THE GUILFORD PRESS
New York London

A Division of Guilford Publications, Inc.
370 Seventh Avenue, Suite 1200, New York, NY 10001
www.guilford.com

Printed in the United States of America

This book is printed on acid-free paper.

The authors have checked with sources believed to be reliable in their efforts to provide information that is complete and generally in accord with the standards of practice that are accepted at the time of publication. However, in view of the possibility of human error or changes in behavioral, mental health, or medical sciences, neither the authors, nor the editors and publisher, nor any other party who has been involved in the preparation or publication of this work warrants that the information contained herein is in every respect accurate or complete, and they are not responsible for any errors or omissions or the results obtained from the use of such information. Readers are encouraged to confirm the information contained in this book with other sources.

Last digit is print number: 9 8 7 6 5 4 3 2 1

Library of Congress Cataloging-in-Publication Data

Names: Beauchamp, Miriam H., editor.
Title: Pediatric neuropsychology : research, theory, and practice / edited by Miriam H. Beauchamp, Robin L. Peterson, M. Douglas Ris, H. Gerry Taylor, Keith Owen Yeates.
Description: Third edition. | New York : The Guilford Press, [2022] |
Includes bibliographical references and index. |
Identifiers: LCCN 2022003459 | ISBN 9781462549443 (cloth)
Subjects: LCSH: Pediatric neuropsychology. | BISAC: PSYCHOLOGY / Neuropsychology | MEDICAL / Psychiatry / Child & Adolescent
Classification: LCC RJ486.5 .P435 2022 | DDC 618.92/8–dc23/eng/20220225
LC record available at *https://lccn.loc.gov/2022003459*

About the Editors

Miriam H. Beauchamp, PhD, is Professor in the Department of Psychology at the University of Montréal, Québec, Canada, and Researcher at the Sainte-Justine Hospital Research Centre, where she leads the ABCs Developmental Neuropsychology Laboratory. Dr. Beauchamp holds the Canada Research Chair in Pediatric Traumatic Brain Injury. She has received early career awards from the International Neuropsychological Society and the International Brain Injury Association, held the inaugural Québec–Bruxelles Chair at the Royal Academy of Sciences in Belgium, and was inducted into the College of New Scholars, Artists, and Scientists of the Royal Society of Canada. In 2017, she was recognized as Québec's most promising early-career researcher. Her research interests include pediatric traumatic brain injury and social neuroscience. She is registered with the Québec Psychology Board and certified in neuropsychological assessment.

Robin L. Peterson, PhD, ABPP-CN, is a pediatric neuropsychologist at Children's Hospital Colorado and Assistant Professor of Physical Medicine and Rehabilitation at the University of Colorado School of Medicine. Dr. Peterson is an investigator with the Colorado Learning Disabilities Research Center, where her research has examined the overlap among different neurodevelopmental disorders. She also has clinical and research interests in pediatric traumatic brain injury and spina bifida. Dr. Peterson is board certified in clinical neuropsychology and pediatric clinical neuropsychology. She previously taught kindergarten and first grade.

M. Douglas Ris, PhD, ABPP-CN, is Distinguished Emeritus Professor and former Head of the Psychology Section in the Department of Pediatrics, Baylor College of Medicine, and former Chief of the Psychology Service at Texas Children's Hospital in Houston. Previously, he founded and directed the Neuropsychology Program and the Pediatric Neuropsychology Postdoctoral Program at Cincinnati Children's Hospital Medical Center. Dr. Ris has held leadership positions in the Society for Clinical Neuropsychology (Division 40 of the American Psychological Association), the American Board of Clinical

Neuropsychology, the International Neuropsychological Society, and the American Association of Postdoctoral Programs in Clinical Neuropsychology. His research interests include the neurodevelopmental effects of exposure to environmental lead and late effects in pediatric brain tumors.

H. Gerry Taylor, PhD, ABPP-CN, is a pediatric neuropsychologist at the Center for Biobehavioral Health (CBH) at the Abigail Wexner Research Institute, Nationwide Children's Hospital, Columbus, Ohio, and Professor of Pediatrics at The Ohio State University. Dr. Taylor heads an initiative at CBH to further understanding of neurodevelopmental outcomes for children with brain-related disorders. He has contributed to research on several neurodevelopmental conditions, including preterm birth, traumatic brain injury, and speech sound disorders, as well as to clinical trials for children with sleep disorders and young adults with Down syndrome. Dr. Taylor is also collaborating on the creation of a parent-based assessment of infant development. His research aims to increase knowledge about child and family consequences of brain-related disorders as well as medical and environmental factors that predict child development.

Keith Owen Yeates, PhD, ABPP-CN, is the Ronald and Irene Ward Chair in Pediatric Brain Injury, Professor and Head of the Department of Psychology, and Adjunct Professor of Pediatrics and Clinical Neurosciences at the University of Calgary, Alberta, Canada. His influential research focuses on the outcomes of childhood brain disorders, especially traumatic brain injury. A recently published bibliometric analysis indicates that Dr. Yeates has authored more of the top 100 most-cited papers in pediatric traumatic brain injury than any other researcher. Dr. Yeates is the inaugural Chair of the Canadian Concussion Network and is Editor-in-Chief of *Neuropsychology*. He has served as President of the Society for Clinical Neuropsychology (Division 40 of the American Psychological Association) and the International Neuropsychological Society.

Contributors

Peter J. Anderson, PhD, Turner Institute for Brain and Mental Health, School of Psychological Sciences, Monash University, Melbourne, Australia

Vicki Anderson, PhD, Clinical Sciences, Murdoch Children's Research Institute; Psychological Sciences, University of Melbourne; and Psychology, Royal Children's Hospital, Melbourne, Australia

Miriam H. Beauchamp, PhD, Department of Psychology, University of Montreal, and Sainte-Justine Hospital Research Centre, Montréal, Québec, Canada

Gemma Bernes, MA, Center for Behavioral Teratology and Department of Psychology, San Diego State University, San Diego, California

Jane Holmes Bernstein, PhD, Department of Psychiatry and Behavioral Sciences, Center for Neuropsychology, Boston Children's Hospital, and Department of Psychiatry, Harvard Medical School, Boston, Massachusetts

Adam R. Cassidy, PhD, LP, ABPP, Department of Psychiatry and Psychology and Department of Pediatric and Adolescent Medicine, Mayo Clinic, Rochester, Minnesota; Department of Psychiatry and Behavioral Sciences, Center for Neuropsychology, and Department of Psychiatry, Boston Children's Hospital, Harvard Medical School, Boston, Massachusetts

Paul T. Cirino, PhD, Department of Psychology, Texas Institute for Measurement, Evaluation, and Statistics (TIMES), University of Houston, Houston, Texas

Kirsty L. Coulter, MS, EdM, Department of Psychological Sciences, University of Connecticut, Storrs, Connecticut

Mary F. S. Dieckhaus, MS, Department of Psychological Sciences, University of Connecticut, Storrs, Connecticut

Deborah Fein, PhD, Department of Psychological Sciences, University of Connecticut, Storrs, Connecticut

Gerard A. Gioia, PhD, Children's National Hospital and George Washington University School of Medicine, Washington, DC

Anne Gordon, PhD, Pediatric Neuroscience Department, Evelina London Children's Hospital, Guy's and St. Thomas' NHS Foundation Trust, and Population Health Sciences, King's College London, London, United Kingdom

Mardee Greenham, PhD, Clinical Sciences, Murdoch Children's Research Institute, Melbourne, Australia

Caroline Greiner de Magalhães, MS, Department of Psychological Sciences, University of Connecticut, Storrs, Connecticut

Tammy Hedderly, MBBS FRCPCH BSc (Hons), TANDeM Clinic, Evelina London Children's Hospital, Guy's and St. Thomas' NHS Foundation Trust, and King's Health Partnership, London, United Kingdom

David Hessl, PhD, MIND Institute, University of California Davis Medical Center, Sacramento, California

Peter K. Isquith, PhD, Department of Psychiatry, Dartmouth Geisel School of Medicine, Hanover, New Hampshire

Lisa A. Jacobson, PhD, NCSP, ABPP, Department of Neuropsychology, Kennedy Krieger Institute, and Department of Psychiatry and Behavioral Sciences, Johns Hopkins University School of Medicine, Baltimore, Maryland

Renée Lajiness-O'Neill, PhD, Department of Psychology, Eastern Michigan University, Ypsilanti, Michigan; Department of Physical Medicine and Rehabilitation, University of Michigan—Ann Arbor, Ann Arbor, Michigan

Rebecca I. LaQuaglia, BS, Department of Psychological and Brain Sciences, Drexel University, Philadelphia, Pennsylvania

Nancy Raitano Lee, PhD, Department of Psychological and Brain Sciences, Drexel University, Philadelphia, Pennsylvania

Mark T. Mackay, MBBS, PhD, Clinical Sciences, Murdoch Children's Research Institute; Neurology, Royal Children's Hospital; and Department of Pediatrics, University of Melbourne, Melbourne, Australia

E. Mark Mahone, PhD, ABPP, private practice, Baltimore, Maryland

Osman Malik, MBBS, MRCPsych, TANDeM Clinic, Evelina London Children's Hospital, Guy's and St. Thomas' NHS Foundation Trust, and King's Health Partnership, London, United Kingdom

Davide Martino, PhD, MD, Department of Clinical Neurosciences, University of Calgary; Alberta Children's Hospital Research Institute; and Hotchkiss Brain Institute, Calgary, Alberta, Canada

Sarah N. Mattson, PhD, Center for Behavioral Teratology and Department of Psychology, San Diego State University, San Diego, California

Carolyn B. Mervis, PhD, Department of Psychological and Brain Sciences, University of Louisville, Louisville, Kentucky

Eileen M. Moore, PhD, Center for Behavioral Teratology and Department of Psychology, San Diego State University, San Diego, California

Bruce F. Pennington, PhD, Department of Psychology, University of Denver, Denver, Colorado

Robin L. Peterson, PhD, ABPP, Children's Hospital Colorado and University of Colorado School of Medicine, Aurora, Colorado

Klajdi Puka, PhD, Institute for Mental Health Policy Research, Center for Addiction and Mental Health (CAMH), Toronto, Ontario, Canada

M. Douglas Ris, PhD, ABPP-CN, Distinguished Emeritus Professor, Department of Pediatrics, Baylor College of Medicine, Houston, Texas

Robert M. Roth, PhD, ABPP, Department of Psychiatry, Geisel School of Medicine at Dartmouth/Dartmouth-Hitchcock Medical Center, Lebanon, New Hampshire

Andrea Schneider, PhD, MIND Institute, University of California Davis Medical Center, Sacramento, California; College of Psychology, California Northstate University, Elk Grove, California

David D. Schwartz, PhD, ABPP, Department of Pediatrics, Baylor College of Medicine, and Texas Children's Hospital, Houston, Texas

Haleigh Scott, PhD, College of Psychology, California Northstate University, Elk Grove, California

Margaret Semrud-Clikeman, PhD, Department of Pediatrics (Emerita), University of Minnesota Medical School, Minneapolis, Minnesota

Rebecca Shields, MS, Human Development Graduate Group, University of California Davis, Davis, California

Yuri Shishido, PhD, Department of Neuropsychology, Children's National Hospital, and George Washington University School of Medicine, Washington, DC

Mary Lou Smith, PhD, Department Psychology, University of Toronto, Mississauga, Ontario, Canada

Catherine Stephan, MS, Department of Psychological and Brain Sciences, Drexel University, Philadelphia, Pennsylvania

Casey E. Swick, MS, Department of Psychology, Eastern Michigan University, Ypsilanti, Michigan

H. Gerry Taylor, PhD, ABPP-CN, Abigail Wexner Research Institute at Nationwide Children's Hospital, and Department of Pediatrics, The Ohio State University, Columbus, Ohio

Rebecca P. Thomas, MA, Department of Psychological Sciences, University of Connecticut, Storrs, Connecticut

Linnea Vaurio, PhD, Department of Psychiatry, NYU Grossman School of Medicine, New York, New York

Rachel M. Wasserman, PhD, Center for Healthcare Delivery Science, Department of Behavioral Health, Nemours Children's Hospital, Orlando, Florida

Erik G. Willcutt, PhD, Department of Psychology and Neuroscience, University of Colorado Boulder, Boulder, Colorado

Keith Owen Yeates, PhD, RPsych, ABPP, FCAHS, FRSC, Departments of Psychology, Pediatrics, and Clinical Neurosciences, University of Calgary; Alberta Children's Hospital Research Institute, University of Calgary; and Hotchkiss Brain Institute, University of Calgary, Calgary, Alberta, Canada

T. Andrew Zabel, PhD, ABPP-CN, Kennedy Krieger Institute and Johns Hopkins University School of Medicine, Baltimore, Maryland

Preface

Pediatric neuropsychology now boasts a rich history of empirical discovery and clinical innovations. The field has made great strides in recognizing that children and adolescents merit theoretical, methodological, and clinical approaches that take into account the complexity of their unique developmental stages.

This edition of *Pediatric Neuropsychology* builds on the foundations, concepts, and disorders covered in the first and second editions, while also introducing conditions not previously addressed. In determining the content and structure of this third edition, the priorities originally established were maintained, in that the aim is to provide a comprehensive yet manageable overview of the most relevant pediatric conditions that have implications for brain–behavior relations. This edition also continues to prioritize coverage of sound empirical evidence while ensuring that the information presented also has clinical relevance.

The first edition, published in 2000, provided extensive coverage of medical and neurological conditions frequently seen in hospital-based neuropsychological practice, such as metabolic diseases, epilepsy, and acquired brain injuries. The content and focus at the time reflected the established presence of neuropsychologists in tertiary care institutions and their expertise in the diagnosis and follow-up of severe conditions such as renal disease, phenylketonuria, or meningitis.

The second edition, published in 2010, again covered disorders such as traumatic brain injury and epilepsy, but also reflected a significant shift by including neurodevelopmental disorders. Some medical conditions, such as phenylketonuria, that were no longer as prevalent in everyday practice because of advances in early detection and treatment, were omitted in favor of extensive coverage of learning disabilities such as dyslexia and dyscalculia, and other prevalent neurodevelopmental disorders such as autism spectrum disorder and attention-deficit/hyperactivity disorder (ADHD).

In this third edition, just over a decade later, we have made further changes to the content of the book after careful consideration of both the current scientific and clinical state of the field. The challenge was to continue to reserve space for conditions that warrant inclusion due to their prevalence and relevance, while also ensuring coverage of new conditions and disorders for which evidence has amassed sufficiently to be discussed from historical, etiological, neuropsychological, and therapeutic perspectives. As a result, the sections on medical/neurological and neurodevelopmental disorders include new topics such as congenital heart disease and movement disorders. A major addition is the introduction of a distinct section on genetic disorders, including fragile X, Williams, 22q deletion, and Down syndromes. Those chapters reflect substantial advances in our understanding of the neuropsychological consequences of these conditions, as well as their underlying etiology through advanced genetic techniques.

Readers familiar with the two previous editions will also notice a new section, "Emergent and Controversial Conditions." Our goal in including these chapters is to showcase conditions that account for a significant number of publications and referrals to clinicians, but have not reached consensus status among neuropsychologists or other medical and diagnostic entities. These chapters are included to stimulate discussion and inspire further work that might resolve their ambiguous status among neuropsychologists.

The result of these changes is a slightly lengthier volume than previous editions. As in the previous editions, each disorder or condition is presented in terms of its history, epidemiology, etiology and neural substrates, neuropsychology, developmental considerations, predictors and moderators, and associated treatment or intervention approaches. Emergent conditions are discussed in terms of their history, debate or controversy, current status in the field, and future directions. Each chapter is written by an expert or group of experts, all of whom consider theory, research, and practice, and provide a balanced and unbiased perspective.

The overall greater number of chapters in this edition seems fitting given that pediatric neuropsychologists today are present both in greater numbers and in more varied settings than ever before, reflecting an expansion of their role and breadth of their expertise, as well as the multifactorial needs of children, adolescents, and their families. No longer limited solely to "brain services" such as neurology or neurosurgery, they now practice alongside colleagues in pediatrics, rehabilitation, oncology, genetics, psychiatry, and neonatology, as well as in highly specialized units, such as concussion or craniofacial clinics. They are also more active outside hospital settings, in private practice, schools, and community care clinics, where they are more likely to encounter less acute but more prevalent conditions, such as ADHD and learning disabilities.

We believe that the content of this book will be of interest to a broad base of neuropsychologists, whether they conduct fundamental or clinical research into the neural, cognitive, and affective underpinnings of these disorders or apply their knowledge to practice, regardless of their place of work or particular population of interest. While written by and for neuropsychologists, we also hope that colleagues from medical fields and allied health disciplines such as speech–language pathology, occupational therapy, physiotherapy, and social work will find information applicable to their own research or practice. Many of the conditions discussed are common in the general and special education settings. Thus, the book can provide valuable information to colleagues working in schools (teachers, special educators, school psychologists, counselors). The book should also be useful to undergraduate and graduate students, as well as to psychology interns, residents, and postdoctoral fellows. It is intended to be suitable as a primary text for graduate courses in neuropsychology, neuroscience, or psychology more broadly.

We would be remiss to not mention the context in which much of the final work leading to the publication of this edition was completed given that when the COVID-19 pandemic was declared worldwide in 2020, some authors were still writing their chapters and the editors were in the midst of reviewing previously submitted chapters. Though COVID-19 itself has thus far largely spared the health of children and adolescents relative to that of adults, its impact on the lives of youth is likely to be more substantial for children diagnosed with the conditions discussed in this book. Emerging evidence highlights an increased impact of COVID-related restrictions on vulnerable populations, including those with disabilities and requiring specialized services for academic achievement, remediation, or psychoeducation. For example, extended school closures, challenges managing and paying attention on virtual learning platforms, reduced access to specialized services, and the psychosocial and mental health effects of physical and social distancing are likely to affect those with preexisting conditions exponentially. Concerns also arise regarding the heightened effects of learning loss, as well as the impact of altered exposure to linguistic and socioaffective stimuli (e.g., masks affecting language learning and social-cognitive development). In future years, we likely will need to consider the effects of the pandemic itself on development and on these groups of children. If nothing else, the pandemic will have provided a lens through which the needs and vulnerabilities of young people living with neuropsychological conditions come into greater focus.

We would like to acknowledge the support and assistance of a number of people without whom this book could not have been completed. First, our appreciation goes to the exceptional group of authors who worked diligently to produce high-quality summaries of their fields, often during some of the most critical stages of the pandemic, when they were faced with increased demands for parenting or caretaking. We thank them for their willingness to incorporate our suggestions and feedback, and their care in following the proposed chapter structure. To those who took on the challenge of tackling the emergent and controversial conditions, a special thanks for embarking with us on this new path and believing that these conditions have a place alongside the more "conventional" disorders. Second, we appreciate the assistance of Rochelle Serwator, Editor at The Guilford Press, who through her good humor, guidance, inspiration, and patience, always manages to get us to the finish line. Finally, we thank our families and friends for their support and encouragement throughout the writing, editing, and publication process.

Contents

PART I
INTRODUCTION

CHAPTER 1

Back to the Future

Phenotypes, Risk, Development, Time, and Reserve as Key Concepts in Pediatric Neuropsychology

Keith Owen Yeates

The first edition of this book, published two decades ago at the beginning of a new millennium, began with an introductory chapter by our late friend and colleague Maureen Dennis (2000), entitled "Childhood Medical Disorders and Cognitive Impairment: Biological Risk, Time, Development, and Reserve." In her chapter, Maureen sketched out an approach to developing an outcome algorithm for childhood medical disorders that conceptualized *cognitive phenotypes* of disorders as determined by the *biological risk* associated with a disorder, as moderated by three key factors: (1) the child's *developmental status*; (2) the *time since onset* of the disorder; and (3) the *reserve* available within the child and their broader environment. Figure 1.1 provides a high-level schematic of this heuristic model.

The concepts outlined by Maureen remain of central importance to the field of pediatric neuropsychology, although major scientific advances since her chapter appeared have broadened and deepened our understanding of them. This chapter revisits the concepts of phenotype, biological risk, development, time, and reserve, and attempts to highlight lessons learned since Maureen's visionary chapter by referencing the remaining chapters in this book, which reflect the empirical evidence accumulated over the past 20 years. In so doing, my hope is not only to acknowledge Maureen and her seminal contributions to the field but also to provide a broad context for understanding the disorders described in the chapters to come.

PHENOTYPE

Maureen defined a cognitive phenotype in terms of mental and behavioral skills. She described phenotypes in terms of both a modal profile, or the typical cognitive strengths and weaknesses associated with a disorder, and variability around that profile, acknowledging the heterogeneity in cognitive outcomes associated with most disorders. She highlighted the possibility of core deficits, or impairments in underlying cognitive processes

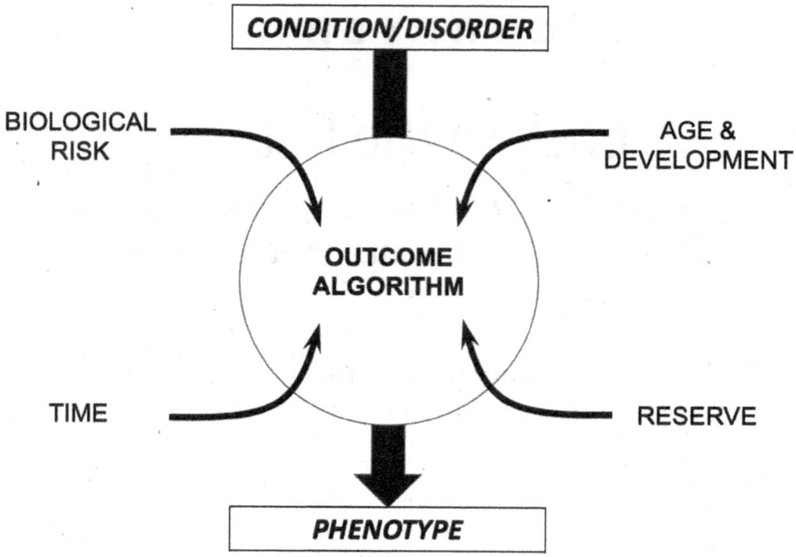

FIGURE 1.1. The relation between condition or disorder and phenotype, as set by biological risk and moderated by development, time, and reserve. Based on Dennis (2000).

that were robust to the severity of the disorder. She discussed the importance of challenge level, noting that evidence of underlying cognitive impairment sometimes becomes apparent only under conditions of high challenge. She also discussed the notion of *cognitive phenocopies,* or phenotypes that are superficially alike but arise from fundamentally different underlying cognitive processes. The model of neurocognitive function in spina bifida that Maureen and her colleagues subsequently set forth epitomizes this approach to cognitive phenotypes (Dennis, Landry, Barnes, & Fletcher, 2006).

Our understanding of phenotypes has been informed by significant scientific developments over the past 20 years. One major advance, as noted in the Preface to the second edition 10 years ago and even further exemplified by the chapters to come, is that the outcomes that characterize childhood disorders are now recognized to extend well beyond cognition to include a broader range of domains, including emotional and social functioning. In that sense, phenotypes can be defined in terms of modal profiles that encompass a broader range of outcomes than the primarily cognitive ones discussed by Maureen. For example, studies of social cognition have found impairments in "theory of mind" to characterize a variety of disorders found in this volume, such as autism spectrum disorder (ASD; Coulter, Skapek, Thomas, & Fein, Chapter 14), traumatic brain injury (TBI; Beauchamp & Yeates, Chapter 5), and Williams syndrome (Mervis & Greiner de Magalhães, Chapter 17). Similarly, complex behavioral phenotypes characterize some disorders, such as the combination of attention-deficit/hyperactivity disorder (ADHD), internalizing symptoms, and social problems seen in association with premature birth (Taylor & Anderson, Chapter 7).

Research has also made it clear that the applicability of the concept of phenotype varies along a continuum, ranging from disorders that are explicitly defined in terms of their phenotype to disorders for which a phenotype may not exist. A major change in the second edition of this book, compared to the first, was the inclusion of neurodevelopmental disorders, as opposed to only medical disorders. Neurodevelopmental disorders are often explicitly defined in terms of cognitive and behavioral characteristics; examples in this edition include ASD (Coulter et al., Chapter 14), ADHD (Willcutt, Chapter 11), and learning disabilities (Cirino, Chapter 13; Peterson & Pennington, Chapter 12). For those disorders, diagnosis and phenotype are closely intertwined, such that phenotypic features, including purported core deficits, are incorporated as diagnostic criteria.

The current edition expands even further the list of included disorders to feature several that are considered provisional or even controversial. Controversies about these disorders arise in part because research suggests they are not clearly associated with a specific phenotype. For instance, the existence of a dysexecutive syndrome seems unlikely given the absence of a unitary executive (Gioia, Isquith, & Roth, Chapter 21), and the defining features of nonverbal learning disabilities continue to be debated (Semrud-Clikeman, Chapter 20).

In contrast to neurodevelopmental disorders, most medical disorders are diagnosed based on underlying biological mechanisms, such as the genetic abnormalities linked to fragile X (Schneider, Scott, Shields, & Hessl, Chapter 16) and 22q11.2 deletion syndrome (Lajiness-O'Neill & Swick, Chapter 18) or the disease processes associated with diabetes (Schwartz & Wasserman, Chapter 10) or brain tumors and cancer (Ris, Chapter 4). Medical disorders may or may not be associated with a neurobehavioral phenotype. In some cases, diagnostic criteria for medical disorders include both phenotypic features and underlying mechanisms, as in the case of fetal alcohol spectrum disorders (Bernes, Moore, Vaurio, & Mattson, Chapter 9). But the purported connection between mechanism and phenotype is sometimes controversial, as in acute-onset neuropsychiatric syndrome (Malik, Martino, & Hedderly, Chapter 22).

For both neurodevelopmental and medical disorders, research suggests that "signature" or core deficits are not discernible in some disorders, such as congenital heart disease (Cassidy, Chapter 8). However, modal profiles likely exist for many disorders, such as fragile X syndrome (Schneider et al., Chapter 16), TBI (Beauchamp & Yeates, Chapter 5), and ADHD (Willcutt, Chapter 11). As Maureen foreshadowed in her discussion of variability, some disorders may be associated with multiple phenotypic profiles, such as ASD (Coulter et al., Chapter 14). Heterogeneity is often a hallmark of other disorders, such as brain tumors (Ris, Chapter 4) and hydrocephalus (Shishido & Zabel, Chapter 2). Even disorders that present with modal profiles, such as Williams syndrome (Mervis & de Magalhães, Chapter 17) and ADHD (Willcutt, Chapter 11), often display substantial heterogeneity. Indeed, some children with disorders that typically lead to significant neurobehavioral deficits show surprisingly positive outcomes, and this type of resilience is becoming a growing focus of research, as seen in premature birth (Taylor & Anderson, Chapter 7) and TBI (Beauchamp & Yeates, Chapter 5).

As Maureen noted in her discussion of phenocopies, some phenotypic features are shared by different disorders, such as processing speed deficits in learning disabilities (Cirino, Chapter 13, and Peterson & Pennington, Chapter 12), brain tumors (Ris, Chapter 4), and diabetes (Schwartz & Wasserman, Chapter 10); math problems in 22q11.2 deletion syndrome (Lajiness-O'Neill & Swick, Chapter 18); and autistic features in fragile

X syndrome (Schneider et al., Chapter 16). Careful parsing of phenotypes is sometimes possible to discern distinct cognitive processes underlying shared phenotypic features, as illustrated by research on speech, language, and reading disabilities (Peterson & Pennington, Chapter 12) and premature birth (Taylor & Anderson, Chapter 7). However, research also underscores the inherent associations between specific cognitive processes that may be responsible for shared phenotypic features across disorders, as exemplified by research on dysexecutive disorders (Gioia et al., Chapter 21) and sluggish cognitive tempo (Jacobson, Chapter 23).

Thus, the concepts of equifinality and multifinality are central to understanding phenotypes (Cicchetti & Rogosch, 1996). *Equifinality* refers to the capacity for different underlying biological and cognitive processes to give rise to similar phenotypes, or, as Maureen noted, phenocopies; *multifinality* refers to the capacity for similar underlying biological and cognitive processes to give rise to a range of phenotypes or to the heterogenous expression of any given phenotype. Further complicating matters is that phenotypes associated with a given disorder also can change over the course of development, sometimes appearing quite different at different ages. This phenomenon, sometimes referred to as *heterotypic continuity*, is exemplified by disorders such as Williams syndrome (Mervis & de Magalhães, Chapter 17), learning disabilities (Cirino, Chapter 13, and Peterson & Pennington, Chapter 12), and 22q11.2 deletion syndrome (Lajiness-O'Neill & Swick, Chapter 18).

The search for phenotypes also must consider practical measurement issues. For example, performance tests and rating scales that purport to measure the same function often display limited agreement, as noted in chapters in this volume on dysexecutive disorders (Gioia et al., Chapter 21) and sluggish cognitive tempo (Jacobson, Chapter 23). These discrepancies can raise questions about the construct validity of not only the measures themselves but also the phenotypes they purport to identify. In other cases, traditional neuropsychological tests suffer from floor effects that hamper the delineation of relative strengths and weaknesses, as in the case of fragile X syndrome (Mervis & de Magalhães, Chapter 17). In the end, measurement concerns suggest that pediatric neuropsychology must not rely entirely on scores on tests and rating scales to "paint by numbers." As highlighted in the concluding chapter of this volume, which focuses on the translation of the knowledge base to clinical cases (Bernstein & Cassidy, Chapter 24), the goal is to develop nuanced portrayals of phenotypes informed by a deep knowledge of neurobehavioral systems, using tests and rating scales as tools to achieve this goal rather than as ends in and of themselves.

BIOLOGICAL RISK

In her introductory chapter, Maureen defined *biological risk* as the cumulative severity of a disorder. She described how severity could encompass a variety of effects, including those related to genotype, metabolism, environmental toxicity, congenital brain dysmorphologies, the primary and secondary effects of acquired brain insult, and treatment morbidity. In the past 20 years, our understanding of biological risk has continued to deepen. We have increasingly come to appreciate that the biological risk associated with most disorders encompasses multiple dimensions. For example, childhood disorders such as stroke (Greenham, Mackay, Gordon, & Anderson, Chapter 6), TBI (Beauchamp & Yeates, Chapter 5), and brain tumors (Ris, Chapter 4) typically involve both diffuse and focal acquired brain insults that have distinct effects on neurobehavioral outcomes. Similarly, medical disorders such as diabetes (Schwartz & Wasserman, Chapter 10) can affect a variety of biological mechanisms, each potentially having specific effects on neuropsychological functioning.

Two major advances over the past 20 years have had a particularly profound impact on our understanding of biological risk. One is the so-called "genetic revolution," the influence of which ranges from the development of "generalist genes" models for neurodevelopmental disorders such as math disability (Cirino, Chapter 13) and speech, language, and reading disabilities (Peterson & Pennington, Chapter 12), to complex polygenic models of disorders such as autistic spectrum disorder (Coulter et al., Chapter 14) and ADHD (Willcutt, Chapter 11), to notions of incomplete or variable phenotypic expression in 22q11.2 deletion syndrome (Lajiness-O'Neill & Swick, Chapter 18) and fragile X syndrome (Schneider et al., Chapter 16). The genetic revolution has driven the call for precision medicine, which has been most evident in research on childhood cancers (Ris, Chapter 4) but is now being extended to other disorders, including TBI (Beauchamp & Yeates, Chapter 5).

The second major advance leading to a deeper understanding of biological risk involves neuroimaging. This advance also was noted in the Preface to the second edition of this volume but is even more apparent now. Examples of how neuroimaging is contributing to research on childhood disorders are ubiquitous in the chapters that follow, for both medical and neurodevelopmental disorders. Two exciting examples include the examination of structural and functional brain networks, as in math disability (Cirino, Chapter 13) or epilepsy (Puka & Smith, Chapter 3), and the use of neuroimaging to predict response to treatment, as in congenital heart disease (Cassidy, Chapter 8). Neuroimaging also has helped distinguish the effects of diffuse versus focal injuries, as reflected in research on the correlates of total brain volume versus specific volumes of the corpus callosum, basal ganglia, and cerebellum in fetal alcohol spectrum disorder (Bernes et al., Chapter 9). Furthermore, neuroimaging has also confirmed that "too much" can be just as characteristic of the brain in childhood disorders as "too little," as reflected in the finding of macrocephaly and increased brain volume in ASD (Coulter et al., Chapter 14) versus microcephaly and decreased brain volume in 22q11.2 deletion syndrome (Lajiness-O'Neill & Swick, Chapter 18). Too much connectivity can also be as problematic as too little, as seen in Down syndrome (Lee, Stephan, & LaQuaglia, Chapter 19). Indeed, some disorders are characterized by both excess and insufficiency in the brain, as reflected in smaller gray matter volumes in cortical regions but larger gray matter volume in the caudate in fragile X syndrome (Schneider et al., Chapter 16). Despite the advances that neuroimaging has yielded in our understanding of many childhood disorders, however, the links between neuroimaging and neurobehavioral outcomes are still tenuous for many disorders, such as ASD (Coulter et al., Chapter 14).

An important caveat about biological risk is that it is not static or fixed. Biological risk can change, both increasing and decreasing as a function of development and time. For instance, congenital heart disease is associated with early and continuing maldevelopment of the brain, especially in the white matter, with the early abnormalities providing a vulnerable substrate for later injury (Cassidy, Chapter 8). Developmental changes in biological risk also can occur as a function of compensatory neural organization in response to injury, as hypothesized in children with premature birth (Taylor & Anderson, Chapter 7). As Maureen highlighted in her chapter, treatment may also increase biological risk, as seen in the effects of radiation and chemotherapy in children with brain tumors (Ris, Chapter 4) or of antiepileptic medication in children with epilepsy (Puka & Smith, Chapter 3).

Biological risk also can vary as a function of demographic factors. In that regard, biological sex plays an important role in the prevalence and expression of a variety of childhood disorders, such as ASD (Coulter et al., Chapter 14), stroke (Greenham et al., Chapter 6), and fragile X syndrome (Schneider et al., Chapter 16). Sex differences in outcomes are not apparent in all disorders, though, such as 22q11.2 deletion syndrome (Lajiness-O'Neill & Swick, Chapter 18). The role of sex as a moderator of outcomes remains uncertain in other disorders, such as TBI (Beauchamp & Yeates, Chapter 5).

AGE AND DEVELOPMENT

In her chapter, Maureen discussed the need to consider age and development at the time of onset of a disorder to understand neuropsychological outcomes. She described a historical dissonance between views that treated early age of onset as both a risk and a protective factor, concluding that the bulk of the evidence suggested early onset is generally associated with worse outcomes. She considered various factors affecting the expression of disorders characterized by fetal onset, early childhood onset, or older age of onset. She highlighted the possibility that certain time windows were associated with heightened vulnerability. She noted that age at onset of a disorder may be associated with not only the level of functioning at any given time but also the rate of decline across time.

The importance of age and development has already been highlighted in the two previous sections, when describing how clinical phenotypes and biological risk can vary by age or development. Further examples of how age at onset affects the expression of childhood disorders are seen in many of the subsequent chapters in this volume, including those on stroke (Greenham et al., Chapter 6), brain tumors (Ris, Chapter 4), and diabetes (Schwartz & Wasserman, Chapter 10). The importance of developmental status is seen specifically in the increasing study of key age-related transitions, such as the entry into adulthood, as discussed in chapters in this volume on congenital heart disease (Cassidy, Chapter 8) and brain tumors (Ris, Chapter 4), as well as the growing interest in adult outcomes of childhood disorders, as described in chapters on epilepsy (Puka & Smith, Chapter 3) and fragile X syndrome (Schneider et al., Chapter 16). Other examples of the important role of development are seen in the varying effect of comorbidities across ages in Down syndrome (Lee et al., Chapter 19) and changes in the heritability of reading skills with age (Peterson & Pennington, Chapter 12).

The growing appreciation of the role of development in childhood disorders over the past two decades has had two important consequences. One, which was noted in the Preface to the second edition, is an increased recognition of the importance of understanding normal development as a context for the study of childhood disorders, as highlighted in the chapter in this volume on math disability (Cirino, Chapter 13). The second is recognition of the need for "lifespan" models of childhood disorders, as discussed in chapters in this volume on diabetes (Schwartz & Wasserman, Chapter 10), brain tumors (Ris, Chapter 4), and ADHD (Willcutt, Chapter 11). Many of these models rest on broader conceptualizations of the developmental origins of health and disease (Silveira, Portella, Goldani, & Barbieri, 2007) or life course health development (Halfon, Larson, Lu, Tullis, & Russ, 2014).

When thinking about age and development as moderators of the outcomes of childhood disorders, an important distinction needs to be drawn between age at onset and age at diagnosis. For some of the disorders discussed in subsequent chapters in this volume, such as epilepsy (Puka & Smith, Chapter 3), neuropsychological morbidity very often precedes diagnosis. In other disorders, diagnosis can be delayed because of uncertainty about diagnostic criteria at younger ages or delays in referral for clinical evaluation, as can occur in ASD (Coulter et al., Chapter 14) or ADHD (Willcutt, Chapter 11). Precise determinations of age of onset are in fact often impossible other than in disorders marked by a specific event, such as TBI (Beauchamp & Yeates, Chapter 5).

TIME

In her chapter, Maureen discussed time since onset as an important moderator of cognitive phenotype. She noted that *time* is not a synonym for *recovery* but may instead involve changes in expression of a disorder or even disease progression and deterioration. She emphasized that time since onset can affect both the level of function and the rate of acquisition, underscoring the need to study developmental trajectories. In this regard, she highlighted the relative paucity of research on the natural course of childhood disorders into adulthood, a topic that, as already noted, is now beginning to receive increased attention. Maureen also stressed the complex interplay between developmental change and recovery from specific disorders.

Maureen's comments on the role of time presaged the increasing attention paid to understanding the outcomes of childhood disorders in terms of trajectories rather than just outcomes at a given time, as highlighted in chapters in this volume on Down syndrome (Lee et al., Chapter 19) and premature birth (Taylor & Anderson, Chapter 7). Her admonishment that *time* is not a synonym for *recovery* foreshadowed discussions of accelerated aging that appear in chapters in this volume on brain tumors and cancer (Ris, Chapter 4) and diabetes (Schwartz & Wasserman, Chapter 10). Similarly, Maureen's appreciation for the complex interplay between development and recovery is reflected in a variety of chapters in this volume, including those on congenital heart disease (Cassidy, Chapter 8), 22q11.2 deletion syndrome (Lajiness-O'Neill & Swick, Chapter 18), and epilepsy (Puka & Smith, Chapter 3). More generally, many of the chapters in this edition highlight changes in the expression of disorders over time, including both neurodevelopmental disorders such as learning disabilities (Cirino, Chapter 13; Peterson & Pennington, Chapter 12) and ASD (Coulter et al., Chapter 14) and medical disorders such as stroke (Greenham et al., Chapter 6) and epilepsy (Puka & Smith, Chapter 3).

Methodologically, the increasing focus on understanding outcomes in terms of trajectories has been reflected in a call for longitudinal rather than cross-sectional studies. Longitudinal studies are becoming more common in some disorders in this volume, such as prematurity (Taylor & Anderson, Chapter 7), brain tumors (Ris, Chapter 4), and TBI (Beauchamp & Yeates, Chapter 5), but are badly needed in others, such as fetal alcohol spectrum disorders (Bernes et al., Chapter 9) and stroke (Greenham et al., Chapter 6). The increase in longitudinal studies of childhood disorders has been paralleled by the application of statistical techniques that explicitly examine trajectories over time, such as mixed models for longitudinal data and developmental trajectory analysis. These techniques have the potential to provide substantial insights into the factors that predict intra-individual change in outcomes over time, at both an individual and group level. One challenge to researchers in the application of these techniques is the inherent confounding of age at onset, time since onset, and age at assessment. These age- and time-related factors are inextricably linked and can only be disentangled through careful research design (Taylor & Alden, 1997).

RESERVE

Maureen defined reserve as all those factors that are available either to buffer dysfunction or to exacerbate it. This definition was broader than some traditional approaches, which focus exclusively on characteristics of the child, and encompassed characteristics of the family or the broader social context of peers and school. Maureen described how pre-insult reserve may involve demographic, cognitive, physical, or socioeconomic factors. She suggested that changes in physical and mental health may alter reserve after the onset of a disorder, and thereby play a key role in cognitive outcomes, highlighting the dynamic nature of reserve. She also indicated that family resources have a critical, and likely bidirectional, relationship to outcomes, and that school and rehabilitation interventions could play an important role as moderators.

Research discussed in the subsequent chapters in this volume highlights both biological and psychological factors that reflect the role of intrapersonal reserve as an important moderator of the outcomes of childhood disorders. For instance, comorbid genetic conditions can moderate the outcomes of medical disorders such as congenital heart disease (Cassidy, Chapter 8). Similarly, psychological resilience appears to be an important factor in predicting the severity of postconcussive symptoms after mild TBI (Beauchamp & Yeates, Chapter 5).

At the same time, extrapersonal factors, particularly parent and family functioning, also play a powerful role in the outcomes of childhood disorders, as discussed in relationship to many disorders, including congenital heart disease (Cassidy, Chapter 8), 22q11.2 deletion syndrome (Lajiness-O'Neill & Swick, Chapter 18), and prematurity (Taylor & Anderson, Chapter 7). Critically, many extrapersonal factors are potentially modifiable; hence, parent- or family-based interventions to foster better child outcomes are becoming more common, as seen in the chapters in this volume on movement disorders (Mahone, Chapter 15), TBI (Beauchamp & Yeates, Chapter 5), and fragile X syndrome (Schneider et al., Chapter 16).

Of course, the existence of an association between parent or family factors and outcomes does not automatically ensure that modifying the environment will change outcomes. Some of the variance in children's outcomes related to parent or family variables may reflect shared genetic influences, as noted in the chapter in this volume on speech, language, and reading disabilities (Peterson & Pennington, Chapter 12). Research designs such as twin and adoption studies can help to tease out the roles of genetic and both shared and nonshared environmental factors as elements of reserve. Additionally, a distinction should be drawn between aspects of children or their environments that account for variation in outcomes, in addition to the effects of a given disorder, versus those that moderate the effects of that disorder. The application of the term *reserve* probably should be limited to situations in which a variable is a moderator, and either buffers or exacerbates the effects of a given disorder, rather than simply helping to account for variance in outcomes.

The recognition of the importance of extrapersonal factors, and the corollary that phenotypes may be more malleable than first appreciated, is reflected in increasing focus in this volume on treatment to modify the outcomes of many childhood disorders, including prematurity (Taylor & Anderson, Chapter 7) and congenital heart disease (Cassidy, Chapter 8). The study of treatment or intervention is becoming more refined, as researchers try to determine which interventions are most effective for which children, consistent with the move to precision medicine. Indeed, many of the subsequent chapters in this volume highlight exciting new research on the moderators of treatment outcomes, such as the timing of intervention in ASD (Coulter et al., Chapter 14) or brain tumors (Ris, Chapter 4). In some cases, though, treatments have been promoted without sufficient empirical support, perhaps especially in the case of controversial diagnoses such as acute-onset neuropsychiatric syndrome (Malik et al., Chapter 22).

One important facet of reserve that was paid relatively little attention in previous editions but is highlighted in the current edition is the potential role of cultural and international variation in what factors reflect reserve and how they operate. Important cultural and international differences are noted in multiple chapters on both neurodevelopmental and medical disorders, including ASD, 22q11.2 deletion syndrome (Lajiness-O'Neill & Swick, Chapter 18), fragile X syndrome (Schneider et al., Chapter 16), diabetes (Schwartz & Wasserman, Chapter 10), epilepsy (Puka & Smith, Chapter 3), and hydrocephalus (Shishido & Zabel, Chapter 2)

The burgeoning research on reserve reflected in this edition calls for broader models that identify intrapersonal and extrapersonal elements of reserve as aspects of risk and resilience that can act to exacerbate or buffer against poor outcomes in childhood disorders. One example of such a model is seen in the chapter in this volume on congenital heart disease (Cassidy, Chapter 8, Figure 8.1). However, because we are dealing with children, such models must also acknowledge that variation in age or developmental status and time since onset of a disorder may modify the nature of risk and resilience factors, as well as their association with outcomes. Indeed, as Maureen noted, the various moderators of the outcomes of childhood disorders do not operate in isolation but instead interact in complex ways. Research has begun to identify how biological risk, age and developmental status, time, and reserve interact, but this will remain a major task for pediatric neuropsychology into the future.

CONCLUSION

At the conclusion of her chapter, Maureen outlined a preliminary approach to an outcome algorithm that would consider the biological risk associated with a given disorder and the level of challenge of any given task, which would together determine a floating impairment threshold that would be raised or lowered by development, time, and reserve as moderators. A schematic of that algorithm is presented in Figure 1.2. As suggested in the preceding sections, the development of an outcome algorithm may be even more challenging than Maureen could have realized given that scientific advances of the past 20 years have underscored the complexity of the key concepts. Nevertheless, the search for algorithms or prediction rules that allow us to forecast the outcomes of childhood disorders remains a worthy aspirational goal.

Achieving this goal implies the need to conduct prospective and longitudinal studies with very large samples, across multiple sites, using common data elements that are collected consistently across all studies. The selection and use of common data elements have been promoted by government funding agencies, such as National Institutes of Health and Canadian Institutes of Health Research (e.g., Hicks et al., 2013; McCauley et al., 2012), as well as by large research consortia. The use of common data elements will foster the pooling of data sets from multiple projects and enable the application of big data techniques such as machine learning to develop robust prediction rules that can be used for prognostic purposes.

The utility of machine learning analyses and other big data approaches is generally higher when informed by expert knowledge, which in this case would involve comprehensive, evidence-based models of outcomes of childhood disorders. As already noted,

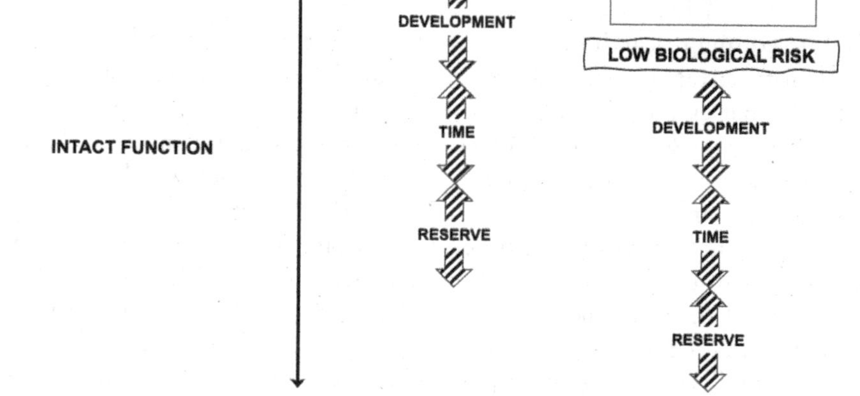

FIGURE 1.2. Outcome algorithm schematic. Based on Dennis (2000).

research in pediatric neuropsychology increasingly depends on lifespan models of childhood disorders that incorporate insights garnered from broader conceptualizations of the developmental origins of health and disease (Silveira et al., 2007) and life course health development (Halfon et al., 2014). These models help to consider the broad range of factors, including biological risk, age and development, time, and reserve involved in the phenotypic expression of a disorder in the individual child. In the future, these models will need to be even broader and incorporate various aspects of diversity to acknowledge how the expression of disorders is also shaped by cultural, racial, and international factors.

In the end, scientific advances should be made in the service of promoting better outcomes for children. Practically speaking, pediatric neuropsychologists will need new assessment approaches and technologies, such as virtual reality and digital health applications, to tap aspects of children's functioning that cannot be readily assessed using traditional tests but are crucial to defining phenotypes. We will continue to need research to determine whether our measures tell us something meaningful about children's brain status or about their everyday functioning, with neurological and ecological validity often being very difficult to achieve in a single measure. In this regard, further study of the contributions of tests versus rating scales is clearly warranted. More broadly, pediatric neuropsychologists have a responsibility to translate insights garnered from research on childhood disorders into rigorous tests of interventions that will help children and their families achieve more optimal outcomes. Indeed, attempts to translate research into clinical practice is another critical goal for the future. We have Maureen Dennis to thank for delineating key concepts that will need to be considered along the way.

REFERENCES

Cicchetti, D., & Rogosch, F. A. (1996). Equifinality and multifinality in developmental psychopathology. *Development and Psychopathology, 8,* 597–600.

Dennis, M. (2000). Childhood medical disorders and cognitive impairment: Biological risk, time, development, and reserve. In K. O. Yeates, M. D. Ris, & H. G. Taylor (Eds)., *Pediatric neuropsychology: Research, theory, and practice* (pp. 3–22). New York: Guilford Press.

Dennis, M., Landry, S. H., Barnes, M., & Fletcher, J. M. (2006). A model of neurocognitive function in spina bifida over the life span. *Journal of the International Neuropsychological Society, 12,* 285–296.

Halfon, N., Larson, K., Lu, M., Tullis, E., & Russ, S. (2014). Lifecourse health development: Past, present, and future. *Maternal and Child Health Journal, 18,* 244–365.

Hicks, R., Giacino, J., Harrison-Felix, C., Manley, G., Valadka, A., & Wilde, E. A. (2013). Progress in developing comment data elements for traumatic brain injury research: Version two—the end of the beginning. *Journal of Neurotrauma, 30,* 1852–1861.

McCauley, S. R., Wilde, E. A., Anderson, V. A., Bedell, G., Beers, S. R., Campbell, T. F., . . . Pediatric TBI Outcomes Workgroup. (2012). Recommendations for the use of common outcome measures in pediatric traumatic brain injury research. *Journal of Neurotrauma, 29,* 678–705.

Silveira, P. P., Portella, A, K., Goldani, M. Z., & Barbieri, M. A. (2007). Developmental origins of health and disease (DOHaD). *Jornal de Pediatria, 83,* 494–504.

Taylor, H. G., & Alden, J. (1997). Age-related differences in outcome following childhood brain insults: An introduction and overview. *Journal of the International Neuropsychological Society, 3,* 555–567.

PART II

MEDICAL AND NEUROLOGICAL DISORDERS

CHAPTER 2

Pediatric Conditions with Hydrocephalus

Yuri Shishido
T. Andrew Zabel

HISTORICAL OVERVIEW

Hydrocephalus is a neurological condition linked to a variety of etiologies that can occur across the lifespan. Broadly defined, it is "an active distension of the ventricular system of the brain related to inadequate passage of cerebrospinal fluid (CSF) from its point of production within the ventricular system to its point of absorption into the systemic circulation" (Rekate, 2009). While historically viewed as a cerebrospinal "plumbing problem," there is a growing appreciation of the complexity associated with the pathogenesis, injury, and intervention of hydrocephalus (McAllister et al., 2015). The complexity of these variables argues against conceptualizing hydrocephalus as a unitary condition with a single cognitive phenotype. Rather, emerging evidence suggests that hydrocephalus and its neuropsychological sequelae are best appreciated within the context of the type of hydrocephalus, the pathology associated with its origin, the developmental period during which it occurred, and the manner in which it is treated or managed (Del Bigio, 2010).

Hydrocephalus was largely considered a terminal condition until the 20th century, at which time new treatment approaches were introduced. Diversion of excess ventricular CSF via a shunt was explored in the 1940s and 1950s, and was successfully accomplished when surgeons at the Hospital of the University of Pennsylvania utilized a shunt valve designed by John Holter, an auto mechanic who created the valve to treat his son who had hydrocephalus (Baru, Bloom, Muraszko, & Koop, 2001). With this initial treatment breakthrough, hydrocephalus became a potentially survivable condition, with patients experiencing increasingly longer lifespans as additional treatment innovations were made. As survivability increased, the investigation into the neuropsychological sequelae of hydrocephalus gained momentum in the 1960s and 1970s, initially focused on IQ (e.g., Mawdsley, Rickham, & Roberts, 1967), and later broadening into various neuropsychological domains. More coherent models were established through the pioneering work of research groups in Toronto (led by Maureen Dennis) and Houston (led by Jack Fletcher) that largely focused on pediatric hydrocephalus within the context of spina bifida.

EPIDEMIOLOGY

Pediatric hydrocephalus is a common neurosurgical condition with a global impact, occurring in approximately 1 in every 1,000 children born in the United States and approximately 5 in every 1,000 births in Africa and Latin America. Approximately 400,000 new cases of pediatric hydrocephalus occur worldwide annually, with Africa, Latin America, and Southeast Asian regions accounting for the majority of new cases (Dewan et al., 2019).

ETIOLOGY, NEUROPATHOLOGY, AND NEURAL SUBSTRATE

Types of Hydrocephalus

Historically, the classification of different types of hydrocephalus has relied upon Walter Dandy's original 1919 characterization of hydrocephalus as either communicating or noncommunicating. The term *communicating hydrocephalus* describes the process in which CSF is free to flow (or communicate) between the lateral, third, and fourth ventricles but is blocked from being absorbed further downstream in the CSF cycle (e.g., absorption into the dural venous sinuses). In contrast, *noncommunicating hydrocephalus* occurs when an obstruction within the ventricular system blocks the flow of CSF and results in increased intracranial pressure (ICP). This classification system remains controversial as pediatric hydrocephalus can present as a disruption of both CSF flow and absorption (e.g., posthemorrhagic hydrocephalus). As such, more recent classification system proposals correspond to the point of and/or completeness of disruption in the CSF cycle (Rekate, 2009).

Neuropathology

The pathophysiology of hydrocephalus is thought to be multifactorial. Disruption of CSF flow or absorption results in ventricular enlargement and stretching, and damage of the periventricular axons and myelin (Del Bigio, 2010). This mechanical injury leads to further injury, as compression of the periventricular white matter has been associated with restriction of periventricular capillaries and subsequent reduction in cerebral blood flow, which further damages white matter. The injury cascade can include ischemia with calcium-mediated exoskeletal damage, as well as downstream injury secondary to the possible accumulation of waste products (Del Bigio, 2006).

Medical treatment such as shunting and endoscopic third ventriculostomy (both discussed below) are used to manage hydrocephalus in children and can reduce the deleterious effects and risk of death associated with ICP, with gradual reductions in ventricular volumes typically observed in the months following these procedures. Animal models suggest that shunting results in the incomplete repair of swollen and fragmented axons associated with hydrocephalic progression, despite apparent reconstitution of the cerebral mantle (Aoyama, Kinoshita, Yokota, & Hamada, 2006). Periventricular axons and myelin are the primary targets of injury in hydrocephalus (Del Bigio, 2006), and children with histories of shunted hydrocephalus frequently present with volume reductions in white matter regions/structures (reductions in the posterior region are larger than in the anterior region). Timing of hydrocephalus is thought to be a key variable, as the early onset of congenital hydrocephalus can disrupt developmental processes such as cell proliferation occurring early in brain development (Del Bigio, 2010).

Conditions Resulting in Hydrocephalus and Developmental Considerations

Congenital

The term *congenital hydrocephalus* refers to a clinical condition that occurs during infancy without an overt extrinsic causal event (Kalyvas et al., 2016) and includes syndromic and/or known genetic conditions that influence early fetal brain development and increase the risk of hydrocephalus.

SPINA BIFIDA

The most common cause of congenital hydrocephalus is spina bifida (i.e., meningocele and myelomeningocele; hereafter, "spina bifida"). Spina bifida is a multifactorial neural tube defect that occurs in approximately 3 per 10,000 live births (Mai et al., 2019). Beginning within the first 3 to 4 weeks of pregnancy, spina bifida involves a failure of the neural tube to close in the region of the embryonic spine. In cases of spina bifida, the neural tube defect allows the meninges (i.e., meningocele) or the meninges and spinal cord (i.e., myelomeningocele) to protrude out of the spinal opening into a sac or cyst (Copp et al., 2015). This process exposes the spinal cord to amniotic fluid and results in neurodegeneration of the cord *in utero*, leading to multiple primary spina bifida-related neurological features, including spinal cord malformation, neurogenic bowel and bladder, and sensory–motor impairment (Stern et al., 2018).

Hydrocephalus is one of several brain abnormalities associated with spina bifida. In typical brain development, a closed neural tube supports distention of the developing ventricular system, which in turn helps determine the shape and size of the posterior fossa formation. When the neural tube of an individual with spina bifida is open, however, fluid drains from the developing ventricular system. Without the structural "scaffolding" provided by CSF distention of the ventricles, the posterior fossa forms in an aberrant and undersized manner (McLone & Dias, 2003). In such cases, the smaller-than-typical posterior fossa cannot contain the growth of the typically sized cerebellum, resulting in herniation of the cerebellar tonsils and vermis, as well as the caudal brainstem, through the foramen magnum (Copp et al., 2015). The resulting structural abnormality is called a Chiari malformation and occurs in approximately 95% of spina bifida cases. Several potential mechanisms of hydrocephalus, including aqueductal occlusion at the level of the foramen magnum, have been linked to the Chiari II malformation (McLone & Dias, 2003), and approximately 90% of individuals with spina bifida and Chiari II malformation have enlarged cerebral ventricles (Del Bigio, 2010). Importantly, in addition to hydrocephalus, numerous disruptions to brain development can occur in spina bifida, including cerebellar and cortical reorganization, distortion of the midbrain and colliculi (i.e., "tectal beaking"), kinking of the spinomedullary junction, and underdevelopment of the corpus callosum (Copp et al., 2015). Because of these extensive brain dysmorphologies, children with spina bifida present with a broad yet distinctive set of neuropsychological strengths and weaknesses.

Dennis and colleagues conceptualized a cognitive phenotype of spina bifida encompassing a pattern of cross- and within-domain strengths and weaknesses associated with the constellation of brain malformations observed in spina bifida (Dennis, Landry, Barnes, & Fletcher, 2006; Dennis & Barnes, 2010). In their model, strengths are evident in associative processes (the ability to form associations between fixed and learned information through repetition), such as decoding, vocabulary, word reading, spelling, and implicit memory. In contrast, weaknesses are observed in assembled processes (the ability to manipulate and integrate information to form coherent, meaningful ideas), such as reading comprehension. In this model, it is injury to the spinal cord, cerebellum, brainstem, and corpus callosum that is thought to represent the primary central nervous system (CNS) insult of spina bifida, while hydrocephalus is viewed as a secondary CNS insult thought to moderate the expression of the spina bifida cognitive phenotype.

DANDY–WALKER SYNDROME

Dandy–Walker syndrome is a congenital brain malformation occurring in approximately 1 in 25,000 to 30,000 live births, which involves the cerebellum and the surrounding fluid-filled spaces (Spennato et al., 2011). Dandy–Walker syndrome is a heterogeneous disorder characterized by a range of brain anomalies, including agenesis or hypoplasia of the cerebellar vermis, with or without enlargement of the posterior fossa due to the cystic dilation of the fourth ventricle. Neuropsychological outcomes of children with Dandy–Walker syndrome vary significantly depending on the severity of CNS abnormalities, neurological conditions, and the effectiveness of treatment of hydrocephalus. Approximately 80% of children with Dandy–Walker syndrome develop hydrocephalus within the first 3 months of life (Spennato et al., 2011), which accounts for 5–10% of congenital hydrocephalus cases. Hydrocephalus occurs due to a blockage of the fourth ventricle secondary to cystic formation and often requires shunting.

CONGENITAL AQUEDUCTAL STENOSIS

Stenosis of the aqueduct of Sylvius accounts for approximately 20% of cases of congenital hydrocephalus (Cinalli et al., 2011), with incidence peaking during the first year of life and adolescence (Hirsch, Hirsch, Sainte Rose, Renier, & Pierre-Khan, 1986). Etiologies of aqueductal stenosis are varied and include syndromic (see "X-Linked Congenital Hydrocephalus" below) and nonsyndromic presentations. Excessive narrowing of the aqueduct can occur secondary to developmental errors, such as congenital atresia, incomplete aqueductal fusion or forking, and gliotic membrane formation. Over time, the disruption posed by stenosis increases ICP, damages the walls of the ventricles, expands ventricular size, and reduces ventricular compliance (Cinalli et al., 2011). Studies involving children with congenital aqueductal stenosis suggest that neurocognitive outcomes vary based on the presence or absence of associated cerebellar abnormalities.

X-LINKED CONGENITAL HYDROCEPHALUS

Mutations of the *L1CAM* gene are the main genetic cause of X-linked hydrocephalus associated with stenosis of the aqueduct of Sylvius, the most common heritable form of hydrocephalus (Tully & Dobyns, 2014). The gene product of *L1CAM* helps guide neuronal migration, and mutation of the gene can result in obstruction of CSF flow by way of narrowing (stenosis) of the CSF canal between the third and fourth ventricles. Of note, the broader phenotypic features of *L1CAM* include physical and cognitive sequelae, such as adducted thumbs, hypoplasia of corticospinal tracts, spasticity, and intellectual disability. Other X-linked syndromes, such as mutation of the *AP1S2* gene (Saillour et al., 2007), have also been linked with variable aqueductal stenosis and congenital hydrocephalus, as well as a broader pattern of intellectual disability and neuroimaging results that are often suggestive of basal ganglia calcification. While sharing a common mechanism of hydrocephalus (i.e., stenosis), these two genetic mutations highlight the difficulty of isolating the general cognitive impact of hydrocephalus and untangling it from the diverse phenotypic features of its genetic context.

Acquired

Acquired hydrocephalus is distinguished from congenital hydrocephalus in that there is a known postnatal factor resulting in disruption of CSF circulation and/or absorption, including hemorrhage, neoplasm, inflammation, or infection (Kalyvas et al., 2016).

POSTHEMORRHAGIC HYDROCEPHALUS

The most common cause of neonatal hydrocephalus is intraventricular hemorrhage (IVH) resulting in posthemorrhagic hydrocephalus. Fifteen to 35% of preterm infants with IVH develop posthemorrhagic hydrocephalus (Flanders, Billinghurst, Flibotte, & Heuer, 2018). Despite a recent decline in the rate of preterm birth, the rate of hospitalization due to IVH and posthemorrhagic hydrocephalus has increased, particularly following grade III IVH or higher. Premature children with IVH and posthemorrhagic hydrocephalus now account for approximately 20% of shunted hydrocephalus in the United States and present with significant mortality and multiple comorbidities (Christian et al., 2016). The mechanism of hydrocephalus secondary to IVH is still unclear. Both noncommunicating (obstructive) and communicating hydrocephalus mechanisms have been proposed, including initial disruption of intraventricular CSF flow posed by blood clots followed by inflammation and obliteration of the arachnoid villi and reabsorption systems of the arachnoid space (Strahle et al., 2012). The neuropsychological prognosis of children with posthemorrhagic hydrocephalus is variable and determined in great part by gestational age, birthweight, and additional medical and neurological complications of prematurity (e.g., pulmonary and hematological complications, congenital heart defects, seizures). In particular, the presence of higher-grade IVH (III/IV) is associated with multiple complications, including hydrocephalus, and significant functional and intellectual deficits (Koschnitzky et al., 2018; Radic, Vincer, & McNeely, 2015).

INFECTION/INFLAMMATION

Hydrocephalus is a common sequela of bacterial meningitis, with estimates of hydrocephalus noted in 7–9% of cases (Huo et al., 2019; Edmond et al., 2010). In such cases, the aqueduct can become obstructed by pus or glial nodules (Cinalli et al., 2011). Viral processes, such as mumps, have also been linked to epididymitis and ependymal cell loss, with peeling thought to occlude the aqueduct in some cases. TORCH infections (i.e., toxoplasmosis, other agents, rubella, cytomegalovirus, and herpes simplex) can disrupt CSF flow within the aqueduct, and both cytomegalovirus and toxoplasmosis can cause inflammation of the arachnoid granulation, which in turn results in hydrocephalus due to impaired CSF absorption (Flanders et al., 2018; McLone et al., 2019).

TECTAL GLIOMA

Tectal glioma or tectal plate tumor is a rare, low-grade, focal brain tumor found in the brainstem, including the superior and inferior colliculi. Tectal glioma often results in obstruction of the aqueduct of Sylvius, hydrocephalus, and increased ICP. The incidence of tectal glioma in youth is unclear, and it is periodically identified incidentally via neuroimaging conducted for head trauma, research protocols, and other diagnostic workups (Perret, Boltshauser, Scheer, Kellenberger, & Grotzer, 2011). Given the indolent course and risk associated with resection in the brainstem, tectal glioma is usually treated by CSF diversion using endoscopic third ventriculostomy or shunting. Currently, the long-term cognitive outcomes of this rare condition are not well understood. Nonetheless, a primary neuropsychological concern for tectal glioma is typically hydrocephalus and the effects of surgical intervention, and not the tumor itself.

NEOPLASMS

Hydrocephalus is a common pre- and postsurgical sequela of pediatric brain tumors, particularly those commonly emerging in the posterior fossa (e.g., medulloblastoma, astrocytoma, and ependymoma; Won et al., 2019). Estimates of hydrocephalus range from 70–90% presurgically, with 10–40% of patients with posterior fossa tumor demonstrating persistent hydrocephalus following resection (Lin & Riva-Cambrin, 2015). Given the heterogeneity in tumor types and their biological behavior across development and treatment, it is difficult to differentiate the cognitive sequelae of hydrocephalus from the cognitive impact of condition-related variables, such as the type of tumor, mass effect, surgical resection, chemotherapy, and radiation.

Neuropsychological Consequences of Hydrocephalus

As would be expected given the multiple etiologies underlying the condition, hydrocephalus is not associated with a specific neuropsychological phenotype. Instead, the neuropsychological presentation of pediatric hydrocephalus is highly variable and dependent on multiple clinical factors, including underlying pathology, age of onset, the effect on brain development, and intervention/treatment. That said, common predictors of neuropsychological outcomes include the severity of hydrocephalus (e.g., CSF accumulation, ventricular enlargement, increased ICP), surgical interventions, and medical/neurological complications (e.g., infection, hemorrhage, epilepsy; McAllister et al., 2015). These factors individually and interactively contribute to the extent of brain/CNS damage and associated disruption posed to the cortical–subcortical structures and associated neural networks.

Inherent in the neuropsychological research of a complex pediatric neurological condition such as hydrocephalus, neuropsychological sequelae are difficult to delineate given confounding etiological factors influencing neuropsychological morbidities that emerge over time. Much of what is known about the cognitive outcomes of hydrocephalus and its neuroanatomical basis has traditionally come from studies of spina bifida or mixed clinical samples. That said, an emerging body of research indicates that the neuropsychological outcomes of hydrocephalus may be best understood in the context of the heterogeneity and overlap across broad functional domains in pediatric disorders with hydrocephalus. Importantly, the ways in which shared and distinct neuropsychological strengths and weaknesses manifest are broadly, but not entirely consistently, congruent with specific functions subsumed under neural systems and brain regions involved in particular disorders with hydrocephalus (Del Bigio, 2010).

Despite considerable heterogeneity, pediatric hydrocephalus commonly presents with deficits in motor, sensory, visual-spatial, attention, memory, and executive function domains, which are thought to negatively affect academic learning, as well as social, emotional, and adaptive functioning. The hallmark of hydrocephalus is the injury posed to the periventricular white matter and its long projection axons, including the corpus callosum, corticospinal tract, and fimbria–fornix pathway. Additional disruption to the development of white and gray matter in the posterior cortical region, as well as callosal and cerebellar abnormalities, all contribute to the disturbance of the frontal/cortical–subcortical systems underlying these cognitive functions (Del Bigio, 2010; Erickson, Baron, & Fantie, 2001). With these general "hallmark features" of hydrocephalus in mind, there are noteworthy similarities and distinctions among various conditions with hydrocephalus with regard to different neuropsychological domains.

Impact of Hydrocephalus by Neuropsychological Domain

General Intellectual Functioning

Hydrocephalus is not independently associated with intellectual disability. Indeed, children with hydrocephalic disorders demonstrate a range of intellectual functioning. Over and above the presence or absence of hydrocephalus, level of intellectual impairment is often a function of the severity of the underlying medical condition itself and/or the related brain dysmorphology contributing to the risk of hydrocephalus. For instance, intellectual disability is frequently noted in youth with early disruption of brain development posed by X-linked causes of hydrocephalus such as mutations of *L1CAM* and *AP1S2* (Saillour et al., 2007; Tully & Dobyns, 2014). Intellectual disability is observed in approximately 50% of children with the most severe type of Dandy–Walker syndrome (i.e., Dandy–Walker malformation; Boddaert et al., 2003; Sasaki-Adams et al., 2008), but is less frequently diagnosed in children with Dandy–Walker variant who have a normally lobulated vermis and do not present with supratentorial malformation. While approximately 20–25% of all children with spina bifida with hydrocephalus are diagnosed with intellectual disability in the United States (Copp et al., 2015), this diagnosis is more frequently made in those children with higher spinal lesions and more complex neurological presentations (Fletcher et al., 2005). Lower Full-Scale IQ scores (e.g., –1 standard deviation [SD]) have also been reported in preterm children with posthemorrhagic hydrocephalus who are shunted (Lacy et al., 2008), but these deficits are more pronounced in children delivered at younger gestational ages. Incidence of intellectual deficits is higher in patients with a history of posthemorrhagic hydrocephalus and higher-grade IVH (III/IV; Koschnitzky et al., 2018; Radic et al., 2015). Finally, the incidence of intellectual impairment in children with hydrocephalus secondary to infection, such as toxoplasmosis, is also high, and the poorer intellectual outcome is associated with increased length of time between toxoplasmosis diagnosis and shunting (McLone et al., 2019).

In contrast to the genetic and congenital conditions noted earlier, which typically disrupt early brain development, hydrocephalus linked to less severe conditions presenting later in development is associated with less severe intellectual impact. This includes hydrocephalus secondary to tectal glioma, which can be treated with a less invasive surgical procedure (i.e., endoscopic third ventriculostomy; Gass et al., 2015; Liu et al., 2018).

Perceptual and Sensorimotor Skills

As would be expected from pathology involving the posterior cortical and subcortical regions, visual-spatial/perceptual and sensorimotor domains represent some of the most consistent areas of deficit across disorders with hydrocephalus. Multiple injuries along the visual system can be observed, including papilledema from the increased ICP, disruption to the geniculo-cortical pathways, and upward gaze palsy (e.g., sundowning) from the compression on the third ventricles (Del Bigio, 2010; Erickson et al., 2001).

With regard to visual-perceptual cognitive systems, there is an indication that youth with spina bifida typically retain the ability to recognize and discriminate objects, suggesting a preserved ventral stream of visual processing (i.e., the "what" pathway). In contrast, the ability to integrate visual-spatial information to identify the spatial location of objects can be significantly compromised, suggesting an impaired dorsal stream (i.e., the "where" pathway; e.g., Dennis & Barnes, 2010). These deficits are further exacerbated when higher demands for attention and motor function are present (Dennis et al., 2006) and can impact a variety of skills, such as handwriting, appreciation of gestalt, and hand–eye coordination.

There has been less research concerning the visual-perceptual functioning of children with etiologies of hydrocephalus other than spina bifida. Children with aqueductal stenosis combined with cerebellar abnormalities perform considerably lower on visual-spatial tasks than those without cerebellar involvement, suggesting a role of the cerebellar abnormality, over and above the hydrocephalus, in the spatial deficits. There is also an indication of persistent visual difficulties (Liu et al., 2018) and impairment of vertical eye movements (Aarsen et al., 2014) in some children with tectal glioma, suggesting a potential disruption of visual pathways posed by the tumor and/or related hydrocephalus.

Language

In children with spina bifida, studies suggest a unique mix of strengths and weaknesses within the language domain, consistent with the associative versus assembled cognitive processing model. Basic language skills at a single-word level, such as expressive–receptive vocabulary, decoding, word reading, and spelling, are frequently intact and are likely supported by a preserved capacity to form associations. In contrast, higher-order language skills requiring assembly-related processes, such as understanding contexts, drawing inferences, and integrating/organizing complex text-based information, are often compromised, as evidenced by weaknesses in verbal and reading comprehension, pragmatic language, and written expression skills among children with spina bifida (Dennis & Barnes, 2010).

Less is known concerning the language skills of children with other etiologies of hydrocephalus, although language delays are common in forms of congenital hydrocephalus (e.g., Dandy–Walker malformation) and early acquired hydrocephalus (e.g., posthemorrhagic hydrocephalus), which have a marked disruption of early brain development (Pinchefsky, Accogli, Shevell, Saint-Martin, & Srour, 2019; Radic et al., 2015). In contrast, language delays and disorders are not typically reported in studies of children with aqueductal stenosis (Hampton et al., 2013).

Attention/Executive Function

Attention and executive function problems are other consistent areas of weakness associated with pediatric hydrocephalus, and children with hydrocephalus are often diagnosed with attention-deficit/hyperactivity disorder (ADHD). However, the attentional and executive function difficulties of children with hydrocephalus may have a different underlying etiology when compared to youth with idiopathic ADHD. Several studies suggest a unique disruption of the posterior/orienting attention network (Posner & Rothbart, 2007) in individuals with spina bifida (but not in aqueductal stenosis; Swartwout et al., 2008), and these findings have been linked to volumes of the tectum and posterior cortex. In spina bifida, it is dysfunction of the posterior attention system that is thought to underlie difficulties with orienting, disengagement, and shifting attention, particularly in individuals who also have tectal beaking (Kulesz et al., 2019; Treble-Barna, Kulesz, Dennis, & Fletcher, 2014). As a result, children with spina bifida can appear "underactivated," potentially less responsive to stimulant medication (Davidovitch et al., 1999), and behaviorally distinct from peers with anterior system dysfunction more consistent with the behavioral symptomatology of developmental ADHD. Of note, Treble-Barna and colleagues (2014) identified disruption of the posterior/orienting attention network in children with Dandy–Walker malformation as well, raising the possibility that abnormalities of the cerebellum, in addition to the midbrain, may contribute to this attentional pattern. Unfortunately, there are no known neuropsychological studies investigating the posterior/orienting attentional network in youth with tectal glioma and hydrocephalus, and the impact of this midbrain condition that occurs later in development has yet to be explored.

The extent to which hydrocephalus disrupts the anterior/executive control attention network remains unclear. Early research suggested deficits in sustained attention in youth with spina bifida (Loss, Yeates, & Enrile, 1998), but more recent studies indicate that the ability to sustain concentration may be preserved in youth with aqueductal stenosis and spina bifida (Rose & Holmbeck, 2007; Swartwout et al., 2008). Once again, differences between the various etiologies of hydrocephalus may be relevant to attentional findings, as a deficit in selective attention has been identified as one of the more pronounced deficits in children with histories of posthemorrhagic ventricular dilation (Holwerda et al., 2016).

Working memory deficits are common across disorders of hydrocephalus. Notable weaknesses in the cognitive aspects of executive function, such as initiation, cognitive inhibition, self-monitoring, and cognitive flexibility, are frequently found in children with spina bifida (Lacy, Baldassarre, Nader, & Frim, 2012; Zabel et al., 2011). In contrast, deficits in the behavioral dimensions of executive function, such as behavioral impulsivity and hyperactivity, are frequently reported among premature children with posthemorrhagic hydrocephalus (Holwerda et al., 2016).

Memory

Memory deficits are frequently found in children with hydrocephalus. The memory problems associated with spina bifida are best appreciated within the context of implicit versus explicit memory. *Implicit memory* refers to learning or facilitation of performance in the absence of conscious recollection and can be measured through priming or demonstration. *Explicit memory* involves conscious recollection of past events or experiences and is typically measured through recall or recognition (Yeates & Enrile, 2005). Implicit memory is often spared in spina bifida, as evidenced by relatively intact language skills at a word-level (e.g., sight-word reading, decoding, spelling), perceptual and semantic priming, and motor procedural learning. In contrast, explicit memory is frequently impaired in both verbal and visual memory domains regardless of test content (e.g., rote word-list learning, story recall, objects or design learning) or format (e.g., free or cued recall, retrieval, or recognition; Dennis et al., 2006).

The deficits in explicit memory seen in children with spina bifida suggest a possible disruption within the medial temporal lobe system. This finding is potentially linked to hydrocephalus, as ventricular enlargement is thought to have cascading effects on the memory system by damaging the periventricular white matter axons in general, and the fimbria–fornix in particular, which connect the hippocampus to the subcortical regions and limbic structures (Del Bigio, 2010). Perhaps more surprisingly, however, is the pattern of preserved implicit memory in spina bifida noted earlier. Implicit memory is supported by a separate memory system involving the motor cortex, subcortical structures, and the cerebellum. The pattern of relative strength in this memory system is unexpected given the overt dysmorphology of the cerebellum (i.e., Chiari malformation) and the disruption of the posterior cortex noted in spina bifida. Further research is needed to delineate brain–behavior relationships for a memory profile in this population (Dennis et al., 2006; Yeates & Enrile, 2005).

In youth with aqueductal stenosis, explicit memory performance has been found to be considerably stronger in those children with normal, versus abnormal, cerebellar magnetic resonance imaging (MRI) findings (Hampton et al., 2013). Interestingly, overt memory deficits are not consistently seen in children with posthemorrhagic hydrocephalus (Holwerda et al., 2016). As is the case in other cognitive domains, the unique contribution of hydrocephalus to memory deficits remains unclear.

Adaptive and Social Functioning

Many medical conditions with hydrocephalus, especially those requiring a shunt placement, become chronic medical conditions that can necessitate an array of medical self-management requirements. These requirements highlight the importance of assessing adaptive functioning in individuals with hydrocephalus, as functional independence involves the patient's ability and willingness to successfully assume responsibilities to manage these demands in a reliable and consistent manner. Lower overall cognitive ability, significant motor deficits, and weakness in executive function generally predict poorer adaptive functioning and functional independence.

Children with spina bifida and hydrocephalus are an example of a medical population with both increased adaptive skill demands and weakness in cognitive skills thought to facilitate functional independence (Tarazi, Mahone, & Zabel, 2007). Individuals with spina bifida often do not ambulate independently due to orthopedic complications (e.g., paraplegia, spasticity, tethered spinal cord, joint contractures) and have neurogenic bowel and bladder (Steinhart et al., 2018). These medical complications then lead to additional self-care requirements, including initiation and completion of self-catheterization several times a day to maintain bladder function and prevent kidney failure. Medical self-management of spina bifida also includes bodily self-inspection to identify pressure ulcers on the feet, legs, and buttocks. Unfortunately, increased executive demands associated with these additional medical self-management requirements, as well as unique patterns of peer and family interaction, create a formidable barrier that makes the transition to self-care and overall functional independence more challenging (Tarazi et al., 2007).

Social skills in youth with spina bifida can also be negatively affected by features of inattention, executive dysfunction (e.g., cognitive inhibition, self-monitoring, set-shifting), and reduced adaptive skills in this population. While social interests, social interaction, and conversational skills are typically preserved, children with spina bifida often present with hypersociability characterized by intrusiveness and overfamiliarity (Erickson et al., 2001). Social interaction can also be disrupted due to difficulty understanding inferences and engaging in the real-time dynamic iteration of back-and-forth conversation that fits the social context. In spina bifida, these difficulties are attributable to difficulties with assembly processes and the manner in which they manifest in verbal discourse (Dennis & Barnes, 2010).

Emotional and Behavioral Adjustment

As to be expected in children with chronic illness, internalizing symptoms (anxiety, somatization, depression) are common across disorders with hydrocephalus (Aarsen et al., 2014; Holwerda et al., 2016; Kelly et al., 2012). These symptoms are often attributed to adjustment challenges related to medical procedures, hospitalizations, and disabilities, and can lead to social isolation, increased dependency, and reduced self-efficacy. Additional externalizing problems (e.g., behavioral dysregulation, impulsivity, hyperactivity), have been reported in some subgroups of children with hydrocephalus, particularly youth with posthemorrhagic hydrocephalus (Erickson et al., 2001; Holwerda et al., 2016).

Academic Achievement

Academic difficulties are common among individuals with hydrocephalus. There is a high rate of special education, lower achievement levels, and a trend toward undereducation or premature termination of education (Erickson et al., 2001; Schmidt, Corn, Wohlfahrt, Melbye, & Munch, 2018). In children with spina bifida, as noted earlier, language skills at a word level, including decoding, sight-word reading, and spelling skills, are typically preserved. In comparison, more complex text-level language subjects, such as reading comprehension and written expression, are often compromised due to difficulties understanding the contextual meaning of texts, drawing inferences, and interpreting texts within preexisting knowledge.

In youth with hydrocephalus in general, the most notable academic weakness is mathematics. Prevalence estimates of math difficulties in children with spina bifida have been as high as 50% (Raghubar & Barnes, 2017; Fletcher et al., 2005). In these children, basic enumeration and calculation skills (e.g., single- and double-digit calculation without regrouping) are typically acquired (albeit slower than the same-age peers), but applied math problem-solving skills that require manipulation of numbers and quantities, mental calculation, and estimation are frequently impaired. Specifically, children with spina bifida typically demonstrate a unique pattern of deficits in math procedural knowledge (e.g., regrouping), automaticity in math facts retrieval, and number sense or estimation. Interestingly, these math deficits are not necessarily associated with visual-spatial deficits but rather are suggestive of working memory and visual learning/memory weaknesses (Barnes et al., 2006). While less is known about math and other etiologies of hydrocephalus, math difficulties have been noted as a common persistent area of difficulty in patients treated for tectal glioma (Liu et al., 2018), as well as children with aqueductal stenosis and cerebellar abnormalities (Hampton et al., 2013).

Predictors and Moderators

CROSS-CULTURAL AND INTERNATIONAL CONSIDERATIONS

The prevalence and incidence of hydrocephalus vary considerably across geographic locations and are greatest in Africa, Latin America, and Southeast Asia. These regions account for three-fourths of new cases, with the majority arising from perinatal and neonatal CNS infection (Warf et al., 2011), while congenital or neurological causes of hydrocephalus are predominant in the United States. These geographical, etiological differences likely reflect a multitude of medical (e.g., access to the maternal–infant medical and neurosurgical care), socioeconomic (e.g., poverty, nutritional deficiencies [folic acid], sanitation, awareness of medical conditions and treatment), and cultural (e.g., social stigma, preference for traditional treatment) factors. Given limited global access to neurosurgical care coupled with the high rates of shunt failure (40% within the first 2 years), the alternative surgical approach of endoscopic third ventriculostomy–choroid plexus cauterization has been pursued and refined over the last two decades through the pioneering work of Benjamin Warf and colleagues in East Africa (Demerdash et al., 2017). Use of this procedure has shown promising results in Africa and Europe, but not to the same extent in the United States and Canada (Texakalidis, Tora, Wetzel, & Chern, 2019), which warrants further research concerning its effectiveness worldwide.

Following the mandatory folic acid fortification of wheat flour in 1998, the birth prevalence of neural tube defects (e.g., spina bifida) has shown a significant decline (by 35%) in the United States and remains stable across all race/ethnicity groups, albeit with the highest rates among Hispanics (Williams et al., 2015). Although the U.S. Food and Drug Administration has allowed folic acid fortification of corn masa flour since 2016, there has been poor implementation of this voluntary fortification program (Kancherla, Averbach, & Oakley, 2019), and it is unclear whether the full benefits of fortification have been achieved in Hispanic populations. Similarly, this question remains a global issue, as regions without full-coverage mandatory folic acid fortification of the food supply (e.g., Asia, Europe) continue to have a higher prevalence of spina bifida (Atta et al., 2016).

Altogether, hydrocephalus is a global neurological condition that warrants global approaches to research, prevention, and treatment. Across the world, efforts are needed to improve access to prevention, cost-effective treatment, and follow-up care that fit regional needs.

Treatment and Intervention

Temporizing Neurosurgical Devices and Procedures

Within the context of neurosurgical management of hydrocephalus, temporizing (nonpermanent) neurosurgical devices and procedures are frequently used treatment options, including ventriculosubgaleal shunts, ventricular access devices, lumbar puncture, and external ventricular drains. These devices are often used by neurosurgeons as a first treatment option for conditions such as posthemorrhagic hydrocephalus in order to avoid the risks (e.g., skin ulceration) associated with ventriculoperitoneal (VP) shunts in very low birth weight infants, as well as the risk of VP shunt failure in general. There may be a cognitive advantage to those children with posthemorrhagic hydrocephalus who are managed with temporizing neurosurgical procedures rather than VP shunting, as they avoid the high risk of complication (e.g., infection) associated with lifetime shunt dependence.

In Utero Surgery

The Management of Myelomeningocele Study was a spina bifida study examining fetal surgery to correct myelomeningocele *in utero*. At 1 year of age, children in the prenatal surgical closure group showed a significant reduction in the need for shunting (40%) compared to those who underwent postnatal surgical correction of myelomeningocele (82%; Moldenhauer & Adzick, 2017). Prenatal surgery for spina bifida repair is now recommended for those fetuses who meet prenatal surgery criteria based on this class I evidence (Tamber et al., 2019). However, as this surgical procedure is targeted toward the correction of spina bifida and upstream variables related to hydrocephalus, it is not an available treatment option for fetuses at risk for hydrocephalus secondary to other etiologies. Longitudinal neurocognitive outcomes from *in utero* corrective surgery are not known at this time.

Shunts

Given that the early onset of hydrocephalus disrupts the development of white matter regions/structures (Del Bigio, 2006, 2010), early shunting is often advocated; however, shunts and shunt revisions are not without potential consequences, and current neurosurgical practice often takes a "wait and see" approach in less acute cases by delaying shunt implantation in order to allow the possibility of spontaneous arrest and avoidance of lifetime shunt dependence. That said, this practice is complicated by emerging evidence suggesting that outcomes may be better in infants with spina bifida when back closure surgery and shunting are conducted simultaneously (i.e., both surgeries occur within the first 72 hours after birth) rather than sequentially (i.e., the time interval between the two surgeries exceeds 72 hours; Kulesz et al., 2019).

Much like John Holter's original shunt design in the 1950s, modern shunts continue to utilize an inflow catheter to drain CSF from the ventricles, a valve mechanism to regulate pressure, and an outflow catheter to divert CSF to the peritoneal cavity (VP shunt) or the right atrium of the heart (i.e., ventriculoatrial [VA] shunt) for absorption into the bloodstream. While early shunting has been found to improve mortality, there is an increased risk of cognitive deficits due to complications from the surgery itself, shunt failure from malfunction (e.g., obstruction, under- and overdrainage of CSF, displacement), or infection, each of which can lead to additional damage to the brain (Vinchon, Rekate, & Kulkarni, 2012).

Despite medical advances in shunt technology, the rate of shunt failure remains high, with 40% of first-time shunts failing within 2 years (McAllister et al., 2015) and an estimated 75% of patients with shunts undergoing at least one revision in their lifetime (Arrington et al., 2016). This alone makes shunting problematic for global use, as the high risk of shunt failure necessitates a proximity of surgical resources to provide revision if required. Studies have associated adverse cognitive effects with shunt revisions in adults, but not consistently for children at present (McAllister et al., 2015). Of note, a recent study linking a greater number of shunt revisions with higher nonverbal IQ in spina bifida, presumably due in part to partial restoration of cortical–subcortical structures and networks, further complicates questions concerning the detrimental impact of shunt failures/revisions (Aoyama et al., 2006; Ware et al., 2020.

At present, efforts to reduce shunt obstruction incidents via improved geometrical design and the addition of anti-fouling coatings have not been successful (McAllister et al., 2015). While efforts are underway to produce "smart shunts" with flow sensors and regulators to reduce shunt failures, technological challenges, such as implantation of low-power draw components, have for the time being prevented the adoption of these types of devices into neurosurgical practice.

Endoscopic Third Ventriculostomy–Choroid Plexus Cauterization

Endoscopic third ventriculostomy (ETV) is a minimally invasive method of CSF diversion in which stereotactic navigation is used to guide an endoscope to the floor of the third ventricle and create a hole to allow CSF to drain into the basal cisterns. Although this approach dates back to the early 20th century, the technique has been increasingly introduced into widespread use via the surgical leadership of Benjamin Warf, who combined ETV with choroid plexus cauterization (CPC) to treat patients with hydrocephalus in East Africa from 2001 to 2004 (Demerdash et al., 2017). CPC, a technique in which electric current is used to burn the tissue in the lateral ventricles to produce less CSF, was initially (unsuccessfully) used by Walter Dandy of Johns Hopkins Hospital (Dandy & Blackfan, 1913). Warf's successful combination of ETV and CPC in the 21st century was found to be a viable alternative to shunting, with ETV-CPC having lower risks of malfunction or postoperative infection than shunts. Moreover, the introduction of the ETV-CPC approach made an effective globally focused treatment available for patients with many forms of hydrocephalus, with reduced need for on-hand surgical resources to rapidly respond to shunt failure (Kulkarni et al., 2016; Warf, 2005). Questions remain regarding the benefits of ETV, however, as long-term post-surgical ventricular volumes frequently remain enlarged despite stoma patency (Hopf, Grunert, Fries, Resch, & Perneczky, 1999; Kulkarni et al., 2016). Moreover, long-term ventricular reduction may be more successful/complete using extracranial CSF shunting compared to ETV (St George, Natarajan, & Sgouros, 2004). While studies examining neurocognitive outcomes following ETV are limited, cases series utilizing reliable change indices suggest that ETV may reverse some of the presurgical cognitive deficits observed in these patients (Hader, Brooks, Partlo, & Hamilton, 2014).

Nonsurgical Treatments

There is enthusiasm behind the potential for nonsurgical treatments for hydrocephalus aimed at modification of blood flow/pulsation, reduced inflammation, and reduced oxidative damage (McAllister et al., 2015). Unfortunately, however, these approaches have to this point had very limited success and have not yet translated into clinical practice (Del Bigio & Di Curzio, 2015).

CONCLUSIONS AND FUTURE DIRECTIONS FOR NEUROPSYCHOLOGY

Hydrocephalus is a multifactorial condition, and its neuropsychological sequelae cannot be generalized into a specific phenotype. Rather, the neuropsychological presentation of hydrocephalus is best appreciated within the context of the underlying pathology, age of onset, effect on brain development, and intervention/treatment. To this end, research efforts are needed to further delineate the potential cognitive phenotypes of the variety of pediatric conditions that cause hydrocephalus. As is evident in this chapter, research on the neuropsychological outcomes of hydrocephalus has primarily involved individuals with spina bifida, with a dearth of research on the remaining disorders. Spina bifida has been a model condition, and the articulation of a cognitive phenotype of spina bifida has helped direct further research and intervention. Comparable attention and efforts involving other conditions with hydrocephalus are now needed in order to better characterize the cognitive profile associated with each of these disorders and delineate brain–behavior relationships. Doing so will support the advancement of evidence-based assessment and intervention for patients across conditions with hydrocephalus.

As evidenced by the groundbreaking work in spina bifida, neuropsychological research can play an important role in hydrocephalus research to promote early and more precise diagnoses that can help with subsequent intervention and resource allocation. While not yet used diagnostically, advances in the field are providing potential biomarkers that could one day shape the course and approach used in treatment and intervention efforts. When this chapter was written, several candidate biomarkers had emerged, including the presence of tectal beaking in children with spina bifida and the presence of cerebellar abnormalities in children with aqueductal stenosis. Both of these physiological correlates have been associated with more significant neuropsychological deficits and should be further investigated to determine their utility in personalized medicine and neuropsychological assessment approaches.

Pediatric conditions with hydrocephalus are now considered lifelong conditions. As such, attention should be given to the manner in which the various conditions interact with educational and vocational systems, as well as how condition-specific impairments interfere with a successful transition into functional independence in adulthood. While spina bifida, aqueductal stenosis, Dandy–Walker syndrome, posthemorrhagic hydrocephalus, and other conditions with hydrocephalus have traditionally been considered the purview of pediatric providers, poor adult outcome indicators highlight the importance of assessment and support across the lifespan. Youth transitional services remain under-resourced across medical, educational, and community settings, which are necessary to promote quality of life (McAllister et al., 2015). Neuropsychology is in a position to act as a conduit for relaying transitional needs from childhood to adulthood and across settings through evidence-based psychoeducation and advocacy for this population.

Finally, the greatest impact of pediatric hydrocephalus continues to lie outside of the United States, raising the need for a global approach to neuropsychological services. Areas of opportunity include the development of internationally based test measures, a broader scope of test administration, incorporation of multilingual/cultural principles into testing, and training of neuropsychologists globally. Importantly, telehealth-based neuropsychological assessment has become a viable service model amid the COVID-19 pandemic, and may represent a potential global platform for cost-, time-, and geographically efficient patient care in the post-COVID-19 era.

REFERENCES

Aarsen, F. K., Arts, W. F. M., Van Veelen-Vincent, M. L. C., Lequin, M. H., & Catsman-Berrevoets, C. E. (2014). Long-term outcome in children with low grade tectal tumours and obstructive hydrocephalus. *European Journal of Paediatric Neurology, 18*(4), 469–474.

Aoyama, Y., Kinoshita, Y., Yokota, A., & Hamada, T. (2006). Neuronal damage in hydrocephalus and its restoration by shunt insertion in experimental hydrocephalus: A study involving the neurofilament-immunostaining method. *Journal of Neurosurgery: Pediatrics, 104*(5), 332–339.

Arrington, C. N., Ware, A. L., Ahmed, Y., Kulesz, P. A., Dennis, M., & Fletcher, J. M. (2016). Are shunt revisions associated with IQ in congenital hydrocephalus?: A meta-analysis. *Neuropsychology Review, 26*(4), 329–339.

Atta, C. A. M., Fiest, K. M., Frolkis, A. D., Jette, N., Pringsheim, T., St Germaine-Smith, C., . . . Metcalfe, A. (2016). Global birth prevalence of spina bifida by folic acid fortification status: A systematic review and meta-analysis. *American Journal of Public Health, 106*(1), e24–e34.

Barnes, M. A., Wilkinson, M., Khemani, E., Boudesquie, A., Dennis, M., & Fletcher, J. M. (2006). Arithmetic processing in children with spina bifida: Calculation accuracy, strategy use, and fact retrieval fluency. *Journal of Learning Disabilities, 39*(2), 174–187.

Baru, J. S., Bloom, D. A., Muraszko, K., & Koop, C. E. (2001). John Holter's shunt1. *Journal of the American College of Surgeons, 192*(1), 79–85.

Boddaert, N., Klein, O., Ferguson, N., Sonigo, P., Parisot, D., Hertz-Pannier, L., . . . Brunelle, F. (2003). Intellectual prognosis of the Dandy-Walker malformation in children: The importance of vermian lobulation. *Neuroradiology, 45*(5), 320–324.

Christian, E. A., Jin, D. L., Attenello, F., Wen, T., Cen, S., Mack, W. J., . . . McComb, J. G. (2016). Trends in hospitalization of preterm infants with intraventricular hemorrhage and hydrocephalus in the United States, 2000–2010. *Journal of Neurosurgery: Pediatrics, 17*(3), 260–269.

Cinalli, G., Spennato, P., Nastro, A., Aliberti, F., Trischitta, V., Ruggiero, C., . . . Cianciulli, E. (2011). Hydrocephalus in aqueductal stenosis. *Child's Nervous System, 27*(10), 1621–1642.

Copp, A. J., Adzick, N. S., Chitty, L. S., Fletcher, J. M., Holmbeck, G. N., & Shaw, G. M. (2015). Spina bifida. *Nature Reviews Disease Primers, 1*(1), Article 15007.

Dandy, W. E., & Blackfan, K. D. (1913). An experimental and clinical study of internal hydrocephalus. *Journal of the American Medical Association, 61*(25), 2216–2217.

Davidovitch, M., Manning-Courtney, Linda, A. H., Watcon, J., Lutkenhoff, M., & Oppenheimer, S. (1999). The prevalence of attentional problems and the effect of methylphenidate in children with myelomenigocele. *Pediatric Rehabilitation, 3*(1), 29–35.

Del Bigio, M. R. (2006). Cellular damage and prevention in childhood hydrocephalus. *Brain Pathology, 14*(3), 317–324.

Del Bigio, M. R. (2010). Neuropathology and structural changes in hydrocephalus. *Developmental Disabilities Research Reviews, 16*(1), 16–22.

Del Bigio, M. R., & Di Curzio, D. L. (2015). Nonsurgical therapy for hydrocephalus: A comprehensive and critical review. *Fluids and Barriers of the CNS, 13*(1), Article 3.

Demerdash, A., Rocque, B. G., Johnston, J., Rozzelle, C. J., Yalcin, B., Oskouian, R., . . . Tubbs, R. S. (2017). Endoscopic third ventriculostomy: A historical review. *British Journal of Neurosurgery, 31*(1), 28–32.

Dennis, M., & Barnes, M. A. (2010). The cognitive phenotype of spina bifida meningomyelocele. *Developmental Disabilities Research Reviews, 16*(1), 31–39.

Dennis, M., Landry, S. H., Barnes, M., & Fletcher, J. M. (2006). A model of neurocognitive function in spina bifida over the life span. *Journal of the International Neuropsychological Society, 12*(2), 285–296.

Dewan, M. C., Rattani, A., Mekary, R., Glancz, L. J., Yunusa, I., Baticulon, R. E., . . . Warf, B. C. (2019). Global hydrocephalus epidemiology and incidence: Systematic review and meta-analysis. *Journal of Neurosurgery, 130*(4), 1065–1079.

Edmond, K., Clark, A., Korczak, V. S., Sanderson, C., Griffiths, U. K., & Rudan, I. (2010). Global and regional risk of disabling sequelae from bacterial meningitis: A systematic review and meta-analysis. *Lancet Infectious Diseases, 10*(5), 317–328.

Erickson, K., Baron, I. S., & Fantie, B. D. (2001). Neuropsychological functioning in early hydrocephalus: Review from a developmental perspective. *Child Neuropsychology, 7*(4), 199–229.

Flanders, T. M., Billinghurst, L., Flibotte, J., & Heuer, G. G. (2018). *Neonatal hydrocephalus. NeoReviews, 19*(8), e467–e477.

Fletcher, J. M., Copeland, K., Frederick, J. A., Blaser, S. E., Kramer, L. A., Northrup, H., . . . Dennis, M. (2005). Spinal lesion level in spina bifida: A source of neural and cognitive heterogeneity. *Journal of Neurosurgery: Pediatrics, 102*(3), 268–279.

Gass, D., Dewire, M., Chow, L., Rose, S. R., Lawson, S., Stevenson, C., . . . Hummel, T. R. (2015). Pediatric tectal plate gliomas: A review of clinical outcomes, endocrinopathies, and neuropsychological sequelae. *Journal of Neuro-Oncology, 122*(1), 169–177.

Hader, W. J., Brooks, B. L., Partlo, L., & Hamilton, M. (2014). Neuropsychological outcome after endoscopic third ventriculostomy. *Canadian Journal of Neurological Sciences, 41*(6), 729–734.

Hampton, L. E., Fletcher, J. M., Cirino, P., Blaser, S., Kramer, L. A., & Dennis, M. (2013). Neuropsychological profiles of children with aqueductal stenosis and spina bifida myelomeningocele. *Journal of the International Neuropsychological Society, 19*(2), 127–136.

Hirsch, J. F., Hirsch, E., Sainte Rose, C., Renier, D., & Pierre-Khan, A. (1986). Stenosis of the aqueduct of Sylvius: Etiology and treatment. *Journal of Neurosurgical Sciences, 30*(1–2), 29–39.

Holwerda, J. C., Van Braeckel, K. N. J. A., Roze, E., Hoving, E. W., Maathuis, C. G. B., Brouwer, O. F., . . . Bos, A. F. (2016). Functional outcome at school age of neonatal post-hemorrhagic ventricular dilatation. *Early Human Development, 96*, 15–20.

Hopf, N. J., Grunert, P., Fries, G., Resch, K. D., & Perneczky, A. (1999). Endoscopic third ventriculostomy: Outcome analysis of 100 consecutive procedures. *Neurosurgery, 44*(4), 795–804.

Huo, L., Fan, Y., Jiang, C., Gao, J., Yin, M., Wang, H., . . . Cao, Q. (2019). Clinical features of and risk factors for hydrocephalus in childhood bacterial meningitis. *Journal of Child Neurology, 34*(1), 11–16.

Kalyvas, A. V., Kalamatianos, T., Pantazi, M., Lianos, G. D., Stranjalis, G., & Alexiou, G. A. (2016). Maternal environmental risk factors for congenital hydrocephalus: A systematic review. *Neurosurgical Focus, 41*(5), Article E3.

Kancherla, V., Averbach, H., & Oakley, G. P. (2019). Nation-wide failure of voluntary folic acid fortification of corn masa flour and tortillas with folic acid. *Birth Defects Research, 111*(11), 672–675.

Kelly, N. C., Ammerman, R. T., Rausch, J. R., Ris, M. D., Yeates, K. O., Oppenheimer, S. G., & Enrile, B. G. (2012). Executive functioning and psychological adjustment in children and youth with spina bifida. *Child Neuropsychology, 18*(5), 417–431.

Koschnitzky, J. E., Keep, R. F., Limbrick, D. D., McAllister, J. P., Morris, J. A., Strahle, J., & Yung, Y. C. (2018). Opportunities in posthemorrhagic hydrocephalus research: Outcomes of the Hydrocephalus Association Posthemorrhagic Hydrocephalus Workshop. *Fluids and Barriers of the CNS, 15*(1), Article 11.

Kulesz, P. A., Ware, A. L., Orkisz, J. S., Williams, V. J., Juranek, J., & Fletcher, J. M. (2019). Are primary and secondary types of brain anomalies exclusive factors affecting the attention networks in individuals with spina bifida? *Neuropsychology, 33*(8), 1057–1064.

Kulkarni, A. V., Riva-Cambrin, J., Holubkov, R.,

Browd, S. R., Cochrane, D. D., Drake, J. M., . . . Wellons, J. C. (2016). Endoscopic third ventriculostomy in children: Prospective, multicenter results from the Hydrocephalus Clinical Research Network. *Journal of Neurosurgery: Pediatrics, 18*(4), 423–429.

Lacy, M., Baldassarre, M., Nader, T., & Frim, D. (2012). Parent Ratings of Executive Functioning in children with shunted hydrocephalus. *Pediatric Neurosurgery, 48*(2), 73–79.

Lacy, M., Pyykkonen, B. A., Hunter, S. J., Do, T., Oliveira, M., Austria, E., . . . Frim, D. (2008). Intellectual functioning in children with early shunted posthemorrhagic hydrocephalus. *Pediatric Neurosurgery, 44*(5), 376–381.

Lin, C.-T., & Riva-Cambrin, J. K. (2015). Management of posterior fossa tumors and hydrocephalus in children: A review. *Child's Nervous System, 31*(10), 1781–1789.

Liu, A. P. Y., Harreld, J. H., Jacola, L. M., Gero, M., Acharya, S., Ghazwani, Y., . . . Qaddoumi, I. (2018). Tectal glioma as a distinct diagnostic entity: A comprehensive clinical, imaging, histologic and molecular analysis. *Acta Neuropathologica Communications, 6*(1), Article 101.

Loss, N., Yeates, K. O., & Enrile, B. G. (1998). Attention in children with myelomeningocele. *Child Neuropsychology, 4,* 7–20.

Mai, C. T., Isenburg, J. L., Canfield, M. A., Meyer, R. E., Correa, A., Alverson, C. J., . . . National Birth Defects Prevention Network (2019). National population-based estimates for major birth defects, 2010–2014. *Birth Defects Research, 111*(18), 1420–1435.

Mawdsley, T., Rickham, P. P., & Roberts, J. R. (1967). Long-term results of early operation of open myelomeningoceles and encephaloceles. *British Medical Journal, 1*(5541), 663–666.

McAllister, J. P., Williams, M. A., Walker, M. L., Kestle, J. R. W., Relkin, N. R., Anderson, A. M., . . . Browd, S. R. (2015). An update on research priorities in hydrocephalus: Overview of the third National Institutes of Health-sponsored symposium "Opportunities for Hydrocephalus Research: Pathways to Better Outcomes." *Journal of Neurosurgery, 123*(6), 1427–1438.

McLone, D. G., & Dias, M. S. (2003). The Chiari II malformation: Cause and impact. *Child's Nervous System, 19*(7–8), 540–550.

McLone, D., Frim, D., Penn, R., Swisher, C. N., Heydemann, P., Boyer, K. M., . . . Karrison, T. (2019, September 6). Outcomes of hydrocephalus secondary to congenital toxoplasmosis. *Journal of Neurosurgery: Pediatrics.* [Epub ahead of print]

Moldenhauer, J. S., & Adzick, N. S. (2017). Fetal surgery for myelomeningocele: After the Management of Myelomeningocele Study (MOMS). *Seminars in Fetal and Neonatal Medicine, 22*(6), 360–366.

Perret, C., Boltshauser, E., Scheer, I., Kellenberger, C. J., & Grotzer, M. A. (2011). Incidental findings of mass lesions on neuroimages in children. *Neurosurgical Focus, 31*(6), Article E20.

Pinchefsky, E. F., Accogli, A., Shevell, M. I., Saint-Martin, C., & Srour, M. (2019). Developmental outcomes in children with congenital cerebellar malformations. *Developmental Medicine and Child Neurology, 61*(3), 350–358.

Posner, M. I., & Rothbart, M. K. (2007). Research on attention networks as a model for the integration of psychological science. *Annual Review of Psychology, 58,* 1–23.

Radic, J. A. E., Vincer, M., & McNeely, P. D. (2015). Outcomes of intraventricular hemorrhage and posthemorrhagic hydrocephalus in a population-based cohort of very preterm infants born to residents of Nova Scotia from 1993 to 2010. *Journal of Neurosurgery: Pediatrics, 15*(6), 580–588.

Raghubar, K. P., & Barnes, M. A. (2017). Early numeracy skills in preschool-aged children: A review of neurocognitive findings and implications for assessment and intervention. *Clinical Neuropsychologist, 31*(2), 329–351.

Rekate, H. L. (2009). A contemporary definition and classification of hydrocephalus. *Seminars in Pediatric Neurology, 16*(1), 9–15.

Rose, B. M., & Holmbeck, G. N. (2007). Attention and executive functions in adolescents with spina bifida. *Journal of Pediatric Psychology, 32*(8), 983–994.

Saillour, Y., Zanni, G., Des Portes, V., Heron, D., Guibaud, L., Iba-Zizen, M. T., . . . Bienvenu, T. (2007). Mutations in the AP1S2 gene encoding the sigma 2 subunit of the adaptor protein 1 complex are associated with syndromic X-linked mental retardation with hydrocephalus and calcifications in basal ganglia. *Journal of Medical Genetics, 44*(11), 739–744.

Sasaki-Adams, D., Elbabaa, S. K., Jewells, V., Carter, L., Campbell, J. W., & Ritter, A. M. (2008). The Dandy–Walker variant: A case series of 24 pediatric patients and evaluation of associated anomalies, incidence of hydrocephalus, and developmental outcomes. *Journal of Neurosurgery: Pediatrics, 2*(3), 194–199.

Schmidt, L. B., Corn, G., Wohlfahrt, J., Melbye, M., & Munch, T. N. (2018). School performance in children with infantile hydrocephalus: A nationwide cohort study. *Clinical Epidemiology, 10*, 1721–1731.

Spennato, P., Mirone, G., Nastro, A., Buonocore, M. C., Ruggiero, C., Trischitta, V., . . . Cinalli, G. (2011). Hydrocephalus in Dandy–Walker malformation. *Child's Nervous System, 27*(10), 1665–1681.

Steinhart, S., Kornitzer, E., Baron, A. B., Wever, C., Shoshan, L., & Katz-Leurer, M. (2018). Independence in self-care activities in children with myelomeningocele: Exploring factors based on the International Classification of Function model. *Disability and Rehabilitation, 40*(1), 62–68.

Stern, C. A., Driscoll, F. B., Ohanian, D., Papadakis, J. L., Zabel, T. A., Zebracki, K., & Holmbeck, G. N. (2018). Spina bifida myelomeningocele. *Neuropsychological Conditions Across the Lifespan*, 24–44.

St George, E., Natarajan, K., & Sgouros, S. (2004). Changes in ventricular volume in hydrocephalic children following successful endoscopic third ventriculostomy. *Child's Nervous System, 20*(11–12), 834–838.

Strahle, J., Garton, H. J. L., Maher, C. O., Muraszko, K. M., Keep, R. F., & Xi, G. (2012). Mechanisms of hydrocephalus after neonatal and adult intraventricular hemorrhage. *Translational Stroke Research, 3*(S1), 25–38.

Swartwout, M. D., Cirino, P. T., Hampson, A. W., Fletcher, J. M., Brandt, M. E., & Dennis, M. (2008). Sustained attention in children with two etiologies of early hydrocephalus. *Neuropsychology, 22*(6), 765–775.

Tamber, M. S., Flannery, A. M., McClung-Smith, C., Assassi, N., Bauer, D. F., Beier, A. D., . . . Mazzola, C. A. (2019). Congress of Neurological Surgeons Systematic Review and Evidence-Based Guideline on the incidence of shunt-dependent hydrocephalus in infants with myelomeningocele after prenatal versus postnatal repair. *Neurosurgery, 85*(3), E405–E408.

Tarazi, R. A., Mahone, E. M., & Zabel, T. A. (2007). Self-care independence in children with neurological disorders: An interactional model of adaptive demands and executive dysfunction. *Rehabilitation Psychology, 52*(2), 196–205.

Texakalidis, P., Tora, M. S., Wetzel, J. S., & Chern, J. J. (2019). Endoscopic third ventriculostomy versus shunt for pediatric hydrocephalus: A systematic literature review and meta-analysis. *Child's Nervous System, 35*, 1283–1293.

Treble-Barna, A., Kulesz, P. A., Dennis, M., & Fletcher, J. M. (2014). Covert orienting in three etiologies of congenital hydrocephalus: The effect of midbrain and posterior fossa dysmorphology. *Journal of the International Neuropsychological Society, 20*(3), 268–277.

Tully, H. M., & Dobyns, W. B. (2014). Infantile hydrocephalus: A review of epidemiology, classification and causes. *European Journal of Medical Genetics, 57*(8), 359–368.

Vinchon, M., Rekate, H., & Kulkarni, A. V. (2012). Pediatric hydrocephalus outcomes: A review. *Fluids and Barriers of the CNS, 9*(1), Article 18.

Ware, A., Kulesz, P., Orkisz, J., Arrington, C., Bowman, R., Fletcher, J. (2020). Long-term intellectual and fine motor outcomes in spina bifida are related to myelomeningocele repair and shunt intervention history. *Journal of the International Neuropsychological Society, 26*(4), 364–371.

Warf, B. C. (2005). Comparison of endoscopic third ventriculostomy alone and combined with choroid plexus cauterization in infants younger than 1 year of age: A prospective study in 550 African children. *Journal of Neurosurgery: Pediatrics, 103*(6), 475–481.

Warf, B. C., Alkire, B. C., Bhai, S., Hughes, C., Schiff, S. J., Vincent, J. R., & Meara, J. G. (2011). Costs and benefits of neurosurgical intervention for infant hydrocephalus in sub-Saharan Africa. *Journal of Neurosurgery: Pediatrics, 8*(5), 509–521.

Williams, J., Mai, C. T., Mulinare, J., Isenburg, J., Flood, T. J., Frohnert, B., & Kirby, R. S. (2015). Updated estimates of neural tube defects prevented by mandatory folic acid fortification—United States, 1995–2011. *Morbidity and Mortality Weekly Report, 64*(1), 5.

Won, S.-Y., Dubinski, D., Behmanesh, B., Bernstock, J. D., Seifert, V., Konczalla, J., . . . Gessler, F. (2020). Management of hydrocephalus after resection of posterior fossa lesions in pediatric and adult patients—Predictors for development of hydrocephalus. *Neurosurgical Review, 43*, 1143–1150.

Yeates, K. O., & Enrile, B. G. (2005). Implicit and explicit memory in children with congenital and acquired brain disorder. *Neuropsychology, 19*(5), 618–628.

Zabel, T. A., Jacobson, L. A., Zachik, C., Levey, E., Kinsman, S., & Mahone, E. M. (2011). Parent- and self-ratings of executive functions in adolescents and young adults with spina bifida. *Clinical Neuropsychologist, 25*(6), 926–941.

CHAPTER 3

Epilepsy

Klajdi Puka
Mary Lou Smith

Epilepsy is defined as a disorder of the brain, characterized by an enduring predisposition to generate epileptic seizures, and, importantly, by the neurobiological, cognitive, psychological, and social consequences of this condition (Fisher et al., 2014). These consequences, commonly referred to as the *comorbidities* of epilepsy, place the disorder centrally within the concern of the field of neuropsychology.

HISTORICAL OVERVIEW

The history of epilepsy dates back many centuries and illustrates many incorrect attributions of the cause of the disorder. In a 2011 review, Magiorkinis, Sidiropoulou, and Diamantis noted the following key highlights. The origin of the term *epilepsy* is the Greek word *epilepsia*, which means "to take hold of (or seize) from above." The oldest account of epilepsy was found on a Babylonian tablet, part of a medical textbook, dating to 2000 B.C.E. or earlier. This document describes many of the different types of seizures and attributes them to supernatural causes, associated with spirits or gods, usually evil in nature. Hippocrates wrote about epilepsy in his fifth-century treatise titled "The Sacred Disease"; despite the title, Hippocrates recognized epilepsy as a brain disorder. Nonetheless, the concepts of the supernatural, including demonic possession, moral or occult afflictions, persisted for a long time, until the Renaissance, when epilepsy was recognized as a manifestation of physical illness. Eventually advances in anatomy, physiology, chemistry and pharmacology contributed to its understanding as a neurological disorder. The foundation of our modern understanding of the pathophysiology of epilepsy is attributed to the British neurologist, Hughlings Jackson, who, in the 1860s proposed that seizures were the result of sudden brief electrochemical discharges in the brain. Soon thereafter, in 1870, the electrical excitability of the cortex was demonstrated by Fritsch and Hitzig.

Neuropsychology, clinical psychology and cognitive neuroscience have all benefited from models of brain–behavior function derived from the study of the epilepsies (Novelly, 1992). The formal study of the neuropsychology of epilepsy dates to the late 19th and early 20th centuries, when there was a transition in thinking of epilepsy as a disease characterized by progressive cognitive decline to recognition that seizures of focal onset could be accompanied by more circumscribed impairments (Loring, 2010). Concepts that are core to the understanding of the organization of the brain, and the development of sensitive neuropsychological test instruments and procedures have been largely derived from the study of patients with epilepsy (Loring, 2010; Novelly, 1992). These concepts include lateralization of cognitive function, the sensorimotor homunculus, brain plasticity, the role of the hippocampus in memory, and the use of intracarotid anaesthetic procedures (the "Wada test") to lateralize language and predict risk to memory after epilepsy surgery. While most of this research was initially established by studying adults, more recent efforts have begun to systematically study the neuropsychology of pediatric epilepsy, as outlined in this chapter (for reviews, see Gonzalez & Wrennall, 2020; Smith & Berl, 2017).

EPIDEMIOLOGY

Epilepsy is a common neurological disorder affecting over 65 million people worldwide and is the third leading contributor to the global burden of disease for neurological disorders (Devinsky et al., 2018). Epilepsy can result from almost any insult affecting brain function and can be secondary to, or co-occur with, various insults/conditions; accordingly, the etiology of epilepsy gives rise to its incidence and prevalence characteristics. Meta-analyses estimate that the worldwide median point prevalence of active epilepsy, median lifetime prevalence, and median incidence rate are 5.40 per 1,000 persons, 7.06 per 1,000 persons, and 56.79 per 100,000 person-years, respectively (Fiest et al., 2017). Notably, there are significant sociodemographic-based disparities: Over 85% of the global burden of epilepsy occurs in 49% of the population living in low- and lower-middle-income countries, where access to treatment and treatment adherence are poor (Newton & Garcia, 2012). Studies evaluating socioeconomic factors report that the median point prevalence of active epilepsy is 4.9 per 1,000 in developed countries, 5.9 per 1,000 in urban areas of developing countries, and 12.7 per 1,000 persons in rural areas of developing countries (Ngugi, Bottomley, Kleinschmidt, Sander, & Newton, 2010). With respect to incidence, a bimodal curve is observed in developed countries, peaking in early childhood and late adulthood (Ngugi et al., 2010). In contrast, developing countries report increased incidence in older children and young adults. Similar socioeconomic-based disparities are also found within developed countries. Observed differences in prevalence and incidence are likely associated with etiologies that are more common in developing countries, such as central nervous system infections and traumatic brain injuries (Newton & Garcia, 2012). In contrast, chronic diseases such as stroke and other vascular diseases contribute to the incidence of epilepsy in high-income countries. Other factors driving this socioeconomic-based disparity include malnutrition, poor prenatal and perinatal care, and poor access to treatment in lower-income countries, as well as classification or record-keeping differences. Common risk factors in high- and low-resource countries include family history and sex, with slightly higher rates in males.

ETIOLOGY, NEUROPATHOLOGY, AND NEURAL SUBSTRATES

Seizures arise from transient abnormal excessive or synchronous neuronal activity and result in a transient behavioral change with objective signs or subjective symptoms, such as muscle stiffening and jerking or loss of awareness. The affected neurons determine the clinical manifestation or the subjective experience of the seizure. The classification of seizures was updated in 2017 by the International League Against Epilepsy (ILAE) to focus on operational classification (not fundamental mechanisms) to promote communication in clinical care, teaching and research (Fisher et al., 2017b). A detailed instruction manual for classifying seizures has also been developed (Fisher et al., 2017a). Some common terms include the following:

- Absence, typical: A sudden onset, interruption of ongoing activities, a blank stare, possibly a brief upward deviation of the eyes
- Tonic: A sustained increase in muscle contracting lasting a few seconds to minutes
- Clonic: Jerking that is regularly repetitive and involves the same muscle groups
- Tonic–clonic: A sequence consisting of tonic followed by a clonic phase
- Myoclonic: Sudden, brief (< 100 msec) involuntary single or multiple contraction(s) of muscle(s) or muscle groups of variable topography
- Atonic: Sudden loss or diminution of muscle tone without apparent preceding myoclonic or tonic event lasting ~1–2 seconds, involving head, trunk, jaw, or limb musculature
- Automatism: A more or less coordinated motor activity usually occurring when cognition is impaired and for which the subject is usually (but not always) amnestic afterward

Characterization of seizures is based on their onset as focal, generalized, or unknown. Focal-onset seizures are those originating within networks limited to one hemisphere of the brain, whereas generalized-onset seizures originate in both hemispheres. Focal-onset seizures also include "focal to bilateral tonic–clonic" seizures, which refer to seizures that originate in one hemisphere and subsequently lead to bilateral tonic–clonic activity. Seizure onset is unknown if it cannot be determined whether the onset is focal or generalized. As part of the classification system, additional classifiers can be added to focal-onset seizures to identify, if possible, whether awareness is retained or impaired at any point during the seizure, and whether the first predominant symptoms are motor or nonmotor. Similarly, generalized-onset seizures can be described using the classifier motor or nonmotor. Though not part of the classification system, additional free-form text is encouraged to clarify the manifestation of individual seizures; to promote common terminology, the ILAE lists common descriptors of behaviors during and after seizures that can be used (Fisher et al., 2017a). These descriptors are categorized as cognitive (e.g., aphasia, dissociation), emotional/affective (e.g., fear, laughing [gelastic]), autonomic (e.g., bradycardia, respiratory changes), automatisms (e.g., eye-blinking, vocalization/speech), motor (e.g., dysarthria, dystonic), auditory (e.g., auditory and olfactory), and laterality (left, right, or bilateral). Last, epilepsy syndromes are also utilized, which refer to a cluster of features incorporating seizure type, electroencephalogram (EEG), and imaging features that tend to occur together (Scheffer et al., 2017). Although there are many well-recognized syndromes, such as childhood absence epilepsy, West syndrome, benign childhood epilepsy with centro-temporal spikes (BECTS), and Dravet syndrome, the ILAE has no formal classification of syndromes (Scheffer et al., 2017).

There is no identifiable cause of seizures in approximately 50% of patients, though seizures can result from almost any insult affecting brain function. The etiology of seizures can be categorized as structural (e.g., stroke, brain tumors), genetic (over 500 genes have been identified), infectious (bacterial or viral), metabolic (e.g., glucose transporter member 1 [*GLUT1*] deficiency), immune (e.g., autoimmune encephalitis), and unknown etiology (Devinsky et al., 2018; Scheffer et al., 2017). A patient's epilepsy may be classified into more than one of these etiology categories. For an in-depth review of epilepsy etiology, see Devinsky et al. (2018). A system of interacting pathogenic and compensatory changes is thought to result in epileptogenesis—the multifactorial process underlying the development and extension of brain tissue that generates spontaneous seizures (Devinsky et al., 2018; Nickels, Zaccariello, Hamiwka, & Wirrell, 2016). In addition, frequent epileptic activity, especially in early life, may lead to synaptic reorganization, increasing the risk of seizures later in life and further exacerbating the dysfunctional activity within the neural circuits, as well as neuropsychological impairments (Nickels et al., 2016). However, it is unclear whether these neural changes arise as a result of neuronal damage or as an adaptive mechanism to compensate for the hyperexcitability of neurons.

Neuroimaging studies show that children with epilepsy have widespread structural and functional changes that extend beyond the epileptogenic (i.e., seizure-causing) zone and are found in both hemispheres even among children with focal seizures (Bonilha et al., 2014; Smith, 2016). Notably, these changes are present at the time of epilepsy diagnosis and have been linked with the duration of epilepsy, suggesting that ongoing seizures may disrupt network organization (Gonzalez & Wrennall, 2019). These changes include cortical and subcortical thinning, reduced white matter integrity, and suboptimal topological organization, including greater network segregation and reduced global integration of networks. These widespread brain changes have been linked with the degree of cognitive impairment and align with the notion that underlying networks, as opposed to isolated regions, play a role in epileptogenesis and related cognitive and psychological impairments (Gonzalez & Wrennall, 2020; Smith, 2016). Accordingly, although some neuropsychological impairments are typically associated with epilepsies originating in specific brain areas, it has become clear that disruption in any part of a network may give rise to impairments.

NEUROPSYCHOLOGICAL CONSEQUENCES

The impact of epilepsy on a person's functioning is recognized to go far beyond the actual seizures, with consequences for physical and mental health, cognitive function, and peer and family relations, all of which can persist in the long term even if seizures are controlled. Studies using population-based cohorts and national administrative data suggest that up to 80% of children with epilepsy may have a cognitive, psychiatric, or other comorbidity or impairment (Aaberg et al., 2016; Reilly et al., 2014b). Notably, cognitive, psychiatric, and social comorbidities are often underdiagnosed and left untreated despite their well-documented co-occurrence with epilepsy (Reilly et al., 2014b). Given that cognitive and psychiatric problems may precede the onset of epilepsy, it is thought that the aberrant neural networks that give rise to seizures also lead to neuropsychological impairments; such impairments are widespread and even reported in epilepsy syndromes previously thought to be benign with respect to cognition (Hermann, Loring, & Wilson, 2017; Kanner, 2017). In childhood, neuropsychological impairments occur in the context of cognitive, emotional, behavioral, and social development, and may therefore be particularly deleterious. Neuropsychological comorbidities have also been associated with increased hospitalizations, emergency department admissions, mortality, treatment-resistant seizures, and increased risk of adverse events in response to anti-seizure medication (ASM) (Kanner, 2017); ASM side effects may include physical and cognitive aspects such sedation, somnolence, psychomotor slowing, reduced vigilance, and language or memory impairment. Therefore, children and youth with epilepsy should receive a comprehensive evaluation by an interdisciplinary team including neurologists/epileptologists, neurosurgeons, neuropsychologists, psychiatrics, and social workers.

General Intellectual Functioning

Cognitive problems are reported by children with epilepsy and their parents to be a main concern of living with epilepsy (Nickels et al., 2016), and have been shown to significantly impact youths' quality of life (QOL; Speechley et al., 2012). Fifty percent of parents report that developmental milestones are not met within the normative time frame, 30% endorse school problems, and 75% indicate their child utilizes special education services (Russ, Larson, & Halfon, 2012). Although the distribution of intellectual quotient (IQ) scores among children with epilepsy is skewed toward lower values, there is considerable variability with some children scoring below the 1st percentile and others scoring above the 99th percentile (Smith, Elliott, & Lach, 2002). Population-based studies suggest that up to 40% of children with epilepsy have a cognitive impairment (IQ < 70) and up to 55% have a mild impairment (IQ < 85) (Reilly et al., 2014b). Even among children with average intelligence, learning disabilities are frequent. Academic problems in reading, spelling, and/or arithmetic are prevalent in up to 72% of children with epilepsy (Reilly et al., 2014a). Although cognitive problems may interfere with the development and attainment of academic skills, academic problems can be distinguished from overall intellectual impairments.

Longitudinal studies indicate that intellectual functioning generally remains stable over time, without progressive deterioration or recovery (Kesselmayer, Morel, Bordenave, Jones, & Hermann, 2019). However, impairments in childhood may lead to progressive lagging behind age-matched peers, as the achievement of new milestones may be delayed. Nonetheless, cognitive deterioration over time has been reported in some cases, particularly among children with more severe epilepsies and specific epilepsy syndromes. However, there is a need for more comprehensive prospective studies of children, particularly over the longer term. There is an indication that children who achieve seizure control show significant improvements in intellectual functioning in the long term, and children with continued seizures show declines relative to healthy peers (Puka, Tavares, & Smith, 2017).

Perceptual and Sensorimotor Skills

Children with epilepsy show perceptual and sensorimotor deficits, though these areas of functioning have received relatively sparse attention in comparison to other neuropsychological deficits (Nickels et al., 2016). This may be because epilepsies originating in the occipital and parietal lobes are less common, and are better characterized by visual auras, eye blinking, alterations in consciousness, motor phenomena, and somatosensory phenomena. In keeping with the concept of epilepsy as a network disorder, it is not surprising that visuospatial and motor impairments have also been demonstrated in epilepsies originating outside the occipital and parietal lobes (MacAllister & Sherman, 2015), Notably, some ASMs may produce motor slowing or tremors as side effects, making assessment of visuomotor skills difficult.

Language

The majority of research on language in children with epilepsy has been in those with BECTS, a common epilepsy syndrome with onset typically between 3 and 10 years of age. A systematic review of the literature on language in BECTS (Teixeira & Santos, 2018) identified a wide range of language deficits involving semantic processing, morphological and syntactic knowledge, comprehension of oral language, phonological processing, and articulation. Predictors of poor language have been inconsistent with respect to age at seizure onset, seizure frequency, and lateralization of epileptic spikes on EEG; duration of epilepsy and number of ASMs are not related to language skills. The presence of bilateral EEG abnormality is associated with greater language impairment, and there is some suggestion that multifocal or temporal spike foci are associated with poorer language skills (Teixeira & Santos, 2018).

Caplan et al. (2009) provided a comprehensive investigation of language in children with average intelligence with complex partial (now called *focal impaired awareness*) seizures or absence epilepsy, who were subdivided into three age groups: 4–8, 8–12, and 12–18 years. After controlling for IQ and sociodemographic variables, the results indicated that the youngest group did not differ from controls. The two older groups had impairments across a wide range of language tasks involving expression, comprehension, vocabulary, reading, and written language. When looking at rate of impairment at the individual level, there was an increase with older age, going from 25% in the youngest group to 50% in the adolescent group. In addition, a different pattern of predictors emerged across age. In the youngest children, duration of epilepsy, absence epilepsy, and psychiatric diagnoses were predictors; in the intermediate age group, IQ and prolonged seizures were important; and in the adolescents, seizure control was related to language skills. The authors suggest that these different patterns may be due to maturational changes in the cognitive abilities associated with language, and in the structural and physiological changes in the brain that occur from early childhood to adolescence.

In children with epilepsy, better language skills are associated with greater volumes in the inferior frontal gyrus, temporal lobe, and posterior superior temporal gyrus gray matter, whereas total brain and dorsolateral prefrontal gray and white matter volumes are positively correlated with language scores in typically developing children (Caplan et al., 2010). For children with epilepsy, deficits were related to smaller anterior superior temporal gyrus gray matter volumes and there was a negative correlation between language scores and dorsolateral prefrontal gray matter volumes (Caplan et al., 2010).

Widespread language deficits have also been found in children with new or recent onset of a range of localization-related epilepsy syndromes (BECTS), temporal lobe epilepsy (TLE), generalized absence, and juvenile myoclonic epilepsy (JME, Jackson et al., 2019). Impairments were found across all subtypes of epilepsy. The BECTS and JME groups were the least affected, and the TLE group showed the most widespread deficits. The data highlighted both discrete and overlapping areas of language impairment across epilepsy syndromes.

Attention

Attentional deficits are present in children with epilepsy (Hermann et al., 2006; MacAllister, Vasserman, Rosenthal, & Sherman, 2014) at the time of epilepsy diagnosis and even preceding the initial onset of seizures (Hermann et al., 2006; Oostrom, Smeets-Schouten, Kruitwagen, Peters, & Jennekens-Schinkel, 2003). Epilepsy can affect various forms of attention, including sustained attention, response inhibition, and attentional vigilance (MacAllister et al., 2014; Srnka, Seidenberg, Hermann, & Jones, 2018). The prevalence of attention deficit hyperactivity disorder (ADHD) has been reported to be 30–40% in clinically referred samples of children with epilepsy and 12.5–15% in a non-targeted, population registry study. These rates are 2.5–5.5 times higher than in otherwise healthy children without seizures (Auvin et al., 2018). The inattentive subtype of ADHD is most common among children with epilepsy, and unlike what is documented in the general population, there is not a preponderance among males. Risk factors for ADHD in children with epilepsy include poor seizure control, treatment with multiple ASMs, and the presence of comorbid developmental disabilities (Auvin et al., 2018).

Memory

Children with epilepsy display memory impairments both relative to test norms and in comparison to healthy peers; in addition, up to 58% of children with epilepsy have been found to have poorer performance in at least one type of memory task than would be expected based on their IQ (Reilly et al., 2015). Memory impairments may be present at the time of seizure onset and before the introduction of ASMs, suggesting that they may result from disruptions to neural substrates, including connections between cortical areas, rather than from seizures themselves (Jackson et al., 2013; Oostrom et al., 2003).

Studies evaluating memory deficits in children with epilepsy have traditionally focused on those with temporal lobe seizures; however, memory dysfunction is common in children with frontal lobe epilepsy and has been documented in other epilepsy syndromes (Menlove & Reilly, 2015; Smith, 2016; Smith & Direnfeld, 2012). Memory deficits are found even in the epilepsy syndromes considered to be benign, and in children with a history of relatively few seizures (Jackson et al., 2013). Children with epilepsy do not always show hemispheric lateralization of memory function but this may emerge with further development (Gonzalez, Mahdavi, Anderson, & Harvey, 2012; Smith & Berl, 2017).

Poor memory may present as abnormally rapid forgetting or impairments in episodic, semantic, or autobiographical memory (Gascoigne et al., 2013, 2014; Smith & Lah, 2011). In qualitative studies of children and adolescents with medically refractory epilepsy, a majority of youth identify memory deficits as a major impediment to progress in school, and also as having an impact on self-esteem (Elliott, Lach, & Smith, 2005; Smith, Elliott, & Lach, 2006).

Executive Functions

Prospective studies of children with new onset epilepsy compared with controls have yielded mixed results in terms of executive functioning, with some showing comparable performance between groups (Rathouz et al., 2014), and others reporting impairments in sustained attention and response inhibition (Oostrom, van Teeseling, Smeets-Schouten, Peters, & Jennekens-Schinkel, 2005). Because the frontal lobes are inextricably associated with executive function, numerous case and group studies have examined executive function specifically in children with frontal lobe epilepsy. This work has documented impaired concentration, attention, response inhibition, cognitive flexibility, organizational skills, problem solving, planning ability, working memory, and motor speed and coordination (Braakman et al., 2011; Smith, 2016).

Executive dysfunction is also present in children with seizures arising outside of the frontal lobe, particularly in those with structural abnormalities in the mesial temporal lobe structures (Rzezak et al., 2007; Smith, 2016). Smith identified that tasks assessing attention, working memory, verbal fluency, rapid decision making, mental flexibility, and resistance to interference have not distinguished between frontal and temporal lobe epilepsy, and tasks on which the frontal lobe group performs significantly less well than children with temporal lobe epilepsy include motor coordination, problem solving, and conceptual formation. However, on tests of response inhibition, planning, and conceptual shifting, some studies indicated similar performance between frontal and temporal lobe groups, and others found worse performance in the former.

Social Cognition

Children with epilepsy show significant impairments relative to typically developing controls in facial emotion perception, including the ability to recognize the basic emotions of happiness, sadness, anger, fear, disgust and surprise. These impairments have been documented across types of epilepsy, including focal (temporal, frontal, or extratemporal/frontal) and generalized epilepsies (Stewart, Catroppa, & Lah, 2016; Stewart, Lah, & Smith, 2019). Impairments in theory of mind (TOM), the ability to attribute mental states to others as well as to oneself, and to understand that the thoughts, intentions, beliefs, and emotions of others may differ from one's own, have been documented in children with focal or generalized epilepsies across a variety of tasks, mainly false-belief and strange or faux pas story tasks (Stewart et al., 2016, 2019).

Social-cognitive skills have been found to be related to younger age of seizure onset and longer duration of epilepsy but not to lateralization of the seizure focus, seizure frequency, and number of ASMs (Stewart et al., 2016, 2019). In a longitudinal study that examined facial emotion expression following focal epilepsy surgical resections, Braams et al. (2015) found that deficits were present before surgery and did not change after surgery, irrespective of site and side of resection and seizure outcome.

Adaptive and Social Functioning

Adaptive functioning refers to how well a person handles common demands in life and how independent one is compared to others of similar age and background. Typically, assessment of adaptive function targets a variety of skills, including communication, socialization, motor function, and daily living skills (skills for personal and household care and for community involvement). A population-based study of early-onset epilepsy (ages 1–7 years) documented delays in adaptive function in 56% of the children (Reilly et al., 2019).

It has long been established that individuals with developmental or intellectual disability often have accompanying delays in adaptive functioning, and this finding holds for children with epilepsy who have intellectual disability, with the latter often exhibiting more pronounced difficulties than those with intellectual disability alone (Reilly et al., 2019). Delays in adaptive function are also found in children with epilepsy who do not have intellectual delays, and can be greater than expected for IQ level (Buelow et al., 2012; Kerr & Fayed, 2017). Adaptive function has important implications for achievement in multiple domains. For example, in preschool children with epilepsy, early social and communication scores predict later school performance (Berg, Caplan, Baca, & Vickrey, 2013), and in older adolescents and young adults with epilepsy, adaptive function predicts life achievement (Shackleton, Kasteleijn-Nolst Trenite, de Craen, Vandenbroucke, & Westendorp, 2003).

A variety of factors may contribute to poor adaptive function. With respect to cognitive variables, in addition to IQ, working memory has been found to influence all domains of adaptive function (Kerr & Fayed, 2017). Children with epileptic encephalopathies and symptomatic etiology, and those with medically refractory seizures are at particular risk for delays in adaptive function (Berg et al., 2004). Younger age at seizure onset, longer duration of epilepsy, the use of multiple ASMs, and the presence of secondarily generalized seizures have been predictive in some but not all studies (Berg et al., 2004; Kerr & Fayed, 2017; Reilly et al., 2019). Sociodemographic factors may also be of importance, as non-White ethnicity and male gender have been associated with lower adaptive function scores (Kerr & Fayed, 2017; Reilly et al., 2019). Finally, lifestyle restrictions, such as reduced opportunities for physical exercise and social interactions, may hamper opportunities to develop and practice adaptive function skills (Wong & Wirrell, 2006).

Children with epilepsy also experience greater social difficulties relative to healthy controls and children with non-neurological chronic conditions (Hamiwka et al., 2009), with almost 50% of parents reporting poor social competence in their children relative to 20% of healthy controls (Russ et al., 2012). In addition, over 40% of children with epilepsy report being bullied, in comparison to 21% of healthy controls and 18% of children with chronic kidney disease (Hamiwka et al., 2009). Relative to healthy control, adults with a history of childhood-onset epilepsy are less likely to be in a romantic relationship, have children, and live independently of their parents, suggesting a persistence of adaptive and social problems (Puka, Tavares, & Speechley, 2019). Poorer social outcomes are predominantly associated with cognitive impairments and not consistently associated with seizure control. Though further research is required to better understand the source and trajectory of social problems, they may be attributable to impaired social cognition, necessary for responding appropriately to social interactions and forming meaningful social relationships.

Emotional and Behavioral Adjustment

With respect to emotional and behavioral adjustment, increasing evidence has shown that the current standard of care does not adequately address patients' needs. The ILAE Child Neuropsychiatry Taskforce reports that 35–50% of children with epilepsy have a comorbid psychiatric/behavioral disorder, with much higher rates among those with structural brain abnormalities and intellectual disability (Besag et al., 2016). Methodological differences in study design, method of assessment, and recruitment setting are thought to account for the variability in reported rates of comorbidities. Nonetheless, children with epilepsy have a three to nine times greater risk for mental health disorders than healthy children and children with non-neurological chronic illness. Despite the widespread nature of these problems, a staggering two-thirds of children are not diagnosed, and consequently do not receive appropriate treatment (Reilly et al., 2014b). As alluded to earlier in this chapter, this is particularly concerning given that these comorbidities are associated with poor disease management and prognosis, increased side effects of ASMs, increased mortality, greater economic burden, poorer outcomes from epilepsy surgery, and poorer QOL (Kanner, 2017).

The most common forms of psychopathology in children with epilepsy include ADHD (30–40%), anxiety (15–36%), depression (8–35%), and oppositional defiant and conduct disorder (13–16%) (Besag et al., 2016). Notably, emotional and behavioral problems may persist over the long term, even among youth who achieve seizure control, and are strong predictors of QOL. Prospective studies find that children with epilepsy have poorer QOL relative to their peers at the time of epilepsy diagnosis and show some improvements over the first 2 years postdiagnosis (Speechley et al., 2012). Notably, children with epilepsy have unique QOL trajectories, with approximately one-third reporting relatively poor QOL over the long term, with the remaining youth showing some improvement over the first 2 years, with scores reaching a plateau over the long-term (Puka et al., 2020). Child comorbidities, epilepsy severity, and family environment at the time of diagnosis have been consistently associated with children's QOL trajectories.

Though more research is required, the relationship between epilepsy and behavioral and emotional problems, particularly depression, has clear neurobiological underpinnings and a shared pathophysiology (Mula, 2019). Depressive symptoms have been associated with TLE, implicating dysfunction in temporal mesial structures, whereas anxiety has been related to dysfunction of the limbic system, especially the amygdala (Gonzalez & Wrennall, 2020). Similarly, dysfunction in the prefrontal lobe may be associated with more behavioral problems.

DEVELOPMENTAL CONSIDERATIONS

A developmental perspective is critical for understanding the neuropsychology of epilepsy. Childhood represents a peak in the age continuum for the onset of epilepsy (Ngugi et al., 2010). A review of types of epilepsy syndromes identified by specific EEG features indicated that of 29 syndromes, 21 were characterized by age of onset prior to adolescence, six typically appeared between adolescence and adulthood, and two had a less specific age relationship (Berg et al., 2010). Abnormalities in cognition, brain structure, and behavior are present at or near the time of diagnosis in children (Hermann, Jones, Jackson, & Seidenberg, 2012). Understanding whether and how all or some of these abnormalities change over time with neural and cognitive maturation, variations in seizure frequency and in response to treatments is challenging, but key to the further advancement of the field. There are substantial differences between childhood-onset epilepsy syndromes, with some characterized by relatively mild impairments, and others characterized by significant arrest in development or regression. Neurodevelopmental disorders such as ADHD, autism, and learning disabilities are disproportionately high among children with epilepsy and may impact on the child's cognitive and behavioral development, and themselves be impacted by the child's epilepsy course over time.

There is evidence to suggest that the pattern of cognitive dysfunction in children with epilepsy may depend on the age of seizure onset. Gonzalez et al. (2014) found that skills in a stage of development at the time of seizure onset were more vulnerable to disruption than were skills that had previously developed and consolidated. In addition, evidence suggesting a key role for developmental stage in the expression of cognitive deficits arise from studies of memory in TLE. Studies of verbal learning and recall suggest that with increasing age, youth with epilepsy show an increasing disparity in performance relative to controls (Gascoigne et al., 2014; Helmstaedter & Elger, 2009). In children with TLE, laterality effects in memory are not seen at young ages but emerge during adolescence (Gonzalez et al., 2012; Helmstaedter & Elger, 2009).

A comprehensive model of neuropsychological functioning in children with epilepsy has been proposed to recognize the interplay between the cognitive and psychological function and intrinsic factors (e.g., genetics and temperament), epilepsy factors and the developmental features that may affect brain function, plasticity and reorganization (Gonzalez & Wrennall, 2020). This model also acknowledges the important roles of parental, family, and environmental characteristics on children's functioning, which is key for understanding the developmental perspective. There is evidence that parental mental health and parental and peer support influence the mental health and QOL of children with epilepsy (Gonzalez & Wrennall, 2020; Goodwin, Wilk, Campbell, & Speechley, 2017). Some family and environmental factors may be modifiable, thus allowing the development of targeted interventions to improve child outcomes.

PREDICTORS AND MODERATORS

Increasing evidence suggests that epilepsy and its neuropsychological comorbidities are an expression of the same underlying aberrant neuronal networks. This view is supported by the finding that neuropsychological comorbidities often precede or co-occur with the first recognized seizures, and is in line with the contemporary view of epilepsy as a network disorder (Wilson & Baxendale, 2014). To understand the neuropsychological manifestations of pediatric epilepsy, the interactions of biological, psychological, social, and/or cultural factors must be considered, and understanding these interactions can support differential treatment pathways (Mula, 2019).

Biological Factors

The extant literature suggests that the underlying neuronal substrates of epilepsy predispose patients to both seizures and neuropsychological impairments, with frequent seizures potentially exacerbating the dysfunction of neuronal networks. In many cases the etiology of seizures is also the cause of neuropsychological impairments, for example, genetic abnormalities (e.g., Rett's disorder, Angelman syndrome), structural brain abnormalities (e.g., malformations of cortical development, hypoxic–ischemic injury), and metabolic abnormalities (e.g., *GLUT1* deficiency, mitochondrial dysfunction) (Nickels et al., 2016). Frequent seizures and epileptic activity are also known to exacerbate neurocognitive dysfunction in syndromes known as *epileptic encephalopathies*, which include, among others, West syndrome, Dravet syndrome, epileptic encephalopathies with electrical status epilepticus in slow-wave sleep (ESES), and Lennox–Gastaut syndrome (Nickels et al., 2016).

Biological factors associated with neuropsychological impairments typically coincide, making it difficult to isolate their independent contribution. Generally, these biological factors include etiology, greater seizure frequency/severity, younger age of seizure onset, longer duration of epilepsy, greater number of ASMs, and ASM side effects (Nickels et al., 2016). Etiology of seizures is inevitably related to seizure frequency and severity, the age of seizure onset, and the chosen ASM regimen. The area from which seizures originate (epileptogenic zone) also contributes to the manifestation of neuropsychological consequences. Improved neuropsychological functioning after seizure control, and deteriorated functioning with recurrent seizures have been reported, particularly over the long-term (Puka et al., 2017), although this association is not consistently found and more research into long-term trajectories is needed.

Psychological and Social Factors

Psychological and social factors have also been found to play an important role in the manifestations of neuropsychological impairments associated with epilepsy and may mitigate the impact of biological factors. Parents' response to their child's illness and ongoing stress, uncertainty, and changed family dynamic are important in maintaining optimal family functioning and in how children will come to understand and cope with epilepsy. Systematic reviews show that up to 50% and 58% of parents are at risk for major depressive disorder and anxiety, respectively (Ferro & Speechley, 2009; Jones & Reilly, 2016). Studies of newly diagnosed children with epilepsy suggest that parental and family factors may have a greater influence on the evolution of neuropsychological impairments than epilepsy-related variables (Austin et al., 2011; Oostrom et al., 2005). Maladaptive parenting and poorer family mastery (e.g., disorganized and less supportive family environment) are associated with poorer neuropsychological performance and academic achievement (Fastenau et al., 2004; Oostrom et al., 2005). Apart from seizure control, few biological factors are consistently associated with children's internalizing and externalizing behavioral problems. In contrast, the child's attitudes toward the illness, external (or unknown) locus of control, hopelessness, parental psychopathology, poor family communications, and other family factors have been associated with internalizing and externalizing problems (Besag et al., 2016). Poor emotional support for children has been associated with increased internalizing problems, whereas restricted child autonomy and poor parenting confidence are associated with more behavioral problems over time (Austin et al., 2011). Few studies have evaluated interactions and mediation mechanisms, but some evidence suggests that family stress and satisfaction with family relationships mediate, while family mastery and extended family support moderate, the negative impact of parental psychopathology on children's emotional well-being (Goodwin et al., 2017).

Cross-Cultural or International Considerations

Historically, epilepsy has been notoriously attributed to various spiritual and religious causes, such as possession by a demon, and is frequently accompanied by considerable stigma. The impact of stigma alone has far-reaching effects, impacting interpersonal relationships and social support, general health, and overall QOL for children with epilepsy and their families (de Boer, Mula, & Sander, 2008). Notably, the experience of epilepsy, symptom reporting, and felt stigma are heavily influenced by cultural backgrounds and beliefs. Cultural background is also associated with socioeconomic status, and both factors are related to access to health care and acceptance of medical professionals. Furthermore, cognitive assessments may present a challenge, as accurate measurement is culture-dependent, typically relying on the experiences of the dominant culture for which the test is primarily intended. Furthermore, minority groups may not be adequately represented in normative samples, diluting validity across populations.

Treatment

Timely treatment of the underlying etiology and achieving seizure control among children with specific syndromes (e.g., *GLUT1* deficiency and ESES) can result in marked improvements in cognition and behavior, and allow cognitive development to progress (Nickels et al., 2016). An integral part of managing children with epilepsy is a comprehensive treatment approach within the context of the family, peer group, and school (Kerr et al., 2011). This requires an interdisciplinary, team-based approach and may include epileptologists, psychiatrists, neuropsychologists, psychologists, nurse practitioners, social workers, and pharmacists. Neuropsychological assessment is recommended to identify and monitor cognitive, emotional, and behavioral symptoms (Jones, 2014; Kerr et al., 2011; Michaelis et al., 2018). In addition, psychological screening of newly diagnosed patients can inform the choice of ASM selection given that a history of psychological symptoms increases the vulnerability to psychological adverse effects of some ASMs. Screening prior to the initiation of ASMs also allows one to determine whether psychological symptoms arising during the course of treatment could be an ASM side effect or an exacerbation of a comorbid problem (Michaelis et al., 2018). Patient and family education, especially once a diagnosis is made, should also receive considerable attention (Critical Care Services Ontario [CCSO], 2015). People with epilepsy and their families frequently misunderstand basic information about epilepsy and its diagnosis, increasing the level of felt stigma and negative attitudes. For children, education and counseling can include information on managing seizures at school, common learning problems, safety, participating in extracurricular activities, dealing with fears, how to access needed resources, and impact on family dynamics.

While there is a lack of randomized pharmacological and nonpharmacological clinical trials for treatment of neuropsychological impairments in children with epilepsy, clinicians are encouraged to base treatment on results of trials on the general pediatric population (Jones, 2014; Michaelis et al., 2018). For children with epilepsy, the potential impact of ASMs on neuropsychological comorbidities should also be considered. Treatment may include psychoeducation, self-management (e.g., focusing on medication adherence, lifestyle changes), or cognitive-behavioral therapy, with a strong family involvement in treatment. In collaboration with the school, school-based programs can also be developed, including strategies to optimize attention, organization, and task completion. Psychotherapy may be tried as a first-line treatment for emotional and behavioral problems, with pharmacotherapy typically considered if comorbid disorders are present, if there is a partial response to therapy, or if symptoms worsen (Jones, 2014). The most efficacious interventions for moderate and severe depression and anxiety include a combination of pharmacotherapy and cognitive-behavioral therapy. A number of ASMs can also be used to treat various psychiatric symptoms. Selective serotonin reuptake inhibitors (SSRIs) for anxiety and depression and psychostimulants for ADHD should not be withheld if clinically indicated, as they are not thought to exacerbate seizures (Besag et al., 2016; Jones, 2014).

TREATMENT AND INTERVENTION

A number of guidelines are available for the management of epilepsy (e.g., CCSO, 2015, 2016) with the goal of providing the best QOL with no seizures and fewest adverse effects from treatment. The first line of treatment is medication (ASMs), of which more than 20 are available. ASMs suppress the propensity for seizures by decreasing neuronal excitability or enhancing inhibitory neurotransmission, and by these same mechanisms can produce neuropsychological side effects. The majority of studies evaluating neuropsychological side effects of ASMs have been conducted in adults as a result of methodological and ethical difficulties in conducting such studies in children; therefore, studies in children tend to be observational. Side effects of ASMs are common, particularly among children with a more severe epilepsy, higher doses of ASMs, polypharmacy, and coexisting neurobehavioral problems, and may include fatigue, cognitive slowing, behavioral changes, altered mood, weight gain, and motor changes. Phenobarbital, topiramate, and valproic acid have been frequently associated with adverse cognitive and behavioral side effects, in contrast to lamotrigine and levetiracetam, which are relatively cognitively inert (Nickels et al., 2016). In addition, medications such as phenobarbital and valproic acid are also known to disrupt sleep, which may further contribute to cognitive impairments. Nonadherence to ASM treatment may also be a concern, and ranges from 43–58% in children (Devinsky et al., 2018; Michaelis et al., 2018). Even a single missed dose can be detrimental and can result in seizure recurrence, poorer QOL, greater health resource utilization, pharmacoresistance, and even death (Devinsky et al., 2018; Michaelis et al., 2018). Despite the introduction of ASMs with novel mechanisms of action, the frequency of drug-resistant epilepsy has remained at approximately 33% (Devinsky et al., 2018). For this subgroup of patients, of whom < 4% are expected to achieve seizure control from continued ASM regimens, treatment options include epilepsy surgery, neurostimulation, and dietary therapies.

Epilepsy surgery involves excision of the area of the brain where seizures originate, is highly effective, and should be considered for all patients after failing to achieve seizure control after two trials of tolerated, appropriately chosen, and appropriately used ASM regimens (Devinsky et al., 2018). On average, the neuropsychological profile of children remains similar in the short term after surgery (Smith, Elliott, & Lach, 2004), with newer long-term studies suggesting improvements in some areas associated with seizure control (Puka et al., 2017).

Approximately one-third of individuals with drug-resistant epilepsy are not eligible for epilepsy surgery because a clear unilateral seizure focus cannot be identified, or the benefits of surgery are outweighed by deficits that would subsequently arise due to surgery. Neurostimulation or dietary therapies may be potential treatment options (CCSO, 2016). Neurostimulation commonly involves the use of a vagal nerve stimulator, a device that stimulates the vagus nerve with electrical impulses. Dietary therapies commonly involve the ketogenic diet—a strict high-fat, low-carbohydrate diet carefully monitored by a dietician. Notably, neurostimulation or dietary therapies are not considered alternatives to epilepsy surgery in eligible patients, because they result in few patients achieving complete seizure control (Devinsky et al., 2018). The ketogenic diet is the treatment of choice for certain conditions such as *GLUT1* deficiency.

CONCLUSIONS AND FUTURE DIRECTIONS

In recent years, a new classification of seizures and subtypes of epilepsy has been proposed that conceptualizes focal and generalized seizures as manifestations of a disease of brain networks (Fisher et al., 2014). Wilson and Baxendale (2014) posited that this change challenges us to rethink the relationship between neuropsychological deficits and epilepsy, arguing that there are differences between what they termed "essential comorbidities" and "secondary effects" of seizures. In this view, the essential comorbidities are assumed to share common mechanisms reflecting the underlying pathology in the network. In the past decade, inroads have been made into investigating the nature of functional connectivity between different brain regions in children with epilepsy and relating such patterns to cognition (Bear, Chapman, & Tregellas, 2019). Future work should focus on furthering such studies to bring light to the cognitive and psychosocial deficits that may be specific to particular epilepsy syndromes and to understanding shared comorbidities across syndromes. Complementing these approaches are the significant strides being made in the understanding of the genetics of childhood-onset epilepsy (Avanzini et al., 2018). These findings may lead to increased understanding of the causes and interrelationships among the cognitive, emotional, and psychosocial features exhibited by children.

Work is required to hone our neuropsychological test instruments to identify those measures that provide the best understanding of the child's current function and reflect the complexities of plasticity or failure of reorganization of brain function, and are sensitive to change with increasing age or changes in epilepsy parameters. In addition, emphasis is sorely needed for systematic research on the best cognitive and psychosocial interventions to maximize the child's development and to avoid the entrenched negative long-term consequences of epilepsy (Hermann et al., 2017).

In order to understand further the developmental aspects of the neuropsychological features of epilepsy, longitudinal studies are required. Ideally, these studies will incorporate information on the spectrum of comorbidities and features of brain structure and physiological function, and will also incorporate key parental, family, and environmental variables. Knowing what changes and when could potentially provide better care and predictions about outcomes. Such work may also help to distinguish between those children whose seizures are well controlled and those who go on to develop medically refractory epilepsies.

REFERENCES

Aaberg, K. M., Bakken, I. J., Lossius, M. I., Lund Soraas, C., Haberg, S. E., Stoltenberg, C., . . . Chin, R. (2016). Comorbidity and childhood epilepsy: A Nationwide Registry Study. *Pediatrics, 138*(3), Article e20160921.

Austin, J. K., Perkins, S. M., Johnson, C. S., Fastenau, P. S., Byars, A. W., deGrauw, T. J., & Dunn, D. W. (2011). Behavior problems in children at time of first recognized seizure and changes over the following 3 years. *Epilepsy and Behavior, 21*(4), 373–381.

Auvin, S., Wirrell, E., Donald, K. A., Berl, M., Hartmann, H., Valente, K., . . . Wilmshurst, J. M. (2018). Systematic review of the screening, diagnosis, and management of ADHD in children with epilepsy: Consensus paper of the Task Force on Comorbidities of the ILAE Pediatric Commission. *Epilepsia, 59*(10), 1867–1880.

Avanzini, G., Mantegazza, M., Terragni, B., Canafoglia, L., Scalmani, P., & Franceschetti, S. (2018). The impact of genetic and experimental studies on classification and therapy of the epilepsies. *Neuroscience Letters, 667,* 17–26.

Bear, J. J., Chapman, K. E., & Tregellas, J. R. (2019). The epileptic network and cognition: What functional connectivity is teaching us about the childhood epilepsies. *Epilepsia, 60,* 1491–1507.

Berg, A. T., Berkovic, S. F., Brodie, M. J., Buchhalter, J., Cross, J. H., van Emde Boas, W., . . . Scheffer, I. E. (2010). Revised terminology and concepts for organization of seizures and epilepsies: report of the ILAE Commission on Classification and Terminology, 2005–2009. *Epilepsia, 51*(4), 676–685.

Berg, A. T., Caplan, R., Baca, C. B., & Vickrey, B. G. (2013). Adaptive behavior and later school achievement in children with early-onset epilepsy. *Developmental Medicine and Child Neurology, 55*(7), 661–667.

Berg, A. T., Smith, S. N., Frobish, D., Beckerman, B., Levy, S. R., Testa, F. M., & Shinnar, S. (2004). Longitudinal assessment of adaptive behavior in infants and young children with newly diagnosed epilepsy: Influences of etiology, syndrome, and seizure control. *Pediatrics, 114*(3), 645–650.

Besag, F., Gobbi, G., Aldenkamp, A., Caplan, R., Dunn, D. W., & Sillanpaa, M. (2016). Psychiatric and Behavioural Disorders in Children with Epilepsy (ILAE Task Force Report): Behavioural and psychiatric disorders associated with childhood epilepsy, syndromes. *Epileptic Disorders, 18*(Suppl. 1), 1–86.

Bonilha, L., Tabesh, A., Dabbs, K., Hsu, D. A., Stafstrom, C. E., Hermann, B. P., & Lin, J. J. (2014). Neurodevelopmental alterations of large-scale structural networks in children with new-onset epilepsy. *Human Brain Mapping, 35*(8), 3661–3672.

Braakman, H. M., Vaessen, M. J., Hofman, P. A., Debeij-van Hall, M. H., Backes, W. H., Vles, J. S., & Aldenkamp, A. P. (2011). Cognitive and behavioral complications of frontal lobe epilepsy in children: A review of the literature. *Epilepsia, 52*(5), 849–856.

Braams, O., Meekes, J., van Nieuwenhuizen, O., Schappin, R., van Rijen, P. C., Veenstra, W., . . . Jennekens-Schinkel, A. (2015). Two years after epilepsy surgery in children: Recognition of emotions expressed by faces. *Epilepsy and Behavior, 51,* 140–145.

Buelow, J. M., Perkins, S. M., Johnson, C. S., Byars, A. W., Fastenau, P. S., Dunn, D. W., & Austin, J. K. (2012). Adaptive functioning in children with epilepsy and learning problems. *Journal of Child Neurology, 27*(10), 1241–1249.

Caplan, R., Levitt, J., Siddarth, P., Wu, K. N., Gurbani, S., Shields, W. D., & Sankar, R. (2010). Language and brain volumes in children with epilepsy. *Epilepsy and Behavior, 17*(3), 402–407.

Caplan, R., Siddarth, P., Vona, P., Stahl, L., Bailey, C., Gurbani, S., . . . Donald Shields, W. (2009). Language in pediatric epilepsy. *Epilepsia, 50*(11), 2397–2407.

Critical Care Services Ontario. (2015). *Provincial guidelines for the management of epilepsy in adults and children.* Toronto: Author.

Critical Care Services Ontario. (2016). *Provincial guidelines for the management of medically refractory epilepsy in adults and children who are not candidates for epilepsy surgery.* Toronto, ON: Author.

de Boer, H. M., Mula, M., & Sander, J. W. (2008). The global burden and stigma of epilepsy. *Epilepsy and Behavior, 12*(4), 540–546.

Devinsky, O., Vezzani, A., O'Brien, T. J., Jette, N., Scheffer, I. E., de Curtis, M., & Perucca, P. (2018). Epilepsy. *Nature Reviews Disease Primers, 4,* Article 18024.

Elliott, I. M., Lach, L., & Smith, M. L. (2005). I just want to be normal: A qualitative study exploring how children and adolescents view the impact of intractable epilepsy on their quality of life. *Epilepsy and Behavior, 7*(4), 664–678.

Fastenau, P. S., Shen, J., Dunn, D. W., Perkins, S. M., Hermann, B. P., & Austin, J. K. (2004). Neuropsychological predictors of academic underachievement in pediatric epilepsy: Moderating roles of demographic, seizure, and psychosocial variables. *Epilepsia, 45*(10), 1261–1272.

Ferro, M. A., & Speechley, K. N. (2009). Depressive symptoms among mothers of children with epilepsy: A review of prevalence, associated factors, and impact on children. *Epilepsia, 50*(11), 2344–2354.

Fiest, K. M., Sauro, K. M., Wiebe, S., Patten, S. B., Kwon, C. S., Dykeman, J., . . . Jette, N. (2017). Prevalence and incidence of epilepsy: A systematic review and meta-analysis of international studies. *Neurology, 88*(3), 296–303.

Fisher, R. S., Acevedo, C., Arzimanoglou, A., Bogacz, A., Cross, J. H., Elger, C. E., . . . Wiebe, S. (2014). ILAE official report: A practical clinical definition of epilepsy. *Epilepsia, 55*(4), 475–482.

Fisher, R. S., Cross, J. H., D'Souza, C., French, J. A., Haut, S. R., Higurashi, N., . . . Zuberi, S. M. (2017a). Instruction manual for the ILAE 2017 operational classification of seizure types. *Epilepsia, 58*(4), 531–542.

Fisher, R. S., Cross, J. H., French, J. A., Higurashi, N., Hirsch, E., Jansen, F. E., . . . Zuberi, S. M. (2017b). Operational classification of seizure types by the International League Against Epilepsy: Position Paper of the ILAE Commission for Classification and Terminology. *Epilepsia, 58*(4), 522–530.

Gascoigne, M., Smith, M. L., Webster, R., Barton, M., Gill, D., & Lah, S. (2013). Autobiographical memory in children with temporal lobe epilepsy. *Journal of the International Neuropsychology Society, 19*(10), 1076–1086.

Gascoigne, M. B., Smith, M. L., Barton, B., Webster, R., Gill, D., & Lah, S. (2014). Accelerated long-term forgetting in children with temporal lobe epilepsy. *Neuropsychologia, 59*, 93–102.

Gonzalez, L. M., Embuldeniya, U. S., Harvey, A. S., Wrennall, J. A., Testa, R., Anderson, V. A., & Wood, A. G. (2014). Developmental stage affects cognition in children with recently-diagnosed symptomatic focal epilepsy. *Epilepsy and Behavior, 39*, 97–104.

Gonzalez, L. M., Mahdavi, N., Anderson, V. A., & Harvey, A. S. (2012). Changes in memory function in children and young adults with temporal lobe epilepsy: A follow-up study. *Epilepsy and Behavior, 23*(3), 213–219.

Gonzalez, L. M., & Wrennall, J. A. (2020). A neuropsychological model for the pre-surgical evaluation of children with focal-onset epilepsy: An integrated approach. *Seizure, 77*, 29–39.

Goodwin, S. W., Wilk, P., Campbell, K. M., & Speechley, K. N. (2017). Emotional well-being in children with epilepsy: Family factors as mediators and moderators. *Epilepsia, 58*(11), 1912–1919.

Hamiwka, L. D., Yu, C. G., Hamiwka, L. A., Sherman, E. M. S., Anderson, B., & Wirrell, E. (2009). Are children with epilepsy at greater risk for bullying than their peers? *Epilepsy and Behavior, 15*(4), 500–505.

Helmstaedter, C., & Elger, C. E. (2009). Chronic temporal lobe epilepsy: A neurodevelopmental or progressively dementing disease? *Brain, 132*(Pt. 10), 2822–2830.

Hermann, B., Jones, J., Sheth, R., Dow, C., Koehn, M., & Seidenberg, M. (2006). Children with new-onset epilepsy: Neuropsychological status and brain structure. *Brain, 129*(Pt. 10), 2609–2619.

Hermann, B., Loring, D. W., & Wilson, S. (2017). Paradigm shifts in the neuropsychology of epilepsy. *Journal of the International Neuropsychological Society, 23*(9–10), 791–805.

Hermann, B. P., Jones, J. E., Jackson, D. C., & Seidenberg, M. (2012). Starting at the beginning: The neuropsychological status of children with new-onset epilepsies. *Epileptic Disorders, 14*(1), 12–21.

Jackson, D. C., Dabbs, K., Walker, N. M., Jones, J. E., Hsu, D. A., Stafstrom, C. E., . . . Hermann, B. P. (2013). The neuropsychological and academic substrate of new/recent-onset epilepsies. *Journal of Pediatrics, 162*(5), 1047–1053.

Jackson, D. C., Jones, J. E., Hsu, D. A., Stafstrom, C. E., Lin, J. J., Almane, D., . . . Hermann, B. P. (2019). Language function in childhood idiopathic epilepsy syndromes. *Brain and Language, 193*, 4–9.

Jones, C., & Reilly, C. (2016). Parental anxiety in childhood epilepsy: A systematic review. *Epilepsia, 57*(4), 529–537.

Jones, J. E. (2014). Treating anxiety disorders in children and adolescents with epilepsy: What do we know? *Epilepsy and Behavior, 39*, 137–142.

Kanner, A. M. (2017). Psychiatric comorbidities in new onset epilepsy: Should they be always investigated? *Seizure, 49*, 79–82.

Kerr, E. N., & Fayed, N. (2017). Cognitive predictors of adaptive functioning in children with symptomatic epilepsy. *Epilepsy Research, 136*, 67–76.

Kerr, M. P., Mensah, S., Besag, F., de Toffol, B., Ettinger, A., Kanemoto, K., . . . Wilson, S. J. (2011). International consensus clinical practice statements for the treatment of neuropsychiatric conditions associated with epilepsy. *Epilepsia, 52*(11), 2133–2138.

Kesselmayer, R. F., Morel, G. M., Bordenave, J. M., Jones, J., & Hermann, B. (2019). Epilepsy and cognition. In M. Mula (Ed.), *The comorbidities of epilepsy* (pp. 245–272). London: Academic Press.

Loring, D. W. (2010). History of neuropsychology through epilepsy eyes. *Archives of Clinical Neuropsychology, 25*(4), 259–273.

MacAllister, W. S., & Sherman, E. M. S. (2015). Evaluation of children and adolescents with epilepsy. In W. B. Barr & C. Morrison (Eds.), *Handbook on the neuropsychology of epilepsy* (pp. 37–62). New York: Springer Science.

MacAllister, W. S., Vasserman, M., Rosenthal, J., & Sherman, E. (2014). Attention and executive functions in children with epilepsy: What, why, and what to do. *Applied Neuropsychology: Child 3*(3), 215–225.

Magiorkinis, E., Sidiropoulou, K., & Diamantis, A. (2011). Hallmarks in the history of epilepsy: From antiquity till the twentieth century. In H. Foyaca-Sibat (Ed.), *Novel aspects on epilepsy* (pp. 131–156). London: IntechOpen.

Menlove, L., & Reilly, C. (2015). Memory in children with epilepsy: A systematic review. *Seizure, 25*, 126–135.

Michaelis, R., Tang, V., Goldstein, L. H., Reuber, M., LaFrance, W. C., Jr., Lundgren, T., . . . Wagner, J. L. (2018). Psychological treatments for adults and children with epilepsy: Evidence-based recommendations by the International League Against Epilepsy Psychology Task Force. *Epilepsia, 59*(7), 1282–1302.

Mula, M. (2019). Epilepsy and mood disorders. In M. Mula (Ed.), *The comorbidities of epilepsy* (pp. 299–314). London: Academic Press.

Newton, C. R., & Garcia, H. H. (2012). Epilepsy in poor regions of the world. *Lancet, 380*(9848), 1193–1201.

Ngugi, A. K., Bottomley, C., Kleinschmidt, I., Sander, J. W., & Newton, C. R. (2010). Estimation of the burden of active and life-time epilepsy: A meta-analytic approach. *Epilepsia, 51*(5), 883–890.

Nickels, K. C., Zaccariello, M. J., Hamiwka, L. D., & Wirrell, E. C. (2016). Cognitive and neurodevelopmental comorbidities in paediatric epilepsy. *Nature Reviews: Neurology, 12*(8), 465–476.

Novelly, R. A. (1992). The debt of neuropsychology to the epilepsies. *American Psychologist, 47*(9), 1126–1129.

Oostrom, K. J., Smeets-Schouten, A., Kruitwagen, C. L., Peters, A. C., & Jennekens-Schinkel, A. (2003). Not only a matter of epilepsy: Early problems of cognition and behavior in children with "epilepsy only"—A prospective, longitudinal, controlled study starting at diagnosis. *Pediatrics, 112*(6, Pt. 1), 1338–1344.

Oostrom, K. J., van Teeseling, H., Smeets-Schouten, A., Peters, A. C., & Jennekens-Schinkel, A. (2005). Three to four years after diagnosis: Cognition and behaviour in children with "epilepsy only": A prospective, controlled study. *Brain, 128*(7), 1546–1555.

Puka, K., Ferro, M. A., Camfield, C. S., Levin, S. D., Smith, M. L., Wiebe, S., . . . Speechley, K. N. (2020). Trajectories of quality of life 10-years following a diagnosis of epilepsy in childhood. *Epilepsia, 61*, 1453–1463.

Puka, K., Tavares, T. P., & Smith, M. L. (2017). Development of intelligence 4 to 11 years after paediatric epilepsy surgery. *Journal of Neuropsychology, 11*(2), 161–173.

Puka, K., Tavares, T. P., & Speechley, K. N. (2019). Social outcomes for adults with a history of childhood-onset epilepsy: A systematic review and meta-analysis. *Epilepsy and Behavior, 92*, 297–305.

Rathouz, P. J., Zhao, Q., Jones, J. E., Jackson, D. C., Hsu, D. A., Stafstrom, C. E., . . . Hermann, B. P. (2014). Cognitive development in children with new onset epilepsy. *Developmental Medicine and Child Neurology, 56*(7), 635–641.

Reilly, C., Atkinson, P., Das, K. B., Chin, R. F., Aylett, S. E., Burch, V., . . . Neville, B. G. (2014a). Academic achievement in school-aged children with active epilepsy: A population-based study. *Epilepsia, 55*(12), 1910–1917.

Reilly, C., Atkinson, P., Das, K. B., Chin, R. F., Aylett, S. E., Burch, V., . . . Neville, B. G. (2014b). Neurobehavioral comorbidities in children with active epilepsy: A population-based study. *Pediatrics, 133*(6), e1586–e1593.

Reilly, C., Atkinson, P., Das, K. B., Chin, R. F., Aylett, S. E., Burch, V., . . . Neville, B. G. (2015). Cognition in school-aged children with "active" epilepsy: A population-based study. *Journal of Clinical and Experimental Neuropsychology, 37*(4), 429–438.

Reilly, C., Atkinson, P., Memon, A., Jones, C., Dabydeen, L., Das, K. B., . . . Scott, R. C. (2019).

Global development and adaptive behaviour in children with early-onset epilepsy: A population-based case-control study. *Developmental Medicine and Child Neurology, 61*(2), 145–151.

Russ, S. A., Larson, K., & Halfon, N. (2012). A national profile of childhood epilepsy and seizure disorder. *Pediatrics, 129*(2), 256–264.

Rzezak, P., Fuentes, D., Guimaraes, C. A., Thome-Souza, S., Kuczynski, E., Li, L. M., . . . Valente, K. D. (2007). Frontal lobe dysfunction in children with temporal lobe epilepsy. *Pediatric Neurology, 37*(3), 176–185.

Scheffer, I. E., Berkovic, S., Capovilla, G., Connolly, M. B., French, J., Guilhoto, L., . . . Zuberi, S. M. (2017). ILAE classification of the epilepsies: Position paper of the ILAE Commission for Classification and Terminology. *Epilepsia, 58*(4), 512–521.

Shackleton, D. P., Kasteleijn-Nolst Trenite, D. G., de Craen, A. J., Vandenbroucke, J. P., & Westendorp, R. G. (2003). Living with epilepsy: Long-term prognosis and psychosocial outcomes. *Neurology, 61*(1), 64–70.

Smith, M. L. (2016). Rethinking cognition and behavior in the new classification for childhood epilepsy: Examples from frontal lobe and temporal lobe epilepsies. *Epilepsy and Behavior, 64*(B), 313–317.

Smith, M. L., & Berl, M. (2017). The role and limitations of neuropsychological evaluation. In A. Arzimanoglou, H. Cross, W. D. Gaillard, H. Holthausen, P. Jayakar, P. Kahane, & G. Mathern (Eds.), *Pediatric epilepsy surgery* (pp. 39–50). Montrouge, France: John Libbey Eurotext.

Smith, M. L., & Direnfeld, E. (2012). Memory in children with epilepsy. In A. Zeman, N. Kapur, & M. Jones-Gotman (Eds.), *Epilepsy and memory* (pp. 102–113). Oxford, UK: Oxford University Press.

Smith, M. L., Elliott, I. M., & Lach, L. (2002). Cognitive skills in children with intractable epilepsy: Comparison of surgical and nonsurgical candidates. *Epilepsia, 43*(6), 631–637.

Smith, M. L., Elliott, I. M., & Lach, L. (2004). Cognitive, psychosocial, and family function one year after pediatric epilepsy surgery. *Epilepsia, 45*(6), 650–660.

Smith, M. L., Elliott, I. M., & Lach, L. (2006). Memory outcome after pediatric epilepsy surgery: Objective and subjective perspectives. *Child Neuropsychology, 12*(3), 151–164.

Smith, M. L., & Lah, S. (2011). One declarative memory system or two?: The relationship between episodic and semantic memory in children with temporal lobe epilepsy. *Neuropsychology, 25*(5), 634–644.

Speechley, K. N., Ferro, M. A., Camfield, C. S., Huang, W., Levin, S. D., Smith, M. L., . . . Zou, G. (2012). Quality of life in children with new-onset epilepsy: A 2-year prospective cohort study. *Neurology, 79*(15), 1548–1555.

Srnka, K., Seidenberg, M., Hermann, B., & Jones, J. (2018). Intraindividual variability in attentional vigilance in children with epilepsy. *Epilepsy and Behavior, 79,* 42–45.

Stewart, E., Catroppa, C., & Lah, S. (2016). Theory of mind in patients with epilepsy: A systematic review and meta-analysis. *Neuropsychology Review, 26*(1), 3–24.

Stewart, E., Lah, S., & Smith, M. L. (2019). Patterns of impaired social cognition in children and adolescents with epilepsy: The borders between different epilepsy phenotypes. *Epilepsy and Behavior, 100*(B), Article 106146.

Teixeira, J., & Santos, M. E. (2018). Language skills in children with benign childhood epilepsy with centrotemporal spikes: A systematic review. *Epilepsy and Behavior, 84,* 15–21.

Wilson, S. J., & Baxendale, S. (2014). The new approach to classification: Rethinking cognition and behavior in epilepsy. *Epilepsy and Behavior, 41,* 307–310.

Wong, J., & Wirrell, E. (2006). Physical activity in children/teens with epilepsy compared with that in their siblings without epilepsy. *Epilepsia, 47*(3), 631–639.

CHAPTER 4

Brain Tumors and Cancer

M. Douglas Ris

HISTORICAL OVERVIEW

The topic of pediatric brain tumors (PBTs) and cancer spans many types of malignant and nonmalignant diseases, the formal classification of which has undergone repeated changes over the past century. From the perspective of neuropsychology, though, clinical and research contributions have been fairly circumscribed and relatively recent, with much of the effort of neuropsychologists concentrating on a limited number of childhood cancers, such as acute lymphoblastic leukemia (ALL) and brain tumors, especially medulloblastoma (MB). This is likely because they are the most common non-central nervous system (CNS) and CNS malignancies of childhood. But, more importantly, great strides have been made in the treatment of these conditions, albeit at the cost of significant long-term, developmental morbidity among growing numbers of survivors. Thus, ALL and brain tumors are the most common such diseases likely to be encountered in clinical neuropsychological practice and, as a field, neuropsychology has the conceptual and clinical tools needed to understand the complex interplay of developmental and risk factors as they affect the brain over time and how this is manifested in altered cognitive, behavioral, social, and adaptive trajectories.

Data from the Central Brain Tumor Registry of the United States (CBTRUS; Ostrom et al., 2019) capture the challenge of a truly comprehensive treatment of this subject. They show 16 types of tumors based on histology that can arise in 16 locations for children and adolescents. This chapter uses a historical progression as a framework to narrow the scope to those conditions that have the most relevance to contemporary neuropsychology and the populations that clinical neuropsychologists are most likely to encounter in specialized and nonspecialized clinical settings. More specifically, in this chapter, MB and gliomas are highlighted. Among non-CNS cancers, ALL is given more extensive treatment. Several other types of brain tumors and cancers are referenced but not covered in as much depth for the reasons stated earlier. In this way, as much *relevant* ground (for neuropsychologists) is covered as possible within the limits of a single chapter.

As will be seen, this is an extremely complex field that is undergoing constant change and advancement, cutting across many health professions/specialties including, but not limited to, pathology, genetics, radiation oncology, oncology, imaging, psychology, neuropsychology, and epidemiology. In this chapter, the major "currents" are examined, such that the reader comes to understand the history and anticipated future developments in the field.

Unlike adults, children with tumors are typically treated under a research protocol. Member institutions of the Children's Oncology Group (COG) are estimated to treat 90% of children and adolescents with cancer in the United States (*http://childrensoncologygroup.org*). As a result, the history of pediatric psycho-oncology and neuropsycho-oncology is, to a great extent, the history of National Cancer Institute (NCI) funded pediatric cancer cooperative groups (COG and its predecessor organizations, the Children's Cancer Group and the Pediatric Oncology Group) which have, over the last 65 years, achieved remarkable success in improving survival for children whose cancer, previously, almost invariably resulted in death (Ris, 2007).[1] This is particularly the case for ALL, in which long-term survival rates are now over 90%. These strides, though, were made through the discovery of chemotherapy agents and radiotherapy (RT) approaches that were also found to be highly toxic, particularly to the CNS. As awareness and concern for the quality of life of these survivors grew, psychologists and neuropsychologists became increasingly involved in these cooperative groups, initially to measure the degree and type of developmental neurotoxicity experienced by these survivors so as to inform refinements in treatment that would reduce toxicities. Consequently, IQ tests were increasingly incorporated into these protocols as "endpoints" of particular interest. Indeed, the precise developmental information this afforded became a key driver toward treatments of much-reduced toxicity and improved outcomes for these children. Psychological testing protocols also led to improved understanding of behavioral and psychosocial risks faced by survivors of pediatric cancer. While these psychometric tools may be considered crude by today's standards, with the heavy reliance on measures of IQ, as we will see later in this chapter, these instruments have proven their worth as psychometrically sound, omnibus measures of demonstrated sensitivity and ecological validity that do not require highly specialized (neuropsychological) expertise—an important consideration for cooperative groups in which many member programs lack such expertise. For these reasons, IQ measures, though less relied upon exclusively, continue to play an important role in the neurodevelopmental monitoring of children treated for cancer.

In understanding the history of pediatric psycho-oncology and neuropsycho-oncology, it is important to keep in mind that brain tumors and cancers in children are statistically rare diseases. Therefore, research programs can only be sustained at a few highly specialized cancer centers, small consortia, or through cooperative groups. These different research platforms come with distinct advantages and disadvantages that frame the type of questions that each can address. For example, cooperative groups are ill-suited to fine-grained, precise neuropsychological measurement and tracking over long periods of time. Individual institutions or small consortia are better able to collect these types of data for correlative imaging research, for example, but are typically unable to assemble samples of sufficient size for highly powered research. Therefore, these approaches should be viewed as complementary, having produced over the course of several decades a body of scientific

[1]In Europe and other countries throughout the world, the International Society of Paediatric Oncology (SIOP) supports collaborate research protocols among over 1,000 member institutions.

literature that is quite impressive and, moreover, impactful on the quality of life (QOL) for growing numbers of children and their families facing life under the "Sword of Damocles" (Koocher & O'Malley, 1981).

EPIDEMIOLOGY

CNS tumors, leukemias, and lymphomas are the three most common malignances in infants, children, and adolescents, accounting for 61% of all childhood malignancies in the United States between 2000 and 2011 according to the Surveillance, Epidemiology, and End Results (SEER) program of the NCI (*www.seer.cancer.gov*).

CNS Tumors

CNS tumors include both nonmalignant and malignant tumors of the brain and spinal cord. Primary malignant CNS tumors are the second most common childhood malignancies, after hematologic malignancies, and are the most common pediatric solid organ tumor. Brain tumors account for approximately 90% of all CNS tumors, and the remaining CNS tumors are found in the spinal cord and cranial nerves. Although progress has been made in the treatment of childhood tumors, significant mortality and morbidity are still associated with malignant brain tumors Among brain tumors, the most common are MB and glioma, particularly gliomas that are considered histologically low grade (World Health Organization: WHO classifications I and II) (Louis et al., 2016).

Types of CNS tumors vary with age, differing in some important respects between those that present in children and in adults. In children, primary CNS tumors predominate, and approximately one-third to one-half are located in the posterior fossa. In contrast, most CNS tumors in adults are metastatic lesions to the cerebral cortex. Two main classification systems are used to categorize childhood CNS tumors: the WHO classification based on tumor histology and molecular parameters, and the International Classification of Childhood Cancer (ICCC) (*https://seer.cancer.gov/iccc*) based on the primary tumor site and morphology. The WHO classification for CNS tumors, which has been universally adopted, was first published in 1979 and subsequently revised five times, most recently in 2021 (Louis et al., 2021). As of the 2016 WHO revision, classification became based not only on histopathological appearance, but also on well-established molecular parameters.

Soon after the publication of the 2016 revision, it became apparent that the science was expanding so rapidly that this revised classification system was already obsolete. Work began immediately on the next revision, which was published in 2021, becoming the fifth edition of the WHO Classification of Tumors of the Central Nervous System (CNS5). CNS5 emphasized even more the role of molecular diagnostics while preserving histology and immunohistochemistry in tumor characterization. Names were simplified, but in some cases, such as medulloblastoma, deeply engrained tumor terminology was retained. Tumor grading, long linked to natural history and survival, has been retained in CNS5. However, Arabic numerals (CNS WHO grades 1–4) have replaced Roman numerals (I–IV), and neoplasms are graded within types rather than across tumor types. Notably, tumor grade may not be applied if it could lead to confusion in clinical application. For example, in medulloblastoma, a grade of 4 might accurately reflect malignancy but mislead in terms of prognosis as this has become a very treatable disease.

For our purposes, new classification systems complicate our application of a large body of existing epidemiological and outcomes research to tumors that have undergone changes in definition. One is forced to move back and forth between taxonomies, treating tumors defined in the modern era as equivalent to their historical predecessors, which, of course, is problematic. This challenge will be with us for some time as it is acknowledged that the CNS5 represents yet another transitional stage toward more precise future classifications (Louis et al., 2021).

In the United States, based on data from the Central Brain Tumor Registry of the United States (Ostrom et al., 2019), the estimated incidence of primary nonmalignant and malignant CNS tumors is 5.6 cases per 100,000 person-years for children and adolescents ≤ 19 years of age. The rate is higher in males compared with females and greatest in White and Asian/Pacific Islander children. About 4,600 children and teenagers are diagnosed with a primary brain or CNS tumor each year, or almost 13 new cases per day. The incidence rate increased for all age groups from 1975 to 1980 and 1987 to 1992. This has been attributed to the increased availability of magnetic resonance imaging (MRI), which likely resulted in improved diagnostic sensitivity rather than an actual increase in incidence. Embryonal CNS tumors (incidence of 0.64 per 100,000 person-years) include MB (the predominant tumor of this group), CNS primitive neuroectodermal tumors (PNETs), and atypical teratoid/rhabdoid tumors (AT/RTs).[2] Tumors of the sellar region (incidence of 0.78 per 100,000 person-years) include pituitary tumors and craniopharyngiomas. These tumors are generally located in the suprasellar area and arise from remnants of Rathke's pouch. By the late teenage years, pituitary tumors surpass all other types in incidence (Ostrom et al., 2019).

The ICCC is used by the Surveillance, Epidemiology, and End Results (SEER) program of the NCI in its epidemiological survey of childhood cancer in the United States. In this classification schema, tumors are categorized by site of origin, then further subdivided into histologic groups: ependymoma, astrocytoma, primitive neuroectodermal tumor (PNET), other gliomas, and miscellaneous. Being based in part on tumor location, the ICCC system preserves information about clinical presentation that can be important for clinical classification and disease management, such as visual deficits in optic pathway gliomas.

ALL is the most common leukemia in children, accounting for approximately 75% of total leukemias. The second most common is acute myeloid leukemia (AML), which accounts for approximately 20% with other subtypes of leukemias (e.g., juvenile

---

[2]Primitive neuroectodermal tumor was part of an earlier proposed WHO update based on the work of Rorke, Gilles, Davis, and Becker (1985) and essentially subsumed MB (also referred to as cerebellar PNET) but also included a supratentorial variant. The most common pituitary tumor is the craniopharyngioma, which accounts for 6–9% of pediatric brain tumors, with a peak incidence of 8–10 years. Though histologically benign, they tend to infiltrate surrounding tissue, often presenting with endocrine problems, visual disturbance, and behavior problems that may be treated with surgery alone or surgery plus focal RT. *Atypical teratoid/rhabdoid Tumors* (AT/RTs) are rare, malignant, and fast-growing tumors that may arise at a young age (3 years) from any part of the brain or spinal cord, with about 50% located in the cerebellum and brainstem, and are treated with surgery, chemotherapy, and radiotherapy.

myelomonocytic leukemia), making up a small minority of leukemias (*www.seer.cancer.gov*). Peak incidence for ALL is in the 2- to 4-year-old range, while that of MB is 5–9 years, and for astrocytoma it is 0–4 years—a difference suspected of having implications for the biobehavioral phenotypes that result, since they impact development at different stages.

Survivorship

Recent estimates indicate that 75% of children diagnosed with a CNS tumor will become 5-year survivors. Consequently, in 2015, an estimated 66,798 people in the United States were alive after a diagnosis of a pediatric CNS tumor (Phillips et al., 2015). Survival for patients with ALL has improved over the years, from 57% in 1975–1979 to 90% in 2003–2009 (SEER). During the same time frames, survival rates for PBT improved from 59 to 75%. Data from SEER indicates that as of 2010, 60,489 survivors of ALL of all ages were alive in the United States (*www.seer.cancer.gov*).

ETIOLOGY, NEUROPATHOLOGY, AND NEURAL SUBSTRATES

Although the etiology of most childhood CNS tumors remains unknown, one established risk factor is exposure to ionizing radiation, in particular high-dose cranial irradiation in patients with ALL, which is associated with a six- and 10-fold increase in the risk of glioma and meningioma, respectively. A genetic predisposition for CNS tumors is associated with several genetic syndromes, including neurofibromatosis types 1 and 2, tuberous sclerosis, Von Hippel–Lindau syndrome, basal cell nevus syndrome, Li- Fraumeni syndrome, and Turcot syndrome.

Medulloblastoma

These tumors typically arise in the cerebellum, invade the vermis, and consist of poorly differentiated epithelial cells. Prior to the 2016 WHO revision, subtypes consisted of histological variants, such as desmoplastic MB that carried a more favorable prognosis, and more aggressive variants—large-cell MB and large-cell anaplastic MB. Often referred to as average or standard risk MB were tumors in patients older than 3 years, with minimal residual tumor, and no evidence of dissemination. Under CNS5, molecularly defined subtypes now include: Medulloblastoma, WNT-activated; Medulloblastoma, SHH-activated and TP53-wildtype; Medulloblastoma, SHH-activated and TP53-mutant; and Medulloblastoma, non-WNT/non-SHH. Treatment of MB tends to be multimodal and include surgery, craniospinal RT, and chemotherapy. Control of disease dissemination was an important breakthrough in improving survival.

Glioma

The majority of gliomas (tumors with glial cells of origin) in children are low- grade gliomas (LGGs) classified as WHO grade 1 or 2. However, some gliomas are high-grade (WHO grade 3 or 4) and very aggressive, with a low survival rate. Specific subtypes of high-grade gliomas include diffuse midline gliomas, intrinsic pontine gliomas, and glioblastoma multiforme (GBM). Many LGGs are pilocytic astrocytomas (PAs) that are often located in the cerebellum. Juvenile pilocytic astrocytoma (JPA) is the most common subtype and accounts for 16% of all PBTs. Other LGGs include oligodendrogliomas, gangliogliomas, optic pathway gliomas, xanthoastrocytomas, and tectal gliomas. Unlike MB, gliomas, particularly LGG, tend not to spread through the craniospinal axis, and so the emphasis has been on local control through surgery and focal RT radiotherapy. In the case of diffuse gliomas, which, prior to the 2016 revision, were grouped with adult diffuse gliomas, CNS5 nomenclature now designates pediatric-specific types such as diffuse midline glioma, H3 K27M-altered, to replace diffuse intrinsic pontine glioma (DIPG).

Acute Lymphocytic Leukemia

ALL develops from immature lymphocytes (white blood cells) in the bone marrow and spreads throughout the blood, infiltrating the lymph system and various organs, including the CNS. CNS-directed therapy, first proposed in the 1960s, is responsible for the greatly improved survival rate. Improvements over the years have included the substitution of high-dose chemotherapy for cranial radiation for standard risk ALL. Three types of therapy are commonly used: chemotherapy, radiation therapy, and stem cell transplant for children at high risk or for children who relapse. Stages of treatment include induction (4–6 weeks), consolidation/intensification (several months), and maintenance (2–3 years). CNS infiltration is rarely detected at initial diagnosis. CNS-directed chemotherapy is associated with a number of neurological toxicities. Some high-risk patients also receive cranial irradiation. Even though the prognosis for pediatric ALL has continuously improved with contemporary treatment protocols, the CNS compartment is involved in roughly one-third of ALL relapses. CNS involvement at relapse occurs mainly in patients who were CNS negative at initial diagnosis (Alsadeq & Schewe, 2017).

The pathophysiology of neuropsychological effects in PBTs has a great deal to do with the treatments used for controlling the disease. Treatments fall into three categories: surgery, RT, and chemotherapy. These are used individually or in various combinations, depending on tumor and patient factors, such as age at treatment. Historically, surgery was the primary treatment for a brain tumor until the benefits of craniospinal RT were established in the early 1950s (Millard & De Braganca, 2016). In recent decades, various applications of adjuvant chemotherapy have been found to contribute to disease control. All three forms of treatment have undergone tremendous improvements over the past several decades, promising even greater long-term survival rates. Nevertheless, all three are implicated in late effects that concern neuropsychologists. Of the three, therapeutic radiation has been studied the most with regard to risk for neurocognitive impairment in survivors.

Radiotherapy

Over the years, steady advances have been made in RT technology and delivery methods aimed at both improving survival and decreasing toxicity. Fundamentally, the goal of all of these advancements has been to deliver the highest dose to the tumor that can be tolerated, while sparing normal tissue in the vicinity of the tumor or along the path of the radiation beam. This can be accomplished by methods that "shape" the radiation dose through smaller doses delivered in multiple planes, such that the maximum dose conforms to the tumor target area (3-D conformal RT, intensity-modulated RT). By distributing total radiation dose over time in various "fractions" and by using forms of radiation with more desirable radiobiological properties (e.g., with proton beam RT), radiation oncology has developed very sophisticated protocols that are effective for many types of tumors and are well-tolerated by patients. For tumors with a propensity to disseminate, such as MB, radiotherapy typically entails a dose to the brain and spinal cord plus a "boost dose" to the area of the tumor—the entire posterior fossa or the tumor bed.

These approaches and many more have been applied, but not all with the same success, and not all with the same implications for the neurodevelopment of survivors (see review of current status of treatment for childhood tumors by Pollack et al., 2019).

The pathophysiology of radiation-induced injury to the CNS is complicated and traditionally takes place in three stages. Within days of radiation therapy, "acute" changes occur, manifested by edema, headache, and drowsiness. Over the course of the subsequent weeks, "early delayed" effects may occur in the form of demyelination, somnolence, attention deficits, and memory deficits. Acute and early effects are considered transient and reversible, and are infrequent with modern RT methods. In contrast, late effects with an onset of about 6 or more months posttreatment are permanent and believed to result from acute and chronic inflammatory response and oxidative stress that cause damage to vascular endothelium, demyelination, gliosis, white matter necrosis, and cognitive impairment (Greene-Schloesser et al., 2012). Currently, the manner in which RT affects mechanisms of plasticity is a major interest of researchers. Radiation-suppression of hippocampal cell proliferation has been documented in animal models (Rodgers, Zawaski, Sahnoune, Leasure, & Gaber, 2016), although such changes at a cellular level cannot be assumed to manifest behaviorally (Peng et al., 2019).

An often overlooked methodological factor in research on RT effects is how dose reconstruction is accomplished. Typically, particularly in the older literature, patients who do and do not receive RT are contrasted—or patients receiving radiation to the whole brain or craniospinal axis might be compared to those who received only focal or restricted-field radiation. Although limited by the technology available at the time, all of these represent rather imprecise ways of capturing radiation exposures, combining patients with significant differences in both dose and volume of brain irradiated. The importance of dose reconstruction is illustrated in a study by Raghubar et al. (2018b), who compared prescribe dose (the most commonly used approach) to more precise physical (mean dose, maximum dose) and biophysical (integral biologically effective dose, generalized equivalent uniform dose) dose reconstruction methods to a target structure (in this case, the hippocampi). Prescribed dose was found to be uncorrelated with other indices and also a poor predictor of learning and memory test performance, whereas the other indices were significantly intercorrelated and predictive of learning and memory test scores. Researchers are increasingly availing themselves of these sophisticated dose–volume reconstruction approaches that promise greater precision when modeling the effects of RT in children with PBTs (Merchant et al., 2006).

Chemotherapy

Chemotherapy protocols for children with brain tumors are tailored to the tumor type and age of the child. Sometimes chemotherapy is given weekly during radiation treatments to enhance the effect of the radiation. Children with MB are usually treated with multiagent chemotherapy. For many other types of tumors, including gliomas, chemotherapy may be used to control residual disease following surgery, or in very young children, to delay treatment with RT.

Until the development of CNS-directed chemotherapy and RT in the 1960s, CNS relapse kept the survival rate for ALL low. Since then, however, refined protocols that are risk-adapted have greatly improved the long-term survival rate of standard-risk ALL. Methotrexate (MTX) has been most implicated and so most studied in regard to neurocognitive late effects. MTX may be delivered intrathecally or intravenously, and intensive MTX therapy has been associated with neurocognitive problems and white matter changes, with significant individual variation. Krull et al. (2008) reported that such variability may be related to certain folate pathway genetic polymorphisms modulating the effects of MTX. Steroids have been used for different purposes in PBTs and ALL. In the former, they control tumor- or surgery-related inflammation, while in ALL they are used as antineoplastic agents. High-dose steroids, such as dexamethasone, have been reported to cause "steroid dementia syndrome" (Wolkowitz, Lupien, & Bigler, 2007) and cognitive deficits (Waber et al., 2000).

As previously noted, psychologists and neuropsychologists have played an essential role in documenting greater neurodevelopmental toxicity associated with certain treatments (e.g., combined intrathecal MTX and cranial radiation) (Maclean et al., 1995). Evaluating these treatments on the basis of both survival and QOL was a turning point that established this as a model for other malignancies. It is commonplace now for treatment protocols to include some form of neuropsychological and/or quality-of-life long-term monitoring of survivors. Whereas improvement in treatment of average-risk ALL is associated with much lower risk for neuropsychological sequelae, risk for relatively mild effects for these children remains. And, for those patients with high-risk ALL necessitating treatments of higher toxicity, neuropsychological risk is significant enough to warrant continued surveillance into survivorship.

Modern neuroimaging has provided a sensitive tool for the identification of altered brain structure and function in ALL. White matter volume was found to be reduced compared to healthy controls, even for those treated with chemotherapy-only, versus those treated with chemotherapy and radiation therapy (Reddick et al., 2006). White matter, but not gray matter, volumes differed significantly between the two treatment groups and between chemotherapy-only and healthy controls. New "connectome" research has been used to study chemotherapy-related white matter effects in ALL. Using diffusion tensor imaging (DTI) data to construct connectomes, Kesler, Gugel, Huston-Warren, and Watson (2016) found lower "small-worldedness" in cancer survivors treated with chemotherapy. This implies decreased connectivity within neighboring brain regions, such that efficiency of local processing is reduced.

Surgery

In PBTs, greater extent of resection is closely associated with improved long-term survival. Modern imaging and surgical technology have permitted increased precision in tumor resection, better demarcation of tumor from nontumor tissue, minimization of mechanical injury to the brain, and improved supportive care and management of complications (e.g., hydrocephalus). Whether or not the desired gross-total resection is achieved, however, is a function of invasiveness and location. For some tumors (e.g., DIPGs[3]), surgery other than biopsy to confirm histology may be inappropriate. Other tumors are located in so-called "eloquent" areas of the brain where only a partial resection is justified, with more aggressive surgery risking major postsurgical morbidity such as paralysis or significant loss of vision. These are often in less accessible areas, such as deep midline structures (e.g., hypothalamus, basal ganglia, tectum). Surgical approach and technique, including endoscopic surgery, varies as a function of tumor characteristics, as well as the preferences of the neurosurgeon. Research on predictors of neuropsychological outcomes has focused less on surgical factors than on chemotherapy and RT factors. One recent exception is the research of Mabbott and associates (2011; Law et al., 2012) on the surgical compromise of circuits associated with cerebellar mutism syndrome (discussed later).

Some tumors are very accessible and well demarcated such that it may be reasonable to speak of a "surgical cure." A noteworthy example is JPAs, which are LGGs often situated in the cerebellar hemispheres. Unlike many other tumors, these may be managed exclusively by the neurosurgery service and not receive the more comprehensive, prospective monitoring available through many cancer centers. Thus, they may only come to the attention of a neuropsychologist if and when concerns (e.g., with school) arise. Terms such as *low-grade* or *benign*, however, can be misleading, as these tumors still carry substantial risk for recurrence, particularly following a subtotal resection. For example, in one study, second or even third surgeries for progressive disease were needed for 28% of patients treated with surgery only (Turner, et al., 2009). Survivors of such tumors are often left with neurological and neuropsychological impairments that impact their development, including adult outcome (Ris et al., 2008, 2019; Beebe et al., 2005).

NEUROPSYCHOLOGICAL CONSEQUENCES

This section selectively samples the extant literature by applying a neuropsychological domain framework that parses the extensive and heterogenous literature by functional domain. A large body of data now attest to the development of late effects in PBT and cancer populations. Foundational capacities (working memory, processing speed, attention) in particular have been the focus of investigation given their importance in providing a firm underpinning and scaffolding for later-emerging skills (Shatz, Kramer, Ablin, & Matthay, 2000; Palmer et al., 2013). Measurement of change over time, though, is highly challenging, and methodological differences in these studies no doubt contribute to variability in findings (see Ris, Grosch, Fletcher, Metah, & Kahalley, 2017, on establishing a baseline; Duda et al., 2020, on reliable change; and Ris & Hiscock, 2013, on the Flynn effect). In particular, investigators have been careful to point out that the "decline" over

[3]DIPGs are high-grade tumors of the brainstem, typically the pons, where 20% of PBTs arise. They are usually not surgically respectable, may respond temporarily to focal RT, and carry a poor prognosis (5–6 months progression-free survival). In contrast, dorsal exophytic brainstem gliomas are low-grade and often treatable with surgery and RT.

time often described in these children is relative and not absolute. In other words, they tend not to lose skills so much as fail to keep pace with the development of their healthy peers, resulting in lagging or declining standardized scores.

Primary Sensory and Motor Deficits

Primary visual, hearing, and motor problems greatly complicate both the assessment of these children and the interpretation of test data.

Visual deficits might present as acuity problems, diplopia (double vision) and other visual effects that may improve over time or by corrective lens or surgery. Children with optic pathway/hypothalamic tumors[4] may present with blindness or visual field impairments (hemianopsia, quadrantanopsia) that may result from tumor infiltration, compression, or surgical section of the optic nerves and pathways.

Sensorineural hearing loss is also commonly encountered, particularly in children who have been treated with platinum-based chemotherapy. Radiation to the cochlea can result in permanent damage and loss of hearing. Recent research suggests that diminished hearing is one of the factors that adversely affects intellectual development in these children (Heitzer et al., 2020b). In comprehensive cancer centers, hearing is routinely tracked for several years after treatment in patients who are at increased risk for hearing loss.

Treatment with vincristine and to a lesser extent vinblastine, frequently causes peripheral neuropathy. This can improve with age, although less improvement is expected for patients treated at an older age (Monje & Fisher, 2011).

General Intellectual Functioning

Early studies on intellectual outcome following standard treatment for MB documented significant decline over several years posttreatment. For example, Hoppe-Hirsch et al. (1990) reported that 75% of patients with MB followed up to 10 years achieved IQs less than 80. Ris, Packer, Goldwein, Jones-Wallace, and Boyett (2001) reported an average decline of 17.4 Full Scale IQ points over 4 years in patients with MB. Vulnerability of younger patients was also evident in these early studies, with Mulhern et al. (1998) reporting a 10–15-point IQ advantage for younger children treated with a lower dose of cranial radiation over those treated with a higher dose.

With improved therapies that both decrease dose (e.g., from a craniospinal dose of 36 Gy to 23.4 Gy in the study by Ris et al., 2001), and volume of brain irradiated, as well as less toxic adjuvant chemotherapy, effect sizes have declined. In a later study of standard-risk patients with MB, Ris et al. (2013) reported a Full Scale IQ (FSIQ) decline of 1.9 points per year.

The benefits of reducing the volume of brain irradiated are not restricted to diseases treated with focal RT (Mabbott et al., 2011), but have also been found to apply to the boost dose in the context of craniospinal radiotherapy for diseases like MB. Moxon-Emre

---

[4]Optic pathway/hypothalamic tumors are low-grade gliomas that tend to occur in younger children and arise from the optic nerve, optic chiasm, or hypothalamus. They have been treated with surgery, focal RT, and chemotherapy with a high survival rate, but they also tend to recur.

et al. (2014) reported better neurocognitive outcomes when the boost was limited to the tumor bed versus the entire posterior fossa.

Kahalley et al. (2019) studied the intellectual outcome following craniospinal proton beam radiotherapy for MB. This technology is increasingly available to children with brain tumors and entails an improved concentration of the highest dose to the tumor site, while greatly reducing the exposure of normal tissue in the path of the radiation beam. Results indicated stable functioning over several years posttreatment in the domains of Global IQ, perceptual reasoning, and working memory. Only processing speed declined. In contrast, patients with MB treated with conventional X-ray RT showed declines in all IQ domains.

For LGGs treated with surgery only, effects on intellectual functioning are measurable but tend to be small and stable in contrast to the decline over time documented in patients treated with radiation (Ris et al., 2008). Craniopharyngiomas, as well, often exhibit no or negligible effects on overall intellectual functioning (Fournier-Goodnight et al., 2017). However, more specific cognitive and sensory deficits may occur.

Treatments for ALL have also undergone significant reductions in toxicity, attenuating long-term intellectual burden. In one study, those treated for ALL with chemotherapy only show better preservation of IQ 3 years posttreatment (FSIQ m = 100.7) than those treated with both cranial radiotherapy and chemotherapy (FSIQ m = 91), although the chemotherapy-only group was still lower than matched healthy controls (FSIQ m = 107.2) (Anderson, Godber, Smibert, Weiskop, & Ekert, 2000). At a mean of 7 years postdiagnosis, Spiegler et al. (2006) did not find a significant difference for children with ALL treated with high-dose MTX versus very high-dose MTX. In a meta-analysis based on 28 studies published between 1980 and 2004 (Campbell et al., 2007), broad intellectual and neurocognitive deficits in ALL survivors were found, but chemotherapy-only patients did not consistently differ from controls. Effects, when seen, were particularly evident in the areas of attention, processing speed, and executive function.

Children with high-risk leukemia or treatment-refractory ALL may be treated with bone marrow transplant (BMT). Annett, Patel, and Phipps (2015, p. S461) summed up the literature on BMT: "Evidence for the impact of CNS-directed therapies for BMT offers relatively weak evidence of interval neuropsychological change although evidence points to younger children (< 3 years) treated with TBI (total body irradiation) as being the subgroup at highest risk."

Academic Skills

Academic failure and need for special education services were documented in early studies, particularly in the case of MB (Hoppe-Hirsch et al., 1990; Dennis, Spiegler, Heatherington, & Greenberg, 1996). Mulhern et al. (1998) reported that 12 of 22 patients with MB required special education services. Dennis et al. (1996) reported that three-fourths of survivors of MB had academic failure or reported learning difficulties, particularly in math. More recent studies based on standardized test performance have likewise found declines relative to peers in all subjects, even with (what was historically) a reduced dose of craniospinal radiation (Ris et al., 2013). Declines in reading for patients with cerebellar mutism syndrome (see "Predictors and Moderators") were particularly evident. Conklin, Li, Xiong, Ogg, and Merchant (2008) found that the academic performance of 87 patients with ependymoma[5] treated with conformal radiotherapy to the tumor was not spared. Reading, in particular, declined over time, with the hypothesized mechanism being compromise of the left ventral visual pathway early in reading development. Holland, Hughes, and Stavinoha (2015) attributed the poor academic performance of their 36 patients with MB to impaired academic fluency based in processing speed deficits.

Adolescent and adult survivors of ALL treated with chemotherapy reported higher rates of learning problems (28%) compared to siblings (14%) in the Childhood Cancer Survivor Study (CCSS)[6]; (Jacola et al. 2016). Those treated with cranial radiation had higher rates of special education placement (45%).

Perceptual–Motor Skills

Pyramidal and extrapyramidal motor systems are often impacted directly by the tumor or indirectly through surgical trauma, chemotherapy, RT, or complications such as hydrocephalus. In patients with MB, Spiegler, Bouffet, Greenberg, Rutka, and Mabbott (2004) found that longitudinal trajectories for motor skills differed from those of other neuropsychological domains in that motor skills tended to be impacted early, then stabilize while cognitive skills tended to show early stability with later decline.

Reduced processing speed (PS) is one of the most commonly reported findings in the late-effects literature. But as in other neuropsychological domains, PS denotes many component abilities, and measures can vary in task parameters resulting in differential sensitivity to neurological insult. For example, much of the literature reporting impaired PS in children treated for brain tumors, particularly those treated with RT, is based on complex measures or composite scores such as the Processing Speed Index (PSI) of the Wechsler scales. Several studies attest to the particular sensitivity of this index, with declines in these scores evident at baseline measured within the first few weeks after surgery (Robinson, Fraley, Pearson, Kuttesch, & Compas, 2013), or defined as the intercept of the statistical models (Moxon-Emre et al., 2014). Jacobson, Mahone, Yeates, and Ris (2019), however, demonstrated differential effects depending upon complexity—that is, simple PS tasks, such as peg placement and reaction time tasks, were less sensitive than PSI to treatment with RT.

Language

Discrete skills and global language development are often relatively preserved in children treated for brain tumors. This is reflected in the relative strength in Verbal Comprehension/Verbal IQ on the Wechsler scales (Ris et al., 2013), as well as the Verbal Domain in

---

[5]Ependymomas can occur as WHO grades 1–3 with subtotal resections often followed by RT, except in very young children (< 12 months). Approximately two-thirds arise in the posterior fossa. Surgery for these tumors can be complicated by their propensity to adhere to the brainstem. Ependymomas also occur at younger ages than MB.

[6]The CCSS is a seminal epidemiological study of survivors of childhood cancer who were diagnosed between 1970 and 1986 and have been followed continuously, along with a comparison group of siblings (Robison et al., 2009).

adults treated as children for LGG (Ris et al., 2019). Nevertheless, verbal intelligence may decline over time, along with other intellectual indices. Individual cases may demonstrate specific receptive or expressive language impairment if the tumor encroaches on classic left-hemisphere language areas or networks. In contrast to language functions, speech production is often affected in a striking manner in patients with posterior fossa tumors, and these deficits may not completely resolve (see "Predictors and Moderators").

Attention

Attention problems have often been reported following treatment for PBTs. These problems may be displayed on commonly used measures of sustained attention, such as the Continuous Performance Task (CPT), or in composite cognitive test scores, such as the Working Memory Index. Problems with inattention were reported for up to 5 years following treatment with RT by Kiehna, Mulhern, Li, Xiong, and Merchant (2006). Similarly, patients treated with RT for MB were reported to have decreased attention and decreased inhibition 1–5 years posttreatment (Reeves et al., 2006). Parent ratings of attention problems tend to be higher than for healthy, same-age peers, although they typically do not reach clinical levels of concern (Willard, Conklin, Huang, Zhang, & Kahalley, 2016). Raghubar et al. (2018b) found decreased attention in patients with PBT treated with and without RT on an auditory attention task, suggesting general effects on attention.

Reddick et al. (2006) found impaired attention in survivors of ALL on a CPT, even in those treated with chemotherapy alone. Unlike most children with attention-deficit/hyperactivity disorder (ADHD), these children do not display overactivity and overt impulsivity, resembling instead the predominantly inattentive presentation of ADHD with "sluggish cognitive tempo" (Becker et al., 2016). However, despite these weaknesses in attention, Kahalley et al. (2011) did not find elevated rates of ADHD (of any subtype) in a sample of children with cancer (PBT and ALL).

Memory

Memory testing often reveals weaknesses following treatment for brain tumors. This may follow resection of a tumor located in the temporal lobe (Whitman et al., 2017). Radiation injury is also suspected to be a factor in the production of specific memory deficits since boost doses in posterior fossa tumors often extend into the temporal lobes.

Particular tumor types, such as craniopharyngiomas and hypothalamic gliomas, may also carry with them an increased risk of memory impairment due to compromised midline memory structures. King et al. (2004) compared patients with tumors in the vicinity of the third ventricle (e.g., hypothalamic hamartomas, craniopharyngiomas) to cerebellar tumors, finding the former group to be impaired on verbal list-learning and delayed recall measures. While Di Pinto, Conklin, Li, and Merchant (2012) did not find impairment in verbal list learning in 57 children treated with conformal RT for LGG and craniopharyngioma, those children who were shunted for hydrocephalus showed adverse effects on learning at baseline and 5 years posttreatment. Nagel et al. (2006) reported verbal retrieval and recognition deficits in a sample of patients with MB during treatment or early posttreatment.

Recently, investigators have explored the relationship between biomarkers of radiation injury and memory functioning. For example, Riggs et al. (2014) found that memory deficits correlated with reduced hippocampal volume and reduced white matter integrity in the uncinate fasciculus. Raghubar et al. (2018a) found that RT dose to both the right and left hippocampi resulted in nonspecific decrements in verbal and visual memory performances.

Executive Functions

Executive functions, a broad category of neuropsychological functions, are highly distributed and networked but assumed to implicate, in particular, the integrity of various regions and connections within and outside of the frontal lobes. As such, they are at risk for disruption secondary to the multiple insults associated with disease, treatments, and complications in PBT. Research on white matter integrity using DTI suggests that the frontal lobes are particularly vulnerable to radiation effects (Qiu, Kwong, Chan, Leung, & Khong, 2007) which may be manifested behaviorally in a wide range of executive function deficits (Spiegler et al., 2004; Wolfe, Madan-Swain, & Kana, 2012).

Working memory (WM) has been studied with both experimental cognitive and clinical methods by Raghubar et al. (2017). On the N-back task, a venerable WM task drawn from cognitive science, patients with PBT treated with RT performed worse than those treated with surgery only. However, the largest group difference was found on the 0-back trial, which is essentially a visual attention task. This was interpreted as consistent with Baddeley's model of WM, with impairment resulting from faulty attentional control in the central executive system (Baddeley, 2003). Conklin et al. (2012) found poorer performance on both experimental and clinical measures of WM in children treated for PBT with conformal RT, with some evidence that the deficits were based in impaired functional networks that include prefrontal brain regions.

Social Cognition

Little empirical research could be found linking PBT and cancer to problems with social cognition, such as those that characterize children with autism spectrum disorders (i.e., deficits in reciprocal social communication and perception). One exception was a study by Bonner et al. (2008), who found facial expression recognition deficits in survivors of PBTs.

More subtle problems of this nature are possible, or even likely, given the broad impact on early brain development and the social isolation that can occur in many of these children, so it may be most prudent to consider this a case of the absence of evidence not necessarily constituting evidence of absence.

Adaptive and Social Functioning

As a group, adaptive and social adjustment are commonly affected in these children and may arise from disruption of neural systems that subserve these functions. As proposed in the social competence model of Yeates et al. (2007) and applied to PBTs by Hocking et al. (2015), brain injury may impact underlying cognitive processes of social information processing, social interaction, and social adjustment. Socioadaptive problems may also be associated with the physical impairments (motor, visual, hearing) and stigmata (alopecia, prominent scars, small stature) that distinguish PBT survivors from their healthy peers, often leading to restrictions that can be the source of embarrassment or even mistreatment. Special education needs, as well, may result in survivors feeling different and being treated so by their peers.

As part of a programmatic investigation of peer relationships (Vannatta et al., 2011), sociometrics and peer nomination methods were used to explore how social competence is affected in children with a range of chronic illnesses, including brain tumors. Overall, children with brain tumors were significantly more likely to score high on the Sensitive/Isolated dimension of the Revised Class Play and low in Leadership–Popularity. Peers also described survivors as higher in Victimization, and survivors self-reported being lower in Surgency (positive affect, energetic) (Salley et al., 2015).

In a longitudinal study of a mixed sample of patients with PBT, the most robust predictors of adaptive functioning 2 years postdiagnosis were premorbid attention and behavior problems (Hoskinson et al., 2018). While standard scores on the ABAS II fell in the average range, the percentage of children exceeding the clinical cutoff was elevated. This was particularly true for Practical Skills. A recent report by Raghubar et al. (2019) suggests that adaptive outcome is more related to sociodemographic factors than to disease or treatment factors. Annual change in IQ did not correlate with annual change in Vineland Adaptive Behavior Scale (VABS) scores in a large sample of children treated with conformal RT for ependymoma, indicating somewhat dissociable causal pathways for perturbed cognitive development and adaptive behavior (Netson, Conklin, Wu, Xiong, & Merchant, 2012).

Emotional and Behavioral Adjustment

In the Hoskinson et al. (2018) study, demographic factors (family income and parent education) predicted behavioral problems on the Behavior Assessment Scale for Children (BASC). Unlike adaptive behavior, parent ratings of emotional–behavioral adjustment were average, without an increased rate of clinical elevations. In contrast, other studies have indicated increased rates of internalizing problems in this population, which may be related to measurement differences across studies (i.e., broadband inventories vs. narrowband questionnaires) (Fuemmelar, Elkin, & Mullins, 2002).

Various aspects of psychosocial risk in pediatric cancer populations were addressed by a COG Psychosocial Late Effects multidisciplinary panel (Bitsko et al., 2016). Their conclusions, based on a review of the literature, were that most survivors experience few psychosocial problems, are not at heightened risk for depression, are at increased risk for symptoms of posttraumatic stress disorder (PTSD) compared to sibs, and are at increased risk for global distress depending on the following risk factors: female gender, unmarried, being a single child, brain tumor diagnosis, diagnosis during adolescence, and receiving more intensive treatment.

In the Jacola et al. (2016) study based in the CCSS, adult survivors of ALL treated with cranial radiotherapy were at higher risk for anxiety–depression, inattention–hyperactivity, and social withdrawal compared to those treated without cranial radiotherapy, who, themselves, were at increased risk compared to sibs for headstrong, attention-hyperactivity, and social withdrawal.

A review of the literature on psychosocial late effects in pediatric cancer (Bitsko et al., 2016, p. 337) summed up the evidence this way: "The majority of studies . . . indicate that survivors experience few psychosocial problems in long-term survivorship. A critical subset, however, are at increased risk . . . secondary to treatment."

DEVELOPMENTAL CONSIDERATIONS

Childhood cancers and brain tumors can occur at any age. Modal ages of diagnosis vary widely from one disease to another. Considering the multiplicity of insults to the developing nervous system distributed over an extended time frame, including well into adulthood (e.g., stroke), a lifespan/chronic illness perspective clearly is required. Concepts of reserve capacity, in particular, are helpful in considering the interaction over time of premorbid factors with disease and treatment factors, as well as complications (Satz, 1993). The "Kennard Principle," based in a mischaracterization of the work of Margaret Kennard (Dennis, 2010, p. 16), whereby "the time to have one's cortical lesion, if one can arrange it, should be early because early lesions seem less disabling than those acquired later in life" (as Teuber provocatively told his students), is actually not supported by the bulk of the literature in PBT and cancer. Rather, substantial evidence indicates that younger children are at higher risk for neurodevelopmental morbidity than older children.

A more elegant account of the relationship between age and plasticity is offered by Dennis et al. (2013), who argue that plasticity may be beneficial or maladaptive, that the plasticity privilege purported to be associated with young age has been overstated, and that plastic change operates in concert with homeostatic mechanisms. For example, in children treated with radiation for brain tumors, the balance between plastic (i.e., change-promoting) and homeostatic (i.e., change-resistant) mechanisms reflects, to some extent, the complex effects of such underlying processes as neuroinflammation.

Growing evidence also indicates that premorbid factors play a significant role in outcome. In the context of PBT, however, operationalizing "premorbid" is complicated (Raghubar et al., 2020), not only because of the distributed (temporally and anatomically) multiplicity of insults mentioned earlier, but also because of our limited understanding of the embryogenesis of PBT. The extent to which tumorigenesis alters regional or global brain development for months or even years before the emergence of clinical signs and symptoms is not yet known but likely varies across diseases.

So-called "growing into a deficit" is another way in which children with cancer may initially appear to be spared, only to exhibit a deficit later relative to their healthy age-peers, akin to what Dennis (1989) has described as a developmental "short-fall." Such a process has been invoked, for example, to explain the delayed emergence of deficits in children with pilocytic astrocytoma (Aarsen et al., 2009).

At the other end of the lifespan, concerns about accelerated cognitive aging have been associated with early insults to the brain (Ris & Hiscock, 2013). Again, such effects might be difficult to tease out in the context of PBT in which insults that occur during childhood (e.g., craniospinal RT) contribute to increased risk of stroke in adulthood. Nevertheless, these diseases and the associated gradient of risk, are likely to continue to impact survivors throughout the lifespan. With improved survival rates, the need for a better understanding of this aging population will become more pressing (Ris et al., 2019).

PREDICTORS AND MODERATORS

Aside from tumor and treatment factors (discussed earlier), factors predictive of increased risk for poorer outcomes include cerebellar mutism syndrome (CMS) and permanent shunt placement.

The hallmark feature of CMS, or posterior fossa syndrome (PFS), is the sudden onset of mutism (or decreased speech production or fluency) within a few days of surgery for a tumor based in the posterior fossa (Gudrunardottir et al., 2016). While mutism is the most striking symptom, other functions may be affected, including alternations in behavior (irritability, lability) and balance (Ris et al., 2013). Marked improvement is typical but may fall short of total resolution. While originally believed to be infrequent, more recent estimates of CMS/PFS are in the range of 20–25% of patients with MB (Robertson et al., 2006). Several studies have now indicated that CMS/PFS is associated with poorer broad neurocognitive outcomes. For example, Ris et al. (2013) found that 22% of patients treated for MB exhibited CMS/PFS and that this was associated with early intellectual and academic deficits. Mabbott and collaborators (Law et al., 2012) have mapped white matter tracts originating in the cerebellum that are implicated in the pathophysiology of the syndrome. Their work indicates that disruption of the right cerebello-thalamo-cerebral (C-T-C) pathway connection to the left cerebral hemisphere may underly the syndrome. Left-handedness, MB histology, and larger tumor size were significant predictors of CMS/PFS. The findings of another MRI study of patients with and without CMS/PFS also pointed to critical involvement of the right C-T-C pathway (Avula et al., 2016). Researchers have proposed that through this injury, the left cerebral hemisphere is deprived of cerebellar modulatory input supporting speech production. However, this proposal does not clearly account for other characteristics of CMS/PFS, such as emotional changes or the impact on nonlanguage cognitive functions.

Hydrocephalus is a common complication when children first present with a brain tumor and often produces symptoms of increased intracranial pressure (i.e., headache, ataxia, blurred retinal discs). In the context of PBT, ventriculomegaly typically arises out of cerebral spinal fluid (CSF) obstruction by a tumor in the fourth ventricle or cerebral aqueduct. Unlike other causes of hydrocephalus associated with congenital malformations, in the case of PBT, the onset may be acute and able to be relieved by resection of the obstructing tumor. Shunting with external drains is common in the acute management of posterior fossa brain tumors (70–80% per Di Rocco, Juca, Zerah, & Sainte-Rose, 2013), with about 30% going on to have a permanent ventriculoperitoneal (VP) shunt placed. Several studies have documented increased risk to neuropsychological development associated with permanent shunting. For example, Hardy, Bonner, Willard, Watral, and Gururangan (2008) found that children with shunted hydrocephalus had lower IQs than those who did not receive shunts.

TREATMENT AND INTERVENTION

The pace of research on the efficacy of interventions to mitigate the neuropsychological and behavioral effects of cancer/PBT and their treatments is accelerating. One of the more established treatments is psychostimulant medication to improve attention and behavioral control. This is based largely on clinical trials conducted at St. Jude Children's Research Hospital. In a series of publications, Conklin and colleagues (2010b) provided strong evidence that methylphenidate at moderate doses (0.6 mg/kg) improves attention in survivors of ALL and PBT, and that improvements are maintained over the course of a year (Conklin et al., 2010b) with low side-effect burden (Conklin et al., 2009). Yet despite improvements in attention across settings (school and home), academic gains were not realized.

Another pharmacological treatment that may hold some promise for survivors of pediatric cancer and brain tumors is metformin, which purportedly stimulates hippocampal neurogenesis and preserves memory functioning in children treated with cranial radiation (Ayoub et al., 2018). The neuroprotective effects of metformin have been investigated in type 2 diabetes, in particular (Ng et al., 2014). However, clinical trials have not yet demonstrated clear efficacy.

Exercise has been shown to ameliorate some of the adverse effects of radiation in both animal models (Sahnoune et al., 2018) and humans. In a controlled trial of 12 weeks of exercise, patients with PBT showed positive changes in white matter integrity, hippocampal volume, and reaction time 1–10 years posttreatment (Riggs et al., 2017).

Under the rubric of "cognitive rehabilitation" are several lines of research, some of which show promise but are as yet unproven. An early and particularly noteworthy attempt to validate such an approach with survivors of childhood cancer was the work of Butler and colleagues and their Cognitive Remediation Program, which demonstrated consistent improvements and generalization to real-world functioning in the area of attention, although effect sizes were modest (e.g., Butler & Mulhern, 2005). More recently, promising results of computerized cognitive training (Cogmed: *www.cogmed.com*) have been reported for children treated for cancer (Conklin et al., 2015).

The most common intervention for childhood survivors of cancer who exhibit chronic neurobehavioral effects is psychoeducational in nature. More specifically, special education resources are garnered to accommodate the individual patterns of exhibited strength and weakness, often using a neuropsychological evaluation as a guide. Anderson, Godber, Smibert, Weiskop, and Ekert (2000) found that greater intensity, higher quality, and tailored educational interventions were associated with improved academic skills in cancer survivors.

While more attention has been paid to neurocognitive and educational needs, rates of some behavioral–emotional problems are elevated in survivors of ALL and PBT (discussed earlier), evidence suggests that this increased risk may be related to premorbid factors. Psychologists may be wary of applying proven treatments for primary behavioral and emotional disorders to similar symptoms exhibited in the context of a neurological condition. While neurological integrity may be an effect modifier, children treated for cancer may be no less likely to respond to such treatments. For example, Treble-Barna, Chapman, Schwartz, and Axelrad (2013) applied an evidence-based intervention for disruptive behavior disorder in the treatment of a child who had undergone right frontotemporal resection for tumor and intractable epilepsy, and demonstrated significant improvement per parent and teacher that was maintained at 2 months posttreatment. Anxiety and symptoms of PTSD, in particular, have been noted in broader cancer populations, and have been treated with some success using evidence-based intervention for PTSD

(Kazak et al., 2004). Poor family functioning appears to be a significant risk factor in these patients (Alderfer, Navsaria, & Kazak, 2009).

Surveillance, Monitoring, and Transition of Care

Chronic illnesses require some form of prospective follow-up so as to detect relapse, complications and other adverse health and adjustment issues for which such patients are at increased risk. How well and how early such problems are detected can greatly affect the health and QOL of patients with chronic illness, including those with PBT and other forms of childhood cancer. Accordingly, neuropsychologists involved in the care of such patients are concerned not only with conducting a single diagnostic evaluation at any particular point in time, but also with how best to track patients over many years to anticipate critical transitions (e.g., from primary to secondary education) and to ensure timely intervention when problems arise (e.g., new deficits secondary to stroke). More so than adult neuropsycho-oncology, working with pediatric populations entails a degree of forward thinking and planning so as to optimize the neuropsychologist's professional contribution to the care of these patients.

Annett, Patel, and Phipps (2015) have proposed some empirically grounded guidelines for the neuropsychological assessment and monitoring of pediatric cancer populations. They conclude that the available evidence supports "regular monitoring of neuropsychological functioning integrated with routine clinical care during and particularly after treatment" (p. S462). They stop short of more explicit guidelines, particularly about the timing of such assessments other than to suggest that the evaluations occur after the completion of treatment and then 2–3 years after treatment or sooner, if significant neuropsychological or functional changes occur.

Baum et al. (2017) elaborated on the range of services provided by neuropsychologists to patients with PBT, distinguishing between neuropsychological monitoring and routine clinical surveillance. *Monitoring* refers to the assessment of change over time in various neurobehavioral domains that inform actual clinical decisions about interventions. *Surveillance* entails regular queries of the patient, parent, and teacher (often through interview or questionnaires) about cognitive and socioemotional functioning.

Effective monitoring and surveillance of survivors may be accomplished through long-term survivor clinics in major cancer centers, although this may not be accessible to many patients. Whether neuropsychologists participate in such clinics/programs or follow survivors apart from such clinics/programs, neuropsychological monitoring and surveillance should be thoughtfully planned and tailored to the individual patient. An important consideration for surveillance and monitoring is risk-adapted intensity. For example, the same amount of neuropsychological resources (frequency, type, and duration of contacts, and extent of formal testing) would not routinely be directed to a condition with a low probability of neuropsychological sequelae as to a condition with a high probability of sequelae. A second consideration is that of critical developmental periods and events. Monitoring and surveillance should take into account developmental timing that would dictate more frequent contacts at younger ages. Critical events such as the transition to high school, when executive function liabilities may surface, also should be considered. Subject and contextual risk factors may also be incorporated into an individualized surveillance/monitoring plan. For example, children with significant premorbid adjustment problems, or those from highly dysfunctional, economically challenged families may be appropriate for more intensive surveillance.

The transition from child/adolescent health systems to adult systems of care is an important aspect of surveillance and monitoring. The potential benefit of systematically incorporating neuropsychology in the transition process for PBT survivors was recently addressed by Heitzer et al. (2020a, 2020b), who proposed a family-centered, multidisciplinary care model that promotes both medical and broader psychosocial transition, with the neuropsychologist playing a key role.

CLINICAL EVALUATION OF THE CHILD OR ADOLESCENT WITH PBT OR CANCER

The clinician involved in the evaluation of patients with childhood cancer and PBT may benefit from the following guidance distilled from the scientific literature and decades of clinical experience in neuropsycho-oncology. Much of this advice may be generalizable to other neurological conditions of childhood, particularly chronic ones:

- Consider the potential impact of the multiple sensory and motor deficits that are common complications in the assessment of these patients and in the interpretation of test findings. Such deficits may or may not be well documented in the medical record. Self- or parent report may also be unreliable in this regard, and patients may be nonadherent to prescribed treatments, such as glasses or hearing aids.
- Since a range of neurobehavioral functions may be affected, a broadband evaluation is often indicated. Well-validated screening tests or batteries are often not available. Instead, rather than a score on a screening test, decisions regarding the allocation of limited and expensive, time-intensive resources, such as a comprehensive neuropsychological evaluation, are better based on presenting complaints (from patient, parent, and teacher), medical history (disease and treatment risk factors), subject risk factors (e.g., age), and contextual risk factors (e.g., family adjustment) to arrive at a determination of net risk that can inform a risk-adapted approach.
- Neurocognitive test results may underestimate functional impairment, so direct assessment of psychosocial (and family) adjustment and adaptive functioning should be routine.
- Fatigue during treatment (Gandy et al., in press) and for years after treatment (Meeske, Katz, Palmer, Burwinkle, & Varni, 2004) is a very common side effect and may interfere with the patient's optimal effort and performance on formal testing. Mitigating the effects of fatigue should be a goal for not only the neuropsychological evaluation but also in regard to the patient's educational and psychosocial adjustment.
- Adverse effects may be delayed, so neuropsychological follow-up in some form is often indicated.
- Parents and patients often require careful explanation of the meaning of scores generated in serial neuropsychological evaluations, particularly the difference between

absolute (raw score) and relative (standardized scores) changes over time. Otherwise, they may erroneously conclude that their child cannot learn or is regressing in skills.

- Communication and coordination with the school is imperative. Sometimes this is undertaken by the neuropsychologist alone or, in large cancer centers, a school liaison team. Typical school personnel have little to no experience with children with cancer and so may make assumptions that are not appropriate for the patient. Standard psychoeducational testing is not sufficient for educational guidance and special education classification decisions. Rather, a neuropsychological evaluation or consultation with an experienced neuropsychologist should be routine.

- Communication with (often several) other providers is also critical to ensure that everyone is "on the same page" and the family is not receiving mixed or confusing messages.

- Prepare early for the transition of care and the attainment of the age of majority. Some cancer centers have formal transition programs. Regardless, the neuropsychologist is often best positioned to understand and guide the processes of increased independence and transferring from child/adolescent-based to adult-based care.

- Treatment options for neurobehavioral sequelae are expanding, placing neuropsychologists in the position of prescribing, informing, or even providing evidence-based treatment.

- Desperate families of cancer survivors sometimes seek out complementary therapies of questionable value that lack empirical support (Myers, Stuber, Bonamer-Rheingans, & Zeltzer, 2005). These interventions may be considered medically harmless, even providing some indirect benefits. However, such interventions can also do harm if they deplete a family's already overtaxed resources (time and money), displace or interfere with proven treatments, add to the discouragement engendered by false promises for improvements, or contribute to an overfocus on a child's deficits rather than the strengthening of competencies in areas of relative strength.

CONCLUSIONS AND FUTURE DIRECTIONS

Pediatric cancer is a challenging but rewarding setting for neuropsychologists who are interested in patient care and research on outcomes. These highly varied diseases are treated through multiple modalities impacting brain function and development at vulnerable ages. Research in this area is often a multidisciplinary team effort involving expertise from neuropsychology, clinical psychology, neuro-oncology, oncology, radiation oncology, neurosurgery, epidemiology, social work, and nursing. Sophisticated statistical methodologies now being applied also require statisticians and methodologists familiar with longitudinal, behavioral research with medical populations.

Work in this area, too, is rewarding in that neuropsychologists have essential and unique expertise to offer that addresses what typically are the overriding questions families have: What long-term effects has the cancer experience had on my child's emotional adjustment and ability to function at school, at home, with peers, in sports, and eventually as an adult? Neuropsychologists can provide an overall conceptualization, integrating information from the various specialties, that is otherwise lacking or presented to parents in fragmented fashion. Families appreciate that someone with the neuropsychologist's unique skill set is part of the team of professionals who will be providing ongoing surveillance and help them grapple with these difficult matters as they occur.

Across the literature on PBT and cancer, one can discern a gradient of biopsychosocial risk as a function of many factors of disease, treatment, and complications intersecting with subject and contextual factors. A few general conclusions can be drawn:

1. The increased risk for these populations spans all neurobehavioral domains.
2. Treatment intensity/toxicity in all modalities is a key factor in determining late effects. This is particularly true for RT.
3. Risk is often a matter of increased rate of problems, compared to healthy controls, that often do not reach diagnostic significance. In group analyses, functioning is often in the range conventionally considered normal or average. Frank psychopathology is not the norm.
4. Relatedly, most children have good outcomes, particularly if the most toxic treatments can be avoided or delayed until later in development.
5. Increased risk may also take the form of neuropathological changes on imaging (particularly in the white matter of the brain) that may not necessarily be manifested at the behavioral level, even on sensitive neuropsychological tests.
6. Risk may change over time in degree and form but is never eliminated, even into late adulthood. Whereas Damocles could flee from the sword suspended by a horsehair, survivors and their families must come to terms with a life that remains more perilous than most.

The trajectory of research thus far, as summarized in this chapter, would suggest that critical insights and discoveries will be forthcoming in the following areas: (1) Continued explication of the highly variable risk to these patients matched with practical, acceptable, cost-effective protocols for long-term neuropsychological surveillance and monitoring that are computerized and Internet-based (Conklin et al., 2013); (2) neuropsychological risk and benefits associated with continuously advancing cancer treatments and technologies; (3) complications that carry the most risk, and how these can be prevented (e.g., CMS/PFS); (4) improved interventions that promote positive cognitive and psychosocial outcomes; (5) a better understanding of linguistic and cultural factors in the neuropsychological management of these diseases (Raghubar et al., 2019); (6) a better understanding of how premorbid factors, including biological and cognitive reserve capacities, influence outcomes, leading to more accurate prediction, early intervention, and optimal allocation of finite resources (Ris & Hiscock, 2013); and (7) application of a lifespan development, chronic disease paradigm that is better suited than the more limited childhood-focus research of the past.

Relatedly, the artificial distinction in health care systems between childhood/adolescence and adulthood is a significant barrier to providing continuity of care for chronic illness populations, including survivors of childhood cancer. There needs to be a sustained, empirically guided reformulation of our health care models to accomplish this transition in a way that promotes continued high-quality care, long-term surveillance, and improved life-outcomes.

REFERENCES

Aarsen, F. K., Paquier, P. F, Arts, W. F., Van Veelen, M. L, Michiels, E., . . . Catsman-Berrevoets, C. E. (2009). Cognitive deficits and predictors 3 years after diagnosis of a pilocytic astrocytoma in childhood. *Journal of Clinical Oncology, 27*(21), 3526–3532.

Alderfer, M. A., Navsaria, N., & Kazak, A. E. (2009). Family functioning and posttraumatic stress disorder in adolescent survivors of childhood cancer. *Journal of Family Psychology, 23*(5), 717–725.

Alsadeq, A., & Schewe, D. M. (2017). Acute lymphoblastic leukemia of the central nervous system: On the role of PBX1. *Haematologica, 102*(4), 611–613.

Anderson, V. A., Godber, T., Smibert, E., Weiskop, S., & Ekert, H. (2000). Cognitive and academic outcome following cranial irradiation and chemotherapy in children: A longitudinal study. *British Journal of Cancer, 82*, 255–262.

Annett, R. D., Patel, S. K., & Phipps, S. (2015). Monitoring and assessment of neuropsychological outcomes as a standard of care in pediatric oncology. *Pediatric Blood and Cancer, 62*, S460–S513.

Avula, S., Spiteri, M., Kumar, R., Lewis, E., Harave, S., . . . Pizer, B. (2016). Post-operative pediatric cerebellar mutism syndrome and its association with hypertrophic olivary degeneration. *Quantitative Imaging in Medicine and Surgery, 6*(5), 535–544.

Ayoub, R., Miller, F., Beera, K., de Medeiros, C., Laughlin, S., Bouffet, E., & Mabbott, D. (2018). Metformin results in hippocampal remodeling and improved memory encoding in paediatric brain tumor survivors treated with cranial radiation: A pilot randomized controlled crossover study. *Neuro-Oncology, 20*, Article i168.

Baddeley, A. (2003). Working memory: Looking back and looking forward. *Nature Reviews Neuroscience, 4*, 829–839.

Baum, K. T., Powell, S. K., Jacobson, L. A., Gragert, M. N., Janzen, L. A., . . . Wilkening, G. N. (2017). Implementing guidelines: Proposed definitions of neuropsychological services in pediatric oncology. *Pediatric Blood and Cancer, 64*, Article e26446.

Becker, S. P., Leopold D. R., Burns, G. L., Jarrett, M. A., Langberg, J. M., . . . Willcutt, E. G. (2016). The internal, external, and diagnostic validity of sluggish cognitive tempo: A meta-analysis and critical review. *Journal of the American Academy of Child and Adolescent Psychiatry, 55*(3), 163–178.

Beebe, D. W., Ris, M. D., Armstrong, F. D., Fontanesi, J., Mulhern, R., Holmes, E., & Wisoff, J. (2005). Cognitive and adaptive outcome in low grade pediatric cerebellar astrocytomas: Evidence of increased risk in national collaborative research studies (CCG9891/POG9130). *Journal of Clinical Oncology, 23*, 5198–5204.

Bitsko, M. J., Cohen, D., Dillon, R., Harvey, J., Krull, K., & Klosky, J. L. (2016). Psychosocial late effects in pediatric cancer survivors: A report from the Children's Oncology Group. *Pediatric Blood and Cancer, 63*(2), 337–343.

Bonner, M. J., Hardy, K. K., Willard, V. W., Anthony, K. K., Hood, M., & Gururangan, S. (2008). Social functioning and facial expression recognition in survivors of pediatric brain tumors. *Journal of Pediatric Psychology, 33*, 1142–1152.

Butler, R. W., & Mulhern, R. K. (2005). Neurocognitive interventions for children and adolescents surviving cancer. *Journal of Pediatric Psychology, 30*, 65–78.

Campbell, L. K., Scaduto, M., Sharp, W., Dufton, L., Van Slyke, D., Whitlock, J. A., & Compas, B. (2007). A meta-analysis of the neurocognitive sequelae of treatment for childhood acute lymphoblastic leukemia. *Pediatric Blood and Cancer, 49*, 65–73.

Conklin, H. M., Ashford, J. M., Howarth, R. A. Merchant, T. E., Ogg, R. J., . . . Xiong, X. (2012). Working memory performance among childhood brain tumor survivors. *Journal of the International Neuropsychological Association, 18*(6), 996–1005.

Conklin, H. M., Ashford, J. M., Di Pinto, M., Vaughan, C. G., Gioia, G. A., . . . Wu, S. (2013). Computerized assessment of cognitive late effects among adolescent brain tumor survivors. *Journal of Neuro-Oncology, 113*(2), 333–340.

Conklin, H. M., Helton, S., Ashford, J., Mulhern, R. K., Reddick, W. E., . . . Khan, R. B. (2010a). Predicting methylphenidate response in long-term survivors of childhood cancer: A randomized, double-blind, placebo-controlled, crossover trial. *Journal of Pediatrics, 35*(2), 144–155.

Conklin, H. M., Lawford, J., Jasper, B. W., Morris, E. B., Howard, S. C., . . . Khan, R. B. (2009). Side effects of methylphenidate in survivors of childhood cancer: A randomized, double-blind, placebo-controlled trial. *Pediatrics, 124*(1), 226–233.

Conklin, H. M., Li, C., Xiong, X., Ogg, R. J., &

Merchant, T. E. (2008). Predicting change in academic abilities after conformal radiation therapy for localized ependymoma. *Journal of Clinical Oncology, 26*, 3965–3970.

Conklin, H. M., Ogg, R. J., Ashford, J. M., Scoggins, M. A., Zou, P., . . . Zhang, H. (2015). Computerized cognitive training for amelioration of cognitive late effects among childhood cancer survivors: A randomized controlled trial. *Journal of Clinical Oncology, 33*(33), 3894–3902.

Conklin, H. M., Reddick, W. E., Ashford, J., Ogg, S., Howard, S. C., . . . Khan, R. B. (2010b). Long-term efficacy of methylphenidate in enhancing attention regulation, social skills, and academic abilities of childhood cancer survivors. *Journal of Clinical Oncology, 28*, 4465–4472.

Dennis, M. (1989). Language and the young damaged brain. In T. E. Boll & B. K. Bryant (Eds.), *Clinical neuropsychology and brain function: Research, measurement, and practice* (pp. 85–124). Washington, DC: American Psychological Association.

Dennis, M. (2010). Margaret Kennard (1899–1975): Not a "principle" of brain plasticity but a founding mother of developmental neuropsychology. *Cortex, 46*(8), 1043–1059.

Dennis, M., Spiegler, B. J., Hetherington, C. R., & Greenberg, M. L. (1996). Neuropsychological sequelae of the treatment of children with medulloblastoma. *Journal of Neuro-Oncology, 29*, 91–101.

Dennis, M., Spiegler, B. J., Juranek, J. J., Bigler, E. D., Snead, O. C., & Fletcher, J. M. (2013). Age, plasticity, and homeostasis in childhood brain disorders. *Neuroscience and Biobehavioral Review, 37*, 1–32.

Di Pinto, M., Conklin, H. M., Li, C., & Merchant, T. E. (2012). Learning and memory following conformal radiation therapy for pediatric craniopharyngioma and low-grade glioma. *International Journal of Radiation Oncology, Biology, Physics, 84*, 363–369.

Di Rocco, F., Juca, C. E., Zerah, M., & Sainte-Rose, C. (2013). Endoscopic third ventriculostomy and posterior fossa tumors. *World Neurosurgery, 79*, e15–e19.

Duda, T. A., Ris, M. D., Yeates, K. O., Mahone, E. M., Haut, J. S., & Raghubar, K. (2020). Reliable change in pediatric brain tumor: A preliminary investigation. *Child Neuropsychology, 26*(1), 15–26.

Fournier-Goodnight, A. S., Ashford, J., Merchant, T. E., Boop, F. A., Indelicato, D. J., . . . Conklin, H. M. (2017). Neurocognitive functioning in pediatric craniopharyngioma: Performance before treatment with proton therapy. *Journal of Neuro-Oncology, 134*(1), 97–105.

Fuemmeler, B., Elkin, T. D., & Mullins, L. L. (2002). Survivors of childhood brain tumors: Behavioral, emotional, and social adjustment. *Clinical Psychology Review, 22*(4), 547–585.

Gandy, K., Chambers, T., Raghubar, K., Okcu, M. F., Chintagumpala, M., . . . Ris, M. D. (in press). A prospective evaluation of fatigue in pediatric brain tumor patients treated with radiation therapy. *Journal of Pediatric Oncology Nursing.*

Greene-Schloesser, D., Robbins, M. E., Peiffer, A. M., Shaw, E. G., Wheeler, K. T., & Chan, M. D. (2012). Radiation-induced brain injury: A review. *Frontiers in Oncology, 2*, 1–18.

Gudrunardottir, T., Morgan, A. T., Lux, A. L., Walker, D. A., Walsh, K. S., . . . Catsman-Berrevoets, C. (2016). Consensus paper on post-operative pediatric cerebellar mutism syndrome: The Iceland Delphi results. *Child's Nervous System, 32*, 1195–1203.

Hardy, K. K., Bonner, M. J., Willard, V. W., Watral, M. A., & Gururangan, S. (2008). Hydrocephalus as a possible additional contributor to cognitive outcome in survivors of pediatric medulloblastoma. *Psycho-Oncology, 17*, 1157–1161.

Heitzer, A. M., Ris, M. D., Raghubar, K., Kahalley, L. S., Hilliard, M. E., & Gragert, M. (2020a). Facilitating transitions to adulthood in pediatric brain tumor patients: The role of neuropsychology. *Current Oncology Reports, 22*, Article 102.

Heitzer, A. M., Villagran, A. M., Raghubar, K., Brown, A. L., Camet, M. L., . . . Kahalley, L. S. (2020b). Effect of sensorineural hearing loss on neurocognitive and adaptive functioning in survivors of pediatric embryonal brain tumor. *Journal of Neuro-Oncology, 146*(1), 147–156.

Hocking, M. C., McCurdy, M., Turner, E., Kazak, A. E., Noll, R. B., Phillip, P., & Barakat, L. P. (2015). Social competence in pediatric brain tumor survivors: Application of a model from social neuroscience and developmental psychology. *Pediatric Blood and Cancer, 62*(3), 375–384.

Holland, A. A., Hughes, C. W., & Stavinoha, P. L. (2015). School competence and fluent academic performance: Informing assessment of educational outcomes in survivors of pediatric medulloblastoma. *Applied Neuropsychology: Child, 4*, 249–256.

Hoppe-Hirsch, E., Renier, D., Lellouch-Tubiana, A., Saint-Rose, C., Pierre-Kahn, A., & Hirsch,

J. F. (1990). Medulloblastoma in childhood: Progressive intellectual deterioration. *Child's Nervous System, 6*, 60–65.

Hoskinson, K. R., Wolfe, K. R., Yeates, K. O., Mahone, M. E., Cecil, K. M., & Ris, M. D. (2018). Predicting changes in adaptive functioning and behavioral adjustment following treatment for a pediatric brain tumor: A report from the Brain Radiation Investigative Study Consortium. *Psycho-Oncology, 27*, 178–186.

Jacobson, L. A., Mahone, E. M., Yeates, K. O., & Ris, M. D. (2019). Processing speed in children treated for brain tumors: Effects of radiation therapy and age. *Child Neuropsychology, 25*, 217–231.

Jacola, L. M., Edelstein, K., Liu, W., Pui, C. H., Hayashi, R., . . . Krull, K. (2016). Cognitive, behavior, and academic functioning in adolescent and young adult survivors of childhood acute lymphoblastic leukaemia: A report from the Childhood Cancer Survivor Study. *Lancet, 3*, 965–972.

Kahalley, L. S., Conklin, H. M., Tyc, V. L., Wilson, S. J., Hinds, P. S., . . . Hudson, M. M. (2011). ADHD and secondary ADHD criteria fail to identify many at-risk survivors of pediatric ALL and brain tumor. *Pediatric Blood and Cancer, 57*(1), 110–118.

Kahalley, L. S., Ris, M. D., Mahajan, A., Okcu, M. F., Chintagumpala, M., . . . Grosshans, D. R. (2019). Prospective, longitudinal comparison of neurocognitive change in pediatric brain tumor patients treated with proton radiotherapy versus surgery only. *Neuro-Oncology, 21*(6), 809–818.

Kazak, A., Alderfer, M., Streisand, R., Simms, S., Rourke, M., . . . Cnarn, A. (2004). Treatment of post-traumatic stress symptoms in adolescent survivors of childhood cancer and their families: A randomized trial. *Journal of Family Psychology, 18*, 493–504.

Kesler, S. R., Gugel, M., Huston-Warren, E., & Watson, C. (2016). Atypical structural connectome organization and cognitive impairment in young survivors of acute lymphoblastic leukemia. *Brain Connectivity, 6*(4), 273–283.

Kiehna, E. N., Mulhern, R. K., Li, C., Xiaong, X., & Merchant, T. E. (2006). Changes in attentional performance of children and young adults with localized primary brain tumors after conformal radiation therapy. *Journal of Clinical Oncology, 24*(33), 5283–5290.

King, T. Z., Fennell, E. B., Williams, L., Algina, J., Boggs, S., Crosson, B., & Leonard, C. (2004). Verbal memory abilities of children with brain tumors. *Child Neuropsychology, 10*(2), 76–88.

Koocher, G. P., & O'Malley, J. E. (1981). *The Damocles Syndrome*. New York: McGraw-Hill.

Krull, K. R., Brouwers, P., Jain, N., Zhang, L., Bomgaars, L., . . . Okcu, M. F. (2008). Folate pathway genetic polymorphisms are related to attention disorders in childhood leukemia survivors. *Journal of Pediatrics, 152*, 101–105.

Law, N., Greenberg, M., Bouffet, E., Taylor, M. D., Laughlin, S., . . . Mabbott, D. J. (2012). Clinical and neuroanatomical predictors of cerebellar mutism syndrome. *Neuro-Oncology, 14*(10), 1294–1303.

Louis, D. N., Perry, A., Reifenberger, G., von Deimling, A., Figarella-Branger, D., . . . Ellison, D. W. (2016). The 2016 World Health Organization classification of tumors of the central nervous system: A summary. *Acta Neuropathologica, 131*, 803–820.

Louis, D. N., Perry, A., Wesseling, P., Brat, D. J., Cree, I. A., Figarella-Branger, D., . . . Ellison, D. W. (2021). The 2021 WHO classification of tumors of the central nervous system: A summary. *Neuro-Oncology*, XX(XX), 1–21.

Mabbott, D. J., Monsalves, E., Spiegler, B. J., Bartels, U., Janzen, L., . . . Bouffet, E. (2011). Longitudinal evaluation of neurocognitive functioning after treatment for central nervous system germ cell tumors in childhood. *Cancer, 117*, 5402–5411.

MacLean, W. E., Noll, R. B., Stehbens, J. A., Kaleita, T. A., Schwartz, E., Whitt, J. K., . . . Hammond, G. D. (1995). Neuropsychological effects of cranial irradiation in young children with acute lymphoblastic leukemia 9 months after diagnosis. The Children's Cancer Group. *Archives of Neurology, 52*, 156–160.

Meeske, K., Katz, E. R., Palmer, S. N., Burwinkle, T., & Varni, J. W. (2004). Parent proxy-report health-related quality of life and fatigue in pediatric patients diagnosed with brain tumors and acute lymphoblastic leukemia. *Cancer, 101*(9), 2116–2125.

Merchant, T. E., Kiehna, E. N., Kun, L. E., Mulhern, R. K., Li, C., . . . Sanford, R. A. (2006). Phase II trial of conformal radiation therapy for pediatric patients with craniopharyngioma and correlation of surgical factors and radiation dosimetry with change in cognitive functioning. *Journal of Neurosurgery, 104*, 94–102.

Millard, N. E., & De Braganca, K. C. (2016). Medulloblastoma. *Journal of Child Neurology, 31*(12), 1341–1353.

Monje, M., &, Fisher, P. G. (2011). Neurological complications following treatment of children with brain tumors. *Journal of Pediatric Rehabilitation Medicine, 4*(1), 31–36.

Moxon-Emre, I., Bouffet, E., Taylor, M. D., Laperriere, N., Scantlebury, N., . . . Mabbott, D. (2014). Impact of craniospinal dose, boost volume, and neurologic complications on intellectual outcome in patients with medulloblastoma. *Journal of Clinical Oncology, 32,* 1760–1768.

Mulhern, R. K., Kepner, J. L., Thomas, P. R., Armstrong, F. D., Friedman, H. S., & Kun, L. E. (1998). Neuropsychologic functioning of survivors of childhood medulloblastoma randomized to receive conventional or reduced-dose craniospinal irradiation: A Pediatric Oncology Group study. *Journal of Clinical Oncology, 16*(5), 1723–1728.

Myers, C., Stuber, M. L., Bonamer-Rheingans, J. I., & Zeltzer, L. K. (2005). Complementary therapies and childhood cancer. *Cancer Control, 12,* 172–180.

Nagel, B. J., Delis, D. C., Palmer, S. L., Reeves, C., Gajjar, A., & Mulhern, R. K. (2006). Early patterns of verbal memory impairment in children treated for medulloblastoma. *Neuropsychology, 20,* 105–112.

Netson, K. L., Conklin, H. M., Wu, S., Xiong, X., & Merchant, T. E. (2012). A 5-year investigation of children's adaptive functioning following conformal radiation therapy in localized ependymoma. *International Journal of Radiation Oncology, Biology, Physics, 84*(1), 217–223.

Ng, P. T., Feng, L., Yap, K. B., Lee, T. S., Tan, C. H., & Winblad, B. (2014). Long-term metformin usage and cognitive function among older adults with diabetes. *Journal of Alzheimer's Disease, 41*(1), 61–68.

Ostrom, Q. T., Cioffi, G., Gittleman, H., Patil, N., Waite, K., Kruchko, C., & Barnholtz-Sloan, J. S. (2019). CBTRUS Statistical Report: Primary brain and other central nervous system tumors diagnosed in the United States in 2012–2016. *Neuro-Oncology, 21*(5), v1–v100.

Palmer, S. L., Armstrong, C., Onar-Thomas, A., Wu, S., Wallace, D., . . . Gajjar, A. (2013). Processing speed, attention, and working memory after treatment for medulloblastoma: An international, prospective, and longitudinal study. *Journal of Clinical Oncology, 31,* 3494–3500.

Peng, S., Yang, B., Duan, M. Y., Liu, Z. W., Wang, W. F., . . . Tang, F. R. (2019). The disparity of impairment of neurogenesis and cognition after acute or fractionated radiation exposure in adolescent BALB/c mice. *Dose–Response, 17*(1), Article 1559325818822574.

Phillips, S. M., Padgett, L. S., Leisenring, W. M., Stratton, K. K., Bishop, K., . . . Mariotto, A. B. (2015). Survivors of childhood cancer in the United States: Prevalence and burden of morbidity. *Cancer Epidemiology, Biomarkers, and Prevention, 24*(4), 653–663.

Pollack, I. F., Agnihotri, S., & Broniscer, A. (2019). Childhood brain tumors: Current management, biological insights, and future directions. *Journal of Neurosurgery in Pediatrics, 23,* 261–273.

Qiu, D., Kwong, D. L. W., Chan, G. C. F., Leung, L. H. T., & Khong, P. K. (2007). Diffusion tensor magnetic resonance imaging finding of discrepant fractional anisotropy between the frontal and parietal lobes after whole-brain irradiation in childhood medulloblastoma survivors: Reflection of regional white matter radiosensitivity? *Journal of Radiation Oncology, Biology, Physics, 69*(3), 846–851.

Raghubar, K. P., Lamba, M., Cecil, K., Yeates, K. O., Mahone, E. M., Limke, C., & Ris, M. D. (2018a). Dose–volume metrics and their relation to memory performance in pediatric brain tumor patients: A preliminary study. *Pediatric Blood and Cancer,* 65(9) Article e27245.

Raghubar, K. P., Mahone, E. M., Yeates, K. O., Cecil, K. M., Makola, M., & Ris, M. D. (2017). Working memory and attention in pediatric brain tumor patients treated with and without radiation therapy. *Child Neuropsychology, 23*(6), 642–654.

Raghubar, K. P., Mahone, E. M., Yeates, K. O., & Ris, M. D. (2018b). Performance-based and parent ratings of attention in children treated for a brain tumor: The significance of radiation therapy and tumor location on outcome. *Child Neuropsychology, 24,* 413–425.

Raghubar, K. P., Orobio, J., Ris, M. D, Heitzer, A. M., Roth, A., . . . Kahalley, L. S. (2019). Adaptive functioning in Hispanic and non-Hispanic pediatric brain tumor survivors. *Pediatric Blood and Cancer,* 66(9), Article e27800.

Raghubar, K. P., Rothhaar, M. D., Yeates, K. O., Mahone, E. M., Grosshans, D. R., Scheurer, M. E., & Ris, M. D. (2020). Premorbid functioning as a predictor of outcome in pediatric brain tumor: An initial examination of the normalcy assumption. *Pediatric Blood and Cancer, 67*(4), Article e28135.

Reddick, W. E., Shan, Z. Y., Glass, J. O., Helton, S., Xiong, X., . . . Mulhern, R. K. (2006). Smaller white-matter volumes are associated with larger deficits in attention and learning among long-term survivors of acute lymphoblastic leukemia. *Cancer, 106*(4), 941–949.

Reeves, C. B., Palmer, S. L., Reddick, W. E., Merchant, T. E., Buchanan, G. M., Gajjar, A., & Mulhern, R. K. (2006). Attention and memory functioning among pediatric patients with medulloblastoma. *Journal of Pediatric Psychology, 31,* 272–280.

Riggs, L., Bouffet, E., Laughlin, S., Laperriere, N., Liu, F., . . . Mabbott, D. J. (2014). Changes to memory structures in children treated for posterior fossa tumors. *Journal of the International Neuropsychological Society, 20,* 168–180.

Riggs, L., Piscione, J., Laughlin, S., Cunningham, T., Timmons, B. W., . . . Mabbott, D. J. (2017). Exercise training for neural recovery in a restricted sample of pediatric brain tumor survivors: A controlled clinical trial with crossover of training versus no training. *Neuro-Oncology, 19*(3), 440–450.

Ris, M. D. (2007). Lessons in pediatric neuropsycho-oncology: What we've learned since Johnny Gunther. *Journal of Pediatric Psychology, 32,* 1029–1037.

Ris, M. D., Beebe, D. W., Armstrong, D., Fontanesi, J., Mulhern, R., Holmes, E., & Wisoff, J. (2008). Cognitive and adaptive outcome in extracerebellar low grade brain tumors in children from a National Collaborative Study (CCG 9891/POG 9130). *Journal of Clinical Oncology, 26,* 4765–4770.

Ris, M. D., Grosch, M., Fletcher, J. M., Metah, P., & Kahalley, L. S. (2017). Measurement of neurodevelopmental changes in children treated with radiation for brain tumors: What is a true "baseline"? *Clinical Neuropsychologist, 31,* 307–328.

Ris, M. D., & Hiscock, M. (2013). Modeling cognitive aging following CNS injury: Reserve and the Flynn Effect. In I. S. Baron & C. Rey-Casserly (Eds.), *Pediatric neuropsychology: Medical advances and lifespan outcomes* (pp. 393–421). New York: Oxford University Press.

Ris, M. D., Leisenring, W. M., Goodman, P., Di, C., Noll, J., Levy, W., . . . Armstrong, G. T. (2019). Neuropsychological and socioeconomic outcomes in adult survivors of pediatric low-grade glioma. *Cancer, 125*(17), 3050–3058.

Ris, M. D., Packer, R., Goldwein, J., Jones-Wallace, D., & Boyett, J. M. (2001). Neurocognitive outcome following reduced-dose radiation therapy plus adjuvant chemotherapy for medulloblastoma: A Children's Cancer Group Study. *Journal of Clinical Oncology, 19,* 3470–3476.

Ris, M. D., Walsh, K., Wallace, D., Armstrong, F. D., Holmes, E., Gajjar, A., Zhou, T., & Packer, R. J. (2013). Intellectual and academic outcome following two chemotherapy regimens and radiotherapy for average-risk medulloblastoma: COG A9961. *Pediatric Blood and Cancer, 60*(8), 1350–1357.

Robertson, P. L., Muraszko, K. M., Holmes, E. J., Spasto, R., Packer, R. J., . . . Allen, C. (2006). Incidence and severity of post-operative cerebellar mutism syndrome in children with medulloblastoma: A prospective study by the Children's Oncology Group. *Journal of Neurosurgery, 105,* 444–451.

Robinson, K., Fraley, C. E., Pearson, M. M., Kuttesch, J. F., & Compas, B. E. (2013). Neurocognitive late effects of pediatric brain tumors of the posterior fossa: A quantitative review. *Journal of the International Neuropsychological Society, 19,* 44–53.

Robison, L. L., Armstrong, G. T., Boice, J. D., Chow, E. J., Davies, S. M., . . . Zeltzer, L. K. (2009). The Childhood Cancer Survivor Study: A National Cancer Institute-supported resource for outcome and intervention research. *Journal of Clinical Oncology, 27,* 2308–2318.

Rodgers, S. P., Zawaski, J. A., Sahnoune, I., Leasure, J. L., & Gaber, M. W. (2016). Radiation-induced growth retardation and microstructural and metabolite abnormalities in the hippocampus. *Neural Plasticity, 2016,* Article 3259621.

Rorke, L. B., Gilles, F. H., Davis, R. L., & Becker, L. E. (1985). Revision of the World Health Organization classification of brain tumors for childhood brain tumors. *Cancer, 56,* 1869–1886.

Sahnoune, I., Inoue, T., Rodgers, S. P., Pederson, S., Zawaski, J. A., . . . Gaber, M. W. (2018). Exercise ameliorates neurocognitive impairments in a translational model of pediatric radiotherapy. *Neuro-Oncology, 20*(5), 695–704.

Salley, C. G., Hewitt, L. L., Patenaude, A. F., Vasey, M. W., Yeates, K. O., Gerhardt, C. A., & Vannatta, K. (2015). Temperament and social behavior in pediatric brain tumor survivors and comparison peers. *Journal of Pediatric Psychology, 40*(3), 297–308.

Satz, P. (1993). Brain reserve capacity on symptom onset after brain injury: A formulation and review of evidence for threshold theory. *Neuropsychology, 7,* 273–295.

Shatz, J., Kramer, J. H., Ablin, A., & Matthay, K. K. (2000). Processing speed, working memory, and IQ: A developmental model of cognitive deficits following cranial radiation therapy. *Neuropsychology, 14,* 189–200.

Spiegler, B., Bouffet, E., Greenberg, M. L., Rutka, J. T., & Mabbott, D. (2004). Change in neurocognitive functioning after treatment with cranial radiation in childhood. *Journal of Clinical Oncology, 22,* 706–713.

Spiegler, B. J., Kennedy, K., Maze, R., Greenberg, M. L., Weitzman, S., Hitzler, J. K., & Nathan, P. (2006). Comparison of long-term neurocognitive outcomes in very young children with acute lymphoblastic leukemia treated with cranial radiation or high-dose or very high-dose intravenous methotrexate. *Journal of Clinical Oncology, 24*(24), 3858–3864.

Treble-Barna, A., Chapman, S., Schwartz, D., & Axelrad, M. (2013). Behavioral intervention for disruptive behavior in a child following frontal and temporal resection for medically intractable epilepsy: A case report. *Clinical Practice in Pediatric Psychology, 1*(4), 355–360.

Turner, C. D., Chordas, C. A., Liptak, C. C., Rey-Casserly, C., Delaney, B. L., . . . Kieran, M. W. (2009). Medical, psychological, cognitive and educational late-effects in pediatric low-grade glioma survivors treated with surgery only. *Pediatric Blood and Cancer, 53,* 417–423.

Vannatta, K., Barrera, M., Gerhardt, C. A., Fairclough, D., Kupst, D., . . . Turner, C. (2011). Social and behavioral adjustment of pediatric brain tumor survivors: Examination of factors that modify risk. *Pediatric Blood and Cancer, 56,* Article 1162.

Waber, D. P., Carpentieri, S. C., Klar, N., Silverman, L. B., Schwenn, M., . . . Sallan, S. E. (2000). Cognitive sequelae in children treated for acute lymphoblastic leukemia with dexamethasone or prednisone. *Journal of Pediatric Hematology/Oncology, 22,* 206–213.

Whitman, L., Scharaga, E. A., Blackmon, K., Wiener, J., Bender, H. A., Weiner, H. L., & MacAllister, W. S. (2017). Material specificity of memory deficits in children with temporal tumors and seizures: A case series. *Applied Neuropsychology: Child, 6*(4), 335–344.

Willard, V. W., Conklin, H. M., Huang, L., Zhang, H., & Kahalley, L. S. (2016). Concordance of parent-, teacher- and self-report ratings on the Conners 3 in adolescent survivors of cancer. *Psychological Assessment, 28*(9), 1110–1118.

Wolfe, K. R., Madan-Swain, A., & Kana, R. K. (2012). Executive dysfunction in pediatric posterior fossa tumor survivors: A systematic literature review of neurocognitive deficits and interventions. *Developmental Neuropsychology, 37*(2), 153–175.

Wolkowitz, O. M., Lupien, S. J., & Bigler, E. D. (2007). The "Steroid Dementia Syndrome": A possible model of human glucocorticoid neurotoxicity. *Neurocase, 13*(3), 189–200.

Yeates, K. O., Bigler, E. D., Dennis, M., Gerhardt, C. A., Rubin, K., . . . Vannatta, K. (2007). Social outcomes in childhood brain disorder: A heuristic integration of social neuroscience and developmental psychology. *Psychological Bulletin, 133,* 535–556.

CHAPTER 5

Traumatic Brain Injury

Miriam H. Beauchamp
Keith Owen Yeates

HISTORICAL OVERVIEW

Traumatic brain injury (TBI) is defined as a disruption to brain function involving an alteration of consciousness and arising from an external mechanical force, such as a blow or jolt to the head or body. Its manifestations and consequences can be observed in a range of domains of functioning (physical–somatic, cognitive, academic–vocational, social-affective, behavioral) and vary in severity from milder injuries, including concussions, to moderate or severe TBI associated with significant intracranial brain lesions. TBIs are a major source of referrals for pediatric neuropsychologists in clinical practice and the topic of multifaceted scientific research across multiple health disciplines.

The literature pertaining to pediatric TBI is extensive and has been the subject of several reviews (Bell & Kochanek, 2013; Coulter & Forsyth, 2019; Lumba-Brown et al., 2018). Mild TBIs (mTBIs; a term considered interchangeable with *concussions*, as used in this chapter) are now recognized as less benign than previously believed. Indeed, a shift has occurred from a focus on injuries that are known to cause significant morbidity and long-term challenges but are relatively rarer (about 10% of TBI), to more attention to mTBI, which may not cause frank brain damage but affects a much larger segment of the pediatric population annually. The field continues to make substantial strides in understanding the complexities of this heterogeneous and multifactorial condition and its associated predictors, moderators, and treatments.

K. O. Yeates, Levin, and Ponsford (2017b) highlight three major scientific advances that have propelled research in the area of TBI over the last 50 years and continue to be of relevance:

1. *Modern neuroimaging techniques:* The advent of computed tomography (CT) scanning in the 1970s enabled the first characterization of the heterogeneity and extent of pathophysiology associated with TBI. In the 1980s, the introduction of magnetic resonance imaging (MRI) significantly expanded the study of brain–behavior relations associated with pediatric TBI. The subsequent introduction of ever more advanced and varied acquisition sequences (e.g., diffusion tensor imaging, susceptibility weighted imaging,

functional and resting-state MRI) and postprocessing analysis software enabled more precise localization and characterization of the extent and nature of brain disruption.

2. *Noninjury influences on TBI:* Research on the effects of demographic and environmental factors (e.g., age, sex, socioeconomic status (SES), family functioning), children's preinjury functioning (e.g., existing neurodevelopmental or psychiatric disorders, preinjury cognitive ability), and, more recently, genetic and epigenetic influences, has led to the recognition that noninjury factors play a significant role in recovery after TBI.

3. *Novel treatments:* Recognition that the pathophysiology and outcome of TBI are extremely complex, and that noninjury factors play an important role in determining outcomes, has shifted much of the treatment focus away from an exclusive search for pharmacological and medical interventions to a more varied, tailored, and symptom-specific approach to management and treatment.

Our aim in this chapter is to build on the historical analysis by Yeates and colleagues (2017b) in three ways: (1) describing the current state of knowledge regarding pediatric TBI and its epidemiology, etiology and neuropathology, and neuropsychological consequences; (2) detailing the developmental factors, predictors, and moderators that affect its outcomes; and (3) summarizing current best practices in terms of treatment and intervention. We conclude by suggesting potential avenues for future work to advance the field.

EPIDEMIOLOGY

TBIs are a leading cause of death and disability among youth, as well as the most common source of acquired brain injury among children and adolescents. They are a major public health problem, resulting in global economic burden at a societal level. Worldwide estimates based on the BIONIC study suggest that TBI-related costs ranged between U.S.$362 and $445 billion in 2017, reflecting 0.5% of annual global expenditures (Feigin et al., 2013; Maas et al., 2017).

Epidemiological studies vary widely in terms of definition of injury, sources of data, data collection techniques, description of cases, and ages of the target population. However, TBI is estimated to affect more than 50 million people worldwide each year, of which a large proportion are children (i.e., TBI sustained before the age of 18 years) (Dewan, Mummareddy, Wellons, & Bonfield, 2016; Maas et al., 2017). For example, in the United States, children with TBI account for 7,000 deaths, 60,000 hospitalizations, and 600,000 emergency department (ED) visits annually. Pediatric TBI spans the globe, though, representing half the pediatric injuries in Iran, 20% of ED trauma admissions in India, and 30% of pediatric injuries in Korea (Dewan et al., 2016). In the United Kingdom, 280 per 100,000 children sustain TBI per year, while in Australia, 486 per 100,000 adolescents do so (Hawley, Ward, Long, Owen, & Magnay, 2003; Mitra, Cameron, & Butt, 2007).

Birth cohort and ED registry data indicate that children between 0 and 5 years of age are at extremely high risk for TBI (Crowe, Anderson, Catroppa, & Babl, 2009; McKinlay et al., 2008). However, the risk of death from TBI is higher in older adolescents. Reported mortality rates again vary widely among countries, with pooled age estimates including 3.6 (Turkey), 13.0 (China), 17.1 (United States), and 21.8 (Switzerland) per 100,000 (Maas et al., 2017). The Centers for Disease Control estimates an annual mortality rate of 4.5 per 100,000 for children 0–14 years of age, but of 24 per 100,000 for 15- to 19-year-olds in the United States (Langlois, Rutland-Brown, & Wald, 2006). Existing statistics may seriously underestimate the true extent of TBI, however, because most injuries are mild, and many of them (possibly up to 80%) go unreported entirely or are treated in outpatient settings and do not result in hospital visits (Maas et al., 2017).

The incidence of TBI varies as a function of demographic factors (e.g., age, sex, race, SES). Boys are about twice as likely to sustain TBI as girls, although the ratio is closer to equal in young children (Langlois et al., 2006). Studies in the United States and the United Kingdom indicate that children from lower SES backgrounds experience higher rates of TBI (see Dewan et al., 2016, for further race and SES details).

Incidence also varies by TBI severity, which is typically classified as mild, moderate, or severe based on a patient's initial clinical presentation. The most common measure of injury severity is the Glasgow Coma Scale (GCS), although other severity indicators, such as duration of loss of consciousness, presence or absence of intracranial lesions, duration of posttraumatic amnesia, and severity of symptoms also have been considered. Only a minority of TBIs are considered moderate or severe, and they are typically those that can result in death, lengthy hospitalizations, and lifelong sequelae. Indeed, the mortality rate is highest among children with severe injuries and is virtually nil among those with mild injuries.

The most common causes of TBI involve unintentional falls and being struck by or against an object, often in sport and recreational settings, followed by motor vehicle collisions. The distribution of causes and mechanisms varies significantly as a function of age and severity. In a sample of 8,233 patients aged 0–17 years who sustained concussion, the most common mechanisms were being struck by an object (31.1%), falls (29.9%), and being struck by a person (21.0%) (Haarbauer-Krupa et al., 2018). The distributions among males and females were similar, but the proportion of concussions owing to falls decreased with advancing age. An estimated 70% of the injuries documented in the sample were sports-related, although this proportion also varied significantly by age, with a clear increase occurring in children 6 years and older. Notably, infants are especially likely to sustain TBI through falls, as well as via inflicted injuries secondary to child abuse. A study in the United States in children younger than 15 years of age found that of 678,503 children admitted for TBI, 3% were victims of nonaccidental trauma; the majority was younger than 6 years of age, and TBI was the most common diagnosis (50%) (Rosenfeld et al., 2020).

NEUROPATHOLOGY

TBIs are associated with multiple forms of neuropathology, including overt damage to brain tissue, reflected in both focal and diffuse lesions, as well as disruptions in brain function at a cellular level. The pathophysiology of TBI begins at the time of impact but continues over a period of days or weeks and sometimes even longer. Research indicates that the brain damage resulting from TBI involves more complex, prolonged, and interwoven processes than were initially recognized (Povlishock & Katz, 2005). Despite pathophysiological commonalities in the effects of different types of TBI, the pediatric brain responds differently to trauma than the mature brain of the adult (Giza, Mink, & Madikians, 2007). For example, children are more likely to display posttraumatic brain swelling, hypoxic–ischemic insult, and diffuse, rather than focal, injuries. The biomechanical properties of the young brain may explain at least some of these differences. Compared to adults, children have a greater head-to-body ratio, less myelination, and greater relative proportion of water content and blood volume in the brain. Once children reach adolescence, TBI-related pathology begins to more closely resemble that seen in adults.

Observable injuries resulting from closed-head trauma can be classified into two broad categories. Primary injuries result directly from the trauma itself, and include skull fractures, contusions and lacerations, and mechanical injuries to nerve fibers and blood vessels. Secondary injuries arise indirectly from the trauma, and in children include brain swelling and edema, hypoxia and hypotension, increased intracranial pressure, and the diffuse lesions associated with these processes.

In most cases, medical management of TBI focuses not on primary injuries but instead on secondary injuries that arise indirectly following the initial trauma. Brain swelling and cerebral edema are two major secondary complications of TBI that are especially common in children (Dinet, Petry, & Badaut, 2019; Kochanek, 2006). They are thought to result from a disruption of the normal relationships between blood, brain tissue, and cerebrospinal fluid, and can cause decreased cerebral blood flow, increased cerebral blood volume, and increased intracranial pressure. The latter perturbations, in turn, can give rise to ischemic and hypoxic injury, as well as to brain herniation and death. Mass lesions involve the accumulation of fluid, usually blood associated with contusion and hemorrhage. Hematomas are blood clots that occur in various locations in and around the brain. Epidural, subdural, and subarachnoid bleeds, as well as intracerebral hematomas and intraventricular hemorrhages, are all potential consequences of TBI (see Pinto, Poretti, Meoded, Tekes, & Huisman, 2012, for a review).

Early posttraumatic seizures, defined as those emerging within the first week after TBI, occur in many children and can involve focal status epilepticus (Arango et al., 2012). About 10–20% of children with severe TBI experience longer-term posttraumatic epilepsy, a condition that is more common in children with penetrating injuries, inflicted injuries, or depressed skull fracture but is not reliably associated with seizures occurring more immediately after injury (Keret et al., 2018).

TBI can be associated with a variety of late effects. Severe TBI often results in a gradual and prolonged process of white matter degeneration and cortical thinning, with associated cerebral atrophy and ventricular enlargement (Bigler, 2013). Though longitudinal studies of neuroimaging outcomes remain scarce, evidence indicates that structural, functional, and metabolic changes can persist in the long term after TBI (Lindsey, Wilde, Caeyenberghs, & Dennis, 2019). More sensitive and advanced neuroimaging techniques and sequences continue to be developed to detect brain changes associated with TBI, including milder injuries (E. L. Dennis, Babikian, Giza, Thompson, & Asarnow, 2018).

The mechanical forces involved in head trauma do not fully account for the diffuse axonal injuries arising from TBI. Instead, reactive axonal changes that occur only gradually lead to brain damage. These reactive changes are mediated by a cascade of biochemical and metabolic reactions that take place following a TBI. These include the production of free radicals and excitatory amino acids, and the disruption of normal calcium homeostasis, as well as changes in glucose metabolism and cerebral blood flow (Giza & Hovda, 2014). These events act in concert to exacerbate the hypoxic–ischemic insult that commonly occurs following TBI. Recent research focuses on the metabolic effects of mTBI given the absence of visible structural lesions in most cases and a need to explain functional brain changes in the absence of structural injury.

NEUROPSYCHOLOGICAL CONSEQUENCES

Consciousness, Alertness, and Orientation

TBI can lead to deficits in a range of neuropsychological domains, with the extent and nature of said deficits depending in part on the severity and location of the brain injury. One more immediate consequence observed in most children with moderate or severe TBI is the experience of a period of fluctuating arousal, as well as disorientation, confusion, and memory loss. These changes in mental status occur during what is usually referred to as the period of posttraumatic amnesia (PTA), which is a common measure of injury severity. Even mTBI can be acutely associated with a transient state of altered consciousness manifested by brief loss of consciousness, confusion, or PTA. After more severe injuries, children may experience more prolonged disorders of consciousness that can be categorized based on levels of neurobehavioral functioning into coma, vegetative state (or "unresponsive wakefulness syndrome"), or minimally conscious state (see Bayne, Hohwy, & Owen, 2017, for a discussion of nomenclature). Recent efforts to characterize the underlying neural substrates of disorders of consciousness have relied on advanced neuroimaging and neurosensory protocols, primarily applied in adults (Di Perri et al., 2018; Padua, Cuccagna, & Pazzaglia, 2019).

Postconcussive Symptoms

mTBI is commonly associated with postconcussive symptoms (PCS). Although PCS tend to improve over time, a substantial minority of children experience persistent PCS for 1 month or longer postinjury (Zemek et al., 2016). PCS typically include a range of physical–somatic (e.g., headache, sleep problems, fatigue, dizziness, hypersensitivity to light or noise), cognitive (e.g., inattention, forgetfulness, slowed processing), and affective symptoms (e.g., irritability, anxiety). Similar symptoms have been reported after moderate to severe TBI (K. O. Yeates et al., 2001).

Sleep–Wake Disturbances

Sleep-wake disturbances are also common after pediatric TBI (Gagner, Landry-Roy, Laine, & Beauchamp, 2015). Reviews indicate that at least 20% of children with TBI experience problems associated with falling or staying asleep, daytime sleepiness, and nightmares (Luther, Poppert Cordts, & Williams, 2020). Sleep problems are associated with increased depression, behavior problems, and poorer quality of life (Botchway, Godfrey, Anderson, & Catroppa, 2019).

Processing Speed

Reaction times and speed of cognitive and linguistic processing can be slowed after pediatric TBI, with corresponding electrophysiological patterns found in frontal regions.

Deficits in processing speed are most pronounced after more severe injuries (Ferraracci, Anzalone, Bridges, Moore, & Decker, 2021), but even those with mTBI frequently exhibit slowed processing speed (Newman, Reesman, Vaughan, & Gioia, 2013).

Intellectual Functioning

The seminal Isle of Wight studies by Rutter and colleagues were among the first to document deficits in intellectual functioning following TBI in children relative to a comparison group of children with orthopedic injuries not involving the head (Chadwick, Rutter, Brown, Shaffer, & Traub, 1981). The magnitude of these deficits was related to injury severity, with little or no change in IQ after mTBI, but significant deficits in both nonverbal and verbal intellectual functioning after moderate to severe injuries. Prospective, longitudinal studies indicate that children with TBI demonstrate significant recovery in IQ over time, with the largest increases occurring among children with more severe injuries (Yeates et al., 2001). Persistent deficits in IQ appear to be especially likely among children with severe TBI and those injured early in life (Anderson, Godfrey, Rosenfeld, & Catroppa, 2012). A meta-analysis encompassing 3,890 children and adults with TBI indicates that children may demonstrate better recovery of IQ after severe TBI than do adults (Königs, Engenhorst, & Oosterlaan, 2016).

Sensory and Motor Skills

Children with moderate to severe TBI often demonstrate corticosensory deficits and fine and gross motor problems. These can include deficits in stereognosis, finger localization, and graphesthesia (Levin & Eisenberg, 1979), as well as olfaction (Bakker, Catroppa, & Anderson, 2016), auditory processing (E. C. Thompson et al., 2018), and vision (Armstrong, 2018). Sustained deficits in fine motor skills, as well as in gait and gross motor skills, are also common after moderate to severe TBI (Kuhtz-Buschbeck et al., 2003). More subtle sensory and motor problems may occur after mTBI. Common symptoms after mTBI include complaints of visual (e.g., seeing double, blurry vision, light sensitivity), auditory (e.g., ringing in the ears, noise sensitivity) and motor (e.g., poor balance, incoordination) problems. Dizziness is also common after mTBI and may be a result of disturbances in vestibulo-ocular function (Wallace & Lifshitz, 2016). Motor deficits may involve subtle changes in balance and gait (Stephens, Salorio, Denckla, Mostofsky, & Suskauer, 2017).

Language

Spontaneous mutism and expressive language deficits are common immediately after severe TBI, but overt aphasic disorders rarely persist following acute recovery. Other, less severe language difficulties are nevertheless common following moderate to severe injuries. Long-term deficits have been identified in syntactical comprehension, sentence repetition, confrontation naming, object description, and verbal fluency (Ewing-Cobbs & Barnes, 2002). Infants, toddlers, and preschool children may be especially vulnerable to the effects of TBI on language development (Crowe, Anderson, Barton, Babl, & Catroppa, 2014). This may include a general impairment in discourse skill, which can be defined as the ability to convey a message by communicating a series of ideas, usually in sentences. Children who sustain TBI before age 6 years may display notable deficits in pragmatic language (Haarbauer-Krupa et al., 2019). Because of the importance of communication skills for success in school, discourse deficits might account for some of the academic difficulties experienced by children with TBI. Pragmatic language problems can also be associated with social communication difficulties (Wiseman-Hakes, Kakonge, Doherty, & Beauchamp, 2020).

Attention

Complaints about attention problems are common following childhood TBI. These problems may be evident acutely even after mTBI. Multiple studies also document significant attention problems after moderate to severe TBI. These occur in virtually all subdomains, including sustained, selective, shifting, and divided attention, although not always to the same extent. Sustained and divided attention appear to be the most vulnerable, as is performance on tasks including a timed component. Attention deficits show some recovery but can persist across time, especially in more severely injured children (Catroppa, Anderson, Godfrey, & Rosenfeld, 2011). Premorbid attention problems, such as a diagnosis of attention-deficit/hyperactivity disorder (ADHD), place children at higher risk for sustaining TBI (Grigorian et al., 2019). Children with preexisting attention difficulties also have poorer outcomes than youth without these difficulties, suggesting a compound effect of TBI on preexisting attention problems (Beauchamp, Aglipay, et al., 2018).

Memory

Frank memory deficits are not often evident on acute neurocognitive testing after mTBI (Brooks, Khan, Daya, Mikrogianakis, & Barlow, 2014). Furthermore, even memory problems that occur in subsets of children with mTBI, such as those hospitalized for their injuries, tend to improve in the weeks following injury (Nance, Polk-Williams, Collins, & Wiebe, 2009). Moderate to severe TBI, on the other hand, frequently result in sustained deficits in explicit memory. General memory scores may be especially depressed in the early postacute period (e.g., 3 months postinjury), with some improvement 1–2 years postinjury, but with high variability across patients, partly related to injury severity (Viot et al., 2019). The effects of moderate to severe TBI on implicit and prospective memory are not well researched. Implicit memory is less likely to be affected (K. O. Yeates & Enrile, 2005), though Lah, Epps, Levick, and Parry (2011) found weaknesses in this domain following early childhood injuries. Time-based prospective memory, on the other hand, may be more vulnerable to pediatric TBI, especially in the presence of accompanying executive deficits (Phillips et al., 2018).

Executive Functions

Deficits in a range of executive functions are reported after childhood TBI, including working memory, inhibitory control, planning, and cognitive flexibility. As in other cognitive domains, mTBI does not appear to be associated with significant long-term deficits in executive functions. However, working memory may be affected early postinjury (Green,

Keightley, Lobaugh, Dawson, & Mihailidis, 2018), and deficits in executive function up to 1 month postinjury have been associated with altered cerebral activation (Khetani, Rohr, Sojoudi, Bray, & Barlow, 2019). Executive dysfunction can persist over many years after moderate to severe TBI, with deficits varying as a function of lesion location and age (Cooper et al., 2014; Resch et al., 2019). The presence and extent of executive deficits after TBI may also depend on mode of assessment. Parental reports of deficits in behavioral regulation and metacognition in everyday setting are common after TBI (Chevignard et al., 2017) but seldom correlate with objective testing. Young children with severe injuries may be particularly vulnerable to executive deficits following TBI (Nadebaum, Anderson, & Catroppa, 2007).

Awareness of Deficits

Deficits in awareness, defined as the lack of recognition of changes in one's functioning and abilities, play an important factor in postinjury adjustment because of their association with self-esteem, emotional and psychosocial outcomes, and aspects of daily functioning such as autonomy and decision making (Lloyd, Ownsworth, Fleming, Jackson, & Zimmer-Gembeck, 2021). Awareness problems are mostly present after severe injuries and typically are associated with memory and executive functions, though the evidence concerning their presence is mixed. Wolfe et al. (2015) found that children with TBI had variable levels of social self-awareness, with less self-awareness related to weaknesses in executive functioning.

Social Cognition and Social Competence

Social cognition following TBI is another area of growing research focus, likely because of research indicating that children with TBI report global difficulties with social functioning and sometimes engage in maladaptive social behaviors. In addition to being perceived as more socially maladjusted, children with TBI report more loneliness, fewer quality friendships and relationships, and less social participation than do children without TBI (Rosema, Crowe, & Anderson, 2012). Social difficulties in younger children may also be reflected in alterations in parent–child relationships, even after mTBI (Lalonde, Gravel, Bernier, & Beauchamp, 2018; Wade et al., 2011).

Attempts to understand the nature of social problems after TBI have focused on specific social-cognitive skills, including theory of mind (TOM), empathy, and moral reasoning (Beauchamp, Vera-Estay, Morasse, Anderson, & Dooley, 2019; M. Dennis et al., 2013; Ryan et al., 2016). A meta-analysis of 11 studies of social cognition after pediatric TBI concludes that more basic skills such as emotion perception and recognition are usually intact, but higher-order social-cognitive functions, such as TOM and pragmatic language, are vulnerable to disruption (On, Ryan, Konjarski, Catroppa, & Stargatt, 2021). In one study, poorer TOM was found in preschool children with mTBI compared to typically developing and orthopedically injured controls, and differences persisted 18 months postinjury, suggesting that young children may be vulnerable to social-cognitive disruption (Bellerose, Bernier, Beaudoin, Gravel, & Beauchamp, 2017). M. Dennis and colleagues (2013) reported difficulties understanding facial emotions in 8- to 12-year-old children with TBI. Other studies have documented post-TBI alterations in electrophysiological patterns underlying emotional face processing in young children (d'Hondt et al., 2017) and a persistence of social-cognitive difficulties into adulthood in children with moderate to severe TBI (McLellan & McKinlay, 2013).

Emotional and Behavioral Adjustment

TBI in childhood is related to increases in a range of emotional and behavioral problems that include both internalizing (e.g., withdrawal, depression) and externalizing symptoms (rule breaking, aggression) (Bellesi, Barker, Brown, & Valmaggia, 2019; Laliberté Durish, Pereverseff, & Yeates, 2018). These problems vary depending on age and severity of injury. Although evidence for postinjury behavioral change is frequently stronger for more severe TBI (Emery et al., 2016), emotional symptoms such as depressed affect, anxiety, and irritability may also be reported as PCS after mTBI. In contrast to physical and cognitive problems after TBI, emotional and behavioral problems are more likely to show a stable or worsening pattern over time (Fay et al., 2009). While new-onset behavioral problems may first occur after TBI, preexisting behavior difficulties and psychiatric disorders are likely compounded by the effects of TBI (Max, 2014).

Academic and Vocational Outcome

Pediatric TBI is frequently associated with declines in academic performance and an increased risk of grade retention, placement in special education, and other indicators of academic difficulties. However, these academic difficulties may not be associated with deficits on formal achievement testing, especially after mTBI (Rozbacher, Selci, Leiter, Ellis, & Russell, 2017). Poor academic performance following TBI is most likely to be apparent in children injured at a young age (Ewing-Cobbs et al., 2006) and in those with more severe injuries (Prasad, Swank, & Ewing-Cobbs, 2017). TBI sustained during childhood can also affect vocational outcomes, with those demonstrating better neuropsychological outcomes more likely to have full-time employment in the long term (Nybo, Sainio, & Muller, 2005).

Concerns also arise regarding academic performance after concussion, as acute and persistent PCS can result in missed days of school and protracted return to the learning environment. A study of elementary school outcomes after early childhood TBI revealed that children who had complicated mTBI had difficulties in academic and language outcomes such as reading comprehension (Haarbauer-Krupa et al., 2019). Recommendations for a gradual return to preinjury academic activities have been developed to optimize management and school reintegration after pediatric concussion (Purcell, Davis, & Gioia, 2019).

Adaptive Functioning and Quality of Life

Children with moderate to severe TBI often display persistent deficits in adaptive functioning (e.g., poorer communication, socialization, and daily living skills) in association with impairments in neuropsychological skills (Shultz et al., 2016). In contrast, mTBI is less likely to result in persistent adaptive deficits. Degeilh, Bernier, Gravel, and Beauchamp (2018), however, reported altered developmental trajectories of adaptive functioning after early childhood mTBI, but only in the social domain. Unsurprisingly, impairments reported in adaptive functioning, especially after moderate to severe TBI, are likely to have an overall impact on quality of life. Multiple lines of evidence indicate that quality of life is significantly reduced after moderate to severe injuries, as well as in some cases of concussion, typically in association with persistent PCS (Novak et al., 2016).

DEVELOPMENTAL CONSIDERATIONS

TBI in children and adolescents occurs in the context of protracted brain development and of collateral emergence and consolidation of a wide range of complex motor, cognitive, and social skills. TBI at any age in childhood can disrupt development. While cognitive and other impairments related to TBI often improve with time and remediation postinjury, some difficulties can persist into adulthood, especially after more severe injuries.

Epidemiological data suggest that mechanisms of injury vary according to age, with younger children sustaining falls primarily, and motor vehicle collisions becoming more prevalent in late adolescence. A link between age and mechanism is also evident in the age-related incidence of inflicted or nonaccidental TBI. While the exact incidence of inflicted TBI in young children is difficult to determine, they clearly occur most often in children under 2 years of age (L. W. Thompson et al., 2019).

Consideration of factors related to age at injury is also relevant in appreciating some of the issues involved in diagnosis of TBI. For example, identifying and tracking the consequences of mTBI in early childhood is inherently challenging, and validated measures of PCS in children under the age of 5 years are only just emerging (Dupont et al., 2021). Clinical guidelines for diagnosing TBI in young children limit the use of CT scanning to identify intracranial lesions because of the risks of associated radiation. A further issue in assessing TBI in infants and toddlers is the lack of standardized measures of specific aspects of cognition and social skills. Clinical evaluations of this age group are often limited to assessments of global developmental outcomes that may not capture the more subtle and variable effects of TBI, especially mTBI. At young ages, observational measures may be more suitable to capture the behavioral effects of TBI, but these typically lack population norms. Different assessment challenges arise in documenting the effects of TBI in adolescents. Questionnaires are the most common means for assessing critical outcomes in older youth, such as changes in behavior and social skills. However, self-report and parent–proxy questionnaires are subjective and thus open to bias, and research suggests limited agreement between the two types of reports (Hajek et al., 2011).

Efforts to understand the biological underpinnings of TBI have shifted somewhat from studying global structural brain changes, such as volumetric differences, to identifying potentially useful blood or genetic biomarkers associated with poor outcome after pediatric TBI (Atif & Hicks, 2019; Kurowski et al., 2019). Despite the potential of these biomarkers to advance understanding of early risk factors and underlying mechanisms of effect, different neurobiological processes may contribute to injury outcomes in younger versus older children, altering the meaning of any single biomarker (Gagner, Tuerk, De Beaumont, Bernier, & Beauchamp, 2021; Treble-Barna et al., 2020). For example, brain-derived neurotropic factor (BDNF) plays a key role in neuronal survival, synaptic plasticity, and neurogenesis, and is associated with several polymorphisms, the protective or risk-enhancing effects of which may vary with age (Casey et al., 2009).

Finally, research in pediatric TBI must consider the demands associated with important life milestones and their potential impact on the ways in which children's functioning is affected by injury. For example, the transition into formal education in early childhood, the increased independence that comes with adolescence, and entry into the job market in early adulthood are likely to influence the types of consequences experienced by youth with TBI (Wehman, Chen, West, & Cifu, 2014).

PREDICTORS AND MODERATORS

The preceding summary of pediatric TBI outcomes is based largely on the results of group comparisons (e.g., children with severe TBI vs. those with orthopedic injuries or typically developing controls). Although the generalizations are valid, they are tempered by the recognition that children with TBI display substantial variability in outcomes, even when they are grouped according to injury severity. These individual differences in outcomes reflect a complex and dynamic interplay among multiple factors, all of which are liable to evolve and change over the course of development. Past research strongly confirms the combined role of preinjury factors, including demographics such as age and sex and premorbid functioning (e.g., presence of attention or learning disabilities or mental health problems), injury characteristics such as severity and presence of specific brain lesions, and environmental factors such as SES and family functioning in determining the outcome of pediatric TBI. More recent work has focused on the contributions of other biological factors, such as genetics, serum biomarkers, and brain structure and function as measured by neuroimaging, as predictors of outcome, as well as on intrinsic psychological factors such as resilience, coping, and temperament. Research on factors associated with persistent PCS after concussion has been a particular fertile area of investigation. Plate 5.1 (see the color insert) proposes a conceptual model of the multiple factors that influence TBI recovery, and a selection of these factors is described here.

Child Factors

Age

As noted earlier, age at injury has a strong association with the outcomes of TBI. Within the school-age range, older age at injury is associated with better outcome after moderate to severe TBI in terms of cognitive functioning or quality of life; however, adolescents appear to report more PCS than do children between 5 and 12 years of age (Zemek et al., 2016). TBI sustained during early childhood (i.e., before age 6) tends to result in the opposite pattern, with infants and toddlers more susceptible to poor outcome than preschoolers (Ségun et al., 2022).

Sex

Sex differences have been reported in both the initial response to and recovery from TBI (Arambula, Reinl, El Demerdash, McCarthy, & Robertson, 2019). Female sex has been associated with prolonged recovery, increased PCS, and poorer functioning after TBI, but not consistently (T. M. Yeates et al., 2021). Different hypotheses have been put forward to account for sex differences, including the possibility of methodological artifacts related to the absence of appropriate comparison groups without TBI or sex-related variations in other factors such as motivation or anxiety.

Medical and Developmental History

Adverse medical or neurodevelopmental conditions that predate TBI are also related to poor outcome. Preexisting problems identified as risk factors for prolonged recovery or poor functioning include neurodevelopmental problems such as learning disabilities or ADHD, a history of mental health problems such as anxiety or depression, and the number, recency, and severity of prior TBI (Zemek et al., 2016).

Individual Psychological Traits

Individual traits, such as temperament (Seguin, Degeilh, Bernier, El-Jalbout, & Beauchamp, 2020) or psychological resilience, can also influence outcomes after TBI. For example, higher psychological resilience has been found to predict fewer persistent PCS in children ages 8–18 years with mTBI (Durish, Yeates, & Brooks, 2018), while a temperament characterized by negative affect is associated with poorer quality of life in young children (18–60 months) with mTBI (Tuerk et al., 2020).

Genes

Few studies have examined genetic contributions to the outcomes of TBI in children, but emerging evidence suggests that genes involved in neural repair or brain plasticity may be associated with outcomes of pediatric TBI. A systematic review of this topic (Kurowski, Martin, & Wade, 2012) found only five genetic association studies, all of which evaluated the apolipoprotein (*APOE*) gene. Studies of BDNF as a moderator of outcome have focused primarily on TBI in adults. A pediatric study (Treble-Barna et al., 2021) provides evidence that some of the unexplained heterogeneity in executive function and behavior in children who sustained TBI between 3 and 7 years of age was related to the cumulative influence of candidate genes involved in the inflammatory response. Despite inconclusive findings in this area, which may reflect the heterogeneity of methods used and the limited size of most study samples, application of genomic approaches is a promising avenue for understanding the complex biology of pediatric TBI (Davidson, Cusimano, & Bendena, 2015).

Environmental Factors

Socioeconomic Status

Multiple lines of evidence indicate that higher parental SES is associated with better TBI outcome. This association may be explained, at least in part, by the relation of higher SES with higher levels of parental education level and income, which confer greater access to resources and are associated with more positive parenting practices (Amram et al., 2015; Liao et al., 2012).

Parental and Family Roles

Research also documents the contribution of parental and family factors, including premorbid family functioning, the quality of the postinjury home environment, and degree of family burden, to outcomes of pediatric TBI (Rashid et al., 2014; Verhaeghe, Defloor, & Grypdonck, 2005). These factors may be particularly important during the early childhood period, when parenting practices and parental mental health (stress, anxiety, depression) are especially salient influences on child development (Beauchamp, Séguin, Gagner, Lalonde, & Bernier, 2021).

Injury Factors

Injury severity is a major determinant of the consequences of TBI, although the other factors discussed earlier account for a substantial variability in outcomes, and often more than injury severity. A dose–response relationship has been established between injury severity and neuropsychological outcome, such that more severe injuries are associated with poorer outcomes. Injury severity has been assessed using a variety of clinical metrics, including level of consciousness (e.g., GCS score), duration of altered consciousness, and length of PTA. Other medical indicators of injury severity include brainstem abnormalities (e.g., pupillary reactivity), seizures, and elevated intracranial pressure. The presence and extent of acute PCS provides an indirect assessment of injury severity in children with mTBI, though these symptoms may also reflect children's premorbid status. Regardless of how severity is assessed, moderate to severe TBI can result in substantial neurobehavioral morbidity. In contrast, the outcomes of mTBI are less clearly related to injury characteristics. Current research aimed at identifying novel biomarkers, whether blood- or brain-based, may provide more sensitive measures of the underlying injury and improve prediction of outcomes in both mild and moderate to severe TBI (Daoud et al., 2014; Papa et al., 2013).

TREATMENT AND INTERVENTION

Biomedical- and Symptom-Targeted Approaches

Evidence for multiple, complex, and heterogeneous predictors and outcomes discussed in this chapter has implications for the study and development of therapies and interventions meant to address the consequences of TBI in children. Clearly, a one-size-fits-all approach is impossible, and the wide range of functional domains that can be variably affected suggests that choices in treatment or remediation need to be tailored to individual profiles of outcomes. A systematic review of randomized clinical trials evaluating interventions in acute settings concludes that few well-designed clinical trials have been conducted to determine the effectiveness of pharmacological, psychoeducational, or follow-up interventions for children with mTBI (Gravel et al., 2013). The scarcity of high-quality, successful clinical studies and randomized controlled trials is reflected in the lack of high-level recommendations for pediatric TBI. Clinical drug, surgery, and hypothermia trials in children with moderate to severe TBI have largely failed, possibly due to the complexity and heterogeneity of the condition (see Appavu, Foldes, & Adelson, 2019, for a review). Despite these setbacks, efforts to develop novel therapies continue and are enriched by ongoing work to identify biomarkers of TBI and driven by the tenets of precision medicine; it seems increasingly clear that no single drug will emerge to address the sequelae of pediatric TBI, but that combinations are likely needed (Kochanek et al., 2020).

Child-Focused Approaches

Rather than searching for a panacea to treat multiple symptoms and impairments, most interventions follow a targeted approach (van Gils et al., 2020). In the acute phase after severe injuries, such treatments are typically medical and may include critical interventions such as neurosurgery or hypothermia (Appavu, Burrows, Foldes, & Adelson, 2019). Treatments for milder injuries may involve managing specific PCS such as headache (Kacperski & Arthur, 2016), nausea (Gravel et al., 2019), attention problems (Kurowski et al., 2014), vestibulomotor difficulties (Wallace & Lifshitz, 2016), or sleep problems (Galland, Elder, & Taylor, 2012; see also Mannix et al., 2019, for pharmacological and nonpharmacological pediatric mTBI therapies). For interventions conducted during inpatient rehabilitation or as part of longer-term outpatient treatment, approaches again tend to target specific domains of functioning, including attention (Virk, Williams, Brunsdon, Suh, & Morrow, 2015), executive function (Sood, Godfrey, Anderson, & Catroppa, 2018), language–communication (Wiseman-Hakes et al., 2020), social–behavioral problems (Narad et al., 2017), family support (Wade et al., 2019), and mental health (Gertler, Tate, & Cameron, 2015). Unfortunately, the results of empirical studies exploring the efficacy and generalizability of these approaches are often mixed and overshadowed by suboptimal study designs and small samples (see Catroppa & Anderson, 2009, for a review of rehabilitation considerations).

Environment-Focused Approaches

The inclusion of family members in the rehabilitation of children with TBI is important, as is the integration of home and school services following discharge from inpatient rehabilitation after severe TBI. Accumulating evidence suggest that parent-based approaches may be useful in addressing behavior problems and improving problem-solving after pediatric TBI (Wade et al., 2019). The management of milder forms of TBI typically involves ruling out more severe injury, directing children to seek appropriate medical follow-up, and educating children and their parents on the expectations and course of recovery (Gravel et al., 2013; Yeo, Yeo, Probert, Sim, & Sirisena, 2020). In some cases, psychological and educational interventions may be needed early in the postinjury period (Al Sayegh, Sandford, & Carson, 2010; Snell, Surgenor, Hay-Smith, & Siegert, 2009). Community and school reintegration is also critical to ensure that children and adolescents with TBI, especially those with more severe injuries, receive adequate longer-term support and follow-up (Clasby, Hughes, Catroppa, & Morrison, 2018).

Return to Activity Guidelines and Exercise after Concussion

The management of concussion is often framed in terms of decisions about return to activity and return to school. A number of existing guidelines provide health care professionals and families with graded steps to help children return safely to their daily activities without severely exacerbating or prolonging PCS or increasing the risk of a second concussion. These guidelines vary somewhat (see, e.g., Lumba-Brown et al., 2018; McCrory et al., 2009), but generally recommend a stepwise progression of increasingly demanding activities after 1 to 2 days of rest, with children progressing through one step per day if they remain asymptomatic or minimally symptomatic. Children whose symptoms worsen significantly are encouraged to drop back to their previous level of activity and resume graduated levels of return after a further 24-hour period of rest. A major change in the management of pediatric concussion is the emerging view that prolonged periods of inactivity and rest are likely to be detrimental to recovery, and that early attempts to reinitiate exercise and other activities may be more beneficial (Grool et al., 2016). Empirical knowledge is still needed to determine the exact timing and amount of rest and exercise that is optimal for recovery and reduction of PCS (Chrisman & Rivara, 2016).

CONCLUSIONS AND FUTURE DIRECTIONS

The field of pediatric TBI has evolved significantly in the past 10 years. Major changes involve an increased focus on mTBI. Although falling along a spectrum, children with mTBI often require different diagnostic, prognostic, management, and therapeutic approaches than children with more severe TBI. Ongoing development of neuroimaging techniques to diagnose TBI and characterize abnormalities in neural structure and function allows clinicians and researchers to assess both observable lesions and more subtle effects on neural functioning. These brain health indicators, together with blood serum and other fluid biomarkers of injury, are becoming increasingly available to inform comprehensive predictive models that consider multiple biological, injury, host (child), and environmental influences on outcome. Single center, cross-sectional study designs are being replaced by research involving multicenter, longitudinal follow-ups aimed at identifying, treating, and tracking a wide range of injury (Bodien et al., 2018; Yeates, Beauchamp, et al., 2017a). The results of these large-scale endeavors are likely to significantly augment what is known about pediatric TBI in the coming years. Longitudinal research, though more prevalent than in the past, continues to be essential in advancing our understanding of the effects of TBI on development across the lifespan and in determining the potential impact of repetitive head injuries, whether in the context of organized sports or simply in recreational activities. Other important research directions include clinical trials to develop and test interventions and evaluation of knowledge translation programs that seek to increase awareness of ways to support children's recovery among child care providers, teachers, coaches, and health care professionals, as well as the injured children and their families.

While group-based results are informative, study designs and analyses capable of teasing out individual trajectories and profiles are increasingly important in understanding the impact of pediatric TBI from patient-centered and precision medicine perspectives. At the same time, awareness is growing with regard to the influence of factors such as sex and gender, race, and SES on the risk for and recovery from pediatric TBI. Further research is needed to capture the range and complexity of individual factors that can influence recovery. Rehabilitation approaches, whether in the context of mTBI or severe TBI, can increasingly rely on cutting-edge technologies such as virtual reality, telehealth, and other online platforms to increase the effectiveness of interventions (e.g., Linden et al., 2016) and improve accessibility (e.g., Wade et al., 2018).

The future of research on pediatric TBI is likely to continue to reflect the three advances described by Yeates and colleagues (2017a): modern neuroimaging techniques, noninjury influences, and novel treatments. Advances in neuroimaging will continue to enhance methods for diagnosis of TBI, as well as the prediction of outcomes. Newer methods (e.g., near-infrared spectroscopy, quantitative susceptibility mapping, spectroscopy, arterial spin labeling, structural covariance analysis) will provide an even more fine-grained appreciation of the subtle and multifaceted structural and functional changes that characterize TBI. With larger studies, shared data repositories, and common data elements, neuroimaging metrics are likely to be studied alongside other biomarkers (e.g., blood serum, cerebrospinal fluid, genetic). Artificial intelligence techniques, such as machine learning, can also be used to construct comprehensive diagnostic and prognostic models. Noninjury influences, including family, friends, and other social, community and school factors, will remain important, but will likely be considered in combination with individual psychological traits and epigenetic influences. Treatment and management techniques will evolve, with increasing attention to the multiple determinants of outcomes and development of more comprehensive diagnostic models. Each child with TBI presents with a unique profile of preexisting characteristics, neural abnormalities, and postinjury environmental influences. We anticipate that models that account for this multiplicity of influences will yield more effective approaches to management and intervention.

REFERENCES

Al Sayegh, A., Sandford, D., & Carson, A. J. (2010). Psychological approaches to treatment of postconcussion syndrome: A systematic review. *Journal of Neurology, Neurosurgery and Psychiatry, 81*(10), 1128–1134.

Amram, O., Schuurman, N., Pike, I., Yanchar, N. L., Friger, M., McBeth, P. B., & Griesdale, D. (2015). Socioeconomic status and traumatic brain injury amongst pediatric populations: A spatial analysis in greater Vancouver. *International Journal of Environmental Research and Public Health, 12*(12), 15594–15604.

Anderson, V., Godfrey, C., Rosenfeld, J. V., & Catroppa, C. (2012). Intellectual ability 10 years after traumatic brain injury in infancy and childhood: What predicts outcome? *Journal of Neurotrauma, 29*(1), 143–153.

Appavu, B., Burrows, B. T., Foldes, S., & Adelson, P. D. (2019). Approaches to multimodality monitoring in pediatric traumatic brain injury. *Frontiers in Neurology, 10,* Article 1261.

Appavu, B., Foldes, S. T., & Adelson, P. D. (2019). Clinical trials for pediatric traumatic brain injury: Definition of insanity? *Journal of Neurosurgery: Pediatrics, 23*(6), 661–669.

Arambula, S. E., Reinl, E. L., El Demerdash, N., McCarthy, M. M., & Robertson, C. L. (2019). Sex differences in pediatric traumatic brain injury. *Experimental Neurology, 317,* 168–179.

Arango, J. I., Deibert, C. P., Brown, D., Bell, M., Dvorchik, I., & Adelson, P. D. (2012). Posttraumatic seizures in children with severe traumatic brain injury. *Child's Nervous System, 28*(11), 1925–1929.

Armstrong, R. A. (2018). Visual problems associated with traumatic brain injury. *Clinical and Experimental Optometry, 101*(6), 716–726.

Atif, H., & Hicks, S. D. (2019, March 8). A review

of microRNA biomarkers in traumatic brain injury. *Journal of Experimental Neuroscience, 13.*

Bakker, K., Catroppa, C., & Anderson, V. (2016). Anosmia and olfactory outcomes following paediatric traumatic brain injury. *Brain Injury, 30*(2), 191–198.

Bayne, T., Hohwy, J., & Owen, A. M. (2017). Reforming the taxonomy in disorders of consciousness. *Annals of Neurology, 82*(6), 866–872.

Beauchamp, M. H., Aglipay, M., Yeates, K. O., Desire, N., Keightley, M., Anderson, P., . . . Zemek, R. (2018). Predictors of neuropsychological outcome after pediatric concussion. *Neuropsychology, 32*(4), 495–508.

Beauchamp, M. H., Séguin, M., Gagner, C., Lalonde, G., & Bernier, A. (2021). The parent model: A pathway approach for understanding parents' role after early childhood mild traumatic brain injury. *Clinical Neuropsychologist, 35,* 846–867.

Beauchamp, M. H., Vera-Estay, E., Morasse, F., Anderson, V., & Dooley, J. (2019). Moral reasoning and decision-making in adolescents who sustain traumatic brain injury. *Brain Injury, 33,* 32–39.

Bell, M. J., & Kochanek, P. M. (2013). Pediatric traumatic brain injury in 2012: The year with new guidelines and common data elements. *Critical Care Clinics, 29*(2), 223–238.

Bellerose, J., Bernier, A., Beaudoin, C., Gravel, J., & Beauchamp, M. H. (2017). Long-term brain-injury-specific effects following preschool mild TBI: A study of theory of mind. *Neuropsychology, 31*(3), 229–241.

Bellesi, G., Barker, E. D., Brown, L., & Valmaggia, L. (2019). Pediatric traumatic brain injury and antisocial behavior: Are they linked? A systematic review. *Brain Injury, 33*(10), 1272–1292.

Bigler, E. D. (2013). Traumatic brain injury, neuroimaging, and neurodegeneration. *Frontiers in Human Neuroscience, 7,* Article 395.

Bodien, Y. G., McCrea, M., Dikmen, S., Temkin, N., Boase, K., Machamer, J., . . . Giacino, J. T. (2018). Optimizing outcome assessment in multicenter tbi trials: Perspectives from track-tbi and the tbi endpoints development initiative. *Journal of Head Trauma Rehabilitation, 33*(3), 147–157.

Botchway, E. N., Godfrey, C., Anderson, V., & Catroppa, C. (2019). A systematic review of sleep-wake disturbances in childhood traumatic brain injury: Relationship with fatigue, depression, and quality of life. *Journal of Head Trauma Rehabilitation, 34*(4), 241–256.

Brooks, B. L., Khan, S., Daya, H., Mikrogianakis, A., & Barlow, K. M. (2014). Neurocognition in the emergency department after a mild traumatic brain injury in youth. *Journal of Neurotrauma, 31*(20), 1744–1749.

Casey, B. J., Glatt, C. E., Tottenham, N., Soliman, F., Bath, K., Amso, D., . . . Lee, F. S. (2009). Brain-derived neurotrophic factor as a model system for examining gene by environment interactions across development. *Neuroscience, 164*(1), 108–120.

Catroppa, C., & Anderson, V. (2009). Traumatic brain injury in childhood: Rehabilitation considerations. *Developmental Neurorehabilitation, 12*(1), 53–61.

Catroppa, C., Anderson, V., Godfrey, C., & Rosenfeld, J. V. (2011). Attentional skills 10 years post-paediatric traumatic brain injury (TBI). *Brain Injury, 25*(9), 858–869.

Chadwick, O., Rutter, M., Brown, G., Shaffer, D., & Traub, M. U. (1981). A prospective study of children with head injuries: II. Cognitive sequelae. *Psychological Medicine, 11*(1), 49–61.

Chevignard, M., Kerrouche, B., Krasny-Pacini, A., Mariller, A., Pineau-Chardon, E., Notteghem, P., . . . Roy, A. (2017). Ecological assessment of everyday executive functioning at home and at school following childhood traumatic brain injury using the BRIEF Questionnaire. *Journal of Head Trauma Rehabilitation, 32*(6), E1–E12.

Chrisman, S. P., & Rivara, F. P. (2016). Physical activity or rest after concussion in youth: Questions about timing and potential benefit. *Journal of the American Medical Association, 316*(23), 2491–2492.

Clasby, B., Hughes, N., Catroppa, C., & Morrison, E. (2018). Community-based interventions for adolescents following traumatic brain injury: A systematic review. *NeuroRehabilitation, 42*(3), 345–363.

Cooper, J. M., Catroppa, C., Beauchamp, M. H., Eren, S., Godfrey, C., Ditchfield, M., & Anderson, V. A. (2014). Attentional control ten years post-childhood traumatic brain injury: The impact of lesion presence, location, and severity in adolescence and early adulthood. *Journal of Neurotrauma, 31*(8), 713–721.

Coulter, I. C., & Forsyth, R. J. (2019). Paediatric traumatic brain injury. *Current Opinion in Pediatrics, 31*(6), 769–774.

Crowe, L. M., Anderson, V., Barton, S., Babl, F. E., & Catroppa, C. (2014). Verbal ability and language outcome following traumatic brain injury in early childhood. *Journal of Head Trauma Rehabilitation, 29*(3), 217–223.

Crowe, L. M., Anderson, A., Catroppa, C., & Babl, F. (2009). Head injuries related to sports and recreation activities in school-age children and adolescents: Data from a referral centre in Victoria, Australia. *Emergency Medicine Australasia, 22*(1), 56–61.

Daoud, H., Alharfi, I., Alhelali, I., Charyk Stewart, T., Qasem, H., & Fraser, D. D. (2014). Brain injury biomarkers as outcome predictors in pediatric severe traumatic brain injury. *Neurocritical Care, 20*(3), 427–435.

Davidson, J., Cusimano, M. D., & Bendena, W. G. (2015). Post-traumatic brain injury: Genetic susceptibility to outcome. *Neuroscientist, 21*(4), 424–441.

Degeilh, F., Bernier, A., Gravel, J., & Beauchamp, M. H. (2018). Developmental trajectories of adaptive functioning following early mild traumatic brain injury. *Developmental Psychobiology, 60*(8), 1037–1047.

Dennis, E. L., Babikian, T., Giza, C. C., Thompson, P. M., & Asarnow, R. F. (2018). Neuroimaging of the injured pediatric brain: Methods and new lessons. *Neuroscientist, 24*(6), 652–670.

Dennis, M., Simic, N., Agostino, A., Taylor, H. G., Bigler, E. D., Rubin, K., . . . Yeates, K. O. (2013). Irony and empathy in children with traumatic brain injury. *Journal of the International Neuropsychological Society, 19*(3), 338–348.

Dewan, M. C., Mummareddy, N., Wellons, J. C., III, & Bonfield, C. M. (2016). Epidemiology of global pediatric traumatic brain injury: Qualitative review. *World Neurosurgery, 91*, 497–509.

d'Hondt, F., Lassonde, M., Thebault-Dagher, F., Bernier, A., Gravel, J., Vannasing, P., & Beauchamp, M. H. (2017). Electrophysiological correlates of emotional face processing after mild traumatic brain injury in preschool children. *Cortex, 17*(1), 124–142.

Dinet, V., Petry, K. G., & Badaut, J. (2019). Brain-immune interactions and neuroinflammation after traumatic brain injury. *Frontiers in Neuroscience, 13*, Article 1178.

Di Perri, C., Amico, E., Heine, L., Annen, J., Martial, C., Larroque, S. K., . . . Laureys, S. (2018). Multifaceted brain networks reconfiguration in disorders of consciousness uncovered by co-activation patterns. *Human Brain Mapping, 39*(1), 89–103.

Dupont, D., Beaudoin, C., Désiré, N., Tran, M., Gagnon, I., & Beauchamp, M. H. (2021, April 30). Report of early childhood traumatic injury observations and symptoms (REACTIONS): Preliminary validation of an observational measure of post-concussive symptoms. *Journal of Head Trauma Rehabilitation.*

Durish, C. L., Yeates, K. O., & Brooks, B. L. (2018). Psychological resilience as a predictor of persistent post-concussive symptoms in children with single and multiple concussion. *Journal of the International Neuropsychological Society, 24*, 759–768.

Emery, C. A., Barlow, K. M., Brooks, B. L., Max, J. E., Villavicencio-Requis, A., Gnanakumar, V., . . . Yeates, K. O. (2016). A systematic review of psychiatric, psychological, and behavioural outcomes following mild traumatic brain injury in children and adolescents. *Canadian Journal of Psychiatry, 61*(5), 259–269.

Ewing-Cobbs, L., & Barnes, M. (2002). Linguistic outcomes following traumatic brain injury in children. *Seminars in Pediatric Neurology, 9*(3), 209–217.

Ewing-Cobbs, L., Prasad, M. R., Kramer, L., Cox, C. S., Jr., Baumgartner, J., Fletcher, S., . . . Swank, P. (2006). Late intellectual and academic outcomes following traumatic brain injury sustained during early childhood. *Journal of Neurosurgery, 105*(4 Suppl.), 287–296.

Fay, T. B., Yeates, K. O., Wade, S. L., Drotar, D., Stancin, T., & Taylor, H. G. (2009). Predicting longitudinal patterns of functional deficits in children with traumatic brain injury. *Neuropsychology, 23*, 271–282.

Feigin, V. L., Theadom, A., Barker-Collo, S., Starkey, N. J., McPherson, K., Kahan, M., . . . Ameratunga, S. (2013). Incidence of traumatic brain injury in New Zealand: A population-based study. *Lancet Neurology, 12*(1), 53–64.

Ferraracci, J., Anzalone, C., Bridges, R. M., Moore, R. D., & Decker, S. L. (2021). QEEG correlates of cognitive processing speed in children and adolescents with traumatic brain injuries. *Applied Neuropsychology: Child, 10*, 247–257.

Gagner, C., Landry-Roy, C., Laine, F., & Beauchamp, M. H. (2015). Sleep–wake disturbances and fatigue after pediatric traumatic brain injury: A systematic review of the literature. *Journal of Neurotrauma, 32*(20), 1539–1352.

Gagner, C., Tuerk, C. B., De Beaumont, L., Bernier, A., & Beauchamp, M. H. (2021). Brain-derived neurotrophic factor Val66Met polymorphism and internalizing behaviors after early mild traumatic brain injury. *Journal of Neurotrauma, 38*, 102–110.

Galland, B. C., Elder, D. E., & Taylor, B. J. (2012). Interventions with a sleep outcome for children with cerebral palsy or a post-traumatic brain injury: A systematic review. *Sleep Medicine Reviews, 16*(6), 561–573.

Gertler, P., Tate, R. L., & Cameron, I. D. (2015). Non-pharmacological interventions for depression in adults and children with traumatic brain injury. *Cochrane Database of Systematic Reviews, 12*, CD009871.

Giza, C. C., & Hovda, D. A. (2014). The new neurometabolic cascade of concussion. *Neurosurgery, 75*(Suppl. 4), S24–S33.

Giza, C. C., Mink, R. B., & Madikians, A. (2007). Pediatric traumatic brain injury: Not just little adults. *Current Opinion in Critical Care, 13*(2), 143–152.

Gravel, J., Boutis, K., Tang, K., Beauchamp, M. H., Freedman, S. B., Dubrovsky, A. S., . . . Zemek, R. (2019). Association between ondansetron use and symptom persistence in children with concussions: A 5p substudy. *CJEM, 21*(2), 204–210.

Gravel, J., D'Angelo, A., Carriere, B., Crevier, L., Beauchamp, M. H., Chauny, J. M., . . . Chaillet, N. (2013). Interventions provided in the acute phase for mild traumatic brain injury: A systematic review. *Systematic Reviews, 2*(63), 1–12.

Green, S. L., Keightley, M. L., Lobaugh, N. J., Dawson, D. R., & Mihailidis, A. (2018). Changes in working memory performance in youth following concussion. *Brain Injury, 32*(2), 182–190.

Grigorian, A., Nahmias, J., Dolich, M., Barrios, C., Jr., Schubl, S. D., Sheehan, B., & Lekawa, M. (2019). Increased risk of head injury in pediatric patients with attention deficit hyperactivity disorder. *Journal of Child and Adolescent Psychiatric Nursing, 32*(4), 171–176.

Grool, A. M., Aglipay, M., Momoli, F., Meehan, W. P., III, Freedman, S. B., Yeates, K. O., . . . Zemek, R. (2016). Association between early participation in physical activity following acute concussion and persistent postconcussive symptoms in children and adolescents. *Journal of the American Medical Association, 316*(23), 2504–2514.

Haarbauer-Krupa, J., Arbogast, K. B., Metzger, K. B., Greenspan, A. I., Kessler, R., Curry, A. E., . . . Master, C. L. (2018). Variations in mechanisms of injury for children with concussion. *Journal of Pediatrics, 197*, 241–248.

Haarbauer-Krupa, J., King, T. Z., Wise, J., Gillam, S., Trapani, J., Weissman, B., & DePompei, R. (2019). Early elementary school outcome in children with a history of traumatic brain injury before age 6 years. *Journal of Head Trauma Rehabilitation, 34*(2), 111–121.

Hajek, C. A., Yeates, K. O., Taylor, H. G., Bangert, B., Dietrich, A., Nuss, K. E., . . . Wright, M. (2011). Agreement between parents and children on ratings of post-concussive symptoms following mild traumatic brain injury. *Child Neuropsychology, 17*(1), 17–33.

Hawley, C., Ward, A., Long, J., Owen, D., & Magnay, A. (2003). Prevalence of traumatic brain injury amongst children admitted to hospital in one health district: A population-based study. *Injury, 34*(4), 256–260.

Kacperski, J., & Arthur, T. (2016). Management of post-traumatic headaches in children and adolescents. *Headache, 56*(1), 36–48.

Keret, A., Shweiki, M., Bennett-Back, O., Abed-Fteiha, F., Matoth, I., Shoshan, Y., & Benifla, M. (2018). The clinical characteristics of post-traumatic epilepsy following moderate-to-severe traumatic brain injury in children. *Seizure, 58*, 29–34.

Khetani, A., Rohr, C. S., Sojoudi, A., Bray, S., & Barlow, K. M. (2019). Alteration in cerebral activation during a working memory task after pediatric mild traumatic brain injury: A prospective controlled cohort study. *Journal of Neurotrauma, 36*(23), 3274–3283.

Kochanek, P. M. (2006). Pediatric traumatic brain injury: Quo vadis? *Developmental Neuroscience, 28*(4–5), 244–255.

Kochanek, P. M., Jackson, T. C., Jha, R. M., Clark, R. S. B., Okonkwo, D. O., Bayır, H., . . . Dixon, C. E. (2020). Paths to successful translation of new therapies for severe traumatic brain injury in the golden age of traumatic brain injury research: A Pittsburgh vision. *Journal of Neurotrauma, 37*(22), 2353–2371.

Königs, M., Engenhorst, P. J., & Oosterlaan, J. (2016). Intelligence after traumatic brain injury: Meta-analysis of outcomes and prognosis. *European Journal of Neurology, 23*(1), 21–29.

Kuhtz-Buschbeck, J. P., Hoppe, B., Golge, M., Dreesmann, M., Damm-Stunitz, U., & Ritz, A. (2003). Sensorimotor recovery in children after traumatic brain injury: Analyses of gait, gross motor, and fine motor skills. *Developmental Medicine and Child Neurology, 45*(12), 821–828.

Kurowski, B. G., Martin, L. J., & Wade, S. L. (2012). Genetics and outcomes after traumatic brain injury (TBI): What do we know about pediatric TBI? *Journal of Pediatric Rehabilitation Medicine, 5*(3), 217–231.

Kurowski, B. G., Treble-Barna, A., Pilipenko, V., Wade, S. L., Yeates, K. O., Taylor, H. G., . . . Jegga, A. G. (2019). Genetic influences on behavioral outcomes after childhood TBI: A novel systems biology-informed approach. *Frontiers in Genetics, 10,* Article 481.

Kurowski, B. G., Wade, S. L., Kirkwood, M. W., Brown, T. M., Stancin, T., & Taylor, H. G. (2014). Long-term benefits of an early online problem-solving intervention for executive dysfunction after traumatic brain injury in children: A randomized clinical trial. *Journal of the American Medical Association Pediatrics, 168*(6), 523–531.

Lah, S., Epps, A., Levick, W., & Parry, L. (2011). Implicit and explicit memory outcome in children who have sustained severe traumatic brain injury: Impact of age at injury (preliminary findings). *Brain Injury, 25*(1), 44–52.

Laliberté Durish, C., Pereverseff, R. S., & Yeates, K. O. (2018). Depression and depressive symptoms in pediatric traumatic brain injury: A scoping review. *Journal of Head Trauma Rehabilitation, 33*(3), E18–E30.

Lalonde, G., Gravel, J., Bernier, A., & Beauchamp, M. H. (2018). Investigating social functioning after early mild TBI: The quality of parent–child interactions. *Journal of Neuropsychology, 12,* 1–22.

Langlois, J. A., Rutland-Brown, W., & Wald, M. M. (2006). The epidemiology and impact of traumatic brain injury: A brief overview. *Journal of Head Trauma Rehabilitation, 21*(5), 375–378.

Levin, H. S., & Eisenberg, H. M. (1979). Neuropsychological outcome of closed head injury in children and adolescents. *Childs Brain, 5*(3), 281–292.

Liao, C. C., Chang, H. C., Yeh, C. C., Chou, Y. C., Chiu, W. T., & Chen, T. L. (2012). Socioeconomic deprivation and associated risk factors of traumatic brain injury in children. *Journal of Trauma and Acute Care Surgery, 73*(5), 1327–1331.

Linden, M., Hawley, C., Blackwood, B., Evans, J., Anderson, V., & O'Rourke, C. (2016). Technological aids for the rehabilitation of memory and executive functioning in children and adolescents with acquired brain injury. *Cochrane Database of Systematic Reviews, 7*(7), CD011020.

Lindsey, H. M., Wilde, E. A., Caeyenberghs, K., & Dennis, E. L. (2019). Longitudinal neuroimaging in pediatric traumatic brain injury: Current state and consideration of factors that influence recovery. *Frontiers in Neurology, 10,* Article 1296.

Lloyd, O. T., Ownsworth, T., Fleming, J., Jackson, M., & Zimmer-Gembeck, M. J. (2021). Impaired self-awareness after pediatric traumatic brain injury: Protective factor or liability? *Journal of Neurotrauma, 38,* 616–627.

Lumba-Brown, A., Yeates, K. O., Sarmiento, K., Breiding, M. J., Haegerich, T. M., Gioia, G. A., . . . Timmons, S. D. (2018). Diagnosis and management of mild traumatic brain injury in children: A systematic review. *JAMA Pediatrics, 172*(11), Article e182847.

Luther, M., Poppert Cordts, K. M., & Williams, C. N. (2020). Sleep disturbances after pediatric traumatic brain injury: A systematic review of prevalence, risk factors, and association with recovery. *Sleep, 43*(10), Article zsaa083.

Maas, A. I. R., Menon, D. K., Adelson, P. D., Andelic, N., Bell, M. J., Belli, A., . . . Yaffe, K. (2017). Traumatic brain injury: Integrated approaches to improve prevention, clinical care, and research. *Lancet Neurology, 16*(12), 987–1048.

Mannix, R., Zemek, R., Yeates, K. O., Arbogast, K., Atabaki, S., Badawy, M., . . . Wisniewski, S. (2019). Practice patterns in pharmacological and non-pharmacological therapies for children with mild traumatic brain injury: A survey of 15 Canadian and United States centers. *Journal of Neurotrauma, 36*(20), 2886–2894.

Max, J. E. (2014). Neuropsychiatry of pediatric traumatic brain injury. *Psychiatric Clinics of North America, 37*(1), 125–140.

McCrory, P., Meeuwisse, W., Johnston, K., Dvorak, J., Aubry, M., Molloy, M., & Cantu, R. (2009). Consensus statement on concussion in sport: The 3rd international conference on concussion in sport held in Zurich, November 2008. *British Journal of Sports Medicine, 43*(Suppl. 1), i76–i84.

McKinlay, A., Grace, R. C., Horwood, L. J., Fergusson, D. M., Ridder, E. M., & MacFarlane, M. R. (2008). Prevalence of traumatic brain injury among children, adolescents and young adults: Prospective evidence from a birth cohort. *Brain Injury, 22*(2), 175–181.

McLellan, T., & McKinlay, A. (2013). Sensitivity to emotion, empathy and theory of mind: Adult performance following childhood TBI. *Brain Injury, 27*(9), 1032–1037.

Mitra, B., Cameron, P., & Butt, W. (2007). Population-based study of paediatric head injury. *Journal of Paediatrics and Child Health, 43*(3), 154–159.

Nadebaum, C., Anderson, V., & Catroppa, C. (2007). Executive function outcomes following traumatic brain injury in young children: A five year follow-up. *Developmental Neuropsychology, 32*(2), 703–728.

Nance, M. L., Polk-Williams, A., Collins, M. W., & Wiebe, D. J. (2009). Neurocognitive evaluation of mild traumatic brain injury in the hospitalized pediatric population. *Annals of Surgery, 249*(5), 859–863.

Narad, M. E., Taylor, H. G., Yeates, K. O., Stancin, T., Kirkwood, M. W., & Wade, S. L. (2017). Internet-based interacting together everyday, recovery after childhood TBI (I-InTERACT): Protocol for a multi-site randomized controlled trial of an internet-based parenting intervention. *Digital Health, 3.*

Newman, J. B., Reesman, J. H., Vaughan, C. G., & Gioia, G. A. (2013). Assessment of processing speed in children with mild TBI: A "first look" at the validity of pediatric impact. *Clinical Neuropsychologist, 27*(5), 779–793.

Novak, Z., Aglipay, M., Barrowman, N., Yeates, K. O., Beauchamp, M. H., Gravel, J., . . . Zemek, R. L. (2016). Association of persistent postconcussion symptoms with pediatric quality of life. *JAMA Pediatrics, 170*(12), Article e162900.

Nybo, T., Sainio, M., & Muller, K. (2005). Middle age cognition and vocational outcome of childhood brain injury. *Acta Neurologica Scandinavica, 112*(5), 338–342.

On, Z. X., Ryan, N. P., Konjarski, M., Catroppa, C., & Stargatt, R. (2021, April 15). Social cognition in paediatric traumatic brain injury: A systematic review and meta-analysis. *Neuropsychology Review.*

Padua, L., Cuccagna, C., & Pazzaglia, C. (2019). Novel sensory paradigms for neuromodulation in disorders of consciousness in traumatic brain injury. *Current Opinion in Neurology, 32*(6), 844–849.

Papa, L., Ramia, M. M., Kelly, J. M., Burks, S. S., Pawlowicz, A., & Berger, R. P. (2013). Systematic review of clinical research on biomarkers for pediatric traumatic brain injury. *Journal of Neurotrauma, 30*(5), 324–338.

Phillips, N. L., Shum, D. H. K., Mandalis, A., Parry, L., Benson, S., Morrow, A., . . . Lah, S. (2018). Time-based prospective memory in children and adolescents with traumatic brain injury: Impact of working memory demands. *Neuropsychology, 32*(5), 575–585.

Pinto, P. S., Poretti, A., Meoded, A., Tekes, A., & Huisman, T. A. (2012). The unique features of traumatic brain injury in children. Review of the characteristics of the pediatric skull and brain, mechanisms of trauma, patterns of injury, complications and their imaging findings—part 1. *Journal of Neuroimaging, 22*(2), e1–e17.

Povlishock, J. T., & Katz, D. I. (2005). Update of neuropathology and neurological recovery after traumatic brain injury. *Journal of Head Trauma Rehabilitation, 20*(1), 76–94.

Prasad, M. R., Swank, P. R., & Ewing-Cobbs, L. (2017). Long-term school outcomes of children and adolescents with traumatic brain injury. *Journal of Head Trauma Rehabilitation, 32*(1), E24–E32.

Purcell, L. K., Davis, G. A., & Gioia, G. A. (2019). What factors must be considered in "return to school" following concussion and what strategies or accommodations should be followed?: A systematic review. *British Journal of Sports Medicine, 53*(4), Article 250.

Rashid, M., Goez, H. R., Mabood, N., Damanhoury, S., Yager, J. Y., Joyce, A. S., & Newton, A. S. (2014). The impact of pediatric traumatic brain injury (TBI) on family functioning: A systematic review. *Journal of Pediatric Rehabilitation Medicine, 7*(3), 241–254.

Resch, C., Anderson, V. A., Beauchamp, M. H., Crossley, L., Hearps, S. J. C., van Heugten, C. M., . . . Catroppa, C. (2019). Age-dependent differences in the impact of paediatric traumatic brain injury on executive functions: A prospective study using susceptibility-weighted imaging. *Neuropsychologia, 124*, 236–245.

Rosema, S., Crowe, L., & Anderson, V. (2012). Social function in children and adolescents after traumatic brain injury: A systematic review 1989–2011. *Journal of Neurotrauma, 29*(7), 1277–1291.

Rosenfeld, E. H., Johnson, B., Wesson, D. E., Shah, S. R., Vogel, A. M., & Naik-Mathuria, B. (2020). Understanding non-accidental trauma in the united states: A national trauma databank study. *Journal of Pediatric Surgery, 55*(4), 693–697.

Rozbacher, A., Selci, E., Leiter, J., Ellis, M., & Russell, K. (2017). The effect of concussion or mild traumatic brain injury on school grades, national examination scores, and school attendance: A systematic review. *Journal of Neurotrauma, 34*(14), 2195–2203.

Ryan, N. P., van Bijnen, L., Catroppa, C., Beauchamp, M. H., Crossley, L., Hearps, S., & Anderson, V. (2016). Longitudinal outcome and recovery of social problems after pediatric traumatic brain injury (TBI): Contribution of brain insult and family environment. *International Journal of Developmental Neuroscience, 49*, 23–30.

Seguin, M., Degeilh, F., Bernier, A., El-Jalbout, R., & Beauchamp, M. H. (2020). It's a matter of surgency: Traumatic brain injury is associated with changes in preschoolers' temperament. *Neuropsychology, 34*(4), 375–387.

Ségun, M., Gagner, C., Tuerk, C., Lacomb Barrios, J., MacKay, P., & Beauchamp, M. H. (2022, January 7). What about the little ones: Systematic review of cognitive and behavioral outcomes following early TBI. *Neuropsychology Review.*

Shultz, E. L., Hoskinson, K. R., Keim, M. C., Dennis, M., Taylor, H. G., Bigler, E. D., . . . Yeates, K. O. (2016). Adaptive functioning following pediatric traumatic brain injury: Relationship to executive function and processing speed. *Neuropsychology, 30*(7), 830–840.

Snell, D. L., Surgenor, L. J., Hay-Smith, E. J., & Siegert, R. J. (2009). A systematic review of psychological treatments for mild traumatic brain injury: An update on the evidence. *Journal of Clinical and Experimental Neuropsychology, 31*(1), 20–38.

Sood, N., Godfrey, C., Anderson, V., & Catroppa, C. (2018). Rehabilitation of executive function in paediatric traumatic brain injury (repeat): Protocol for a randomized controlled trial for treating working memory and decision-making. *BMC Pediatrics, 18*(1), Article 362.

Stephens, J., Salorio, C., Denckla, M., Mostofsky, S., & Suskauer, S. (2017). Subtle motor findings during recovery from pediatric traumatic brain injury: A preliminary report. *Journal of Motor Behavior, 49*(1), 20–26.

Thompson, E. C., Krizman, J., White-Schwoch, T., Nicol, T., LaBella, C. R., & Kraus, N. (2018). Difficulty hearing in noise: A sequela of concussion in children. *Brain Injury, 32*(6), 763–769.

Thompson, L. W., Bass, K. D., Agyei, J. O., Naseem, H. U., Borngraber, E., Wang, J., & Reynolds, R. M. (2019). Incidence of nonaccidental head trauma in infants: A call to revisit prevention strategies. *Journal of Neurosurgery: Pediatrics, 20,* 1–8.

Treble-Barna, A., Pilipenko, V., Wade, S. L., Jegga, A. G., Yeates, K. O., Taylor, H. G., . . . Kurowski, B. G. (2020). Cumulative influence of inflammatory response genetic variation on long-term neurobehavioral outcomes after pediatric traumatic brain injury relative to orthopedic injury: An exploratory polygenic risk score. *Journal of Neurotrauma, 37,* 1491–1503.

Treble-Barna, A., Wade, S. L., Pilipenko, V., Martin, L. J., Yeates, K. O., Taylor, H. G., & Kurowski, B. G. (2021, April 13). Brain-derived neurotrophic factor Val66Met and behavioral adjustment following early childhood traumatic brain injury. *Journal of Neurotrauma, 39*(1–2), 114–121.

Tuerk, C., Gagner, C., Dégeilh, F., Bellerose, J., Lalonde, G., Landry-Roy, C., . . . Beauchamp, M. H. (2020). Quality of life 6 and 18 months after mild traumatic brain injury in early childhood: An exploratory study of the role of genetic, environmental, injury, and child factors. *Brain Research, 1748,* Article 147061.

van Gils, A., Stone, J., Welch, K., Davidson, L. R., Kerslake, D., Caesar, D., . . . Carson, A. (2020). Management of mild traumatic brain injury. *Practical Neurology, 20*(3), 213–221.

Verhaeghe, S., Defloor, T., & Grypdonck, M. (2005). Stress and coping among families of patients with traumatic brain injury: A review of the literature. *Journal of Clinical Nursing, 14*(8), 1004–1012.

Viot, S., Câmara-Costa, H., Laurence, W., Francillette, L., Toure, H., Brugel, D., . . . Chevignard, M. (2019). Assessment of memory functioning over two years following severe childhood traumatic brain injury: Results of the TGE cohort. *Brain Injury, 33*(9), 1208–1218.

Virk, S., Williams, T., Brunsdon, R., Suh, F., & Morrow, A. (2015). Cognitive remediation of attention deficits following acquired brain injury: A systematic review and meta-analysis. *NeuroRehabilitation, 36*(3), 367–377.

Wade, S. L., Cassedy, A. E., Taylor, H. G., McNally, K. A., Kirkwood, M. W., Stancin, T., . . . Kurowski, B. G. (2019). Adolescent quality of life following family problem-solving treatment for brain injury. *Journal of Consulting and Clinical Psychology, 87*(11), 1043–1055.

Wade, S. L., Cassedy, A., Walz, N. C., Taylor, H. G., Stancin, T., & Yeates, K. O. (2011). The relationship of parental warm responsiveness and negativity to emerging behavior problems following traumatic brain injury in young children. *Developmental Psychology, 47*(1), 119–133.

Wade, S. L., Taylor, H. G., Yeates, K. O., Kirkwood, M., Zang, H., McNally, K., . . . Zhang, N. (2018). Online problem solving for adolescent brain injury: A randomized trial of 2 approaches. *Journal of Developmental and Behavioral Pediatrics, 39*(2), 154–162.

Wallace, B., & Lifshitz, J. (2016). Traumatic brain injury and vestibulo-ocular function: Current challenges and future prospects. *Eye and Brain, 8,* 153–164.

Wehman, P., Chen, C. C., West, M., & Cifu, G. (2014). Transition planning for youth with traumatic brain injury: Findings from the National Longitudinal Transition Survey-2. *NeuroRehabilitation, 34*(2), 365–372.

Wiseman-Hakes, C., Kakonge, L., Doherty, M., & Beauchamp, M. H. (2020). A conceptual framework of social communication: Clinical applications to pediatric traumatic brain injury. *Seminars in Speech and Language, 41*(2), 143–160.

Wolfe, K. R., Bigler, E. D., Dennis, M., Gerhardt, C. A., Rubin, K., Taylor, H. G., . . . Yeates, K. O. (2015). Self-awareness of peer-rated social attributes in children with traumatic brain injury. *Journal of Pediatric Psychology, 40*(3), 272–284.

Yeates, K. O., Beauchamp, M. H., Craig, W., Doan, Q., Zemek, R., Bjornson, B., . . . Schneider, K. J. (2017a). Advancing Concussion Assessment in Pediatrics (A-CAP): A prospective, concurrent cohort, longitudinal study of mild traumatic brain injury in children: Protocol study. *BMJ Open, 7*(7), Article e017012.

Yeates, K. O., & Enrile, B. G. (2005). Implicit and explicit memory in children with congenital and acquired brain disorder. *Neuropsychology, 19*(5), 618–628.

Yeates, K. O., Levin, H. S., & Ponsford, J. (2017b). The neuropsychology of traumatic brain injury: Looking back, peering ahead. *Journal of the International Neuropsychological Society, 23*(9–10), 806–817.

Yeates, K. O., Taylor, H., Barry, C., Drotar, D., Wade, S., & Stancin, T. (2001). Neurobehavioral symptoms in childhood closed-head injuries: Changes in prevalence and correlates during the first year postinjury. *Journal of Pediatric Psychology, 26*(2), 79–91.

Yeates, T. M., Taylor, H. G., Bigler, E. D., Minich, N. M., Tang, K., Cohen, D. M., . . . Yeates, K. O. (2021, April 5). Sex differences in the outcomes of mild traumatic brain injury in children presenting to the emergency department. *Journal of Neurotrauma, 39*(1–2), 93–101.

Yeo, P. C., Yeo, E. Q. Y., Probert, J., Sim, S. H. S., & Sirisena, D. (2020). A systematic review and qualitative analysis of concussion knowledge amongst sports coaches and match officials. *Journal of Sports Science & Medicine, 19*(1), 65–77.

Zemek, R., Barrowman, N., Freedman, S. B., Gravel, J., Gagnon, I., McGahern, C., . . . Osmond, M. H. (2016). Clinical risk score for persistent postconcussion symptoms among children with acute concussion in the ed. *Journal of the American Medical Association, 315*(10), 1014–1025.

CHAPTER 6

Stroke

Mardee Greenham
Mark T. Mackay
Anne Gordon
Vicki Anderson

HISTORICAL OVERVIEW

Stroke is an acute cerebrovascular event that may occur during any stage of development, including the prenatal and perinatal periods, as well as throughout childhood. Contrary to commonly held views, children do not recover better than adults following a stroke and may experience more generalized functional consequences (Simonetti et al., 2015). Furthermore, the lifelong individual, family, and societal burden of stroke early in life is likely to be greater than that in adults, because infant and child stroke survivors face many more years living with disability. The key difference between children and adults is that pediatric stroke results primarily in disruption to developing brain networks and a changed ability to achieve rather than a loss of functional independence. The extent and severity of deficits across motor, sensory, cognitive, social, and behavioral domains may not be apparent in the short term following stroke, particularly in newborns and preschool children, who typically grow into their deficits (Gordon et al., 2015; Westmacott, Askalan, Macgregor, Anderson, & DeVeber, 2010).

While pediatric stroke is considered relatively rare compared to stroke in the adult population, it is increasingly recognized as an important cause of childhood disability. Stroke is among the top 10 causes of death in children in developed countries; it is more common than childhood brain tumors (Murphy, 2000), and has a 10% fatality rate. Pediatric stroke is commonly associated with a range of comorbidities, including cardiac disease, arteriopathies (disorder of the cerebral arteries), prothrombotic disorders (risk of blood coagulation/thrombosis), sickle cell anemia, and arteriovenous malformation (AVM). Despite known risk factors, causal relationships are not well established, with around one-fifth of stroke cases being idiopathic. To date, pediatric stroke research has primarily examined acute treatment, immediate outcomes, diagnosis, and etiology (De Schryver, Kappelle, Jennekens-Schinkel, & Boudewyn Peters, 2000; deVeber, 2003; Ganesan et al., 2000; Ganesan, Prengler, McShane, Wade, & Kirkham, 2003). In contrast, research documenting outcomes, impairment rates, and prognostic considerations for recovery is scarce, despite anecdotal clinical observations suggesting that significant functional impairments (e.g., mobility, communication, and educational deficits) are present in many survivors. Of note, for survivors, such ongoing sequelae suggest that this condition can be classified as a chronic illness.

Due to variable etiology, lesion location, and size (deVeber, 2003; Ganesan et al., 2003; Kirton, Westmacott, & deVeber, 2007), the pediatric stroke population is a heterogeneous group, characterized by diverse functional and cognitive deficits of varying severity. It is also likely that the presence and severity of psychosocial deficits are equally diverse and dependent on multiple factors, both stroke-related (e.g., etiology, lesion size, and location) and non-stroke-related (e.g., environment, child's premorbid temperament).

The economic burden of pediatric stroke on families and health services has recently been reported. Higher stroke costs correlate with more impairment and poorer quality of life (Hamilton, Huang, Seiber, & Lo, 2015). In a retrospective study, Gardner, Hills, Sidney, Johnston, and Fullerton (2010) estimated the 5-year direct medical cost of perinatal and childhood stroke to be $110,921, representing a 15-fold cost increase compared to healthy controls. Costs were higher for childhood stroke ($135,611) than for perinatal stroke ($51,719) and higher for hemorrhagic stroke than for arterial ischemic stroke. In addition to these medical costs, families experience substantial out-of-pocket expenses related to lost wages, transportation, and nonreimbursed health care.

EPIDEMIOLOGY

There are two main stroke subtypes, arterial ischemic stroke (AIS) and hemorrhagic stroke (HS). AIS occurs when blood supply to an area of the brain is interrupted, for example, by thrombus, vasospasm, or dissection of the vascular wall. The interruption of blood flow results in a reduction in the supply of oxygen and nutrients, causing neuronal cell death, which is also referred to as *infarction*. Contrasting with adults, atherosclerosis is a rare cause for childhood AIS. A diverse range of risk factors have been identified in association with AIS in children, including vasculopathy, infection (Hills, Johnston, Sidney, Zielinski, & Fullerton, 2012), trauma (Hills et al., 2012), cardiac disorders consisting predominantly of congenital heart disease (Fox, Sidney, & Fullerton, 2015) and hematological disorders (Maguire, deVeber, & Parkin, 2007), (Amlie-Lefond et al., 2009; Hay & Missiuna, 1998; Sylvestre, Nadeau, Charron, Larose, & Lepage, 2013; Wrotniak, Epstein, Dorn, Jonesc, & Kondilisc, 2006); however, approximately half of children who suffer an AIS were previously healthy at the time of the index event (Ganesan et al., 2003).

Multiple risk factors converge in > 50% of children with AIS (Mackay et al., 2011), but at least 10% remain idiopathic. Rates of recurrent AIS range from 6 to 35% (deVeber, MacGregor, Curtis, & Mayank, 2000; Ganesan, Prengler, Wade, & Kirkham, 2006; Simonetti et al., 2015). Population-based data suggest that 5-year recurrence rates approach 50% (deVeber et al., 2000; Fullerton, Wu, Sidney, & Johnston, 2007). Presence of arteriopathy is the most important predictor of recurrent AIS, with rates of > 65% reported (deVeber et al., 2000; Fullerton et al., 2007; Ganesan et al., 2006). Other factors linked to recurrence include genetic thrombophilia (Ganesan et al., 2006; Sträter et al., 2002), previous transient ischemic attack, bilateral infarction, immunodeficiency, and leucocytosis (Ganesan et al., 2006). AIS occurs more commonly in boys, with a reported male:female ratio of around 1.5:1 (Golomb, 2009). While the reason for this difference is not clearly understood, it has been suggested that estrogen, which is higher in girls than in boys, may play a role due to its vasodilatory and anti-inflammatory effects (Reeves et al., 2008).

HS (subarachnoid/intracerebral) involves the rupture of an artery and often leads to more diffuse brain lesions, as bleeding can result in pressure injuries to the brain, as well as interruption of pathways connecting neural networks. The common causes of nontraumatic HS are arteriovenous malformations, hematological abnormalities, and brain tumors, with other etiologies including cavernous hemangioma, vasculopathy, vasculitis, and infections (Jordan & Hillis, 2007). Fewer data are available on risk factors for recurrent HS. In a large population-based cohort study (2.3 million children), 116 cases of nontraumatic HS were identified over 11 years, with a 5-year cumulative recurrence rate of 10% (Fullerton et al., 2007). Almost two-thirds of bleeds occurred within the first 6 months of diagnosis. No child with idiopathic HS had a recurrent event, whereas 13% of children with structural abnormalities (e.g., AVMs or tumors) and medical etiologies (e.g., thrombocytopenia or hypertension) had recurrent events.

The reported mortality for AIS ranges from 7 to 28% (deVeber et al., 2000; Simonetti et al., 2015; Simonetti et al., 2015), and from 6 to 54% for HS (Blom et al., 2003). In a U.S. study reporting stroke mortality between 1979 and 1998, 4,881 deaths could be attributed to pediatric stroke, giving average annual mortality rates of 0.09 per 100,000 person years for AIS, 0.14 for intracerebral hemorrhage, and 0.11 for subarachnoid hemorrhage (Fullerton, Chetkovich, Wu, Smith, & Johnston, 2002). Risk of death is higher in infants, males, African Americans, and children living in the Stroke Belt (an eight-state region in the southeastern United States with a disproportionately high stroke mortality rate) (Fullerton et al., 2002; Mallick, Ganesan, & O'Callaghan, 2010). Declining mortality rates have been observed in HS, possibly related to improvements in critical care, with far smaller decreases in AIS mortality rates (Fullerton et al., 2002). This may be partially due to the comorbidities associated with AIS, such as heart disorders, which also have an increased risk of mortality.

In the pediatric stroke literature, the population is generally categorized into *perinatal stroke*, occurring between 28 weeks of gestation and 28 days of age, or *childhood stroke*, occurring between ages 29 days and 18 years. Incidence of childhood stroke is between 1.3 and 13 per 100,000 (Mallick et al., 2010). Stroke incidence rates are much higher during the perinatal period, in which stroke has been reported to affect as many as 1 in every 1,200 live births (Dunbar & Kirton, 2020). Of note, these figures may underestimate true stroke rates, as clinical signs for diagnosis are often difficult to detect in neonates. Advances in neuroimaging techniques and increasing awareness of stroke in children have led to a rise in diagnoses in recent years. While recurrence is rare in perinatal stroke, it is estimated that up to one-third of those with childhood stroke experience a further stroke during the following few years (Fullerton et al., 2007; Ganesan et al., 2006), explained by the risk associated with comorbid medical conditions such as cardiac disorders and sickle cell disease.

ETIOLOGY, NEUROPATHOLOGY, AND NEURAL SUBSTRATES

Clinical presentation in children and infants with stroke varies and is influenced by the age of the child and arterial circulation. Children typically present with focal neurological deficits, and hemiparesis is the most common presenting symptom, occurring in up to 94% of cases (Mackay et al., 2011; Tsze & Valente, 2011). Seizures are also common, occurring in up to 50% of cases (Younkin, 2002), and 30% of children present with headaches at or shortly after the onset of symptoms (Steinlin, 2012). Infants (< 1 year of age) most commonly present with seizures and altered mental states, such as lethargy. Toddlers often demonstrate irritability, sleepiness, feeding difficulties, cold extremities (Tsze & Valente, 2011) and focal weakness (Zimmer, Garg, Williams, & Golomb, 2007).

A proportion of neonates are not diagnosed acutely, referred to in the literature as presumed perinatal strokes. These infants are not observed to exhibit clinical signs in the perinatal period but generally present at around 6 to 12 months of age when parents begin to notice asymmetry in body movement, developmental delays or the onset of seizures.

Depending on the cerebral artery affected, brain lesions caused by stroke can vary in severity, size and location (cortical, subcortical or both). For example, infarcts in the middle cerebral artery often lead to lesions in the dorsolateral cortex, basal ganglia and white matter, whilst infarcts in the anterior cerebral artery can cause lesions to the orbitofrontal, temporal and parietal cortices. The basal ganglia, cerebellum and the rostral midbrain structures are also common lesions sites (Amarenco, Bogousslavsky, Caplan, Donnan, & Hennerici, 2009; Ganesan et al., 2000, 2003).

There are three major arteries that supply blood to the cerebral hemispheres: the middle cerebral artery (MCA), and the anterior cerebral artery (ACA), derived from the internal carotid arteries, and the posterior cerebral artery (PCA), derived from the vertebral arteries (see Plate 6.1 in the color insert; Vanderah, 2019). The MCA territory is the most common location for infarcts in adults, as well as children and infants (Kirton & deVeber, 2011).

The MCA is the largest terminal branch of the internal carotid artery and supplies blood to part of the frontal lobe and the lateral surface of the temporal and parietal lobes. Depending on the site of occlusion (superior, inferior, or deep territory branches, or the stem of the MCA, affecting all branches), an MCA territory infarct may affect the motor cortex, as well as Broca's and Wernicke's areas. Clinical presentation can include weakness in the face and upper or lower limbs (hemiplegia), altered vision and aphasia (Ciccone, Cappella, & Borgna-Pignatti, 2011). The ACA is the second terminal branch of the internal carotid artery and supplies most of the medial surface of the brain's cortex, including the frontal and prefrontal cortices and medial parts of the primary motor and sensory cortices. ACA infarcts primarily present with leg weakness but can also cause grasp reflex, behavioral abnormalities, and transcortical aphasia (Mauro, Murphy, Thomson, Venbrux, & Morgan, 2014). The PCA supplies the infero-medial temporal and occipital lobes. In children symptoms of occlusions of this artery territory can include visual field defects (Ciccone et al., 2011).

Recent advances in neuroimaging have identified arteriopathies (disease of the artery) as the most common cause of AIS, detected in around half of children (Amlie-Lefond et al., 2009; Fullerton et al., 2007; Mackay et al., 2011). In a sample of 277 children from the International Pediatric Stroke Study, the top three arteriopathy subtypes were focal cerebral arterial stenosis with no apparent cause (25%), moyamoya (22%), and arterial dissection (20%) (Amlie-Lefond et al., 2009). These were followed by vasculitis (12%), sickle cell disease (8%), and post-varicella angiopathy (7%).

Cardiac disease is the second most common cause of AIS, accounting for up to one-third of cases (deVeber et al., 2000; Ganesan et al., 2003; Mackay et al., 2011). Stroke can occur both spontaneously in these children or during or within 72 hours of cardiac surgery or catheterization (Tsze & Valente, 2011). Abnormal cardiac anatomy or changes in perfusion during surgery lead to abnormal blood flow and may predispose children to the formation of intracardiac thrombi and subsequent embolization to the brain (Golomb, 2009). Strokes before and after cardiac surgery can also relate to the effects of anticoagulation medication necessary for surgery.

Other risk factors include hemoglobinopathies, hereditary conditions that cause abnormalities of the hemoglobin molecule or the rate of hemoglobin synthesis. Sickle cell disease (SCD) comprises a group of autosomal recessive disorders that cause blood cells to distort into a sickle or crescent shape. SCD is the most common hemoglobinopathy associated with AIS, and 11% of children with the disease will have a stroke (Earley et al., 1998). SCD occurs primarily in individuals of African, Mediterranean, Indian, and Middle Eastern heritage (Reid, Charace, & Lubin, 1995). The prevalence is about 1–2% among African descendants in Europe and the United States, and 4% in West Africa (Ware, de Montalembert, Tshilolo, & Abboud, 2017). Thrombophilias, a group of blood coagulation disorders associated with increased risk of clotting, have been reported to be present in 20–50% of cases, but the importance of thrombophilia in AIS remains uncertain (Friedman, 2009). Major infections such as sepsis, meningitis, and encephalitis have long been recognized as risk factors for stroke, but minor infections, including varicella, borrelia, mycoplasma, enterovirus, and parvovirus, are now being recognized as risk factors (Amlie-Lefond & Fullerton, 2010). Inflammation of the blood vessels, caused by the infection, can lead to progressive stenosis or intraluminal thrombosis (Amlie-Lefond & Fullerton, 2010).

Poststroke epilepsy occurs in approximately 15–20% of children with childhood AIS (deVeber et al., 2000) and up to 17% of HS (Blom et al., 2003). Larger cortical lesions are associated with higher risk of developing seizures (deVeber, MacGregor, Curtis, & Mayank, 2000; Yang, Park, & Hartlage, 1995). Emerging data from the International Pediatric Stroke study suggest the incidence of a first remote seizure is 1% per month, with a cumulative 13% incidence of active epilepsy by 1 year following AIS (Fox, Glass, Sidney, Lowenstein, & Fullerton, 2013). Younger age, multifocal or cortical infarction, involvement of the MCA territory, presence of focal cerebral arteriopathy, and presence and duration of symptomatic seizures at the time of diagnosis are associated with increased risk of epilepsy (Fox et al., 2013; Kopyta, Sarecka-Hujar, & Skrzypek, 2015). Children with epilepsy complicating AIS have poorer cognitive outcomes (De Schryver et al., 2000).

NEUROPSYCHOLOGICAL CONSEQUENCES

General Intellectual Functioning

Group studies investigating general intellectual function in children following stroke have revealed that mean IQ scores are generally within the average range but skewed toward the lower end and significantly lower than those of typically developing control groups and standardized test norms (Everts et al., 2008; Gomes, Spencer-Smith, Jacobs, Coleman, & Anderson, 2012; Hajek et al., 2014; Max et al., 2002; O'Keeffe et al., 2014; Pavlovic et al., 2006; Westmacott, MacGregor, Askalan, & deVeber, 2009). Our group has also explored general intellectual function, using a resilience framework and has found that the majority of stroke survivors demonstrated age-appropriate cognitive skills 12 months postinjury, cautioning overemphasis of poor outcomes. Identified risk factors included perinatal timing, MCA territory infarction, and presence of seizures poststroke (Anderson et al., 2020), suggesting that children with these characteristics may warrant further follow-up.

Perceptual and Sensorimotor Skills

Limited research evaluating visuospatial processing indicates subtle deficits following pediatric stroke. Max (2004) reported low-average performance on the Developmental Test of Visual-Motor Integration in children with both left- (n = 13) and right-sided (n = 16) AIS or HS (perinatal or childhood onset) (Max, 2004). A study of 99 children with childhood-onset AIS also revealed low-average performance on measures of visuo-constructive skills (Studer et al., 2014). Similarly, Allman and Scott (2013) reported subtle impairments in visuo-constructive skills and non-dominant hand dexterity in 44 children with childhood onset AIS (Allman & Scott, 2013). A study comparing outcomes of children (perinatal or childhood onset) and adults with similar unilateral stroke lesions reported significantly poorer visuoconstructive performance in the children compared to the adults (Mosch, Max, & Tranel, 2005).

Studies of children with perinatal stroke also suggest subtle spatial deficits. In a study using a spontaneous grouping task, children ages 3 to 4 years (n = 20) showed impairment regardless of lesion laterality compared to healthy controls (Stiles & Nass, 1991). Children with right-hemisphere lesions showed difficulty organizing objects into coherent spatial groups, while those with left-sided lesions had problems with logical relations within the spatial array. Studies investigating visuospatial processing in children following perinatal stroke suggest compensation for deficits by adopting alternative processing strategies (Stiles, Stern, Trauner, & Nass, 1996; Vicari, Stiles, Stern, & Resca, 1998). At 4 to 6 years of age, the accuracy of children with left-hemisphere lesions on a block construction task was comparable to age-matched healthy controls; however, the procedures used were greatly simplified, comparable to that of younger children. Children with right-sided stroke also showed delay, but different patterns were observed. At age 4, the accuracy of constructions for children with right-sided lesions was very poor, but the procedures used were comparable to those of age-matched controls. By age 6, the accuracy of children with right-hemisphere lesions was similar to that of controls, but like children with left-sided lesions, they used simpler procedures. By using a less complicated construction strategy, children with right-hemisphere lesions were able to compensate for spatial deficits and generate accurate constructions. Similar findings have been reported in a study of 6- to 13-year-olds with perinatal stroke using the Rey–Osterrieth Complex Figure (Akshoomoff, Feroleto, Doyle, & Stiles, 2002). On the copying task, regardless of hemisphere affected, children with stroke performed more poorly than controls; this was particularly evident in the younger children (age 6). By age 10, copying accuracy had improved but immature and piecemeal strategies were used. The lack of difference between children with left- and right-hemisphere lesions is likely due to the underlying task demands placing equal emphasis on segmentation and integration. While children with left- and right-sided lesions performed similarly on the copying task, differences between the lesion groups were reported on the memory task. Children with right-hemisphere stroke used a piecemeal strategy, as they had on the copying task, whereas children with left-sided lesions adopted a different strategy for the memory task. They organized their memory reproductions around the core triangle and produced relatively few additional details. Compensation strategies were demonstrated in the coping task, while the additional demands of the memory task were characteristic of a left-hemisphere visuospatial processing deficit.

Language

Speech and language outcomes have not been widely explored; however, one study reported aphasia symptoms in 30% of children 12 months following AIS (Cnossen et al., 2010). In adults, language impairments commonly occur following left-hemisphere lesions, but the association between lesion laterality and language outcomes in children may be dependent on age at stroke onset. Children with perinatal-onset stroke have been reported to display initial expressive and receptive language delay, with relatively normal language skills by school age (Bates, 1998; Bates et al., 1997; Dick, Wulfeck, Krupa-Kwiatkowski, & Bates, 2004; Vicari et al., 2000). Bates and colleagues (1997) reported delayed language onset in a group of children with perinatal stroke. Children with right-sided perinatal stroke showed delays in word comprehension and gesture from 10 to 17 months of age, while children with left temporal lobe lesions demonstrated expressive language delays from 10 to 31 months. Studies involving children with perinatal-onset stroke after 5 years of age have shown average to low-average language skills, with no lesion laterality effect (Bates et al., 2001; Reilly, Bates, & Marchman, 1998). These findings suggest that regardless of lesion laterality, perinatal-onset stroke results in delays during the early stage of language learning, but these difficulties are overcome once the fundamental properties of language have been acquired. However, lesion laterality has been shown to play a greater role in language outcome following childhood-onset stroke. A study comparing children with perinatal-onset (n = 7) and childhood-onset (n = 5) left-hemisphere strokes revealed that children with perinatal stroke had similar language function to controls, while childhood-onset stroke resulted in significantly poorer expressive and receptive language skills (Ilves et al., 2014). Gout and colleagues (2005) also reported language impairments in six of nine children with childhood-onset left-hemisphere lesions, including naming difficulties, reduced fluency, repetition difficulties, and written language difficulties. However, they reported that younger age at onset, as well as posteriorly located lesions, was associated with poorer language outcome (Gout et al., 2005). Another study comparing children with left (n = 10) and right (n = 7) basal ganglia infarcts found no group differences but did note greater variation in performance of the children with left-hemisphere stroke (Rowan et al., 2007).

Attention

Few studies have comprehensively examined attentional skills in children following stroke, and only a handful have employed age-normed, child-specific tools. Emerging evidence suggests that problems in this area are common. O'Keeffe and colleagues (2014) identified significant weaknesses in attentional skills following AIS, reporting impairment rates of 51% for sustained attention (Test of Everyday Attention for Children [TEA-Ch]: Walk/Don't Walk) and 67% on a selective attention task (TEA-Ch: Sky Search) (O'Keeffe et al.,

2014), while Everts et al. (2008) reported divided attention deficits following AIS. In a study from our team (Hajek et al., 2014), we found that children with AIS performed significantly worse than chronic illness (asthma) controls on measures of sustained attention (TEA-Ch: Walk/Don't Walk) and switching attention (TEA-Ch: Creature Counting). Elias and Moura-Ribeiro (2013) reported poorer auditory selective attention in children with AIS compared to healthy controls. Elias et al. (2014) later described elevated rates of attention-deficit/hyperactivity disorder (ADHD) following stroke, supporting the earlier findings of Max et al. (2003), who reported that 46% of children with stroke had ADHD, compared to just 17% of orthopedic controls.

Memory

Studies examining memory following pediatric stroke have shown variable results, but some suggest vulnerability to subtle deficits. Block, Nanson, and Lowry (1999) reported that children with childhood-onset unilateral AIS (n = 11) showed subtle weaknesses on measures of verbal learning and functional memory compared to healthy controls (n = 11). Children with AIS remembered fewer words across trials on the California Verbal Learning Test (CVLT), but no differences were found for short- and long-delay free recall. Poorer performances on the Rivermead Behavioural Memory Test were also reported for children with AIS compared to controls. Lansing et al. (2004) reported similar subtle verbal memory deficits in a sample of 26 children with unilateral AIS or HS (perinatal or childhood onset). Compared to orthopedic controls, the stroke group remembered fewer words across trials and showed poorer performance on both long-delay free and cued recall. They were also less able to utilize an efficient verbal learning and memory strategy (semantic clusters) and were more susceptible to retroactive interference. Other studies using the CVLT have reported no difference between children with stroke and controls (Chapman, Max, Gamino, McGlothlin, & Cliff, 2003; Everts et al., 2008; Schatz et al., 1999). In a study involving 31 children with AIS or HS (21 perinatal onset; 10 childhood onset) and 31 healthy controls, Kolk, Ennok, Laugesaar, Kaldoja, and Talvik (2011) reported impairments on Memory for Faces and Sentence Repletion. Other studies have indicated no deficits using the Wechsler Memory Scales in children with HS (Blom et al., 2003) or the Rey–Osterreith Complex Figure in children with AIS or HS (Everts et al., 2008).

Executive Functions

Early studies reported mixed findings for executive function outcomes poststroke. For example, Max et al. (2003) found no difference between children with stroke and orthopedic controls on tasks of verbal fluency, suggesting largely intact verbally based executive function. In contrast, De Schryver et al. (2000) divided children with stroke into those with and without a diagnosis of ADHD, and compared their results on the Wisconsin Card Sorting Task (WCST), a measure of cognitive flexibility and set shifting. They found that children with stroke + ADHD performed more poorly, while those without ADHD achieved results similar to normative levels. Similarly, Schatz et al. (1999) explored planning skills, using the Tower of Hanoi, with children with stroke and sibling controls, with the stroke group demonstrating poorer performance. On balance, this work points to vulnerabilities in specific executive functions following stroke but has not explored the breadth of executive skills.

Evidence from more recent studies suggests that children with stroke may be vulnerable to more global deficits in executive function. In a study examining 28 children with AIS or HS, and investigating multiple aspects of executive function, Long et al. (2011) reported that mean performance levels for these children fell below normative expectations on tasks tapping attentional control, cognitive flexibility, and information processing, with scores toward the lower end of the average range. These authors also explored rates of impaired executive skills and found that 46% of their sample exhibited impaired attentional control, including sustained attention and inhibitory control, and between 40 and 70% showed cognitive flexibility deficits (working memory, mental flexibility and divided attention). Everyday executive function was also affected, with 25% of participants being rated as having clinically significant executive function impairment based on parent ratings, and 25–61% based on teacher ratings. Similar findings were reported in a study involving 49 children with AIS. O'Keeffe et al. (2014) described low-average scores on measures of sequencing, switching, working memory, and cognitive flexibility, with group means significantly below normative expectations, and with 30% of their sample functioning in the impaired range. Parent and teacher ratings of everyday executive function also identified problems.

Psychosocial Function

Psychosocial problems are some of the most distressing and enduring symptoms reported by families following child brain insult (Anderson, Catroppa, Haritou, Morse, & Rosenfeld, 2005; Anderson, Northam, Hendy, & Wrennal, 2001; Bohnert, Parkerb, & Warschauskyc, 1997), yet this is a relatively unexplored domain in the pediatric stroke literature. In a review of psychosocial outcomes following pediatric stroke, Gomes, Rinehart, Greenham, and Anderson (2014) identified 11 studies reporting on social function, 11 on psychological function, and six addressing both domains. They reported that while the research was limited, there was a trend for elevated social and psychological problems, lower levels of social participation, and reduced peer acceptance. Findings suggested an overall moderate degree of impairment, with some children showing few or no difficulties. Clinically, problems in these domains can be present in the context of normal intellectual ability (Lo et al., 2014) and may not emerge until children are discharged from hospital or rehabilitation centers and need to reintegrate into school and the community.

A limited literature has described a variety of psychological impairments, including internalizing (anxiety, inattention, psychosomatic complaints) and externalizing (aggression, hyperactivity, emotional regulation, impulsivity) problems (Gomes et al., 2014). In a study of 133 children, 2–16 years poststroke, parents reported significantly poorer emotional well-being in their children following stroke, compared to healthy controls (Neuner et al., 2011). Gordon, Ganesan, Towell, and Kirkham (2002) also found parent-reported emotional problems in 25% of a smaller sample of 17 children, 2 years following stroke. Another study of 16 children found parent-reported externalizing behavior problems (emotional lability, temper tantrums, and aggressive outbursts) in 44% of their sample (Steinlin, Roellin, & Schrot, 2004). Everts et al. (2008) found that parent-reported symptoms of ADHD (learning difficulties, attention problems, anxiety, and impulsivity) were present in 50% of their sample (n = 14), 1 month to 14 years poststroke. Max and colleagues (2002, 2003) reported psychiatric disorders, based on standardized measures from parents and children, in a sample of children with stroke (n = 29) and a matched chronic illness control group. They found that 59% of the children with stroke developed psychiatric disorders compared to only 14% of controls. The disorders with the highest rate of prevalence in this sample were ADHD (49%), anxiety disorder (31%), mood disorders (21%) and personality change (17%).

Other researchers have reported reduced social and peer relationship scores on parent-report quality-of-life measures (De Schryver et al., 2000; Friefeld, Yeboah, Jones, & deVeber, 2004; Gordon et al., 2002; Neuner et al., 2011; O'Keeffe, Ganesan, King, & Murphy, 2012). In a study comparing children with AIS to those with chronic asthma and healthy controls, we found higher rates of psychosocial problems, and most particularly internalizing problems and reduced social participation, in children with stroke. These problems were associated with poorer quality of home environment (e.g., parent mental health) and reduced family function (Anderson et al., 2014; Greenham et al., 2017b). Hurvitz, Warschausky, Berg, and Tsai (2004) reported outcomes of survivors 12 years post AIS and HS. They found that despite a high level of employment and college attendance, financial independence and independent living were relatively low. Daily living skills, communication, and socialization were in the moderately low range. Other researchers have reported significant reductions in family and school participation, using self- and parent-report measures of participation and quality of life (De Schryver et al., 2000; Gordon et al., 2002; Hurvitz et al., 2004).

A prospective, longitudinal study from our group revealed poorer than expected psychosocial function at 6 and 12 months poststroke, characterized by emotional difficulties, inattention, and hyperactivity (Greenham et al., 2017b). These difficulties were associated with older age at stroke onset, acute neurological impairment, and poor parent mental health, suggesting the importance of environmental factors in the psychosocial domain. Furthermore, follow-up at 5 years poststroke identified that ongoing psychosocial problems were again predicted by not only older age at stroke onset but also poorer cognitive and psychological function at 12 months poststroke and concurrent excessive fatigue (Greenham et al., 2017a; Greenham et al., 2018). Of note, there was no link between these outcomes and any motor, language, or cognitive outcomes.

Motor Function

Physical and motor impairment following pediatric stroke is common. Long-term follow-up studies have reported motor impairment ranging from mild clumsiness to significant hemiparesis in 50% to 80% of children (Boardman et al., 2005; Cnossen et al., 2010; Cooper et al., 2017, 2019; De Schryver et al., 2000; deVeber et al., 2000; Ganesan et al., 2000). Hemiplegia is reported in three-fourths of children (de Veber et al., 2000).

Lesion size and location are significant predictors of motor outcome in both perinatal and later acquired stroke, yet these factors differ for the two age-at-onset groups. Hemiparesis in the perinatal population is often associated with multiple lesion-site locations (basal ganglia, cerebral cortex, and internal capsule), while in later-onset stroke, just one or two of these areas can result in hemiparesis (Boardman et al., 2005; Mercuri et al.,

1999, 2004). There is a significant difference in the prevalence of hemiplegia in perinatal and later acquired stroke. Hemiplegia affects around one-third of children with perinatal-onset stroke (Mercuri et al., 2004), while the prevalence in later acquired stroke is estimated to be three-fourths (deVeber et al., 2000; Salih, Abdel-Gader, Al-Jarallah, Kentab, & Al-Nasser, 2006).

The severity of motor deficits varies, but most children will gain or regain independent mobility (Ganesan et al., 2000; Golomb et al., 2003; Lanska, Lanska, Horwitz, & Aram, 1991). However, even mild motor impairment may limit a child's ability to participate in activities and affect self-confidence (Hay & Missiuna, 1998; Sylvestre et al., 2013; Wrotniak et al., 2006). In a prospective, longitudinal study ($n = 50$), Gordon et al. (2015) identified sensorimotor impairments as the most significant consequence of stroke, both acutely and at 6 months poststroke, with older children more affected.

Hemorrhagic Stroke

Studies examining outcomes following stabilization of recovery have focused on pediatric AIS, with only a handful of publications addressing HS, despite this subtype accounting for almost half of childhood strokes (Fullerton, Wu, Zhao, & Johnston, 2003). Following HS, poor outcomes (including cognitive and motor outcomes) have been reported in 25–52% of children in a retrospective case series (Blom et al., 2003; Lo, Hajek, Pappa, Wang, & Zumberge, 2013; Meyer-Heim & Boltshauser, 2003). In a U.S. study of 19 children, Lo et al. (2013) described mild to moderate neurological impairments and significantly lowered quality of life in the majority of survivors. Predictors of poorer neurological outcomes include younger age (Meyer-Heim & Boltshauser, 2003), depressed conscious state at presentation in some (Meyer-Heim & Boltshauser, 2003) but not other studies (Lo et al., 2013), intracerebral hemorrhage volume (Lo et al., 2013) and presence of vascular anomaly (Lo et al., 2013). A Dutch study describing long-term outcome in 31 survivors of HS found that over half had physical impairments with paresis or cerebellar ataxia, and a similar proportion of children showed cognitive deficits when compared to premorbid academic functioning (Blom et al., 2003). These findings are consistent with an earlier U.S. study of 26 patients reporting motor and cognitive deficits in 38% and 50% of survivors, respectively (Broderick, Talbot, Prenger, Leach, & Brott, 1993).

Few studies have examined cognitive outcome in detail following HS, and the majority reporting in this domain rely on measures of neurological function that fail to capture the subtlety of cognitive deficits. Murphy, Compas, Gindville, Reeslund, and Jordan (2017) examined cognitive function, using Wechsler Intelligence Scales, over 2 years in seven children following HS. They reported that while verbal comprehension and perceptual reasoning skills improved over the 2-year period, the same trajectory was not observed for more "dynamic" processing skills, including processing speed and working memory. Processing speed scores were in the average range at 1 and 2 years poststroke, but the interquartile ranges showed low performance. Raw scores for working memory showed improvement over time; however, age-normed percentiles revealed that these children did not progress at age-expected rates, and their performances remained well below those of their peers at both 1 and 2 years poststroke. This finding is consistent with other, early brain insult research indicating that deficits may emerge or worsen with time as a child develops and cognitive demands increase (Anderson, Spencer-Smith, & Wood, 2011).

Sickle Cell Disease

Children with SCD are at increased risk of both AIS and HS, and may experience a "silent stroke," defined as an infarction/ischemic changes in brain tissue identified on brain imaging in the absence of clinical symptoms or signs of neurological dysfunction (Daly, Kral, & Tarazi, 2011). It is estimated that by the age of 14 years, 11% of children with SCD experience an overt stroke, and 14% show radiological evidence of a clinically silent stroke (Moser et al., 1996). While overt strokes are an obvious cause of neurological abnormalities and cognitive impairment in children with SCD, cognitive deficits are common in children who have no evidence of focal brain injury (Steen et al., 2005). The rigid geometry of the sickle- or crescent-shaped red blood cells in SCD compromises their ability to flow through the bloodstream, reducing the delivery of oxygen and nutrients to the brain, and resulting in endothelial injury that promotes thrombosis. Children with infarcts have demonstrated lower Full Scale IQ (FSIQ), Verbal IQ (VIQ), and Performance IQ (PIQ) compared to children SCD without abnormalities on magnetic resonance imaging (MRI) (Thompson et al., 2003; Watkins et al., 1998), yet even in the absence of cerebrovascular damage, children with SCD show poorer IQ performance compared with healthy controls (Steen et al., 2005). Qualitative MRI studies suggest that conventional MRI may be insensitive to subtle neurological damage in these patients (Steen et al., 1998; Steen, Xiong, Mulhern, Langston, & Wang, 1999). Children with SCD have also been shown to have impairments across neuropsychological domains (Berkelhammer et al., 2007). Deficits in attention and executive functions are among the most commonly reported symptoms in children with SCD and are more pronounced in children with infarcts compared with those with no evidence of cerebral damage (Brown et al., 2000; Watkins et al., 1998). One study revealed that 53% of children with silent infarct had impaired attention and executive function, compared to 13% without evidence of infarct and 0% of healthy siblings (Schatz, Brown, Pascual, Hsu, & DeBaun, 2001). Memory deficits have been documented in children with SCD, although impairments in this domain appear limited to children with clinical infarcts (Berkelhammer et al., 2007). While language abilities are affected in children with infarction, as well as those with normal MRI, deficits appear to be related to neurological integrity and are associated with lesion volume and left-sided infarcts (Cohen, Branch, McKie, & Adams, 1994; Schatz et al., 1999). Inconsistent findings have been reported on visuomotor skills, with some studies reporting impairment only in children with clinical infarct (Armstrong et al., 1996) and others finding impairment regardless of infarct (Grueneich et al., 2004; Schatz et al., 2001). Children with SCD are at elevated risk of academic problems. Schatz and colleagues (2001) reported impaired academic achievement in 37% of children with silent infarct and 27% of children with no evidence of infarct. Furthermore, they found that 58% of children with silent infarct and 27% of children without infarct experience grade retention or received special education services.

DEVELOPMENTAL CONSIDERATIONS

Pediatric stroke occurs during a time of rapid brain development and has the potential to cause impairment in already developed skills and disrupt the development of emerging skills and the neural networks underpinning them. Although research on the long-term outcomes of pediatric stroke is limited, pediatric traumatic brain injury research shows that the full effects of acquired injuries are often not seen until later in development, when the gap between the child and their peers widens (Anderson & Moore, 1995; Dennis, 1989; Eslinger, Biddle, Pennington, & Page, 1999). Whereas adult stroke results in loss of function, pediatric stroke results in both loss of function and reduced capacity to acquire new abilities and knowledge (e.g., literacy). Clinically, survivors of pediatric stroke commonly experience permanent disability, requiring ongoing therapy, monitoring, and educational support. Residual neurological impairments have been reported in 50–60% of children following AIS (deVeber et al., 2000; Mallick et al., 2016; Simonetti et al., 2015). These impairments, including motor and visual deficits, as well as language, cognitive and behavioral problems, have the potential to impact a child's ability to engage in activities and interact socially with others.

PREDICTORS AND MODERATORS

Larger lesion volume (Everts et al., 2008; Hajek et al., 2014; Hetherington, Tuff, Anderson, Miles, & deVeber, 2005; Westmacott et al., 2010) and lesions involving both cortical and subcortical regions (Westmacott et al., 2010) have been associated with poorer intellectual outcomes. For example, in a study from our group, Long et al. (2011) documented significantly poorer results for child stroke associated with large lesion size than for those with small or medium-size lesions across multiple domains of executive function, including attentional control, goal setting, cognitive flexibility, and information processing. In contrast, there is limited or no evidence that lesion location is related to outcomes poststroke. Inconsistent findings have been reported on the effect of lesion laterality. Allman and Scott (2013) reported better neuropsychological outcomes following right-sided strokes, while other researchers have found no laterality effect (Max et al., 2004; McLinden, Baird, Westmacott, Anderson, & deVeber, 2007; Westmacott et al., 2010).

In children with perinatal-onset stroke, Ricci et al. (2008) reported language delay and significantly lower VIQ compared to PIQ, regardless of lesion laterality. However, Allman and Scott (2013) found that left-hemisphere strokes occurring during infancy led to significantly poorer performance on tasks typically associated with right-hemisphere functioning (e.g., perceptual reasoning), and relatively normal language function. They suggested this may be explained by the "crowding hypothesis" (Lidzba, Staudt, Wilke, Grodd, & Krägeloh-Mann, 2006), which postulates that early left-hemisphere lesions may result in the reorganization of language to the right hemisphere.

The early brain insult literature suggests that cognitive outcome is affected by age at insult, with possible periods of vulnerability and plasticity that relate to growth spurts within the brain (Anderson et al., 2009). Within the pediatric AIS literature, age-at-onset outcomes vary between studies. Some researchers have found that younger age at onset, particularly the perinatal period up to 1 year of age, has been associated with weaker performance across cognitive measures (Allman & Scott, 2013; Max et al., 2004; Pavlovic et al., 2006; Westmacott et al., 2010). Others have reported nonlinear findings, suggesting periods of greater vulnerability. Allman and Scott (2013) found poorer outcomes in children who suffered a stroke before age 1 and after 6 years of age, while those with onset between 1 and 6 years showed a relatively preserved profile. Pavlovic et al. (2006) reported better outcomes in children who had a stroke between 5 and 10 years of age and comparatively poorer outcomes in those with onset before or after this period. Cognitive outcomes vary widely between studies, possibly due to largely cross-sectional design and differing methodology, such as varying age range of cohorts and wide range in time since diagnosis.

TREATMENT AND INTERVENTION

Although stroke-specific intervention research is scarce, guidelines providing recommendations for pediatric stroke rehabilitation have been developed in Australia (Greenham et al., 2021), the United Kingdom (*Stroke in Childhood*, 2017) and Canada (Hebert et al., 2016). Due to minimal stroke-specific literature, pediatric rehabilitation clinicians utilize generic approaches applicable across childhood-acquired brain injury. Psychoeducation is an integral aspect of this approach, providing accurate information about pediatric stroke, its recovery path, available resources, and school reintegration. More direct neuropsychological rehabilitation approaches for children with stroke fall into two broad categories, substitution and restoration of function, to minimize the consequences of neurobehavioral impairments and maximize the opportunity to utilize the child's strengths. In general, specific programs are not usually adopted; rather, interventions are customized to the child's needs, acknowledging neurobehavioral variability in children with brain dysfunction. In many instances, adaptation and compensatory approaches are instituted in conjunction with specific interventions, for example, reading intervention or speech therapy. Thus, the child works on specific deficits but within an environment where he or she can utilize cognitive strengths, or develop strategies to circumvent problem areas.

CONCLUSIONS AND FUTURE DIRECTIONS

Until recently, the pediatric stroke literature has focused predominately on epidemiology, etiology, diagnosis, and risk factors, with reported clinical outcomes often limited to neurological impairment. While outcome literature is emerging, studies have largely been retrospective and cross-sectional in nature. There has also been wide variation in measures used, as well as the use of insensitive measures that are unable to detect subtle impairments and changes. Age at the time of stroke and time since stroke to follow-up vary widely between studies, making comparison difficult. Given the relative rarity of pediatric stroke, the majority of outcome studies are limited by small sample sizes and wide age ranges. There is limited reporting of the clinical, radiological, and environmental factors that may influence outcome and potentially identify children who are likely to benefit most from early therapy interventions. Furthermore, it is only recently that prospective, longitudinal studies have been undertaken to examine the trajectory of recovery of children following stroke.

These substantial gaps in knowledge mean there is little consensus to assist in guiding rehabilitation. Larger, prospective, multicenter studies are required, using consistent diagnostic definitions and adequate, developmentally appropriate outcome measures in order to generate better outcome data (Saver et al., 2012). Future research should compare neurological and functional outcomes in children with cryptogenic stroke to those with preexisting conditions such as congenital heart disease or SCD, to guide the development of targeted interventions to improve outcomes. Further investigation of other variables that potentially influence outcome such as age and lesion characteristics may also assist in identifying children most at risk. Additionally, longitudinal studies are essential, particularly in infants and younger children in whom it is more difficult to predict outcome, and neurological deficits are not immediately apparent at the time of diagnosis.

Pediatric stroke provides a useful model of the impact of focal brain damage early in life, and highlights the diversity of functional profiles that may occur following such an event. While there are numerous gaps in the outcome literature for these children, the weight of evidence suggest that they will have an elevated risk of long-term impairment spanning multiple functional domains, including mobility, communication, and academic achievement, which will impact their ability to participate in all aspects of activity across the lifespan. Additional impairments have been documented across a range of neurocognitive (attention, executive function, memory and learning, information processing) and socioemotional skills (behavior, social cognition), related to both stroke and nonstroke factors.

The presence of such wide-ranging difficulties supports the need for (1) multidisciplinary involvement is assessment, diagnosis, and treatment, and (2) comprehensive testing of all aspects of physical, speech, neurocognitive and socioemotional skills. Furthermore, employing a holistic view of the child poststroke that considers stroke-related factors and comorbidities, as well as environmental influences (access to rehabilitation, family function, parent mental health) is essential to achieving a meaningful understanding of the child's strengths, weaknesses, and treatment needs.

The persistent nature of impairments, and the potential for new problems to emerge as children fail to meet developmental expectations, indicates the need for long-term follow-up and monitoring of children poststroke, particularly at important developmental transitions such as school entry, adolescence, and transition to adulthood.

REFERENCES

Akshoomoff, N. A., Feroleto, C. C., Doyle, R. E., & Stiles, J. (2002). The impact of early unilateral brain injury on perceptual organization and visual memory. *Neuropsychologia, 40*(5), 539–561.

Allman, C., & Scott, R. B. (2013). Neuropsychological sequelae following pediatric stroke: A nonlinear model of age at lesion effects. *Child Neuropsychology, 19*(1), 197–107.

Amarenco, P., Bogousslavsky, J., Caplan, L. R., Donnan, G. A., & Hennerici, M. G. (2009). Classification of stroke subtypes. *Cerebrovascular Diseases, 27*(9), 493–501.

Amlie-Lefond, C., Bernard, T. J., Sébire, G., Friedman, N. R., Heyer, G. L., Lerner, N. B., . . . International Pediatric Stroke Study Group. (2009). Predictors of cerebral arteriopathy in children with arterial ischemic stroke: Results of the International Pediatric Stroke Study. *Circulation, 119*(10), 1417–1423.

Amlie-Lefond, C., & Fullerton, H. J. (2010). Rashes, sniffles, and stroke: A role for infection in ischemic stroke of childhood. *Infectious Disorder Drug Targets, 10*(2), 67–75.

Anderson, V., Catroppa, C., Haritou, F., Morse, S., & Rosenfeld, J. (2005). Identifying factors contributing to child and family outcome 30 months after traumatic brain injury in children. *Journal of Neurology Neurosurgery and Psychiatry, 76*(3), 401–408.

Anderson, V., Darling, S., Mackay, M., Monagle, P.,

Greenham, M., Cooper, A., . . . Gordon, A. L. (2020). Cognitive resilience following paediatric stroke: Biological and environmental predictors. *European Journal of Paediatric Neurology, 25,* 52–58.

Anderson, V., Gomes, A., Greenham, M., Hearps, S., Gordon, A. L., Rinehart, N., . . . Mackay, M. (2014). Social competence following pediatric stroke: Contributions of brain insult and family environment. *Social Neuroscience, 9*(5), 471–483.

Anderson, V., & Moore, C. (1995). Age at injury as a predictor of outcome following pediatric head injury. *Child Neuropsychology, 1*(3), 187–202.

Anderson, V., Northam, E., Hendy, J., & Wrennal, J. (2001). *Developmental neuropsychology: A clinical approach.* East Sussex, UK: Psychology Press.

Anderson, V., Spencer-Smith, M., Leventer, R., Coleman, L., Anderson, P., Williams, J., . . . Jacobs, R. (2009). Childhood brain insult: Can age at insult help us predict outcome? *Brain, 132,* 45–56.

Anderson, V., Spencer-Smith, M., & Wood, A. (2011). Do children really recover better?: Neurobehavioural plasticity after early brain insult. *Brain, 134*(8), 2197–2221.

Armstrong, F. D., Thompson, R. J., Jr., Wang, W., Zimmerman, R., Pegelow, C. H., Miller, S., . . . Vass, K. (1996). Cognitive functioning and brain magnetic resonance imaging in children with sickle cell disease: Neuropsychology Committee of the Cooperative Study of Sickle Cell Disease. *Pediatrics, 97,* 864–870.

Bates, E. (1998). Plasticity, localization and language development. In S. Broman & J. M. Fletcher (Eds.), *The changing nervous system: Neurobehavioral consequences of early brain disorders* (pp. 214–253). New York: Oxford University Press.

Bates, E., Reilly, J. S., Wulfeck, B., Dronkers, N., Opie, M., Fenson, J., . . . Herbst, K. (2001). Differential effects of unilateral lesions on language production in children and adults. *Brain and Language, 79*(2), 223–265.

Bates, E., Thal, D., Trauner, D., Fenson, J., Aram, D., Eisele, J., & Nass, R. D. (1997). From first words to grammar in children with focal brain injury. *Developmental Neuropsychology, 13*(3), 275–343.

Berkelhammer, L. D., Williamson, A. L., Sanford, S. D., Dirksen, C. L., Sharp, W. G., Margulies, A. S., & Prengler, R. A. (2007). Neurocognitive sequelae of pediatric sickle cell disease: A review of the literature. *Child Neuropsychology, 13,* 120–131.

Block, G. W., Nanson, J. L., & Lowry, N. J. (1999). Attention, memory, and language after pediatric ischemic stroke. *Child Neuropsychology, 5,* 81–91.

Blom, I., De Schryver, E. L., Kappelle, L. J., Rinkel, G. J., Jennekens-Schinkel, A., & Peters, A. C. (2003). Prognosis of haemorrhagic stroke in childhood: A long-term follow-up study. *Developmental Medicine and Child Neurology, 45*(4), 233–239.

Boardman, J. P., Ganesan, V., Rutherford, M. A., Saunders, D. E., Mercuri, E., & Cowan, F. (2005). Magnetic resonance image correlates of hemiparesis after neonatal and childhood middle cerebral artery stroke. *Pediatrics, 115*(2), 321–326.

Bohnert, A. M., Parkerb, J. G., & Warschauskyc, S. A. (1997). Friendship and social adjustment of children following a traumatic brain injury: An exploratory investigation. *Developmental Neurpsychology, 13*(4), 477–486.

Broderick, J., Talbot, G. T., Prenger, E., Leach, A., & Brott, T. (1993). Stroke in children within a major metropolitan area: The surprising importance of intracerebral hemorrhage. *Journal of Child Neurology, 8*(3), 250–255.

Brown, R. T., Davis, P. C., Lambert, R., Hsu, L., Hopkins, K., & Eckman, J. (2000). Neurocognitive functioning and magnetic resonance imaging in children with sickle cell disease. *Journal of Pediatric Psychology, 25,* 503–513.

Chapman, S. B., Max, J. E., Gamino, J. F., McGlothlin, J. H., & Cliff, S. N. (2003). Discourse plasticity in children after stroke: Age at injury and lesion effects. *Pediatric Neurology, 29*(1), 34–41.

Ciccone, S., Cappella, M., & Borgna-Pignatti, C. (2011). Ischemic stroke in infants and children: Practical management in emergency. *Stroke Research and Treatment, 2011,* Article 736965

Cnossen, M. H., Aarsen, F. K., Akker, S. L., Danen, R., Appel, I. M., Steyerberg, E. W., & Catsman-Berrevoets, C. E. (2010). Paediatric arterial ischaemic stroke: Functional outcome and risk factors. *Developmental Medicine and Child Neurology, 52*(4), 394–399.

Cohen, M. J., Branch, W. B., McKie, V. C., & Adams, R. J. (1994). Neuropsychological impairment in children with sickle cell anemia and cerebrovascular accidents. *Clinical Pediatrics, 33,* 517–524.

Cooper, A., Anderson, V., Greenham, M., Hearps, S., Hunt, R. W., Mackay, M. T., . . . Gordon, A. L. (2019). Motor function daily living skills 5 years after paediatric arterial ischaemic stroke: A prospective longitudinal study. *Developmental Medicine and Child Neurology, 61*(2), 161–167.

Cooper, A., Anderson, V., Hearps, S., Greenham, M., Ditchfield, M., Coleman, L., . . . Gordon, A. (2017). Trajectories of motor recovery in the first year following pediatric arterial ischaemic stroke. *Pediatrics, 140*(2), Article e20163870.

Daly, B., Kral, M. C., & Tarazi, R. A. (2011). The role of neuropsychological evaluation in pediatric sickle cell disease. *Clinical Neuropsychologist, 25*(6), 903–925.

Dennis, M. (1989). Language and the young damaged brain. In T. Boll & B. K. Bryant (Eds.), *Clinical neuropsychology and brain function: Research, measurement and practice* (pp. 85–124). Washington, DC: Psychological Association.

De Schryver, E. L., Kappelle, L. J., Jennekens-Schinkel, A., & Boudewyn Peters, A. C. (2000). Prognosis of ischemic stroke in childhood: A long-term follow-up study. *Developmental Medicine and Child Neurology, 42*(5), 313–318.

deVeber, G. (2003). Risk factors for childhood stroke: Little folks have different strokes. *Annals of Neurology, 53*(2), 149–150.

deVeber, G., MacGregor, D., Curtis, R., & Mayank, S. (2000). Neurologic outcome in survivors of childhood arterial ischemic stroke and sinovenous thrombosis. *Journal of Child Neurology, 15*(5), 316–324.

deVeber, G., MacGregor, D., Curtis, R., & Mayank, S. (2000). Neurologic outcome in survivors of childhood arterial ischemic stroke and sinovenous thrombosis. *Journal of Child Neurology, 15*(5), 316–324.

Dick, F., Wulfeck, B., Krupa-Kwiatkowski, M., & Bates, E. (2004). The development of complex sentence interpretation in typically developing children compared with children with specific language impairments or early unilateral focal lesions. *Developmental Science, 7*(3), 360–377.

Dunbar, M. J., & Kirton, A. (2020). The incidence of perinatal stroke is 1:1200 live births: A population-based study in Alberta Canada. *Stroke, 51*, Article A51.

Earley, C. J., Kittner, S. J., Feeser, B. R., Gardner, J., Epstein, A., Wozniak, M. A., . . . Buchholz, D. (1998). Stroke in children and sickle cell disease: Baltimore–Washington Cooperative Young Stroke Study. *Neurology, 51*, 169–176.

Elias, K. M., & Moura-Ribeiro, M. V. (2013). Stroke caused auditory attention deficits in children. *Arquivos de Neuro-Psiquiatria, 71*(1), 11–17.

Elias, K. M., Oliveira, C. C., Airoldi, M. J., Franco, K. M. D., Rodrigues, S. D. D., Ciasca, S. M., & Moura-Ribeiro, M. V. L. (2014). Central auditory processing outcome after stroke in children. *Arquivos de Neuro-Psiquiatria, 72*(9), 680–686.

Eslinger, P., Biddle, K., Pennington, B., & Page, R. (1999). Cognitive and behavioural development up to 4 years after early right frontal lobe lesion. *Developmental Neuropsychology, 15*(2), 157–191.

Everts, R., Pavlovic, J., Kaufmann, F., Uhlenberg, B., Seidel, U., Nedeltchev, K., . . . Steinlin, M. (2008). Cognitive functioning, behavior, and quality life after stroke in childhood. *Child Neuropsychology, 14*, 323–338.

Fox, C. K., Glass, H. C., Sidney, S., Lowenstein, D. H., & Fullerton, H. J. (2013). Acute seizures predict epilepsy after childhood stroke. *Annals of Neurology, 74*(2), 249–256.

Fox, C. K., Sidney, S., & Fullerton, H. J. (2015). Community-based case–control study of childhood stroke risk associated with congenital heart disease. *Stroke, 46*(2), 336–340.

Friedman, N. R. (2009). Pediatric stroke: Past, present and future. *Advances in Pediatrics, 56*, 271–299.

Friefeld, S. J., Yeboah, O., Jones, J. E., & deVeber, G. (2004). Health-related quality of life and its relationship to neurological outcome in child survivors of stroke. *CNS Spectrums, 9*(6), 465–475.

Fullerton, H. J., Chetkovich, D. M., Wu, Y. W., Smith, W. S., & Johnston, S. C. (2002). Deaths from stroke in US children, 1979 to 1998. *Neurology, 59*(1), 34–39.

Fullerton, H. J., Wu, Y. W., Sidney, S., & Johnston, S. C. (2007). Recurrent hemorrhagic stroke in children: A population-based cohort study. *Stroke, 38*, 2658–2662.

Fullerton, H. J., Wu, Y. W., Zhao, S., & Johnston, S. C. (2003). Risk of stroke in children: Ethnic and gender disparities. *Neurology, 61*(2), 189–194.

Ganesan, V., Hogan, A., Shack, N., Gordon, A. L., Isaacs, E., & Kirkham, F. J. (2000). Outcome after ischaemic stroke in childhood. *Developmental Medicine and Child Neurology, 42*(7), 455–461.

Ganesan, V., Prengler, M., McShane, M. A., Wade, A. M., & Kirkham, F. J. (2003). Investigation of risk factors in children with arterial ischemic stroke. *Annals of Neurology, 53*(2), 167–173.

Ganesan, V., Prengler, M., Wade, A., & Kirkham, F. J. (2006). Clinical and radiological recurrence after childhood arterial ischemic stroke. *Circulation, 114*(20), 2170–2177.

Gardner, M. A., Hills, N. K., Sidney, S., Johnston, S. C., & Fullerton, H. J. (2010). The 5-year direct medical cost of neonatal and childhood stroke in a population-based cohort. *Neurology, 74*(5), 372–378.

Golomb, M. R. (2009). Stroke in neonates and children. In J. Biller (Ed.), *Stroke in children and young adults* (2nd ed., pp. 69–80). Philadelphia: Saunders.

Golomb, M. R., de Veber, G. A., MacGregor, D. L., Domi, T., Whyte, H., Stephens, D., & Dick, P. (2003). Independent walking after neonatal arterial ischemic stroke and sinovenous thrombosis. *Journal of Child Neurology, 18*, 530–536.

Gomes, A., Rinehart, N., Greenham, M., & Anderson, V. (2014). A critical review of psychosocial outcomes following childhood stroke (1995–2012). *Developmental Neuropsychology, 39*(1), 9–24.

Gomes, A., Spencer-Smith, M. M., Jacobs, R. K., Coleman, L., & Anderson, V. A. (2012). Attention and social functioning in children with malformations of cortical development and stroke. *Child Neuropsychology, 18*(4), 392–403.

Gordon, A. L., Anderson, V., Ditchfield, M., Coleman, L., Mackay, M. T., Greenham, M., . . . Monagle, P. (2015). Factors associated with six-month outcome of pediatric stroke. *International Journal of Stroke, 10*(7), 1068–1073.

Gordon, A. L., Ganesan, V., Towell, A., & Kirkham, F. J. (2002). Functional outcome following stroke in children. *Journal of Child Neurology, 17*(6), 429–434.

Gout, A., Seibel, N., Rouvière, C., Husson, B., Hermans, B., Laporte, N., . . . Sébire, G. (2005). Aphasia owing to subcortical brain infarcts in childhood. *Journal of Child Neurology, 20*(12), 1003–1008.

Greenham, M., Anderson, V., Cooper, A., Hearps, S., Ditchfield, M., Coleman, L., . . . Gordon, A. L. (2017a). Early predictors of psychosocial functioning 5 years after pediatric stroke. *Developmental Medicine and Child Neurology, 59*(10), 1034–1041.

Greenham, M., Anderson, V., Hearps, S., Ditchfield, M., Coleman, L., Mackay, M. T., . . . Gordon, A. L. (2017b). Psychosocial function in the first year following childhood stroke. *Developmental Medicine and Child Neurology, 59*(10), 1027–1033.

Greenham, M., Gordon, A. L., Cooper, A., Ditchfield, M., Coleman, L., Hunt, R. W., . . . Anderson, V. (2018). Social functioning following pediatric stroke: Contribution of neurobehavioral impairment. *Developmental Neuropsychology, 43*(4), 312–328.

Greenham, M., Knight, S., Rodda, J., Scheinberg, A., Anderson, V., Fahey, M. C., . . . Victorian Subacute Childhood Stroke Advisory Committee. (2021). Australian clinical consensus guideline for the subacute rehabilitation of childhood stroke. *International Journal of Stroke, 16*, 311–320.

Grueneich, R., Ris, M. D., Ball, W., Kalinyak, K. A., Noll, R., & Vannatta, K. (2004). Relationship of structural magnetic resonance imaging, magnetic resonance perfusion, and other disease factors to neuropsychological outcome in sickle cell disease. *Journal of Pediatric Psychology, 29*, 83–92.

Hajek, C. A., Yeates, K. O., Anderson, V., Mackay, M., Greenham, M., Gomes, A., & Lo, W. (2014). Cognitive outcomes following arterial ischemic stroke in infants and children. *Journal of Child Neurology, 29*(7), 887–894.

Hamilton, W., Huang, H., Seiber, E., & Lo, W. (2015). Cost and outcome in pediatric ischemic stroke. *Journal of Child Neurology, 30*(11), 1483–1488.

Hay, J., & Missiuna, C. (1998). Motor proficiency in children reporting low levels of participation in physical activity. *Canadian Journal of Occupational Therapy, 65*(2), 64–71.

Hebert, D., Lindsay, M. P., McIntyre, A., Kirton, A., Rumney, P. G., Bagg, S., . . . Garnhum, M. (2016). Canadian stroke best practice recommendations: Stroke rehabilitation practice guidelines, update 2015. *International Journal of Stroke, 11*(4), 459–484.

Hetherington, R., Tuff, L., Anderson, P., Miles, B., & DeVeber, G. (2005). Short-term intellectual outcome after arterial ischemic stroke and sinovenous thrombosis in childhood and infancy. *Journal of Child Neurology, 20*(7), 553–559.

Hills, N. K., Johnston, S. C., Sidney, S., Zielinski, B. A., & Fullerton, H. J. (2012). Recent trauma and acute infection as risk factors for childhood arterial ischemic stroke. *Annals of Neurolology, 72*(6), 850–858.

Hurvitz, E., Warschausky, S., Berg, M., & Tsai, S. (2004). Long-term functional outcome of pediatric stroke survivors. *Topics in Stroke Rehabilitation, 11*(2), 51–59.

Ilves, P., Tomberg, T., Kepler, J., Laugesaar, R., Kaldoja, M., Kepler, K., & Kolk, A. (2014). Different plasticity patterns of language function in children with perinatal and childhood stroke. *Journal of Child Neurology, 29*(6), 756–764.

Jordan, L. C., & Hillis, A. E. (2007). Hemorrhagic stroke in children. *Pediatric Neurology, 36*(2), 73–80.

Kirton, A., & deVeber, G. (2011). Pediatric stroke syndromes. In R. M. Kliegman, B. F. Stanton, J. W. St. Geme, N. F. Schor, & R. E. Behrman (Eds.), *Nelson textbook of pediatrics* (19th ed., pp. 2080–2085). Philadelphia: Saunders.

Kirton, A., Westmacott, R., & deVeber, G. (2007). Pediatric stroke: Rehabilitation of focal injury in the developing brain. *NeuroRehabilitation, 22*(5), 371–382.

Kolk, A., Ennok, M., Laugesaar, R., Kaldoja, M. L., & Talvik, T. (2011). Long-term cognitive outcomes after pediatric stroke. *Pediatric Neurology, 2*, 101–109.

Kopyta, I., Sarecka-Hujar, B., & Skrzypek, M. (2015). Post-stroke epilepsy in Polish paediatric patients. *Developmental Medicine and Child Neurology, 57*(9), 821–828.

Lansing, A. E., Max, J. E., Delis, D. C., Fox, P. T., Lancaster, J., Manes, F. F., & Schatz, A. (2004). Verbal learning and memory after childhood stroke. *Journal of the International Neuropsychological Society, 10*(5), 742–752.

Lanska, M. J., Lanska, D. J., Horwitz, S. J., & Aram, M. A. (1991). Presentation, clinical course, and outcome of childhood stroke. *Pediatric Neurology, 7*, 333–341.

Lidzba, K., Staudt, M., Wilke, M., Grodd, W., & Krägeloh-Mann, I. (2006). Lesion-induced right-hemispheric language and organization of nonverbal functions. *NeuroReport, 17*(9), 929–933.

Lo, W. D., Gordon, A., Hajek, C., Gomes, A., Greenham, M., Perkins, E., . . . Mackay, M. (2014). Social competence following neonatal and childhood stroke. *International Journal of Stroke, 9*(8), 1037–1044.

Lo, W. D., Hajek, C. A., Pappa, C., Wang, W., & Zumberge, N. (2013). Outcomes in children with hemorrhagic stroke. *JAMA Neurology, 70*(1), 66–71.

Long, B., Anderson, V., Jacobs, R., Mackay, M., Leventer, R., Barnes, C., & Spencer-Smith, M. (2011). Executive function following child stroke: The impact of lesion size. *Developmental Neuropsychology, 36*(8), 971–987.

Mackay, M., Wizniter, M., Benedict, S., Lee, K., deVeber, G., Ganesan, V., & Group, I. P. S. S. (2011). Arterial ischemic stroke risk factors: The international pediatric stroke study *Annals of Neurology, 69*(1), 130–140.

Maguire, J. L., deVeber, G., & Parkin, P. C. (2007). Association between iron-deficiency anemia and stroke in young children. *Pediatrics, 120*(5), 1053–1057.

Mallick, A. A., Ganesan, V., Kirkham, F. J., Fallon, P., Hedderly, T., McShane, T., . . . Amin, S. (2016). Outcome and recurrence 1 year after pediatric arterial ischemic stroke in a population-based cohort. *Annals of Neurology, 79*(5), 784–793.

Mallick, A. A., Ganesan, V., & O'Callaghan, F. J. (2010). Mortality from childhood stroke in England and Wales, 1921–2000. *Archives of Disease in Childhood, 95*(1), 12–19.

Mauro, M. A., Murphy, K. P. J., Thomson, K. R., Venbrux, A. C., & Morgan, R. A. (2014). Cerebral functional anatomy and rapid neurologic examination. In M. A. Mauro, K. P. J. Murphy, K. R. Thomson, A. C. Venbrux, & R. A. Morgan (Eds.), *Image-guided interventions* (2nd ed., pp. 670–676). New York: Elsevier.

Max, J. (2004). Effect of side of lesion on neuropsychological performance in childhood stroke. *Journal of the International Neuropsychological Society, 10*, 698–708.

Max, J., Mathews, K., Manes, F., Robertson, B., Fox, P., Lancaster, J., & Collings, N. (2003). Attention deficit hyperactivity disorder and neurocognitive correlates after childhood stroke. *Journal of the International Neuropsychological Society, 9*(6), 815–829.

Max, J., Matthews, K., Lansing, A., Robertson, B., Fox, P., Lancaster, J., . . . Smith, J. (2002). Psychiatric disorders after childhood stroke. *Journal of the Academy of Child and Adolescent Psychiatry, 41*(5), 555–562.

Max, J., Robin, D. A., Taylor, H. G., Yeates, K. O., Fox, P. T., Lancaster, J. L., . . . Austermann, S. (2004). Attention function after childhood stroke. *Journal of the International Neuropsychological Society, 10*, 976–986.

McLinden, A., Baird, A. D., Westmacott, R., Anderson, P. E., & deVeber, G. (2007). Early cognitive outcome after neonatal stroke. *Journal of Child Neurology, 22*(9), 1111–1116.

Mercuri, E., Barnett, A., Rutherford, M., Guzzetta, A., Haataja, L., Cioni, G., . . . Dubowitz, L. (2004). Neonatal cerebral infarction and neuromotor outcome at school age. *Pediatrics, 113*(1), 95–100.

Mercuri, E., Rutherford, M., Cowan, F., Pennock, J., Counsell, S., Papadimitriou, M., . . . Dubowitz, L. (1999). Early prognostic indicators of outcome in infants with neonatal cerebral infarction: A clinical, electroencephalogram, and magnetic resonance imaging study. *Pediatrics, 103*(1), 39–46.

Meyer-Heim, A. D., & Boltshauser, E. (2003). Spontaneous intracranial haemorrhage in children: Aetiology, presentation and outcome. *Brain and Development, 25*(6), 416–421.

Mosch, S., Max, J., & Tranel, D. (2005). A matched lesion analysis of childhood versus adult-onset brain injury due to unilateral stroke: Another perspective on neural plasticity and recovery of social functioning. *Cognitive and Behavioral Neurology, 18*, 5–17.

Moser, F. G., Miller, S. T., Bello, J. A., Pegelow, C. H., Zimmerman, R. A., Wang, W. C., . . . Kinney, T. R. (1996). The spectrum of brain MR abnormalities in sickle-cell disease: A report from the Cooperative Study of Sickle Cell Disease. *American Journal of Neuroradiology, 17*, 965–972.

Murphy, L. K., Compas, B. E., Gindville, M. C., Reeslund, K. L., & Jordan, L. C. (2017). Cognitive functioning over 2 years after intracerebral hemorrhage in school-aged children. *Developmental Medicine and Child Neurology, 59*(11), 1146–1151.

Murphy, S. L. (2000). Deaths: Final data for 1998. *National Vital Statistics Report, 48*(11), 1–105.

Neuner, B., von Mackensen, S., Krumpel, K., Manner, D., Friefeld, S., Nixdorf, S., . . . Nowak-Göttl, U. (2011). Health-related quality of life in children and adolescents with stroke, self-reports, and parent/proxies reports: Cross-sectional investigation. *Annals of Neurology, 70*, 70–78.

O'Keeffe, F., Ganesan, V., King, J., & Murphy, T. (2012). Quality of life and psychosocial outcome following childhood arterial ischaemic stroke. *Brain Injury, 26*, 1072–1083.

O'Keeffe, F., Liégeois, F., Eve, M., Ganesan, V., King, J., & Murphy, T. (2014). Neuropsychological and neurobehavioral outcome following childhood arterial ischemic stroke: Attention deficits, emotional dysregulation, and executive dysfunction. *Child Neuropsychology, 20*(5), 557–582.

Pavlovic, J., Kaufmann, F., Boltshauser, E., Capone Mori, A., Gubser Mercati, D., Haenggeli, C. A., & Steinlin, M. (2006). Neuropsychological problems after paediatric stroke: Two year followup of Swiss children. *Neuropediatrics, 37*, 13–19.

Reeves, M. J., Bushnell, C. D., Howard, G., Gargano, J. W., Duncan, P. W., Lynch, G., . . . Lisabeth, L. (2008). Sex differences in stroke: Epidemiology, clinical presentation, medical care, and outcomes. *Lancet Neurology, 7*, 915–926.

Reid, C. D., Charace, S., & Lubin, B. (1995). *Management and therapy of sickle cell disease.* Darby, PA: Diane.

Reilly, J. S., Bates, E., & Marchman, V. (1998). Narrative discourse in children with early focal brain injury. *Brain and Language, 61*(3), 335–375.

Ricci, D., Mercuri, E., Barnett, A., Rathbone, R., Cota, F., Haataja, L., . . . Cowan, F. (2008). Cognitive outcome at early school age in term-born children with perinatally acquired middle cerebral artery territory infarction. *Stroke, 39*(2), 403–410.

Rowan, A., Vargha-Khadem, F., Calamante, F., Tournier, J. D., Kirkham, F. J., Chong, W. K., . . . Gadian, D. G. (2007). Cortical abnormalities and language function in young patients with basal ganglia stroke. *NeuroImage, 36*(2), 431–440.

Salih, M. A., Abdel-Gader, A. G., Al-Jarallah, A. A., Kentab, A. Y., & Al-Nasser, M. N. (2006). Outcome of stroke in Saudi children. *Saudi Medical Journal, 27*(Suppl. 1), S91–S96.

Saver, J. L., Warach, S., Janis, S., Odenkirchen, J., Becker, K., Benavente, O., . . . Schwamm, L. (2012). Standardizing the structure of stroke clinical and epidemiologic research data: The National Institute of Neurological Disorders and Stroke (NINDS) Stroke Common Data Element (CDE) project. *Stroke, 43*(4), 967–973.

Schatz, J., Brown, R. T., Pascual, J. M., Hsu, L., & DeBaun, M. R. (2001). Poor school and cognitive functioning with silent cerebral infarcts and sickle cell disease. *Neurology, 56*, 1109–1111.

Schatz, J., Craft, S., Koby, M., Siegel, M., Resar, L., Lee, R., . . . DeBaun, M. (1999). Neuropsychological deficits in children with sickle-cell disease and cerebral infarction: Role of lesion site and volume. *Child Neuropsychology, 5*(2), 92–103.

Simonetti, B. G., Cavelti, A., Arnold, M., Bigi, S., Regényi, M., Mattle, H. P., . . . Fischer, U. (2015). Long-term outcome after arterial ischemic stroke in children and young adults. *Neuology, 84*(19), 1941–1947.

Steen, R. G., Fineberg-Buchner, C., Hankins, G., Weiss, L., Prifitera, A., & Mulhern, R. K. (2005). Cognitive deficits in children with sickle cell disease. *Journal of Child Neurology, 20*, 102–107.

Steen, R. G., Reddick, W. E., Mulhern, R. K., Langston, J. W., Ogg, R. J., Bieberich, A. A., . . . Wang, W. (1998). Quantitative MRI of the brain in children with sickle cell disease reveals abnormalities unseen by conventional MRI. *Resonance Imaging, 8*, 535–543.

Steen, R. G., Xiong, X., Mulhern, R. K., Langston, J. W., & Wang, W. C. (1999). Subtle brain abnormalities in children with sickle cell disease: Relationship to blood hematocrit. *Annals of Neurology, 45,* 279–286.

Steinlin, M. (2012). A clinical approach to arterial ischemic childhood stroke: Increasing knowledge over the last decade. *Neuropediatrics, 43,* 1–9.

Steinlin, M., Roellin, K., & Schrot, G. (2004). Long-term follow-up after stroke in childhood. *European Journal of Pediatrics 163,* 245–250.

Stiles, J., & Nass, R. (1991). Spatial grouping activity in young children with congenital right or left hemisphere brain injury. *Brain and Cognition, 15*(2), 201–222.

Stiles, J., Stern, C., Trauner, D., & Nass, R. (1996). Developmental change in spatial grouping activity among children with early focal brain injury: Evidence from a modeling task. *Brain and Cognition, 31*(1), 46–62.

Sträter, R., Becker, S., von Eckardstein, A., Heinecke, A., Gutsche, S., Junker, R., . . . Nowak-Göttl, U. (2002). Prospective assessment of risk factors for recurrent stroke during childhood—a 5-year follow-up study. *Lancet, 360*(9345), 1540–1545.

Stroke in childhood: Clinical guideline for diagnosis, management and rehabilitation. (2017). London: The Royal College of Paediatrics and Child Health.

Studer, M., Boltshauser, E., Capone Mori, A., Datta, A., Fluss, J., Mercati, D., . . . Steinlin, M. (2014). Factors affecting cognitive outcome in early pediatric stroke. *Neurology, 82*(9), 784–792.

Sylvestre, A., Nadeau, L., Charron, L., Larose, N., & Lepage, C. (2013). Social participation by children with developmental coordination disorder compared to their peers. *Disability and Rehabilitation, 35*(21), 1814–1820.

Thompson, R. J., Armstrong, F. D., Link, C. K., Pegelow, C. H., Moser, F., & Wang, W. C. (2003). A prospective study of the relationship over time of behavior problems, intellectual functioning, and family functioning in children with sickle cell disease: A report from the cooperative study of sickle cell disease. *Journal of Pediatric Psychology, 28,* 59–65.

Tsze, D. S., & Valente, J. H. (2011). Pediatric stroke: A review. *Emergency Medicine International, 2011,* Article 734506.

Vanderah, T. W. (2019). *Nolte's essentials of the human brain.* New York: Elsevier Books.

Vicari, S., Albertoni, A., Chilosi, A. M., Cipriani, P., Cioni, G., & Bates, E. (2000). Plasticity and reorganization during language development in children with early brain injury. *Cortex, 36*(1), 31–46.

Vicari, S., Stiles, J., Stern, C., & Resca, A. (1998). Spatial grouping activity in children with early cortical and subcortical lesions. *Developmental Medicine and Child Neurology, 40*(2), 90–94.

Ware, R. E., de Montalembert, M., Tshilolo, L., & Abboud, M. R. (2017). Sickle cell disease. *Lancet, 390*(10091), 311–323.

Watkins, K. E., Hewes, D. E., Connelly, A., Kendall, B. E., Kingsley, D. P., Evans, J. E., . . . Kirkham, F. J. (1998). Cognitive deficits associated with frontal-lobe infarction in children with sickle cell disease. *Developmental Medicine and Child Neurology, 40,* 536–543.

Westmacott, R., Askalan, R., Macgregor, D., Anderson, P., & DeVeber, G. (2010). Cognitive outcome following unilateral arterial ischaemic stroke in childhood: Effects of age at stroke and lesion location. *Developmental Medicine and Child Neurology, 52*(4), 386–393.

Westmacott, R., MacGregor, D., Askalan, R., & deVeber, G. (2009). Late emergence of cognitive deficits after unilateral neonatal stroke. *Stroke, 40,* 2012–2019.

Wrotniak, B. H., Epstein, L. H., Dorn, J. M., Jonesc, K. E., & Kondilisc, V. A. (2006). The relationship between motor proficiency and physical activity in children. *Pediatrics, 118*(6), 1758–1765.

Yang, J. S., Park, Y. D., & Hartlage, P. L. (1995). Seizures associated with stroke in childhood. *Pediatric Neurology, 12*(2), 136–138.

Younkin, D. P. (2002). Diagnosis and treatment of ischemic pediatric stroke. *Current Neurology and Neuroscience Reports, 2*(1), 18–24.

Zimmer, J. A., Garg, B. P., Williams, L. S., & Golomb, M. R. (2007). Age-related variation in presenting signs of childhood arterial ischemic stroke. *Pediatric Neurology, 37*(3), 171–175.

CHAPTER 7

Premature Birth

H. Gerry Taylor
Peter J. Anderson

INTRODUCTION

Definitions

Premature birth is defined by a gestational age (GA) of < 37 weeks. The degree of prematurity is the most critical of many factors that contribute to developmental outcomes of prematurity. For this reason, preterm birth is typically subclassified as extremely preterm (EPT; GA < 28 weeks), very preterm (VPT; GA 28 to 31 6/7 weeks), moderate preterm (MPT; GA 32 to 33 6/7 weeks), and late preterm (LPT; 34 to 36 6/7 weeks) (Martin, Hamilton, Osterman, Driscoll, & Drake, 2018; Wilson-Costello & Payne, 2019). Prematurity is closely related to birthweight, and in the past, low birthweight (LBW) has been used as a proxy for prematurity due to an inability to accurately estimate GA. LBW (< 2,500 g) is also subclassified as extremely LBW (ELBW, < 1,000 g) and very LBW (VLBW, < 1,500 g) (Mandy, Weisman, & Kim, 2019). Some samples comprise children selected on the basis of prematurity and birthweight such as those born EPT and/or ELBW (EPT/ELBW) or VPT and/or VLBW (VPT/VLBW). Although short- and long-term outcomes are less favorable the lower the child's GA or birthweight, evidence suggests adverse consequences across the full range of these two classifications (Richards et al., 2016).

Because preterm/LBW children are born prior to completion of term gestation, their age is often corrected for the degree of prematurity by subtracting the number of weeks the child was born prior to the due date from the child's chronical age. Corrected age is frequently applied through the first 2 or 3 years of life, especially in clinical follow-up, though correction for older children can be justified by differences between scores based on corrected versus chronological age on tests of developmental outcome (Wilson-Ching, Pascoe, Doyle, & Anderson, 2014). Another consideration is whether children's birthweight is lower than expected for GA, in which case they are referred to as being small for GA (SGA). Preterm children born SGA, typically defined by birthweight < 10th percentile for GA, have poorer outcomes than preterm/LBW children whose weight is appropriate for GA (Miller, Huppi, & Mallard, 2016). Although some children are constitutionally SGA, with low weight consistent with genetically determined physical size, others meet criteria for fetal growth restriction, or intrauterine growth retardation (IUGR), which is defined by signs of fetal pathology, most typically symptoms of placental insufficiency as identified by an abnormal umbilical artery Doppler flow in pregnancy or an elevated ratio of the pulsatility index (maximum–minimum blood flow velocity/average velocity) for the umbilical artery relative to that for the middle cerebral artery. IUGR is classified as early- or late-onset depending on whether it occurs in the second or third trimester of pregnancy and can be accompanied by asymmetric fetal growth in the brain relative to the rest of the body, a condition referred to as "brain sparing."

Significance and Chapter Overview

Premature birth is common and has significant consequences for health and development, including high rates of brain abnormalities and developmental disabilities, especially for those with more extreme degrees of prematurity (Richards et al., 2016). Based on a 2010 survey of live births from 171 countries, approximately 11%, or about 15 million children, were born preterm (Blencowe et al., 2012). Rates were as low as 5% in parts of Europe and as high as 18% in some African countries. Care for preterm children in the United States totals over $26 billion per year, or an average of nearly $52,000 per child (McCabe, Carrine, Russell, & Howse, 2014). Costs of neonatal intensive care alone are estimated to be $13.4 billion per year, representing 20% of newborn health care costs in the United States. Preterm infants average 13 days of neonatal hospitalization compared to 1.5 days for term infants (Purisch & Gyamfi-Bannerman, 2017). Stays in the neonatal intensive care unit (NICU) for less mature children are much longer, with estimates of about 2 months for VPT children and 3 months for EPT infants (Stoll et al., 2015). Medical costs of preterm birth across the first year are about 10 times those for full-term infants, or approximately $32,000 versus $3,000 per child (Purisch & Gyamfi-Bannerman, 2017). Societal goals of research in this area include prevention, improved quality of care, and early identification of neurodevelopmental problems (McCabe et al., 2014).

The neuropsychologist's role in evaluating and managing these children is to identify developmental strengths and weaknesses, provide guidance to families and physicians with regard to needs for follow-up and interventions to improve outcomes, increase awareness of risk and protective factors, and contribute to knowledge of brain–behavior relationships and underlying neurogenetic and environmental mechanisms. Chapter objectives are to assist neuropsychologists and other health and educational trainees and professionals engaged in research and practice with preterm/LBW children. Specific aims are to review research on epidemiology, historical trends in treatment and outcomes, neuropathological correlates, developmental outcomes and predictors, and interventions. Because research has focused primarily on VPT/VLBW or EPT/ELBW children, the chapter not only highlights findings from these subsets of the preterm/LBW population but also summarizes research on MPT and LPT samples. The final section of the chapter considers methodological issues in conducting research, potentially fruitful directions for future study, and clinical implications. Emphasis is placed on updated trends in survival and on new information regarding developmental outcomes, predictors, and underlying brain abnormalities.

EPIDEMIOLOGY

According to a report from the Division of Vital Statistics, nearly 4 million births occurred in the United States in 2016 (Martin et al., 2018). The percentage of children born preterm was 9.85%, which included 7.09% with GA 34–36 weeks, 1.17% with GA 32–33 weeks, 0.92% with GA 28–31 weeks, and 0.68% with GA < 28 weeks. Rates of preterm birth were higher in African Americans compared to non-Hispanic White and Hispanic women (14 vs. 9%). Similarly, the percent of children born in the LBW range was 8.17%, including 5.17% weighing 2,000–2,499 g, 1.59% weighing 1,500–1,999 g, 0.74% weighing 1,000–1,499 g, and .66% weighing < 1,000 g. Rates were again higher for African Americans than for non-Hispanic Whites or Hispanic women (14 vs. 7%).

Survival following preterm birth is lower for infants born with more extreme prematurity or IUGR. According to 2013 U.S. estimates, 62.5% of infants with GA < 28 weeks survived compared to 96.4% with GA 28–31 weeks, 98.4% with GA 32–33 weeks, and 99.3% with GA 34–36 weeks, though the survival rate for even the latter LPT subset was lower than the 99.8% survival rate for term birth (Mandy et al., 2019). In a multisite study of infants with GA 22–28 weeks and birthweight 401–1,500 g, survival ranged from 9% at GA 22 weeks to 94% at GA 28 weeks (Stoll et al., 2015). Rates of preterm birth and survival also vary across countries and hospitals, with higher survival associated with provision of active, specialized care for infants born at the limits of viability (Mandy et al., 2019).

Survival is frequently classified as either "disability-free" or accompanied by neurodevelopment impairment in later infancy or toddlerhood, defined as cerebral palsy (CP), a hearing or vision disorder, or scores falling below expectations for corrected age on a test of early development. Both disability-free and overall survival are lower in preterm infants with lower GA, neonatal complications, and major congenital anomalies, such as congenital heart disease or chromosomal abnormalities (Mandy et al., 2019).

Most premature births occur spontaneously following early labor or rupture of the membranes (Mandy et al., 2019; Purisch & Gyamfi-Bannerman, 2017). Although the causes are often unknown, risks for spontaneous early deliveries are a previous preterm birth, multiple gestations (twins or multiples), maternal illness such as infections, hypertension, and diabetes, and placental–cervical–uterine abnormalities. Maternal stress and related activation of the maternal or fetal hypothalamic–pituitary–adrenal axis is another risk factor (Mathewson et al., 2017). Approximately 15–20% of the broader spectrum of preterm infants are multiple gestations, with somewhat higher rates for those with more extreme prematurity (Adams-Chapman et al., 2018; Purisch & Gyamfi-Bannerman, 2017). Elective or "indicated" preterm deliveries account for a minority of preterm births and are related to factors such as concerns for the mother or for fetal development, such as preeclampsia/eclampsia, IUGR, maternal hypertension, and placental abruption. In some instances, delivery of early term or LPT infants are not medically indicated, though this practice is discouraged and has decreased in recent years with associated decreases in early births (McCabe et al., 2014; Richards et al., 2016).

HISTORICAL TRENDS

Major advances have been made in the care of preterm infants since the advent of neonatal intensive care in the 1960s (Rogers & Hintz, 2016). As resuscitation and intravenous therapies were not available for infants born prior to that period, few infants with more extreme prematurity survived. A number of new therapies were implemented between 1940 and 1960, some of which led to high rates of adverse outcomes. Examples include nutritional deprivation, overuse of oxygen for jaundice, leading to retinopathy and blindness, and use of antibiotics that caused deafness. Single- and multisite follow-up studies conducted in the 1950s and 1960s revealed sensorimotor and neurodevelopmental problems in a majority of LBW survivors.

Practice changes undertaken with the advent of neonatal intensive care included improved delivery room care, assisted ventilation, phototherapy to treat jaundice, monitoring of oxygen saturation and vital signs, intravenous administration of fluids and nutrition, and drugs for patent ductus arteriosus (failure of closure of fetal artery joining aorta to pulmonary artery) and apnea (temporary cessation in breathing). These and other new treatments led to substantial increases in survival and reduced rates of complications, especially for children with more extreme prematurity. Additions to neonatal care in the latter 1980s and 1990s included antenatal steroids to promote lung development and surfactant for lung health. Survival increased dramatically during this period but without substantial change in neonatal or developmental outcomes. Survival has continued to improve marginally since the 1990s with efforts to prevent hypothermia, reduction in administration of the postnatal steroid dexamethasone, decreased use of invasive forms of mechanical ventilation and greater application of noninvasive ventilation, and the introduction of newer therapies such as caffeine and antenatal magnesium sulfate (Mandy et al., 2019; Mathewson et al., 2017; Wilson-Costello & Payne, 2019). The most dramatic improvements in survival have been for infants with the lowest GAs.

Studies suggest ongoing improvement in survival in more extremely preterm infants, with an increase in the total number of disability-free births but with little change in the proportion of surviving infants with moderate to severe disability and similar levels of adverse developmental outcomes (Johnson & Marlow, 2017). Follow-up of geographic EPT/ELBW cohorts born in Australia in 1991–1992, 1997, and 2005 failed to reveal reduced rates of developmental delay over this period despite advances in obstetric and neonatal care (Doyle, Roberts, & Anderson, 2011). In fact, more recent follow-up of Australian birth cohorts suggest a trend for EPT/ELBW children born in the 2000s to have higher rates of problems in motor skills, executive function, and academic achievement at 8 years' corrected age than those born in the 1990s (Burnett et al., 2018; Spittle, Cameron, Doyle, & Cheong, 2018a). A U.S. study offers a more mixed picture of trends in survival and morbidity from 2011 to 2014 for infants with GA ≤ 27 weeks (Adams-Chapman et al., 2018). In this study, decreasing rates of severe CP and moderate to severe neurodevelopmental impairment across birth years were accompanied by increasing rates of mild CP. Rates of preterm birth in the United States have also declined over time, from 13% in 2006 to 11% in 2013 (McCabe et al., 2014) and 10% in 2016.

NEUROPATHOLOGY AND OTHER COMPLICATIONS OF PREMATURITY, AND THEIR ASSOCIATIONS WITH OUTCOMES

Cranial ultrasonography is the standard of care for identifying neonatal neuropathology in preterm/LBW neonates, but it is less sensitive to brain abnormalities than magnetic resonance imaging (MRI; Ment, Hirtz, & Huppi, 2009a). Several MRI abnormalities are commonly found: (1) germinal matrix hemorrhage and intraventricular hemorrhage (GMH–IVH), ranging from hemorrhage confined to the germinal matrix (Grade I) to hemorrhage taking up 10–50% of lateral ventricles (Grade II), hemorrhage occupying

> 50% of ventricles with ventricular expansion (Grade III), and periventricular hemorrhagic infarction involving the white matter (Grade IV); (2) white matter abnormalities, including cystic periventricular leukomalacia (PVL; white matter necrosis in the area surrounding the lateral ventricles), diffuse noncystic maldevelopment of the white matter, and reduced fractional anisotrophy; (3) reduced cortical, subcortical, and cerebellar white and gray matter volumes; (4) less differentiation of white and gray matter and delayed cortical folding; and (5) diminished connectivity between white matter tracts (Batalle et al., 2017; de Vries & Leijser, 2019; Ment et al., 2009b). Whereas GMH–IVH tends to occur most frequently in children with more extremely low GA, reduced brain volumes and disruptions in white matter maturation are present in many children with VPT in the absence of frank brain injury.

Brain abnormalities are evident throughout childhood and into adulthood, with reduced volumes of gray and white matter and altered patterns of activation on functional MRI (fMRI) (Ment et al., 2009b). Volume reductions are especially prominent in white matter, the cerebellum, and subcortical and periventricular gray matter. Abnormalities in left-hemisphere language lateralization raise the possibility of compensatory neural organization (Karolis et al., 2017). Figure 7.1 illustrates some of the brain abnormalities evident in survivors of extremely preterm neonates.

Major neonatal complications of preterm birth/LBW besides ICH-IVH are bronchopulmonary dysplasia (BPD; typically defined as placement on supplementary oxygen for at least 36 days corrected age), necrotizing enterocolitis (NEC; deterioration of the intestinal tissues), early- and late-onset sepsis (symptoms of infection appearing either within or after the first 72 hours after birth), retinopathy of prematurity (abnormal development of blood vessels in the retina), apnea, patent ductus arteriosus, and receipt of postnatal steroids to treat severe lung disease (Adams-Chapman et al., 2018; Stoll et al., 2015). Associations of reduced brain volumes or white matter abnormalities with BPD, NEC, and sepsis, and of slower early postnatal cerebellar growth with brain insults and morphine exposure, confirm the vulnerability of postnatal brain development in preterm infants (Dubner et al., 2019; Zwicker et al., 2016).

Brain abnormalities in preterm/LBW infants have multiple etiologies. Fetal antecedents include stress and related neuroendocrine effects on the fetal brain, chronic placental

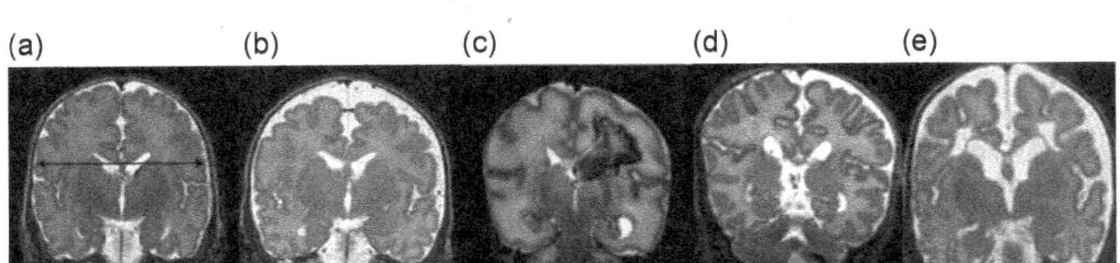

FIGURE 7.1. Coronal images from brain MRI in the neonatal period, characterizing different forms of neuropathology related to preterm birth: (a) typical preterm with arrow showing measurement of biparietal width; (b) impaired growth as demonstrated by the increased extracerebral space and interhemispheric distance; (c) Grade IV IVH; (d) unilateral cerebellar hemorrhage; and (e) bilateral cystic PVL associated with marked impaired growth. Images courtesy of Terrie E. Inder, MBChB, Department of Pediatric Newborn Medicine, Brigham and Women's Hospital, Boston, Massachusetts.

insufficiency and associated fetal hypoxemia or suboptimal nutrition, maternal–fetal inflammatory processes, IUGR, and drug or other toxic exposures (Kuban et al., 2019; Mathewson et al., 2017). Postnatal etiologies include the vulnerability of the preterm brain (and of white matter precursors referred to as pre-oligodendrocytes) to exposures such as medical interventions and to inflammation and hypoxic–ischemic injury related to neonatal complications (e.g., infections, NEC, BPD) and the inability of the extrauterine preterm brain to regulate growth promoting or protective processes. Genetic and epigenetic factors also play a role as additional predictors of outcome and moderators of the effects of pre- and perinatal risk factors (Ment et al., 2014).

Perinatal neurological abnormalities related to subsequent developmental problems include brain lesions, volume reductions, and loss of white matter integrity, as well as more molar indications of poor brain growth, as reflected in early postnatal head growth, biparietal width, interhemispheric distance, and small head circumference (Kidokoro et al., 2014). Early outcomes are better for children with less severe brain insults, but even infants with Grade I/II IVH do less well than infants without IVH (Mukerji, Shah, & Shah, 2015). Some studies document associations of abnormalities in specific brain regions or circuits with specific types of cognitive deficits (Anderson et al., 2017). Research also confirms associations of developmental outcomes with BPD, NEC, and sepsis, administration of postnatal dexamethasone, neonatal pain and morphine exposure, retinopathy of prematurity, elevations in inflammatory proteins, and reduced levels of neurotrophins (Dubner et al., 2019; Kuban et al., 2019; Molloy, Anderson, Anderson, & Doyle, 2016; Rand, Austin, Inder, Bora, & Woodward, 2016; Zwicker et al., 2016).

DEVELOPMENTAL OUTCOMES

Infancy and Toddlerhood

The *Bayley Scales of Infant Development, Second Edition* (Bayley II; Bayley, 1993) or *Bayley Scales of Infant and Toddler Development, Third Edition* (Bayley III; Bayley, 2006) are commonly used assessments of early developmental disability. In a 2009–2011 Canadian birth cohort of infants with GA < 29 weeks followed to 21 months corrected age (Synnes et al., 2017), 46% had some degree of impairment, and 17% had significant impairment. Delays in development are the most common reason for impairment, with lesser rates of CP and a prevalence of hearing and vision disorders of ≤ 5% (Johnson & Marlow, 2017). Follow-up of a 2005 Australian cohort with GA < 28 weeks at a corrected age of 2 years (Doyle et al., 2010) revealed delays in 47.9% on the Bayley III, relative to an expected rate of 16% (< –1 *SD* below the mean). By comparison, CP was diagnosed in 9.8% and deafness in 2.5%, with no cases of blindness. A review of early outcomes of EPT birth found rates of severe neurodevelopment impairment ranging from 17 to 59% and rates of CP ranging from 7 to 14% (Jarjour, 2015). Other studies document deficits during infancy and toddlerhood in cognitive, language, and motor skills, as well as high rates of speech therapy and early interventions (Vohr, 2014; Wang, Howe, Lin, & Hsu, 2014). Language problems include smaller vocabularies, more limited use of words, and weaker grammatical skills (Vandormael, Schoenhals, Huppi, Filippa, & Tolsa, 2019).

Effects of preterm birth on physical health that begin to emerge in this period include increased blood pressure and other cardiovascular anomalies, obstructive lung disease and respiratory problems, reduced insulin sensitivity and renal volume, seizures, eating and sleeping problems, and substandard growth (Crapnell, Woodward, Rogers, Inder, & Pineda, 2015; Douglas et al., 2017; Hack et al., 2014; Luu, Rehman Mian, & Nuyt, 2017; Stangenes et al., 2018). Relative to expectation for corrected age, EPT and VPT infants and toddlers also have behavior problems, including lower levels of persistence and attention, difficulties making transitions, more internalizing symptoms, and poorer socioemotional competence and behavioral self-regulation (Woodward, Lu, Morris, & Healey, 2017). Parent-reported symptoms of autism spectrum disorder (ASD) may also be evident, though in many cases these symptoms may reflect other neurodevelopmental impairments (Johnson & Marlow, 2017).

Preschool Period

Developmental problems persist into the preschool period, extending from approximately 3–5 years of age. VPT groups have deficits relative to term controls in global cognition and on measures of executive function assessing attention, inhibition, working memory, cognitive flexibility, and verbal fluency (Baron, Kerns, Muller, Ahronovich, & Litman, 2012a). Delays in receptive and expressive language are manifest in lower levels of verb production and social use of language compared to term-born peers (Foster-Cohen, Friesen, Champion, & Woodward, 2010). Rates of developmental coordination disorder, defined as motor deficits not accounted for by a medical or neurological condition or overall developmental impairment, are also higher in preterm/LBW children than in their full-term peers (Rogers & Hintz, 2016).

The American Academy of Pediatrics (High, 2008) defines children's *academic or school readiness* in terms of health and physical development, socioemotional adjustment, and age-appropriate approaches to learning as exemplified by motivation and self-control, communication skills, and cognition and general knowledge. Studies of children 3–5 years of age document deficits relative to term controls in several of these areas (Aylward, 2014; Baron, Erickson, Ahronovich, Baker, & Litman, 2011; Woodward et al., 2009). Delays in at least one area of school readiness were found in 44% of Australian VPT 5-year-olds compared to 16% of term controls (Roberts, Lim, Doyle, & Anderson, 2011). Similarly, three times as many New Zealand VPT children compared to term controls had generalized delays in school readiness skills at age 4 years (Pritchard, Bora, Austin, Levin, & Woodward, 2014). Deficits in self-regulation and socioemotional functioning in VPT infants and toddlers are also evident in the preschool period (Woodward et al., 2017).

Early School Age

Cognitive, learning, and behavior problems are also documented at early school age (6–8 years). In a U.S. sample comprised primarily of kindergarten students, VPT children had lower scores than those born at term on composite measures of early reading and language and of early number and nonverbal skills (Shah, Kaciroti, Richards, & Lumeng, 2016). Studies examining outcomes in kindergarten and the early primary grades confirm deficits relative to term controls in children with more extreme prematurity across multiple neuropsychological domains, including overall cognitive ability, language, visuospatial and nonverbal reasoning skills, motor skills, memory, and executive function (Orchinik et al., 2011).

Deficits are evident in overall cognition and in motor and visuomotor abilities, phonological processing, and memory, even when excluding children with more severe intellectual disability (Hasler & Akshoomoff, 2019; Omizzolo et al., 2014). Controlling for global cognitive ability or acquired verbal knowledge reveals evidence for selective weaknesses in spatial location memory, perceptual-motor skills, and executive function (Baron et al., 2012b; Orchinik et al., 2011). In a Swedish study of 6½-year-olds, developmental coordination disorder was identified in 37.1% of EPT children compared to 5.5% of term controls (Bolk, Farooqi, Hafstrom, Aden, & Serenius, 2018). Learning problems in VPT children are found on formal tests of academic achievement and curriculum-based assessments and are most prominent in mathematics (Pritchard et al., 2009). School observations documenting more teacher attention and off-task behavior in EPT/ELBW children compared to classmate controls also point to problems in classroom learning (Wong et al., 2014).

Evidence for the preterm behavioral phenotype of attention-deficit/hyperactivity disorder (ADHD), internalizing symptoms, and social problems emerge by early school age (Johnson & Marlow, 2011). Psychiatric interview of parents in an Australian study revealed nearly three times the rate of psychiatric disorders in 7-year-old VPT children compared to term controls (24 vs. 9%) (Treyvaud et al., 2013), with group differences in rates of ADHD, anxiety, and ASD. Another study employing a structured psychiatric interview and parent and teacher ratings of behavior found more symptoms of ADHD, socioemotional problems, and executive dysfunction in EPT/ELBW kindergarten children compared to classmate controls (Scott et al., 2012). Other less favorable outcomes for VPT or ELBW children relative to term controls include higher parent ratings of executive dysfunction and lower parent perceptions of child satisfaction with health, comfort, and achievement (Hack et al., 2011; Hasler & Akshoomoff, 2019).

Middle School Age and Adolescence

Research on outcomes at middle school age and adolescence documents lower IQs in preterm/LBW children compared to their term-born peers. Anderson (2014) reported IQ reductions of about 11 points across studies, with larger differences for preterm children with lower GA. Weaknesses in language, memory, attention and executive function, processing speed, and motor skills are also evident (Johnson & Marlow, 2017; Nguyen et al., 2018; Vohr, 2014). In a study of 12-year-olds, Luu et al. (2009) found language impairment in 22–24% of children with birthweight 600–1,250 g compared to 2–4% of term controls. Estimated rates of motor deficits are three to four times higher in preterm children than in the general population (Williams, Lee, & Anderson, 2010). EPT children also have deficits in visual acuity, stereopsis, and convergence (Molloy et al., 2013). Language processing, executive function, and visual-constructive skills may be more impaired than receptive vocabulary, object recognition, and sustained attention (Geldof, van Wassenaer, de Kieviet, Kok, & Oosterlaan, 2012; Wilson-Ching et al., 2013).

Older preterm/LBW youth obtain lower scores than controls on tests of literacy and mathematics, lower teacher ratings of academic performance, and higher rates of special education services (Johnson & Marlow, 2017). Compared to controls, EPT/ELBW youth have higher rates of learning disability, defined by low scores on achievement tests in the absence of sensorimotor or cognitive disability, and deficits in mathematics skills even when researchers control for global cognitive abilities or exclude children with lower IQ

(Akshoomoff et al., 2017; Litt et al., 2012; Simms et al., 2015). Poor achievement is associated with lower IQ and weaknesses in executive function, processing speed, visual memory, visuospatial skills, and phonological processing (Litt et al., 2012; Simms et al., 2015).

The preterm behavior phenotype continues to be evident in adolescence (Johnson & Marlow, 2017; Taylor, Margevicius, Schluchter, Andreias, & Hack, 2015). Behavior ratings of executive dysfunction are also higher in VPT adolescents than in term controls (Luu et al., 2009). ADHD is less closely associated with externalizing problems in preterm youth than in other children with ADHD, with more symptoms of inattention than hyperactivity (Franz et al., 2018; Johnson & Marlow, 2011). Studies have documented nearly double the rate of anxiety disorders in VPT/VLBW adolescents compared to controls (Somhovd, Hansen, Brok, Esbjorn, & Greisen, 2012) and nearly three times the rate of psychiatric disorders in EPT 11-year-olds compared to their peers (Johnson et al., 2011b). VPT/EPT children also have more deficits in social communication, higher rates of ASD, and lower perceptions of health status than their full-term peers (Johnson et al., 2011a; Joseph et al., 2017; Baumann, Bartmann, & Wolke, 2016). Social problems include more difficulties in establishing friendships, increased social rejection, and lower social satisfaction compared to term-born peers (Ritchie, Bora, & Woodward, 2018).

Adulthood

VPT/VLBW adults score less well than term-born controls on measures of IQ, executive function, memory and learning, and processing speed (Aanes, Bjuland, Skranes, & Lohaugen, 2015; Breeman, Jaekel, Baumann, Bartmann, & Wolke, 2015; Strang-Karlsson et al., 2010). Preterm adults are also more likely that full-term controls to have higher blood pressure, increased insulin resistance, reduced bone density, more asthma, and higher rates of cerebral palsy and sensory impairments (Doyle & Anderson, 2010; Raju, Buist, Blaisdell, Moxey-Mims, & Saigal, 2017). Mental health problems are similar to those evident in adolescence and include ADHD, internalizing problems, and social difficulties (Mathewson et al., 2017; Raju et al., 2017). Personality styles of adults born preterm are characterized by less risk taking, social engagement, and interpersonal communication and greater worry or neuroticism (Eryigit Madzwamuse, Strauss, Baumann, Bartmann, & Wolke, 2015).

Compared to their full-term peers, VPT/VLBW adults are more likely to live with their parents, less likely to complete high school or attend college or university, and have lower levels of employment, income, self-esteem, and health-related quality of life (Baumann et al., 2016). These "real life" limitations are more marked in VPT/VLBW adults with lower GA or neurosensory impairments, earlier disabilities, or impaired executive function (Kroll et al., 2017). Nonetheless, the vast majority of adults with preterm birth/LBW, including those with more extreme prematurity, have independent lives with educational and vocational attainments similar to their term-born peers (Saigal et al., 2016b).

PREDICTORS OF OUTCOME AND LONGITUDINAL CHANGE

Longitudinal follow-up of preterm/LBW children is useful in determining the utility of earlier assessments as predictors of later outcomes, identifying age-specific consequences of prematurity, and examining the effects of prematurity on developmental change. In addition to neonatal and genetic risk factors, lower socioeconomic status (SES) is a well-established correlate of less positive neurodevelopmental and health outcomes (Doyle et al., 2015). SES typically comprises more "distal" family characteristics, such as parent education, income, occupation, minority status, single versus two-parent household, and composites of these or similar variables. Other more "proximal" environmental risk factors include less sensitive and supportive parenting styles, less stimulating home settings, higher parent burden and distress, fewer opportunities for human interactions in the NICU, and bullying (Day et al., 2016; Jaekel, Pluess, Belsky, & Wolke, 2015a; Taylor, Minich, Schluchter, Espy, & Klein, 2019a; Treyvaud et al., 2016; Woodward et al., 2014). These factors are associated with a wide range of early and later developmental outcomes independently of biological risks (Doyle et al., 2015; Taylor et al., 2019a). Some studies suggest that social advantages may buffer the negative consequences of preterm birth or that disadvantaged environments may exacerbate these effects (Benavente-Fernandez et al., 2019; Jaekel et al., 2015a).

Problems in learning and behavior are also related to both prior and concurrent neurodevelopmental functioning and health status. Cognitive weaknesses are concurrently associated with symptoms of ADHD, poorer classroom performance, and lower academic achievement (Scott et al., 2012; Taylor et al., 2018; Wong et al., 2014). Children with chronic health problems also have poorer academic achievement (Litt & McCormick, 2016). Associations of earlier developmental outcomes to later ones suggest cross-age continuity. Examples include associations of early weaknesses in executive functioning with later learning and behavior problems (Woodward et al., 2017); early neuromotor assessments with later hand functioning and school-age measures of motor ability, working memory, and processing speed (Wang et al., 2014); poorer motor ability, lower IQ, and more problems with peer relationships in early childhood with ADHD at 11 years (Johnson et al., 2016); and poorer fluid intelligence at 8 years with more externalizing symptoms in young adulthood (Lahat, van Lieshout, Saigal, Boyle, & Schmidt, 2015). Scores on the Bayley and other early childhood assessments are related to later cognitive abilities, though low Bayley scores early in life frequently fail to predict poor functioning later in childhood (Breeman et al., 2015; O'Shea et al., 2018).

Research on longitudinal change in the same or similar outcome measures in preterm/LBW cohorts have yielded mixed findings. Some studies suggest that catch-up to term-born controls is possible in receptive vocabulary, verbal reasoning, and reading skills (Litt et al., 2012; Luu, Vohr, Allan, Schneider, & Ment, 2011), while others indicate slower development of visuomotor skill and executive functioning and a worsening of quality of life (Baumann et al., 2016; Taylor, Minich, Klein, & Hack, 2004). Most longitudinal research suggests similar deficits across age relative to term controls (Mangin, Horwood, & Woodward, 2017; Saigal et al., 2016a).

Application of cluster-analytic and latent growth modeling methods reveal subgroups of VPT children with different growth trajectories relative to term controls. Some children display stable weaknesses over time, while others show catch-up growth or fall increasingly behind age standards (Clark et al., 2013; Luu et al., 2011; Nguyen et al., 2018). Higher medical and social risks and smaller brain volumes are associated with less optimal growth. Additional longitudinal research reveals poorer learning progress in EPT/ELBW children with cognitive weaknesses or symptoms of ADHD in kindergarten (Taylor et al.,

2018, 2019b), slower gains in cognitive abilities from 18 months to 5 years in children with birthweights 500–1,250 g (Manley et al., 2015), and slower growth in executive function from 3–5 years in LBW children exposed to less sensitive parenting (Camerota et al., 2015).

Long-term outcomes can be conceptualized as the residual effects of early disruptions in neural development, as postulated by the "developmental origins of health and disease" model (Heindel et al., 2015). According to this model, compromised neurobiological status in the perinatal period has residual effects that are manifest in different ways across development. A more inclusive model is one that acknowledges the contributions of postnatal experiences, ongoing neural development, and previously attained cognitive skills, academic achievement, and social-behavioral adjustment to children's subsequent longitudinal course. As Illustrated in Figure 7.2, the latter model conceives of development as an evolving process, with outcomes at each age dependent on previous achievements but also susceptible to new influences. The model is consistent with developmental "cascades" in which earlier outcomes help shape later ones, but with longitudinal trajectories subject to multiple contextual factors. Application of this framework helps explain the variable and at times atypical developmental pathways taken by preterm/LBW children (Sansavini, Guarini, & Caselli, 2011).

OUTCOMES OF MODERATE AND LATE PRETERM BIRTH

MPT and LPT infants comprise as many as 75–80% of all infants born preterm (6–11% of all births) and represent the subset of the preterm population showing the most rapid increases in birth rates (Khan et al., 2015). Compared to term-born infants, these infants have higher rates of mortality, greater length of neonatal hospitalization and NICU admissions, and early medical morbidities and rehospitalizations than children born at term (Baron, Litman, Ahronovich, & Baker, 2012c). Because of their larger numbers relative to less mature infants, they account for most of the costs of preterm care, with utilization of health and social services in the first 2 years costing four times more than care for term infants (Khan et al., 2015; McCabe et al., 2014).

The consequences of MPT/LPT birth are less pronounced than those associated with VPT birth but include weakness on measures of intelligence, language, memory, visuomotor and visuospatial skills, fine motor dexterity, and attention, as well as lower levels of academic achievement, more health problems and internalizing symptoms, and poorer social and communication skills (Baron et al., 2012c; Johnson et al., 2015a). Although some deficits may resolve with age (Baron, Weiss, Litman, Ahronovich, & Baker, 2014b), adverse effects are documented in infancy, childhood and adolescence, and adulthood (Baron et al., 2014b; Heinonen et al., 2015).

Poorer outcomes of MPT/LPT births are also associated with higher social risk, medically indicated births, preeclampsia, male sex, decreased growth in head circumference in the first year of life, and short stature (Dotinga et al., 2016; Johnson et al., 2015a). It is unclear whether neonatal complications of MPT/LPT births contribute to negative outcomes independently of GA and how many of these children are adversely affected (Baron et al., 2014a). A latent class analysis of profiles of socioemotional impairments in 2-year-olds found that only 7% of an MPT/LPT group displayed a profile that was similar to the

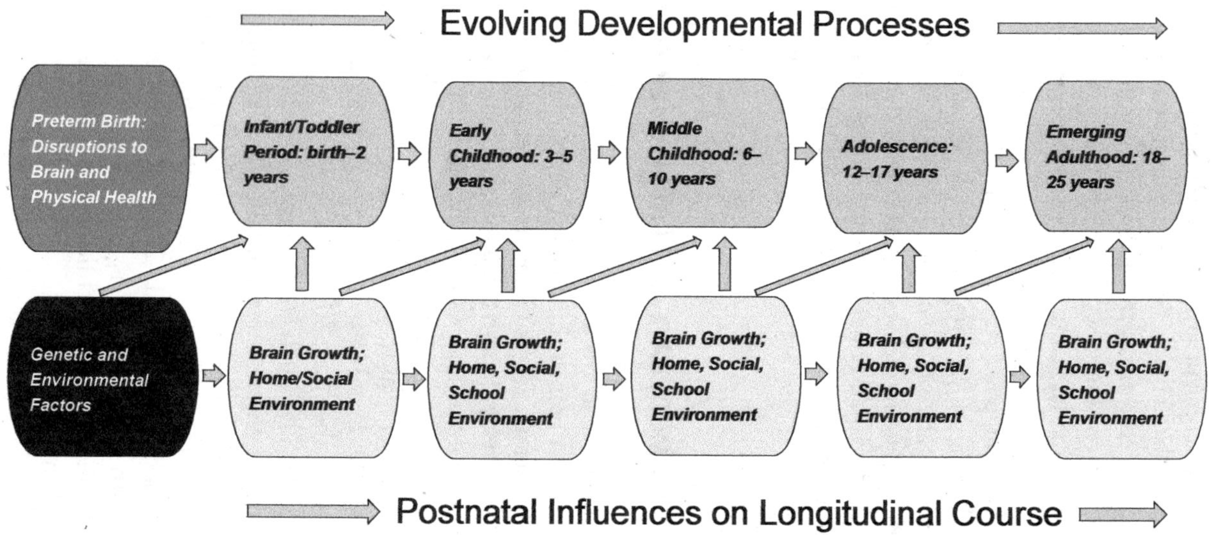

FIGURE 7.2. Model of longitudinal outcomes as manifestations of evolving developmental processes.

preterm behavioral phenotype but distinct from profiles also observed in term controls (Johnson et al., 2018).

DEVELOPMENTAL INTERVENTIONS

A majority of research on interventions to promote positive outcomes for preterm/LBW children have focused on those delivered in the NICU or during early childhood. The major goal of these interventions is to reduce the adverse effects of prematurity through "developmentally informed care," referring to approaches that provide infants with environmental supports to minimize stress and foster development in ways that consider their special needs and capabilities (Browne, 2011). These interventions are primarily preventive and include working with caregivers in the NICU to reduce potentially harmful environmental exposures, while providing appropriate levels of stimulation, promoting behavioral regulation, continuing to build positive parent–child relationships after discharge, and fostering children's early development through parent- and professional-based therapies (Colditz et al., 2019). Therapies are also provided for specific impairments, such as CP and motor delays (Hughes, Redsell, & Glazebrook, 2016). Benefits of these approaches include reduced neonatal mortality and morbidity with Kangaroo mother care (Boundy et al., 2016) and improved development and behavior for VPT infants whose parents received family-centered care (Spittle & Treyvaud, 2016). One study found evidence of improved white matter integrity at term age equivalent in infants with GA < 30 weeks whose parents were in a NICU parenting program compared to those whose parents were not in the program (Milgrom et al., 2010).

Positive effects of early intervention can result in selective improvements in treated vs. untreated preterm children (Colditz et al., 2019; Spittle, Orton, Anderson, Boyd, & Doyle, 2015). A meta-analysis found that the effects of early interventions on motor skills in preterm infants are present up to 24 months' chronological age but diminish with advancing age, and that programs focused on motor-based activities had more positive effects compared to more generic interventions (Hughes et al., 2016). Studies of early developmental interventions also reveal decreasing benefits over time and suggests that these interventions may be more helpful for children at higher social risk (Spittle, Treyvaud, Lee, Anderson, & Doyle, 2018b).

Other potential interventions for preterm/LBW children are (1) treatment of caregiver psychological distress and burden; (2) occupational, physical, and speech–language therapies; and (3) preschool and school-age programs to enhance academic achievement, cognitive skills, and social-behavioral adjustment. Psychological distress and internalizing symptoms are higher in parents of younger VPT children than in parents of term-born controls but become less pronounced in later childhood (Pace et al., 2016). Because parent distress and maladjustment are associated with poorer child outcomes, mental health treatment of parents may be an important component of intervention (Woodward et al., 2014). Although we are not aware of research designed to isolate the effects of different approaches to intervention, one study found that longer and more intense community-based early intervention services were associated with higher teacher ratings of kindergarten skills (Litt, Glymour, Hauser-Cram, Hehir, & McCormick, 2018). However, preterm/LBW children who attend preschool remain behind in school readiness (Chen, Claessens,

& Msall, 2014) and those with delayed school entry may fare worse in academic achievement than those who enter school at a time that is appropriate for their chronological age (Jaekel, Strauss, Johnson, Gilmore, & Wolke, 2015b).

Lack of teacher awareness of preterm/LBW children's behavioral, attentional, and learning difficulties argues for school-age educational and behavioral programs, as well as increased teacher education (Johnson, Gilmore, Gallimore, Jaekel, & Wolke, 2015b). Research on programs to enhance children's cognitive skills report short-term effects on these skills but little generalization to related but nontrained abilities. Notably, a randomized controlled trial of CogMed Working Memory Training with 7-year-old EPT/ELBW children failed to reveal positive effects of this program compared to a placebo intervention on measures of academic achievement, attention and executive function, or behavior (Anderson et al., 2018).

RESEARCH METHODS AND FUTURE DIRECTIONS

Research methods vary considerably in studies of preterm/LBW children (Anderson, 2014). An ideal study would be one in which (1) the birth cohort is well defined (e.g., by GA) and represents a population of children; (2) the sample includes an age-matched control group from a similar background as the preterm/LBW group, and deficits in the latter group are identified relative to outcomes for controls rather than normative standards; (3) both groups are followed across age beginning in infancy with limited attrition; (4) assessments are age-appropriate, with corrections for GA made in evaluating younger preterm children, and include reliable and validated measures of diverse aspects of development (multiple neuropsychological skills, achievement, behavior); (5) information is obtained from multiple sources, including direct testing and observations, diagnostic interviews, ratings of development, behavior, achievement, and quality of life, and with efforts to avoid potential sources of bias (e.g., keeping examiners or observers uninformed of birth status of examinees); (6) data on prenatal and neonatal medical risk factors, potential genetic influences, and the family, school, and social environment allow examination of sources of variability in outcome; and (7) appropriate statistical techniques are applied and include procedures for examining the contributions of individual and subgroup differences to group means. Although these requirements are aspirational, knowledge of developmental outcomes of prematurity is limited to the extent that existing studies have failed to meet these criteria. A further challenge is the evolving nature of neonatal intensive care, raising the possibility that outcomes from earlier birth cohorts may not apply to current ones. One of the aims of outcomes research is to determine whether innovations in neonatal care benefit children's longer-term development. Positive effects may be subtle or obscured by failure to focus on the children most likely to benefit or by increased survival of higher-risk infants.

Application of rigorous methods is critical to advancement of knowledge in several areas:

1. Researchers have long recognized that a subset of preterm/LBW children, including those with more extreme degrees of prematurity, are relatively free of the long-term

developmental impairments evident in group comparisons of preterm cohorts to controls (Anderson, 2014). A study following young school-age EPT/ELBW children and term-born classmates controls at school found that some participants in the EPT/ELBW group met criteria for *resilience,* as defined by the absence of academic deficits or behavior problems (Taylor et al., 2019a). Resilience was identified in close to half (43–55%) of the EPT/ELBW group across three school years and was associated with more advantaged family environments and higher scores on neuropsychological tests. An important direction for future research is to shed light on potential compensatory mechanisms by examining neural, genetic, and environmental characteristics of children with more rather than less favorable outcomes.

2. More precise early predictors of shorter- and longer-term developmental outcomes are needed to identify high-risk children. Implementation of newer imaging methods may increase the predictive validity of early neuroimaging. In keeping with the concept of development origins of health and disease, research on genomic and fetal–maternal–placental risk and protective factors is likewise warranted (Miller et al., 2016), as are studies of the factors related to outcomes of MPT/LPT births (Samra, McGrath, & Wehbe, 2011).

3. Despite a surfeit of evidence for developmental deficits in preterm/LBW children, we lack comprehensive knowledge of the nature and comorbidity of these impairments. Tests intended to assess specific cognitive abilities typically place demands on multiple skills (Anderson, 2014). Similarly, scores on many standardized tests of mathematics achievement reflect composites of multiple mathematics skills (Taylor, Espy, & Anderson, 2009). More research is needed to identify component deficits, as illustrated by studies examining the basis of deficits on visuomotor tasks (De Kieviet et al., 2013) and the effects of extreme prematurity on individual number skills (Tatsuoka et al., 2016). Identifying component deficits will inform the search for underlying neural mechanisms of effect and enhance knowledge of associations of cognitive and academic impairments. A more general goal is to further knowledge of patterns of comorbidity of cognitive, learning, and behavior deficits and their neural basis.

4. We have much to learn about how prematurity affects development. Consistent with the "developmental processes" model depicted in Figure 7.2, environmental influences contribute to both brain and developmental outcomes, and these outcomes, in turn, affect subsequent neurodevelopment. Further research is required to elucidate the parenting styles, socialization experiences, and educational opportunities associated with developmental change and explore their effects on neural development. Special emphasis might be placed on periods of transition, such as the relation of school readiness in preschool children to later learning abilities or development of social adjustment during adolescence (Doyle et al., 2014).

5. Finally, finding better ways to identify and treat the cognitive, learning, and behavior consequences of prematurity is imperative. Doing so will require testing of interventions informed by research on longitudinal change and efforts to develop additional preventive interventions, including ones that extend early interventions to older ages. Treatments for existing cognitive, educational, and behavioral problems in preterm/LBW children are critical and will need to be tailored to their specific needs. Programs designed for the broader child population also deserve consideration. An example of such

a program is Tools of the Mind, an instructional program that promotes the development and utilization of self-regulatory skills in the learning process (Blair & Raver, 2014). Finding effective ways to identify the children with these problems will require systems for monitoring their progress. Comprehensive assessments for children with extreme prematurity are justified by their high rates of impairment. Early interventions that prevent or lessen later impairments also have a sound economic rationale (O. Doyle, Harmon, Heckman, & Tremblay, 2009). Unfortunately, little if any research has been conducted on best practices for monitoring the later development of these children or the much larger population of MPT/LPT births (L. W. Doyle et al., 2014; Johnson & Marlow, 2017).

SUMMARY AND CLINICAL IMPLICATIONS

Approximately 1 in 10 infants in the United States is born prematurely, as defined by a GA < 37 weeks or < 2,500 g birthweight. Comparisons with term-born children reveal more neonatal complications, brain abnormalities, and developmental impairments across the preterm/LBW spectrum. However, adverse consequences vary with the degree of prematurity and are the most severe and pervasive in the 1–2% of infants with GA < 28 weeks or < 1,000 g birthweight. Despite increases in survival of the latter subset of infants in past decades, with some reduction in rates of CP, developmental outcomes have remained largely unchanged. For this reason, neuropsychologists, other health professionals, and educators are increasingly likely to encounter these children in their clinical practices and classrooms.

A small minority of preterm/LBW children have global developmental impairments, but most are either typically developing or have more moderate and frequently uneven profiles of cognitive ability, academic achievement, and social-behavioral adjustment. Problems in executive function, visuospatial and motor skills, memory, and mathematics are especially common in EPT/ELBW children, though weaknesses in language processing skills are also evident. A behavioral phenotype comprised of symptoms of ADHD (primarily inattentive subtype), internalizing problems, and social difficulties is well documented. Deficits are found on measures of infant development and persist into adulthood. These deficits can be conceptualized as the residual effects of early biological, genetic, and environmental factors in combination with subsequent experience-dependent growth processes. Methodologically rigorous research will be required to identify early biomarkers of risk and factors that contribute to individual differences in developmental outcome, explore mechanisms that account for resilience, better understand the nature and neural basis of comorbid deficits, and design better approaches to developmental monitoring and intervention.

Existing research supports the need for health care professionals to identify problems early and monitor outcomes over time, recognize that consequences vary across children and can often be selective, and provide recommendations for immediate interventions, as well as anticipatory guidance. Parents and teachers are well-advised to seek evaluations for any concerns and follow through on age-appropriate interventions, whether they be parenting programs, special therapies, or efforts to boost socialization skills. At the societal level, this research argues for the need for educational and health care policies to ensure better monitoring of outcomes and continuity of care.

REFERENCES

Aanes, S., Bjuland, K. J., Skranes, J., & Lohaugen, G. C. C. (2015). Memory function and hippocampal volumes in preterm born very-low-birth-weight (VLBW) young adults. *NeuroImage, 105,* 76–83.

Adams-Chapman, I. Heyne, R. J., DeMauro, S. B., Duncan, A. F., Hintz, S. R., Pappas, A., . . . Higgins, R. D. for the Follow-up Study of the Eunice Kennedy Shriver National Institute of Child Health and Human Development Neonatal Research Network. (2018). Neurodevelopmental impairment among extremely preterm infants in the Neonatal Research Network. *Pediatrics, 141*(5), Article e20173091.

Akshoomoff, N., Joseph, R. M., Taylor, H. G., Allred, E. N., Heeren, T., O'Shea, T. M., & Kuban, K. C. K. (2017). Academic achievement deficits and their neuropsychological correlates in children born extremely preterm. *Journal of Developmental and Behavioral Pediatrics, 38,* 627–637.

Anderson, P. J. (2014). Neuropsychological outcomes of children born very preterm. *Seminars in Fetal and Neonatal Medicine, 19,* 90–96.

Anderson, P. J., Lee, K. J., Roberts, G., Spencer-Smith, M. M., Thompson, D. K., Seal, M. L., . . . Pascoe, L. (2018). Long-term academic functioning following CogMed Working Memory Training for children born extremely preterm: A randomized controlled trial. *Journal of Pediatrics, 202,* 92–97.

Anderson, P. J., Treyvaud, K., Neil, J. J., Cheong, J. L. Y., Hunt, R. W., Thompson, D. T., . . . Inder, T. E. (2017). Associations of newborn brain magnetic resonance imaging with long-term neurodevelopmental impairments in very preterm children. *Journal of Pediatrics, 187,* 58–65.

Aylward, G. P. (2014). Neurodevelopmental outcomes of infants born prematurely. *Journal of Developmental and Behavioral Pediatrics, 35*(6), 394–407.

Baron, I. S., Brandt, J., Ahronovich, M. D., Baker, R., Erickson, K., & Litman, F. R. (2012b). Selective deficit in spatial location memory in extremely low birth weight children at age six: The PETIT Study. *Child Neuropsychology, 18*(3), 299–311.

Baron, I. S., Erickson, K., Ahronovich, M. D., Baker, R., & Litman, F. R. (2011). Neuropsychological and behavioral outcomes of extremely low birth weight at age three. *Developmental Neuropsychology, 36*(1), 5–21.

Baron, I. S., Kerns, K. A., Muller, U., Ahronovich, M. D., & Litman, F. R. (2012a). Executive function in extremely low birth weight and late-preterm preschoolers: Effects of working memory and response inhibition. *Child Neuropsychology, 18*(6), 586–599.

Baron, I. S., Litman, F. R., Ahronovich, M. D., & Baker, R. (2012c). Late preterm birth: A review of medical and neuropsychological childhood outcomes. *Neuropsychological Review, 22,* 438–450.

Baron, I. S., Weiss, B. A., Baker, R., Khoury, A., Remsburg, I., Thermolice, J. W., . . . Ahronovich, M. D. (2014a). Subtle adverse effects of late preterm birth: A cautionary note. *Neuropsychology, 28*(1), 11–18.

Baron, I. S., Weiss, B. A., Litman, F. R., Ahronovich, M. D., & Baker, R. (2014b). Latent mean differences in executive function in at-risk preterm children: The delay-deficit dilemma. *Neuropsychology, 28,* 541–551.

Batalle, D., Hughes, E. J., Zhang, H., Tournier, J.-D., Tusor, N., Aljabar, P., . . . Counsell, S. J. (2017). Early development of structural networks and the impact of prematurity on brain connectivity. *NeuroImage, 149,* 379–392.

Baumann, N., Bartmann, P., & Wolke, D. (2016). Health-related quality of life into adulthood after very preterm birth. *Pediatrics, 137*(4), Article e20153148.

Bayley, N. (1993). *Bayley Scales of Infant Development, 2nd Edition.* San Antonio, TX: Psychological Corporation.

Bayley, N. (2006). *Manual for the Bayley Scales of Infant and Toddler Development, 3rd Edition.* San Antonio, TX: Psychological Corporation.

Benavente-Fernandez, I., Synnes, A., Grunau, R. E., Chau, V., Ramraj, C., Glass, T., . . . Miller, S. P. (2019). Associations of socioeconomic status and brain injury with neurodevelopmental outcomes of very preterm children. *JAMA Network Open, 2*(5), Article e192914.

Blair, C., & Raver, C. C. (2014). Closing the achievement gap through modification of neurocognitive and neuroendocrine function: Results from a cluster randomized controlled trial of an innovative approach to the education of children in kindergarten. *PLoS ONE, 9*(11), e112393.

Blencowe, H., Cousens, S., Oestergaard, M. Z., Chou, D., Moller, A.-B., Narwal, R., . . . Lawn, J. E. (2012). National, regional, and worldwide estimates of preterm birth rates in the year 2010 with time trends since 1990 for selected countries: A systematic analysis and implications. *Lancet, 379*(9832), 2162–2172.

Bolk, J., Farooqi, A., Hafstrom, M., Aden, U., & Serenius, F. (2018). Developmental coordination disorder and its association with developmental comorbidities at 6.5 years in apparently healthy children born extremely preterm. *JAMA Pediatrics, 172*(8), 765–774.

Boundy, E. O., Dastjerdi, R., Spiegelman, D., Fawzi, W. W., Missmer, S. A., Lieberman, E., . . . Chan, G. J. (2016). Kangaroo mother care and neonatal outcomes: A meta-analysis. *Pediatrics, 137*(1), Article e20152238.

Breeman, L. D., Jaekel, K., Baumann, N., Bartman, P., & Wolke, D. (2015). Preterm cognitive function into adulthood. *Pediatrics, 136*(3), 415–423.

Browne, J. V. (2011). Developmental care for high-risk newborns: Emerging science, clinical application, and continuity from newborn intensive care unit to community. *Clinical Perinatology, 38,* 719–729.

Burnett, A. C., Anderson, P. J., Lee, K. J., Roberts, G., Doyle, L. W., & Cheong, J. L. Y. for the Victorian Infant Collaborative Study Group. (2018). Trends in executive functioning in extremely preterm children across three birth eras. *Pediatrics, 141*(1), Article e20171958.

Camerota, M., Willoughby, M. T., Cox, M., & Greenberg, M. T., & the Family Life Project Investigators. (2015). Executive function in low birth weight preschoolers: The moderating effect of parenting. *Journal of Abnormal Child Psychology, 43,* 1551–1562.

Chen, J.-H., Claessens, A., & Msall, M. E. (2014). Prematurity and school readiness in a nationally representative sample of Australian children: Does typically occurring preschool moderate the relationship? *Early Human Development, 90,* 73–79.

Clark, C. A. C., Fang, J., Espy K. A., Filipek, P. A., Juranek, J., Bangert, B., . . . Taylor, H. G. (2013). Relation of neurological structure to persistently low academic achievement in children of differing birth weights. *Neuropsychology, 27,* 364–377.

Colditz, P. B., Boyd, R. N., Winter, L., Pritchard, M., Gray, P. H., Whittingham, K., . . . Sanders, M. R. (2019). A randomized trial of Baby Triple P for Preterm Infants: Child outcomes at 2 years of age. *Journal of Pediatrics, 210,* 48–54.

Crapnell, T. L., Woodward, L. J., Rogers, C. E., Inder, T. E., & Pineda, R. G. (2015). Neurodevelopmental profile, growth, and psychosocial environment of preterm infants with difficult feeding behavior at age 2 years. *Journal of Pediatrics, 167,* 1347–1353.

Day, K. L., Schmidt, L. A., Vaillancourt, T., Saigal, S., Boyle, M. H., & Van Lieshout, R. J. (2016). Long-term psychiatric impact of peer victimization in adults born at extremely low birth weight. *Pediatrics, 137*(3), Article e20153383.

De Kieviet, J. F., Stoof, C. J. J., Geldof, C. J. A., Smits, J., Piek, J. P., Lafeber, H. N., . . . Oosterlaan, J. (2013). The crucial role of the predictability of motor response in visuomotor deficits in very preterm children at school age. *Developmental Medicine and Child Neurology, 55,* 624–630.

de Vries, L. S., & Leijser, L. M. (2019). *Germinal matrix hemorrhage and intraventricular hemorrhage (GMH-IVH) in the newborn: Pathogenesis, clinical presentation, and diagnosis.* Retrieved June 11, 2019, from *www.uptodate.com.*

Dotinga, B. M., Eshuis, M. S., Bocca-Tjeertes, I. F., Kerstjens, J. M., Van Braeckel, K. N. J. A., Reijneveld, S. A., & Bos, A. F. (2016). Longitudinal growth and neuropsychological functioning at age 7 in moderate and late preterms. *Pediatrics, 138*(4), Article e20153638.

Douglas, L. M., Heeren, T. C., Stafstrom, C. E., DeBassio, W., Allred, E. N., Leviton, A., . . . Kuban, K. (2017). Cumulative incidence of seizures and epilepsy in ten-year-old children born before 28 weeks' gestation. *Pediatric Neurology, 73,* 13–19.

Doyle, L. W., & Anderson, P. J. (2010). Adult outcome of extremely preterm infants. *Pediatrics, 126,* 342–351.

Doyle, L. W., Anderson, P. J., Battin, M., Bowen, J. R., Brown, N., Callanan, C., . . . Woodward, W. J. (2014). Long term follow up of high risk children: Who, why and how? *BMC Pediatrics, 14,* Article 279.

Doyle, L. W., Cheong, J. L. Y., Burnett, A., Roberts, G., Lee, K. J., & Anderson, P. J., for the Victorian Infant Collaborative Study Group. (2015). Biological and social influences on outcomes of extreme-preterm/low-birth weight adolescents. *Pediatrics, 136*(6), e1513–e1520.

Doyle, L. W., Roberts, G., & Anderson, P. J. (2011). Changing long-term outcomes for infants 500–999 g birth weight in Victoria, 1979–2005. *Archives of Diseases of Children Fetal and Neonatal Edition, 96,* F443–F447.

Doyle, O., Harmon, C. P., Heckman, J. J., & Tremblay, R. E. (2009). Investing in early human development: Timing and economic efficiency. *Economics and Human Biology, 7,* 1–6.

Dubner, S. E., Dodson, C. K., Marchman, V. A.,

Ben-Shachar, M., Feldman, H. M., & Travis, K. E. (2019, April 22). White matter mircrostructure and cognitive outcomes in relation to neonatal inflammation in 6-year-old children born preterm. *NeuroImage Clinical, 23.*

Eryigit-Madzwamuse, S., Strauss, V., Baumann, N., Bartmann, P., & Wolke, D. (2015). Personality of adults who were born very preterm. *Archives of Disease in Children Fetal and Neonatal Edition, 100,* F524–F529.

Foster-Cohen, S. H., Friesen, M. D., Champion, P. R., & Woodward, L. J. (2010). High prevalence/low severity language delay in preschool children born very preterm. *Journal of Developmental and Behavioral Pediatrics, 31,* 658–667.

Franz, A. P., Bolat, G. U., Bolat, H., Matijasevich, A., Santos, I. S., Silveira, R. C., . . . Moreira-Maia, C. R. (2018). Attention-deficit/hyperactivity disorder and very preterm/very low birth weight: A meta-analysis. *Pediatrics, 141*(1), Article e20171645.

Geldof, C. J. A., van Wassenaer, A. G., de Kieviet, J. F., Kok, J. H., & Oosterlaan, J. (2012). Visual perception and visual-motor integration in very preterm and/or very low birth weight children: A meta-analysis. *Research in Developmental Disabilities, 33*(2), 726–736.

Hack, M., Forrest, C. B., Schluchter, M., Taylor, H. G., Drotar, D., Holmbeck, G., & Andreias, L. (2011). Health status of extremely low-birth-weight children at 8 years of age. *Archives of Pediatrics and Adolescent Medicine, 165*(10), 922–927.

Hack, M., Schluchter, M., Margevicius, S., Andreias, L., Taylor, H. G., & Cuttler, L. (2014). Trajectories and correlates of growth among extremely low birth weight adolescents. *Pediatric Research, 75*(2), 358–366.

Hasler, H. M., & Akshoomoff, N. (2019). Mathematics ability and related skills in preschoolers born very preterm. *Child Neuropsychology, 25*(1–2), 162–178.

Heindel, J. J., Balbus, J., Birnbaum, L., Brune-Drisse, M. N., Grandjean, P., Gray, K., . . . Hanson, M. (2015). Developmental origins of health and disease: Integrating environmental influences. *Endocrinology, 156*(10), 3416–3421.

Heinonen, K., Ericksson, J. G., Lahti, J., Kajantie, E., Pesonen, A.-K., Tuovinen, S., . . . Raikkonen, K. (2015). Late preterm birth and neurocognitive performance in late adulthood: A birth cohort study. *Pediatrics, 135*(4), e818–e825.

High, P. C. (2008). School readiness. *Pediatrics, 121,* e1008–e1015.

Hughes, A. J., Redsell, S. A., & Glazebrook, C. (2016). Motor development interventions for preterm infants: A systematic review and meta-analysis. *Pediatrics, 138*(4), Article e20160147.

Jaekel, J., Pluess, M., Belsky, J., & Wolke, D. (2015a). Effects of maternal sensitivity on low birth weight children's academic achievement: A test of differential susceptibility vs. diathesis stress. *Journal of Child Psychology and Psychiatry, 56*(6), 693–701.

Jaekel. J., Strauss, V. Y-C., Johnson, S., Gilmore, C., & Wolke, D. (2015b). Delayed school entry and academic performance: A natural experiment. *Developmental Medicine and Child Neurology, 57,* 652–659.

Jarjour, E. T. (2015). Neurodevelopmental outcome after extreme prematurity: A review of the literature. *Pediatric Neurology, 52,* 143–152.

Johnson, S., Evans, T. A., Draper, E. S., Field, D. J., Manktelow, B. N., Marlow, N., . . . Boyle, E. M. (2015a). Neurodevelopmental outcomes following late and moderate prematurity: A population-based cohort study. *Archives of Disease in Children, 100,* F301–F308.

Johnson, S., Gilmore, C., Gallimore, I., Jaekel, J., & Wolke, D. (2015b). The long-term consequences of preterm birth: What do teachers know? *Developmental Medicine and Child Neurology, 57,* 571–577.

Johnson, S., Hollis, C., Hennessy, E., Kochhar, P., Wolke, D., & Marlow, N. (2011a). Screening for autism in preterm children: Diagnostic utility of the Social Communication Questionnaire. *Archives of Disease of Children, 96,* 73–77.

Johnson, S., Hollis, C., Kochhar, P., Hennessy, E., Wolke, D., & Marlow, N. (2011b). Psychiatric disorders in extremely preterm children: Longitudinal findings at age 11 years in the EPICure Study. *Journal of the American Academy of Child and Adolescent Psychiatry, 49*(5), 453–463.

Johnson, S., Kockhar, P., Hennessy, E., Marlow, N., Wolke, D., & Hollis, C. (2016). Antecedents of attention-deficit/hyperactivity disorder symptoms in children born extremely preterm. *Journal of Developmental and Behavioral Pediatrics, 37*(4), 285–297.

Johnson, S., & Marlow, N. (2011). Preterm birth and childhood psychiatric disorders. *Pediatric Research, 69,* 11R–18R.

Johnson, S., & Marlow, N. (2017). Early and long-term outcome of infants born extremely preterm. *Archives of Diseases in Children, 102,* 97–102.

Johnson, S., Waheed, G., Manktelow, B. N., Field, D. J., Marlow, N., Draper, E. S., & Boyle, E. M. (2018). Differentiating the preterm phenotype:

Distinct profiles of cognitive and behavioral development following late and moderately preterm birth. *Journal of Pediatrics, 193*, 85–92.

Joseph, R. M., O'Shea, T. M., Allred, E. N., Heeren, T., Hirtz, D., Paneth, N., . . . Kuban, K. C. (2017). Prevalence and associated features of autism spectrum disorder in extremely low gestational age newborns at age 10 years. *Autism Research, 10*(2), 224–232.

Karolis, V. R., Froudist-Walsh, S., Kroll, J., Brittain, P. J., Tseng, C.-E. J., Nam, K.-W., . . . Nosarti, C. (2017). Volumetric grey matter alternations in adolescents and adults born very preterm suggest accelerated brain maturation. *NeuroImage, 163*, 379–389.

Khan, K. A., Petrou, S., Dritsaki, M., Johnson, S., Manktelow, B., Draper, E. S., . . . Boyle, E. M. (2015). Economic costs associated with moderate and late preterm birth: A prospective population-based study. *BJOG: An International Journal of Obstetrics and Gynaecology, 122*, 1495–1505.

Kidokoro, H., Anderson, P. J., Doyle, L. W., Woodward, L. J., Neil, J. J., & Inder, T. E. (2014). Brain injury and altered brain growth in preterm infants: Predictors and prognosis. *Pediatrics, 134*, e444–e453.

Kroll, J., Karolis, V., Brittain, P. J., Tseng, C.-E. J., Froudist-Walsh, S., Murray, R. M., & Nosarti, C. (2017). Real-life impact of executive function impairments in adults who were born very preterm. *Journal of the International Neuropsychological Society, 23*, 381–389.

Kuban, K. C. K., Jara, H., O'Shea, T. M., Heeren, T., Joseph, R. M., Fichorova, R. N., . . . Paneth, N., for the ELGAN Study Investigators. (2019). Association of circulating proinflammatory and anti-inflammatory protein biomarkers in extremely preterm born children with subsequent brain magnetic resonance imaging volumes and cognitive function at age 10 years. *Journal of Pediatrics, 210*, 81–90.

Lahat, A., van Lieshout, R. J., Saigal., S., Boyle, M. H., & Schmidt, L. A. (2015). Small for gestational age and poor fluid intelligence in childhood predict externalizing behaviors among young adults born at extremely low birth weight. *Development and Psychopathology, 27*, 181–188.

Litt, J. S., & McCormick, M. C. (2016). The impact of special health care needs on academic achievement in children born prematurely. *Academic Pediatrics, 16*(4), 350–357.

Litt, J. S., Glymour, M., Hauser-Cram, P., Hehir, T., & McCormick, M. S. (2018). Early intervention services improve school-age functional outcome among neonatal intensive care unit graduates. *Academic Pediatrics, 18*(4), 468–474.

Litt, J. S., Taylor, H. G., Margevicius, S., Schluchter, M., Andreias, L., & Hack, M. (2012). Academic achievement of adolescents born with extremely low birth weight. *Acta Paediatrica, 101*, 1240–1245.

Luu, T. M., Ment, L. R., Schneider, K. C., Katz, K. H., Allan, W. C., & Vohr, B. R. (2009). Lasting effects of preterm birth and neonatal brain hemorrhage at 12 years of age. *Pediatrics, 123*(3), 1037–1044.

Luu, T. M., Rehman Mian, M. O., & Nuyt, A. M. (2017). Long-term impact of preterm birth: Neurodevelopmental and physical health outcomes. *Clinics in Perinatology, 44*(2), 305–314.

Luu, T. M., Vohr, B. R., Allan, W., Schneider, K. C., & Ment, L. R. (2011). Evidence for catch-up in cognition and receptive vocabulary among adolescents born very preterm. *Pediatrics, 128*, 313–322.

Mandy, G. T., Weisman, L. E., & Kim, M. S. (2019). *Incidence and mortality of the preterm infant.* Retrieved July 7, 2019, from *www.uptodate.com.*

Mangin, K. S., Horwood, L. J., & Woodward, L. J. (2017). Cognitive development trajectories of very preterm and typically developing children. *Child Development, 88*(1), 282–298.

Manley, B. J., Roberts, R. S., Doyle, L. W., Schmidt, B., Anderson, P. J., Barrington, K. J., . . . Davis, P. G., on behalf of the Caffeine for Apnea of Prematurity (CAP) Trial Investigators. (2015). Social variables predict gains in cognitive scores across the preschool years in children with birth weights 500 to 1250 grams. *Journal of Pediatrics, 166*, 870–876.

Martin, J. A., Hamilton, B. E., Osterman, M. J. K., Driscoll, A. K., & Drake, P. (2018). Births: Final data for 2016. *National Vital Statistics Reports, 67*(1), 1–55.

Mathewson, K. J., Chow, C. H. T., Dobson, K. G., Pope, E. I., Schmidt, L. A., & Van Lieshout, R. J. (2017). Mental health of extremely low birth weight survivors: A systematic review and meta-analysis. *Psychological Bulletin, 143*(4), 347–383.

McCabe, E. R. B., Carrino, G. E., Russell, R. B., & Howse, J. L. (2014). Fighting for the next generation: U.S. prematurity in 2030. *Pediatrics, 134*(6), 1193–1199.

Ment, L. R., Aden, U., Lin, A., Kwon, S. H., Choi, M., Hallman, M., . . . Bauer, C. R., for the Gene Targets for IVH Study Group (2014). Gene-environment interactions in severe intraventricular hemorrhage of preterm neonates. *Pediatric Research, 75*(1), 241–250.

Ment, L. R., Hirtz, D., & Huppi, P. S. (2009a). Imaging biomarkers of outcome in the developing preterm brain. *Lancet, 8,* 1042–1055.

Ment, L. R., Kesler, S., Vohr, B., Katz, K. H., Baumgartner, H., Schneider, K. C., . . . Reiss, A. L. (2009b). Longitudinal brain volume changes in preterm and term control subjects during late childhood and adolescence, *Pediatrics, 123*(2), 503-511.

Milgrom, J., Newnham, C., Anderson, P. J., Doyle, L. W., Gemmill, A. W., Lee, K., . . . Inder, T. (2010). Early sensitivity training for parents of preterm infants: Impact on the developing brain. *Pediatric Research, 67,* 330–335.

Miller, S. L., Huppi, P. S., & Mallard, C. (2016). The consequences of fetal growth restriction on brain structure and neurodevelopmental outcomes. *Journal of Physiology, 594,* 807–823.

Molloy, C. S., Anderson, P. J., Anderson, V. A., & Doyle, L. W. (2016). The long-term outcome of extremely preterm (< 28 weeks' gestational age) infants with and without severe retinopathy of prematurity. *Journal of Neuropsychology, 10,* 276–294.

Molloy, C. S., Wilson-Ching, M., Anderson, V. A., Roberts, G., Anderson, P. J., & Doyle, L. W., for the Victoria Collaborative Study Group. (2013). Visual processing in adolescents born extremely low birth weight and/or extremely preterm. *Pediatrics, 132*(3), e704–e712.

Mukerji, A., Shan, V., & Shah, P. S. (2015). Periventricular/intraventricular hemorrhage and neurodevelopmental outcomes: A meta-analysis. *Pediatrics, 136*(6), 1132–1143.

Nguyen, T.-N.-N., Spencer-Smith, M., Haebich, K. M., Burnett, A., Scratch, S. E., Cheong, J. L. Y., . . . Anderson, P. J. (2018). Language trajectories of children born very preterm and full term from early to late childhood. *Journal of Pediatrics, 202,* 86–91.

Omizzolo, C., Scratch, S. E., Stargatt, R., Kidokoro, H., Thompson, D. K., Lee, K. J., . . . Anderson, P. J. (2014). Neonatal brain abnormalities and memory and learning outcomes at 7 years in children born very preterm. *Memory, 22*(6), 605–615.

O'Shea, T. M., Joseph, R. M., Allred, E. N., Taylor, H. G., Leviton, A., Heeren, T., . . . Kuban, K. C. K. for the ELGAN Study Investigators. (2018). Accuracy of the Bayley-II Mental Development Index at 2 years as a predictor of cognitive impairment at school age among children born extremely preterm. *Journal of Perinatology, 38,* 908–916.

Orchinik, L. J., Taylor, H. G., Espy, K. A., Minich, N., Klein, N., Sheffield, T., & Hack, M. (2011). Cognitive outcomes for extremely preterm/extremely low birth weight children in kindergarten. *Journal of the International Neuropsychological Society, 17,* 1067–1079.

Pace, C. C., Spittle, A. J., Molesworth, C. M.-L., Lee, K. J., Northam, E. A., Cheong, J. L. Y, . . . Anderson, P. J. (2016). Evolution of depression and anxiety symptoms in parents of very preterm infants during the newborn period. *JAMA Pediatrics, 170*(9), 863–870.

Pritchard, V. E., Bora, S., Austin, N. C., Levin, K. J., & Woodward, L. J. (2014). Identifying very preterm children at educational risk using a school readiness framework. *Pediatrics, 143*(3), e825–e832.

Pritchard, V. E., Clark, C. A. C., Liberty, K., Champion, P. R., Wilson, K., & Woodward, L. J. (2009). Early school-based learning difficulties in children born very preterm. *Early Human Development, 85,* 215–224.

Purisch, S. E., & Gyamfi-Bannerman, C. (2017). Epidemiology of preterm birth. *Seminars in Perinatology, 41,* 387–391.

Raju, T. N. K., Buist, A. S., Blaisdell, C. J., Moxey-Mims, M., & Saigal, S. (2017). Adults born preterm: A review of general health and system-specific outcomes. *Acta Paediatrica, 106,* 1409–1437.

Rand, K. M., Austin, C., Inder, T. E., Bora, S., & Woodward, L. J. (2016). Neonatal infection and later neurodevelopmental risk in the very preterm infant. *Journal of Pediatrics, 170,* 97–104.

Richards, J. L., Drews-Botsch, C., Sales, J. M., Flanders, W. D., & Kramer, M. R. (2016). Describing the shape of the relationship between gestational age at birth and cognitive development in a nationally representative U.S. Birth Cohort. *Paediatric and Perinatal Epidemiology, 30,* 571–582.

Ritchie, K., Bora, S., & Woodward, L. J. (2018). Peer relationship outcomes of school-age children born very preterm. *Journal of Pediatrics, 201,* 238–244.

Roberts, G., Lim, J., Doyle, L. W., & Anderson, P. J. (2011). High rates of school readiness difficulties at 5 years of age in very preterm infants compared with term controls. *Journal of Developmental and Behavioral Pediatrics, 32,* 117–124.

Rogers, E. E., & Hintz, S. R. (2016). Early neurodevelopmental outcomes of extremely preterm infants. *Seminars in Perinatology, 40,* 497–509.

Saigal, S., Ferro, M. A., Van Lieshout, R. J., Schmidt, L. A., Morrison, K. M., & Boyle, M. H. (2016a). Health-related quality of life trajectories of extremely low birth weight survivors into adulthood. *Journal of Pediatrics, 179,* 68–73.

Saigal, S., Kay, K. L., Van Lieshout, R. J., Schmidt, L. A., Morrison, K. M., & Boyle, M. H. (2016b). Health, wealth, social integration, and sexuality of extremely low-birth-weight prematurely born adults in the fourth decade of life. *JAMA Pediatrics, 170*(7), 678–686.

Samra, H. A., McGrath, J. M., & Wehbe, M. (2011). An integrated review of developmental outcomes and late-preterm birth. *Journal of Obstetric, Gynaecologic and Neonatal Nursing, 40,* 399–411.

Sansavini, A., Guarini, A., & Caselli, M. C. (2011). Preterm birth: Neuropsychological profiles and atypical developmental pathways. *Developmental Disabilities Research Reviews, 17,* 102–113.

Scott, M. N., Taylor, H. G., Fristad, M. A., Klein, N., Espy, K. A., Minich, N., & Hack, M. (2012). Behavior disorders in extremely preterm/extremely low birth weight children in kindergarten. *Journal of Developmental and Behavioral Pediatrics, 33,* 202–213.

Shah, P. E., Kaciroti, N., Richards, B., & Lumeng, J. C. (2016). Gestational age and kindergarten school readiness in a national sample of preterm infants. *Journal of Pediatrics, 178,* 61–67.

Simms, V., Gilmore, C., Cragg, L., Clayton, S., Marlow, N., & Johnson, S. (2015). Nature and origins of mathematics difficulties in very preterm children: A different etiology than developmental dyscalculia. *Pediatric Research, 77,* 389–395.

Somhovd, M. J., Hansen, B. M., Brok, J., Esbjorn, B. H., & Greisen, G. (2012). Anxiety in adolescents born preterm or with very low birthweight: A meta-analysis of case–control studies. *Developmental Medicine and Child Neurology, 54*(11), 988–994.

Spittle, A. J., Cameron, K., Doyle, L. W., & Cheong, J. L. for the Victorian Infant Collaborative Study Group. (2018a). Motor impairment trends in extremely preterm children: 1991–2005. *Pediatrics, 141*(4), Article e20173410.

Spittle, A. J., Orton, J., Anderson, P., Boyd, R., & Doyle, L. W. (2015). Early developmental intervention programmes provided post-hospital discharge to prevent motor and cognitive impairments in preterm infants. *Cochrane Database of Systematic Reviews, 11,* CD005495.

Spittle, A. J., & Treyvaud, K. (2016). The role of early developmental intervention to influence neurobehavioral outcomes of children born preterm. *Seminars in Perinatology, 40,* 542–548.

Spittle, A. J., Treyvaud, K., Lee, K., Anderson, P. J., & Doyle, L. W. (2018b). The role of social risk in an early preventative care programme for infants born very preterm: A randomized controlled trial. *Developmental Medicine and Child Neurology, 60,* 54–62.

Stangenes, K. M., Hysing, M., Fevang, S. K., Elgen, I. B., Halvorsen, T., Markestad, T., & Bjorvatn, B. (2018). Prenatal and neonatal factors predicting sleep problems in children born extremely preterm or with extremely low birthweight. *Frontiers in Pediatrics, 6,* Article 178.

Stoll, B. J., Hansen, N. I., Bell, E. F., Walsh, M. C., Carlo, W. A., Shandaran, S., . . . Higgins, R. D. for the Eunice Kennedy Shriver National Institute of Child Health and Development Neonatal Research Network. (2015). Trends in care practices, morbidity, and mortality of extremely preterm neonates, 1993–2012. *Journal of the American Medical Association, 314*(10), 1039–1051.

Strang-Karlsson, S., Andersson, S., Paile-Hyvarinen, M., Darby, D., Hovi, P., Raikkonen, K., . . . Kajantie, E. (2010). Slower reaction times and impaired learning in young adults with birth weight < 1500 g. *Pediatrics, 125,* e74–e82.

Synnes, A., Luu, T. M., Moddermann, D., Church, P., Lee, D., Vincer, M., . . . Lee, S. K. on behalf of the Canadian Neonatal Network and the Canadian Neonatal Follow-up Network. (2017). Determinants of developmental outcomes in a very preterm Canadian cohort. *Archives of Disease in Children Fetal and Neonatal Edition, 102,* F235–F243.

Tatsuoka, C., McGowan, B., Yamada, T., Espy, K. A., Minich, N., & Taylor, H. G. (2016). Effects of extreme prematurity on numerical skills and executive function in kindergarten children: An application of partially ordered classification modeling. *Learning and Individual Differences, 49,* 332–340.

Taylor, H. G., Espy, K. A., & Anderson, P. J. (2009). Mathematics deficiencies in children with very low birth weight or very preterm birth. *Developmental Disabilities Research Reviews, 15,* 52–59.

Taylor, H. G., Klein, N., Espy, K. A., Schluchter, M., Minich, N., Stilp, R., & Hack, M. (2018). Effects of extreme prematurity and kindergarten neuropsychological skills on early academic progress. *Neuropsychology, 32*(7), 809–821.

Taylor, H. G., Margevicius, S., Schluchter, M., Andreias, L., & Hack, M. (2015). Persisting behavior problems in extremely low birth weight adolescents. *Journal of Developmental and Behavioral Pediatrics, 36,* 178–187.

Taylor, H. G., Minich, N. M., Klein, N., & Hack, M. (2004). Longitudinal outcome of very low birth weight: Neuropsychological findings. *Journal of the International Neuropsychological Society, 10,* 149–163.

Taylor, H. G., Minich, N., Schluchter, M., Espy, K. A., & Klein, N. (2019a). Resilience in extremely preterm/extremely low birth weight kindergarten children. *Journal of the International Neuropsychological Society, 25,* 362–374.

Taylor, H. G., Orchinik, L., Fristad, M. A., Minich, N., Klein, N., Espy, K. A., . . . Hack, M. (2019b). Associations of attention deficit hyperactivity disorder (ADHD) at school entry with early academic progress in children born prematurely and full-term controls. *Learning and Individual Differences, 69,* 1–10.

Treyvaud, K., Doyle, L. W., Lee, K. J., Ure, A., Inder, T. E., Hunt, R. W., & Anderson, P. J. (2016). Parenting behavior at 2 years predicts school-age performance at 7 years in very preterm children. *Journal of Child Psychology and Psychiatry, 57*(7), 814–821.

Treyvaud, K., Ure, A., Doyle, L. W., Lee, K. J., Rogers, C. E., Kidokoro, H., . . . Anderson, P. J. (2013). Psychiatric outcomes ag age seven for very preterm children: Rates and predictors. *Journal of Child Psychology and Psychiatry, 54*(7), 772–779.

Vandormael, C., Schoenhals, L., Huppi, P. S., Filippa, M., & Tolsa, C. B. (2019). Language in preterm born children: Atypical development and effects of early interventions on neuroplasticity. *Neural Plasticity, 2019,* 6873270.

Vohr, B. (2014). Speech and language outcomes of very preterm infants. *Seminars in Fetal and Neonatal Medicine, 19,* 78–83.

Wang, T.-N., Howe, T.-H., Lin, K.-C., & Hsu, Y.-W. (2014). Hand function and its prognostic factors of very low birth weight preterm children up to a corrected age of 24 months. *Research in Developmental Disabilities, 35,* 322–329.

Williams, J., Lee, K. J., & Anderson, P. J. (2010). Prevalence of motor-skill impairment in preterm children who do not develop cerebral palsy: A systematic review. *Developmental Medicine and Child Neurology, 52,* 232–237.

Wilson-Ching, M., Molloy, C. S., Anderson, V. A., Burnett, A., Roberts, G., Cheong, J. L., . . . Anderson, P. J. (2013). Attention difficulties in a contemporary geographic cohort of adolescents born extremely preterm/extremely low birth weight. *Journal of the International Neuropsychological Society, 19*(10), 1097–1108.

Wilson-Ching, M., Pascoe, L., Doyle, L. W., & Anderson, P. J. (2014). Effects of correcting for prematurity on cognitive test scores in childhood. *Journal of Paediatrics and Child Health, 50,* 182–188.

Wilson-Costello, D., & Payne, A. (2019). *Long-term neurodevelopmental outcome of preterm infants: Epidemiology and risk factors.* Retrieved May 5, 2019, from *www.uptodate.com.*

Wong, T., Taylor, H. G., Klein, N., Espy, K. A., Anselmo, M. G., Minich, N., & Hack, M. (2014). Kindergarten classroom functioning of extremely preterm/extremely low birth weight children. *Early Human Development, 90,* 907–914.

Woodward, L. J., Bora, S., Clark, C. A. C., Montgomery-Honger, A., Pritchard, V. E., Spencer, C., & Austin, N. C. (2014). Very preterm birth: Maternal experiences of the neonatal intensive care environment. *Journal of Perinatology, 34,* 555–561.

Woodward, L. J., Lu, Z., Morris, A., & Healey, D. (2017). Self-regulatory skills during early childhood are associated with later mental health and educational achievement in very preterm and typically developing children. *Clinical Neuropsychologist, 31*(2), 404–422.

Woodward, L. J., Moor, S., Hood, K. M., Champion, P. R., Foster-Cohen, S., & Inder, T. E. (2009). Very preterm children show impairments across multiple neurodevelopmental domains by age 4 years. *Archives of Diseases of Children Fetal and Neonatal Edition, 94,* F339–F344.

Zwicker, J. G., Miller, S. P., Grunau, R. E., Chau, V., Brant, R., Studholme, C., . . . Tam, E. W. Y. (2016). Smaller cerebellar growth and poorer neurodevelopmental outcomes in very preterm infants exposed to neonatal morphine. *Journal of Pediatrics, 172,* 81–87.

CHAPTER 8

Congenital Heart Disease

Adam R. Cassidy

The human heart begins beating 3 weeks after conception. Its distinctive four chambers and accompanying vessels are formed by 8–10 weeks' gestation, making it the body's first functional organ. Congenital heart disease (CHD) describes a diverse constellation of conditions, ranging from mild to critical, wherein heart development does not proceed as expected. In some instances, these deviations are small and relatively benign, and may be left to resolve on their own. Others require early and intensive intervention(s) to surgically manufacture the conditions necessary for life. This chapter focuses on these "critical" forms of CHD and their impact on brain and behavioral development.

HISTORICAL OVERVIEW

The majority of children born with even the most critical forms of CHD such as hypoplastic left heart syndrome (HLHS) and dextro-transposition of the great arteries (d-TGA) are now surviving well into adulthood (Spector et al., 2018; Warnes et al., 2001). This was not the case a few decades ago. As recently as the early 1980s, a diagnosis of HLHS was considered fatal, and it was not yet known whether newborns with d-TGA could survive the arterial switch operation that was needed to reconfigure their transposed aorta and pulmonary artery. Survival rates for HLHS now exceed 80%, and the neonatal arterial switch operation remains the standard of care for the treatment of d-TGA. In this way, the history of CHD traces a course not unlike that of leukemia, extreme prematurity, and several other major medical conditions with which pediatric neuropsychologists are familiar: Driven by monumental advances in medical and surgical care, what once was fatal is no longer.

And now that critical CHD is no longer uniformly fatal, the balance of attention among clinicians and researchers has shifted toward understanding and optimizing outcomes for the growing population of CHD survivors. Whether independently or as a member of a dedicated cardiac neurodevelopmental follow-up clinic, pediatric neuropsychologists are being called on with increasing regularity to contribute to the care of children, adolescents, and young adults with CHD.

EPIDEMIOLOGY

CHD ranks among the most prevalent congenital conditions, affecting an estimated 9 per 1,000 live births (Hoffman & Kaplan, 2002). In the United States alone, this equates to approximately 40,000 children born with CHD per year. Roughly 6 per 1,000 children have either moderate or severe CHD; and, 3 per 1,000 are born with a critical form of CHD requiring early and intensive surgical intervention(s) to sustain life (Hoffman & Kaplan, 2002). Descriptions of several common CHD types and frequently encountered cardiac procedures are provided in Tables 8.1 and 8.2, respectively.

CHD survival rates correlate with disease severity/complexity. Long-term survival is thought to be around 95% for simple forms of CHD (e.g., atrial septal defect, ventricular septal defect); 90% for moderate-severity CHD (e.g., coarctation of the aorta, tetralogy of Fallot); and, 80% for the most severe and complex forms of CHD (e.g., single-ventricle conditions) (Warnes et al., 2001). Looking at early- (1982–1992) versus later-era (1998–2003) 15-year standardized mortality ratios, which provide an index of long-term mortality relative to the general population, survival has improved over time for all forms of CHD, particularly the most severe forms such as d-TGA (11.0 vs. 3.8) and single-ventricle conditions (53.7 vs. 31.3) (Spector et al., 2018).

ETIOLOGY, NEUROPATHOLOGY, AND NEURAL SUBSTRATES

Etiology

The etiology of CHD is thought to be multifactorial. Both genetic and environmental factors have been implicated and seem to functionally converge in undermining protein networks involved in early heart development (Lage et al., 2012). Recent advances in genomewide and high-throughput genetic sequencing have greatly enhanced our knowledge of the underlying causes of CHD (Morton, Quiat, Seidman, & Seidman, 2021; Russell, Chung, Kaltman, & Miller, 2018). An estimated 28% of congenital heart defects have an identified genetic etiology (Russell et al., 2018). Of these, 6% involve *chromosomal abnormalities* (e.g., trisomies 13, 18, and 21; Turner syndrome); 10% involve *copy number variants* (e.g., 22q11.2/DiGeorge syndrome, 7q11.23/Williams–Beuren syndrome, 1p36 and 8p23.1 deletion syndromes); and, 12% involve *single-gene defects* such as the RASopathies (e.g., Noonan syndrome, Costello syndrome), ciliopathies (e.g., Bardet-Biedl syndrome, Alstrom syndrome, McKusick–Kaufman syndrome), chromatin modifier-related syndromes (e.g., Holt–Oram syndrome), and other nonsyndromic de novo variants (Russell et al., 2018). Interestingly, exome sequencing of individuals with CHD and their unaffected parents has shown that approximately 10% of CHD is caused by coding variants not present in either parent (i.e., de novo variants); and, this estimate rises to about 20% when comorbid neurodevelopmental deficits and/or extracardiac anomalies are also present (Homsy et al., 2015).

In addition to genetic factors, advanced maternal age (Miller, Riehle-Colarusso, Siffel, Frías, & Correa, 2011), assisted reproductive techniques (e.g., *in vitro* fertilization; Tararbit et al., 2014), and *in utero* exposure to certain maternal illnesses/infections (e.g., phenylketonuria, rubella, diabetes, influenza, febrile illnesses), drugs/substances (e.g., cigarette smoking, alcohol, fluoxetine), and/or environmental contaminants (e.g., vehicle exhaust,

TABLE 8.1. Description of Selected CHD Subtypes (Presented Alphabetically) and Associated Genetic Conditions

Defect	Type	Description	Associated genetic conditions/syndromes
Aortic valve stenosis	Systemic outflow obstructive lesion	Malformation of aortic valve (bicuspid, unicuspid, or dysplastic)	Williams (though usually associated with supravalvar AS)
Atrial septal defect (ASD)	2V shunt lesion	Defect in the wall (septum) between the left and right atrium	VACTERL; CHARGE; Down (T21); fetal alcohol syndrome; Holt–Oram
Atrio-ventricular (AV) canal defect	2V shunt lesion, may be associated with more complex SV defect	Defect in the formation of the endocardial cushions. Incomplete: primum ASD with cleft mitral valve. Complete: primum ASD and large inlet VSD, single, common atrioventricular valve	Down (T21); Noonan; heterotaxy
Coarctation of the aorta (CoA)	Systemic obstructive lesion	Narrowing of the aortic arch, usually discrete. Can occur in isolation or with other left-sided lesions (anomalies of the mitral and aortic valve)	Down (T21); Turner; Alagille
Dextro-transposition of the great arteries (d-TGA)	Conotruncal anomaly	Ventricular arterial discordance (i.e., the aorta originates from the RV and the pulmonary artery from the LV)	
Double inlet left ventricle (DILV)	SV with conotruncal abnormality with pulmonary or systemic outflow obstruction	Mitral and tricuspid valves drain into the LV, usually with atrioventricular discordance and transposed great arteries	
Ebstein anomaly	Severe valvular defect	Inferior displacement of the septal leaflets of the tricuspid valve that are abnormally tethered to the right ventricular septum	
Hypoplastic left heart syndrome (HLHS)	SV with systemic outflow obstruction	Underdeveloped or severely dysfunctional LV, usually with mitral valve and aortic valve stenosis or atresia and aortic arch hypoplasia	Jacobsen; Turner
Patent ductus arteriosus (PDA)	Shunt lesion	Failure of the ductus arteriosus to close	Down (T21); CHARGE; Rubinstein–Taybi; also associated with premature birth and rubella

Pulmonary valve stenosis (PS)	Pulmonary outflow obstructive lesion	Thickened pulmonary valve, abnormal leaflets	Noonan; Williams (including supravalvar and branch PS)
Pulmonary atresia with intact ventricular septum	SV (or 2V) with pulmonary outflow obstruction	Pulmonary valve atresia with underdeveloped RV, tricuspid valve may be small with stenosis or regurgitation. RV-dependent coronary circulation may be present.	
Tetralogy of Fallot (TOF)	Conotruncal anomaly	Four anatomic abnormalities, including (1) VSD, (2) anterior shift of the aorta over the VSD, (3) subpulmonary and pulmonary valve stenosis or atresia, and (4) RV hypertrophy (occurs later if not repaired)	Alagille; CHARGE; Down (T21); DiGeorge (22q11.2); VACTERL
Total anomalous pulmonary venous return (TAPVR)	Multiple variants; can occur with obstruction	Pulmonary veins drain anomalously into a systemic vein which enters the right atrium	
Tricuspid atresia	SV usually with pulmonary outflow obstruction (though may be associated with systemic outflow obstruction or no outflow obstruction)	Tricuspid valve is atretic with underdeveloped RV, VSD may be present, great arteries normal or transposed	
Truncus arteriosus	Conotruncal anomaly	Failed separation of aortic and pulmonary arteries such that there is a single arterial trunk, usually with a VSD. Can have an associated interrupted aortic arch	DiGeorge (22q11.2)
Ventricular septal defect (VSD)	Shunt lesion	Defect in the wall (septum) between ventricles	VACTERL; CHARGE; Down (T21); Noonan; DiGeorge (22q11.2); trisomies 13 and 18

Note. SV, single-ventricle; 2V, two-ventricle/biventricle; ASD, atrial septal defect; LV, left ventricle; RV, right ventricle; VSD, ventricular septal defect. Obstructive lesions refer to lesions that involve narrowing of blood vessels or blood flow within the heart. Shunt lesions refer to lesions in which directional blood flow patterns are atypical. Conotruncal anomalies refer to malformations of the heart's outflow tracts. Adapted from Cassidy et al. (2018, 863). Copyright 2017 by Informa UK Limited, trading as Taylor & Francis Group. Reprinted with permission.

TABLE 8.2. Frequently Encountered Cardiac Procedures, Surgeries, and Mechanical Support Devices

Procedure/device	Shorthand	Description
Cardiac catheterization	Cardiac cath	Invasive (non-open-heart) procedure used to examine heart structure and function, and measure oxygen and pressure in each chamber of the heart. A thin tube (i.e., catheter or long IV) is inserted into a blood vessel in the groin, neck, or arm, and threaded to the heart.
Cardiac MRI	–	Noninvasive procedure that uses a strong magnetic field to create detailed images of the structure of the heart and blood vessels.
Cardiac stress test	Stress test	Noninvasive test during which a patient is asked to walk on a treadmill/ride bike while his/her vital signs and cardiac status are monitored; used to evaluate heart function under the stress of exercise
Echocardiogram	Echo; cardiac ultrasound	Non-invasive clinical test that uses ultrasound (i.e., high-frequency sound waves) to create pictures of the heart and blood vessels. It is used to assess heart structure, function, and blood flow.
Extracorporeal membrane oxygenation	ECMO	Mechanical support device, reserved for use among the most critical patients, wherein a cardiopulmonary bypass machine moves blood from the patient to an external "lung," where it is oxygenated and carbon dioxide is removed, before returning it to the patient. Sedation is required to prevent the child from moving and to keep the apparatus positioned appropriately.
Heart transplantation (orthotopic heart transplant)	–	Invasive surgical procedure wherein a patient's heart is removed and replaced with a donor heart. Most commonly performed in the case of end-stage heart failure.
Implanted cardioverter–defibrillator	ICD	Surgically implanted device, similar but slightly larger in size than a pacemaker, which detects ventricular arrhythmias and is capable of sending out either a low-energy electrical pulse to return the heart to a more appropriate rhythm or a high-energy pulse in the case of a more severe arrhythmia.

Pacemaker	—	Small, battery-powered device implanted in the chest or abdomen. Wires with electrodes are extended from the pacemaker and attached directly on to the heart. Pacemakers monitor the heart's rhythm and, when necessary, send out an electrical pulse to reestablish a normal heart rate and/or rhythm.
Ventricular assist device	VAD	Mechanical support device, used most often is the case of heart failure to support blood flow from one or both lower heart chambers (ventricles) while awaiting surgery or transplant.
Two-ventricle repair	—	Surgical operation that restores a normal circulation. Examples include 1. Arterial switch for TGA 2. Transannular patch and VSD closure for TOF 3. ASD/VSD and repair of AV valve for endocardial cushion defect 4. ASD or VSD closure for septal defect 5. RV to pulmonary artery conduit placement with VSD closure for TOF/PA or truncus 6. Arch repair for coarctation of the aorta
Single ventricle palliation; usually staged, with final operation the Fontan procedure	—	1. Norwood with shunt for HLHS, BT shunt for tricuspid atresia or pulmonary atresia with hypoplastic right heart, pulmonary artery band for complex SV with no aortic/pulmonary obstruction (soon after birth) 2. SVC to pulmonary artery connection—bidirectional Glenn or hemi-Fontan (4–12 months) 3. Systemic venous baffle (SVC and IVC to PA)—Fontan (18 months to 3 years)

Note. TGA, transposition of the great arteries; VSD, ventricular septal defect; TOF, tetralogy of Fallot; ASD, atrial septal defect; AV, aortic valve; RV, right ventricle; PA, pulmonary atresia; HLHS, hypoplastic left heart syndrome; BT, Blalock–Taussig; SV, single-ventricle; SVC, superior vena cava; IVC, inferior vena cava. From Cassidy et al. (2018, p. 864).

agricultural pesticides) have also been linked to CHD (Gao et al., 2017; Hoang, Marengo, Mitchell, Can, & Agopian, 2017; Jenkins et al., 2007; Nicoll, 2018).

Neuropathology and Neural Substrates

The brain and the heart develop in tandem, the result of partially overlapping genetic programs, shared embryonic cell lineages, and transacting physiologies that bind them together from very early in the fetal period (McQuillen & Miller, 2010). As early as the second or third prenatal trimester, brain maturation is atypical among fetuses with critical CHD (Clouchoux et al., 2013; Limperopoulos et al., 2010; Ortinau et al., 2019; Schellen et al., 2015; Sun et al., 2015; Wu et al., 2021). Compared to healthy controls, fetuses with complex CHD exhibit impaired neuronal/axonal health and relative declines in total brain volume during the third trimester (Limperopoulos et al., 2010), with continued divergence from expected brain growth trajectories across the transition from prenatal to postnatal environments (Ortinau et al., 2018b). Relative declines in third trimester cortical–subcortical gray and cortical white matter volumes have also been noted among fetuses with HLHS (Clouchoux et al., 2013). Prominent delays in cortical gyrification were evident even earlier, beginning at 25 weeks' gestation, and, in fact, predated drop-offs in brain volume in this cohort, suggesting that delays in cortical folding may be a harbinger of later arrests in brain growth (Clouchoux et al., 2013). Delays in total brain, gray matter, and subcortical volumes have since been reported even earlier than 25 weeks' gestation in fetuses with tetralogy of Fallot (TOF; Schellen et al., 2015). Ortinau and colleagues (2019) reported second-trimester alterations in Sylvian fissure and early-emerging sulci, predominantly within the left hemisphere. And in a recent study, clinically-elevated levels of stress and anxiety among women carrying fetuses with CHD were not only highly prevalent (65% and 44% for stress and anxiety, respectively) but were also associated with reduced hippocampal and cerebellar volumes in fetuses at 21–40 weeks' gestation (Wu et al., 2021).

As in the fetal period, abnormalities in axonal/neuronal health have been documented postnatally among infants with complex CHD (Miller et al., 2007). At birth, the pattern of brain maturation seen in newborns with d-TGA and HLHS is equivalent to what would be seen 4 weeks earlier in gestation (Licht et al., 2009). Prior to cardiac surgery, conventional magnetic resonance imaging (MRI) studies have observed total (von Rhein et al., 2015a) and regional alterations in brain size within the thalamus and basal ganglia (Owen et al., 2013), as well as the frontal lobe and brainstem (Ortinau et al., 2012); reduced cortical surface area and cortical folding, particularly within the right lateral sulcus and left orbitofrontal cortex, cingulate cortex, and central sulcus (Ortinau et al., 2013); impaired dendritic arborization (Kelly et al., 2019); and, incomplete closure of the operculum (Licht et al., 2009). Findings regarding the operculum—a structure known to be involved in feeding and language development—are particularly notable in light of evidence that pre- to postsurgical growth in left temporal auditory and language areas (i.e., Heschl's gyrus, anterior planum temporale) is correlated with 12-month language abilities among infants with CHD (Jakab, Meuwly, Feldmann, von Rhein, & Kottke, 2019).

Volumetric and structural brain abnormalities are also highly prevalent among adolescents with complex CHD. Quantitative volumetric MRI studies have revealed reduced total brain, white matter, and subcortical gray matter volumes (Rivkin et al., 2013; von Rhein et al., 2014), particularly within the striatum and pallidum, and more widely distributed across parietal, medial frontoparietal, cingulate, and temporal areas (Watson et al., 2016). Hippocampal alterations (Fontes et al., 2019; Munoz-Lopez et al., 2017), abnormal left-hemisphere sulcal patterns (Morton et al., 2020), and reduced posterior cerebellar volume (Semmel, Dotson, Burns, Mahle, & King, 2018) have also been reported during adolescence and young adulthood.

According to a recent systematic review and meta-analysis (Bolduc, Lambert, Ganeshamoorthy, & Brossard-Racine, 2018), adolescents with CHD were 15.6 times more likely than healthy controls to present with a brain abnormality on MRI. The risk was especially high for adolescents with single-ventricle physiology, who were much more likely to present with a brain abnormality than adolescents with two-ventricle physiology. Furthermore, of the abnormalities detected, brain mineralization was particularly common (found in 23–60% of adolescents), likely the sequelae of subtle hemorrhagic injury sustained much earlier in life.

Throughout development, white matter dysmaturity and injury are among the most common neuropathological findings associated with critical CHD (Beca et al., 2013; Claessens et al., 2019; Guo et al., 2018; Mahle et al., 2002; Miller et al., 2007; Ortinau et al., 2012; Rivkin et al., 2013). In a longitudinal study of 153 infants with CHD, white matter injury was present in 20% of infants prior to surgery, and an additional 42% after surgery (Beca et al., 2013). Despite some indication that white matter lesions may resolve over time (Andropoulos et al., 2010; Mahle et al., 2002), evidence of widespread reductions in fractional anisotropy (Rivkin et al., 2013) and associated neurobehavioral difficulties in a cohort of adolescents with d-TGA (Rollins et al., 2014) suggest that disturbances in white matter microstructural integrity do, in fact, persist, and may be permanent. Looking at the connectome, alterations in white matter network topology have also been documented among these adolescents, including increased modularity and small-worldness, as well as a trend-level reduction in global network efficiency, and were indeed found to mediate a range of cognitive outcomes (Panigrahy et al., 2015; Schmithorst et al., 2016).

Furthermore, brain dysmaturity and risk for white matter injury are not independent. Rather, brains that are less structurally and microstructurally mature seem to provide a vulnerable substrate within which white matter injury is more likely to occur. Across several cohorts of infants with complex CHD, overall brain immaturity has been identified as an independent predictor of both presurgical and newly acquired postsurgical white matter injury (Andropoulos et al., 2010; Beca et al., 2013; Dimitropoulos et al., 2013) and, in at least one study, presurgical brain immaturity was associated with more severe white matter injury following surgery (Andropoulos et al., 2010). The risk for intraventicular hemorrhage (IVH) was also higher among infants with CHD, most notably among those who were also born preterm, and indeed the more preterm the delivery, the higher the risk for IVH (Ortinau, Anadkat, Smyser, & Eghtesady, 2018a).

Why is white matter particularly vulnerable to disruption in CHD? The third-trimester timing of deflection from typical brain maturation trajectories may provide some insight. In the final 3 months leading up to birth, the fetal brain undergoes prodigious growth and change marked by axon path finding, synapse formation, and the refinement of cortical networks. To fuel this massive undertaking, approximately one-fourth of the combined ventricular output from the fetal heart is pumped to the brain; and one-half of all oxygen consumed by the fetus is consumed within the brain (Sun et al., 2015). Around this same time in gestation, the population of cells that will ultimately go on to become mature, white matter-producing oligodendrocytes consists overwhelmingly of premyelinating oligodendrocytes that are extremely vulnerable to hypoxic–ischemic injury (Volpe, Kinney, Jensen, & Rosenberg, 2011). Disruptions in cerebral oxygen delivery and consumption are common among third-trimester fetuses with complex CHD (Sun et al., 2015) and, as demonstrated in a recent sheep model, even when adequate delivery of calories/nutrients to the brain is maintained, fetal hypoxia is associated with white matter hypervascularity, lower neuronal density, and impaired myelination (Lawrence et al., 2019; also see Stinnett et al., 2017). Similar to healthy controls, myelination in infants with CHD progresses in a posterior-to-anterior and central-to-peripheral fashion (Claessens et al., 2019). However, unlike the central predominance of white matter injury more commonly seen in preterm infants, in whom the peak of white matter injury occurs earlier in gestation, white matter injury in individuals with CHD seems to have a predilection for later-myelinating anterior and posterior regions, including the corona radiata/centrum semiovale, posterior periventricular white matter, and corticocortical white matter tracts (Guo et al., 2018; Rivkin et al., 2013)—consistent with the third-trimester timing of altered development in CHD.

In summary, as advanced neuroimaging modalities have permitted ever-greater insights into brain structure, function, and network organization, it has become increasingly clear that critical CHD poses a serious threat to typical brain development. Developing white matter tracts are particularly vulnerable, likely the result of *in utero* alterations in brain growth and maturation (i.e., dysmaturity) that conspire in creating a neural foundation within which injury is more likely to occur.

NEUROPSYCHOLOGICAL CONSEQUENCES

Having established that brain development is undermined by critical CHD, we now turn to a discussion of functional outcomes informed by a neuropsychological level of analysis (see also Cassidy et al., 2018). First, to briefly address a misconception: that all or even most children with CHD present with a cohesive, distinctive, predictable neurobehavioral "signature." While it is indeed the case that most children with isolated (i.e., nonsyndromic) critical CHD do not exhibit broad-based general cognitive deficits, there seems to be considerable heterogeneity in individual neuropsychological profiles (Cassidy et al., 2018; Sanz et al., 2021). Moreover, although weaknesses in executive function, attention, visuospatial processing, and social cognition are perhaps among the most commonly reported neurobehavioral challenges for children with CHD, the notion that any singular profile of strengths and weaknesses represents a pathognomonic signature that reliably distinguishes individuals with CHD from those with other neurodevelopmental disorders (or who are typically developing) is not well-supported, nor is such a signature likely to be identified in a population as diverse as the CHD population.

General Intellectual Functioning

Global impairment in general intellectual functioning is uncommon among children and adolescents with CHD. Most demonstrate intelligence quotient (IQ) scores within the average to low-average range for age, although this depends in part on the severity of their CHD, as well as what specific components of IQ are considered. In a meta-analysis examining Full Scale IQ scores by CHD subtype (Karsdorp, Everaerd, Kindt, & Mulder, 2007), trivial-to-small mean effects, on the order of approximately 2 to 3 standard score points below normative standards, were found for children with d-TGA or TOF. In contrast, a large mean effect of approximately 12 standard score points below normative standards was detected for children with HLHS (Karsdorp et al., 2007) and has since been replicated in a more recent meta-analysis (Siciliano et al., 2019). There is also some indication that effect size magnitudes may vary depending on the source of comparator data. Murphy et al. (2017), for example, reported that in comparison to healthy siblings, Full Scale IQ scores were nearly two-thirds of a standard deviation lower among adolescents and young adults with d-TGA or TOF. If replicated, this finding suggests that study designs that fail to account for demographic and other shared environmental factors may underestimate the true magnitude of cognitive differences seen in individuals with CHD.

When IQ is further divided by domain, effects on Performance IQ are reliably stronger than they are on Verbal IQ (Karsdorp et al., 2007; Mills, McCusker, Tennyson, & Hanna, 2017). In a meta-analysis of 18 unique cohorts of adolescents and young adults with CHD requiring invasive interventions, whereas verbal reasoning abilities were not significantly different from population expectations (~2 standard score points), nonverbal reasoning abilities were one-third of a standard deviation (5 standard score points) below the norm (Mills et al., 2018). A similar pattern held for children with d-TGA and HLHS (Karsdorp et al., 2007); however, the magnitude of the differences was much greater among children with HLHS, who were found on average to have Verbal IQ scores approximately 6–9 points below the norm and Performance IQ scores approximately 13 points below the norm (Karsdorp et al., 2007; Siciliano et al., 2019).

Perceptual and Sensorimotor Skills

Visuospatial/perceptual processing and visuomotor integration abilities are highly sensitive to disruption by CHD. Basic visual-perceptual processing abilities, including visual discrimination, figure-ground perception, and visual closure, among others, were found to be below expected population means in adolescents with d-TGA, TOF, or single-ventricle conditions requiring the Fontan procedure (Bellinger et al., 2011, 2015a, 2015b). Across several studies, children and adolescents with various forms of CHD scored lower than controls and/or expected population norms on tasks of visuomotor integration (Brosig et al., 2013; Kirshbom et al., 2005; Mahle et al., 2000; Tindall, Rothermel, Delamater, Pinsky, & Klein, 1999); and, in one study of adolescents with CHD, those with identified MRI abnormalities exhibited greater difficulty with visuomotor integration than those with normal MRI scans (von Rhein et al., 2011).

Managing more complex visuospatial materials can also be challenging for children and adolescents with CHD, as shown, for example, by their copy productions of the Rey-Osterrieth Complex Figure (ROCF). Using the ROCF Developmental Scoring System (ROCF-DSS; Bernstein & Waber, 1996)—a process-oriented method of scoring the ROCF that is more sensitive than other scoring methods for detecting differences among individuals with CHD (von Rhein et al., 2015b)—more than half of 8-year-old children with d-TGA scored within the lowest organizational level, a rate twice that of healthy controls (Bellinger, Bernstein, Kirkwood, Rappaport, & Newburger, 2003a). Problems with complex visuospatial organization, as measured using the ROCF-DSS, have also been documented in adolescents with TOF (Bellinger et al., 2015a) and single-ventricle cardiac conditions (Bellinger et al., 2015b). On average, these adolescents seemed to be drawn toward the more incidental elements of the figure rather than to underlying organizational features. Nearly half (47%) of adolescents with single-ventricle conditions (vs. 25–34% of adolescents with d-TGA, TOF, and healthy controls) adopted a highly linear, part-oriented approach to copying the figure, which in turn was associated with lower scores on higher-level reading comprehension and math problem-solving tasks (Bean Jaworski et al., 2018). Interestingly, 8-year performance on the ROCF-DSS has also been shown to predict reading and math outcomes during adolescence, when practitioners were 16 years of age (Fasano-McCarron et al., 2021).

Language

Atypical speech and language development have been documented in children with CHD, as has an increased incidence of hearing loss (Grasty et al., 2018). The acquisition of early language milestones may also be delayed (Andropoulos et al., 2014; Mussatto et al., 2014). Deficits in early oral–motor control and speech articulation and a higher prevalence of "apraxia of speech," referring to impaired oral–motor planning, were noted in 4-year-old children with d-TGA, particularly those who underwent the arterial switch operation using deep hypothermic circulatory arrest as the primary method of vital organ support (Bellinger et al., 1999). Receptive and expressive naming abilities were also lower than expected population means (Bellinger et al., 1999). At 8-years of age, these children continued to present with oral–motor and speech deficits, as well as relative weaknesses in phonological awareness and sentence formulation (Bellinger et al., 2003b). Difficulties with phonological processing, lexical access (i.e., speeded naming), and following verbal instructions have also been reported (Miatton, De Wolf, François, Thiery, & Vingerhoets, 2007b, 2007c; Sarrechia et al., 2015), and in a pilot study of school-age children with mixed forms of CHD, moderate to large effect-size differences were noted for lexical and grammatical processing and immediate sentence repetition (Sommariva et al., 2020).

Attention

Problems with attention are commonly reported in children and adolescents with CHD (Bellinger et al., 2011, 2015a, 2015b; Brosig, Mussatto, Kuhn, & Tweddell, 2007; Mahle et al., 2000; Miatton, De Wolf, François, Thiery, & Vingerhoets, 2007a; Murphy et al., 2017; Shillingford et al., 2008). Performance deficits have been documented in several aspects of attention as well, particularly sustained and divided attention (Bellinger et al., 2003b; Kirshbom et al., 2005; Miatton et al., 2007c; Mills et al., 2018; Sarrechia et al., 2016). Moreover, deficits in executive attention (but not more basic attentional alerting or orienting) were found in 7-year-olds with TOF using Posner and Petersen's Attention Network Test (Hövels-Gürich et al., 2007) and are consistent with growing evidence of prominent executive function challenges among children with complex CHD.

Memory

Children and adolescents with complex CHD appear to be at risk for memory difficulties, although a consistent profile of memory impairment(s) has yet to emerge. As early as 3 months of age, infants with CHD show signs of relative deficits in memory on a mobile kicking task (Chen, Harrison, & Heathcock, 2015). Among older children and adolescents, whereas some studies reported relatively lower verbal than visual memory abilities (Miatton et al., 2007b, 2007c; Pike et al., 2016; Sarrechia et al., 2016), others reported greater weaknesses in visual than verbal memory abilities (Brosig et al., 2013; Tindall et al., 1999). Still others reported no differences (Kirshbom et al., 2005; Wotherspoon et al., 2020). A meta-analysis of adolescents and young adults with CHD identified moderate overall reductions in verbal memory (g = –.43, p = .013), but unfortunately did not examine visual memory as a key outcome measure (Mills et al., 2018).

In the largest detailed examination of memory outcomes to date, Cassidy, Newburger, and Bellinger (2017) found that adolescents with d-TGA or TOF performed below expected population means on a range of tasks from the Children's Memory Scale. Adolescents with CHD were more likely than controls to perform within the impaired range (i.e., ≥1.5 SD below the mean) on immediate and delayed visual memory composites (17–31% for CHD vs. 2–3% for controls). On verbal memory composites, frequencies of impaired scores were also somewhat higher among adolescents with CHD (17–29%) versus controls (10–16%), although the relative odds of earning an impaired verbal memory composite score were comparable across groups.

Executive Functions

Executive function (EF) skills are among the most sensitive to compromise by critical CHD (Mills et al., 2018; Feldman et al., 2021; Jackson et al., 2021). Beginning in infancy, alterations in basic homeostatic and self-regulatory capacities are highly prevalent in newborns with CHD and may complicate the formation of secure attachment relationships and increase parent stress (Butler et al., 2019), as well as disrupt early serve-and-return dynamics and autonomy-supportive parenting behaviors that facilitate EF development (Distefano, Galinsky, McClelland, Zelazo, & Carlson, 2018; National Scientific Council on the Developing Child, 2004).

Throughout preschool and early/middle childhood, relative deficits in core (i.e., inhibitory control, working memory, cognitive flexibility/shifting) and higher-level EFs (e.g., planning, organization/integration of information, problem-solving) have been documented across several studies (Bellinger et al., 2003a; Calderon et al., 2010; Calderon, Jambaqué, & Bonnet, 2014b; Gaynor et al., 2010; Hövels-Gürich et al., 2007; Miatton et al., 2007c). Some of the earliest evidence of EF vulnerability in CHD came from the 8-year follow-up of the Boston Circulatory Arrest Study, which revealed weaknesses in inhibitory control, working memory, phonetic verbal fluency, and novel problem solving among children with corrected d-TGA (Bellinger et al., 2003b). More recent studies have confirmed and extended these findings. Performance-based problems with inhibitory control and cognitive flexibility have since been documented as early as 4 years of age (Calderon et al., 2012; Gaynor et al., 2010) and seem to remain fairly stable over the transition from kindergarten to early elementary school (Calderon et al., 2014b). Working memory deficits have also been documented in preschool and early school-age children with d-TGA (Calderon et al., 2012, 2010), and in a longitudinal structural equation model, a combined working memory/inhibitory control latent factor was found to mediate associations between processing speed and reading and math outcomes in children with d-TGA both concurrently in childhood and 8 years later, during adolescence (Cassidy, White, DeMaso, Newburger, & Bellinger, 2016). On the Behavior Rating Inventory of Executive Function (BRIEF), the parents of early school-age children with CHD endorsed difficulties in at least one real-world EF ability at more than twice the rate of controls (65 vs. 30%), with working memory and cognitive flexibility capacities identified as among the most problematic (Cassidy, 2020; Sanz et al., 2017). Parent ratings of EF have also been found to predict psychosocial quality of life (Sanz et al., 2018) and school performance (Gerstle, Beebe, Drotar, Cassedy, & Marino, 2016).

Throughout adolescence, parents and teachers continue to endorse clinically elevated EF concerns in more than half of individuals with d-TGA, TOF, or single-ventricle cardiac conditions versus 15–29% of healthy controls (Cassidy, White, DeMaso, Newburger, & Bellinger, 2015). Notably, despite rating themselves more positively on the self-report BRIEF compared to ratings from parent and teacher versions of this measure, the application of a more relaxed cutoff score of ≥ 60 revealed that these adolescents did in fact see themselves as having more trouble with cognitive flexibility and emotion regulation than their healthy peers (Cassidy et al., 2015), suggesting perhaps more awareness of their EF challenges than had previously been appreciated. These adolescents also performed more poorly than controls on a range of standardized clinical tasks, including Sorting, Word Context, Tower, Design Fluency, and Verbal Fluency subtests from the Delis–Kaplan Executive Function System (D-KEFS). Problems with cognitive flexibility and problem solving were particularly prominent across all three CHD groups (Cassidy et al., 2015; see also Cassidy, 2020), as were marked weaknesses with organization and integration on the ROCF (Bean Jaworski et al., 2018). Diagnostically, rates of attention-deficit/hyperactivity disorder (ADHD)—a disorder often characterized by deficits in EF—were also found to be high relative to controls and the general population, present in 19% for adolescents with d-TGA or TOF without a comorbid genetic condition, 34% of adolescents with single-ventricle conditions who underwent the Fontan procedure, and 39% of adolescents with TOF and a comorbid genetic condition (DeMaso et al., 2014, 2017; Holland et al., 2017).

Social Cognition

The possibility that children with CHD may be at risk for problems with social cognition was first raised by Bellinger (2008), who observed difficulties with aspects of social communication in children with d-TGA. At 4-years of age, these children were more limited in their use of symbolic language during free play than their healthy peers, and at 4- and 8-years of age, their elicited personal narratives were less emotionally complex and often failed to adequately meet the information needs of the listener. Taken together, these observations suggest difficulties understanding complex emotions and accurately inferring others' mental states (i.e., "theory of mind")—hypotheses that have since been affirmed in several studies using experimental measures such as false-belief tasks and the Reading the Mind in the Eyes Test (Abda et al., 2019; Bellinger et al., 2011, 2015a, 2015b; Calderon, Angeard, Pinabiaux, Bonnet, & Jambaqué, 2014a; Calderon et al., 2010; Sarrechia et al., 2015).

Further confirmation of social-cognitive deficits comes from an increased prevalence of autism spectrum disorder diagnoses associated with CHD. Studies have reported anywhere from a two- to fivefold increase in autism spectrum diagnoses among children with CHD (Razzaghi, Oster, & Reefhuis, 2015; Tsao et al., 2017), although it is important to note that these estimates were drawn from health survey and insurance databases rather than formal clinical assessments (Calderon, Bellinger, & Newburger, 2019).

Adaptive and Social Functioning

Prior studies, though limited in number, highlight a range of adaptive functioning limitations in children with CHD. Persistent delays, particularly in conceptual and social skills, have been documented in a cohort of children with CHD followed from infancy/toddlerhood through preschool (Alton et al., 2015). Five-year-olds who underwent fetal aortic valvuloplasty for evolving HLHS were rated by their parents on the Adaptive Behavior Assessment System, Second Edition (ABAS-II) as having lower overall functional independence, with specific weaknesses noted in practical self-care, household, self-directed, and community navigation skills (Laraja et al., 2017). And among young children with CHD who underwent the Fontan procedure, 26% exhibited pre- to post-Fontan declines of > 1 standard deviation on the ABAS-II (Ricci et al., 2018). These declines were particularly prevalent in children who experienced a peri-Fontan stroke or were older at the time of surgery.

Children with CHD have also been described by parents and teachers as being less socially competent than their peers and siblings (McCusker, Armstrong, Mullen, Doherty, & Casey, 2013; Miatton et al., 2007a; Spijkerboer, Utens, Bogers, Verhulst, & Helbing, 2008). Social withdrawal, rejection–exclusion, victimization (e.g., teasing, bullying), and difficulty establishing and maintaining age-appropriate peer relationships have been noted as well (McCusker et al., 2013; Miatton et al., 2007a) and may be linked in part to disease-related factors such as limitations in physical activity and stamina that hinder participation in sports, body image concerns related to surgical scars or diminutive stature, and displacement from the home to pursue medical/surgical care (Chong et al., 2018).

Emotional and Behavioral Adjustment

Data from multiple sources highlight an increased risk for emotional and behavioral maladjustment among children and adolescents with CHD. According to a recent meta-analysis (Abda et al., 2019), 1 out of 4 children or adolescents with CHD was rated by his or her parent as having at least one emotional or behavioral problem. Moreover, in studies that used the parent-report Child Behavior Checklist (CBCL), pooled prevalence rates of internalizing and externalizing concerns among children and adolescents with CHD were 24.9% and 14.7%, respectively (Abda et al., 2019). Rates of diagnosable lifetime anxiety disorders, as determined by structured clinical interview, are particularly high during adolescence, especially among adolescents with single-ventricle cardiac anatomy (35%) and those with TOF and a comorbid genetic condition (43%), as well as in 12–15% of adolescents with either d-TGA or isolated TOF (DeMaso et al., 2017, 2014; Holland et al., 2017). Interestingly, in these same cohorts, adolescents who approached complex visuospatial information (i.e., the ROCF) in a highly part-oriented fashion were more than twice as likely as their more holistic peers to meet diagnostic criteria for an anxiety disorder (lifetime odds ratio [OR] = 2.2, p = .02, 95% confidence interval [CI] = 1.1–4.1; current OR = 2.7, p = .03, 95% CI = 1.1–6.5), but were at no greater risk for ADHD, disruptive behavior, or mood disorders; and, of the 25 adolescents with CHD and a diagnosable current anxiety disorder, 15 (60%) were part-oriented in their approach to the ROCF (Cassidy, Bernstein, Bellinger, Newburger, & DeMaso, 2019).

DEVELOPMENTAL CONSIDERATIONS

CHD alters development via a series of cascading events that unfold over time and across neurobehavioral systems. Over the lifespan, individuals with CHD will come up against the same developmental challenges and strive to meet the same milestones as their typically developing peers and, like their peers, they will confront those challenges as best they can within the bounds of their own unique neurobehavioral circumstances and broader support systems. Transitions, of which there are many for individuals with CHD (e.g., from inpatient to outpatient settings; early intervention to the school system; childhood to adolescence; adolescence to young adulthood; pediatric to adult medical care), represent periods of vulnerability during which extra support and intervention may be needed (Cassidy et al., 2021). During infancy and early childhood (0–3 years), early intervention services geared toward addressing motor, feeding, speech–language, social, and adaptive skills delays should be provided to all children with critical CHD, and referral to early intervention should be considered standard-of-care at the time of discharge after cardiac surgery. Later childhood and adolescence can be particularly challenging with regard to both personal identity and development of interpersonal relationships. As social and academic demands increase and it becomes more difficult to compensate for even subtle neurobehavioral and self-regulatory weaknesses, children and adolescents with CHD may find it difficult to make effective academic progress and keep up with their peers without more intensive educational supports (Oster, Watkins, Hill, Knight, & Meyer, 2017). Physical activity restrictions and body image concerns may become increasingly problematic during this time as well (Daliento et al., 2005), further complicating interpersonal relationships and amplifying an already-present sense of "being different" that has existed for many individuals with CHD since early childhood.

With overall adulthood survival rates greater than 85%, the composition of the CHD population has changed dramatically in recent years. There are now more adults than children living with CHD (Marelli, Miller, Marino, Jefferson, & Newburger, 2016). Relative to the general population, adults with CHD present with higher rates of atrial fibrillation, hypertension, disordered glucose metabolism, coronary artery disease, and other cardiovascular and metabolic conditions that increase their risk for stroke and dementia (Marelli et al., 2016), as well as a host of neurobehavioral (Ilardi, Ono, McCartney, Book, & Stringer, 2017) and psychosocial issues (Kovacs et al., 2009) that may limit educational and employment opportunities (Opić et al., 2015) and disrupt the continuity of cardiac follow-up care. Rates of dementia, particularly early-onset dementia (i.e., prior to 65-years of age), are also elevated among adults with CHD (Bagge et al., 2018). Thus, it is reasonable to conclude that CHD is no longer a predominantly pediatric condition, but rather a lifespan condition that requires the coordinated efforts of specialists across the full spectrum of pediatric, adult, and rehabilitation neuropsychology.

PREDICTORS AND MODERATORS

Neuropsychological outcomes in children and adolescents with CHD are highly variable, affected by myriad transacting biological, familial, psychological, social, contextual, and as-yet-unknown factors that emerge and change over the course of development. Except for select cases involving some genetic syndromes (e.g., trisomy 18, trisomy 21, 22q11.2

deletion) and/or serious medical/neurological complications (e.g., prolonged cardiac arrest, stroke), it is not possible to predict individual neuropsychological outcomes with even modest specificity, and heterogeneity often prevails even in those select cases. This will almost certainly improve as developmentally informed longitudinal studies, incorporating multiple levels of analysis, shed new light on the mechanisms underlying short- and longer-range outcomes.

As in many other complex medical conditions, socioeconomic and sociodemographic factors such as income, race, insurance, and parental education are typically among the strongest predictors of outcomes in children with CHD (Bucholz et al., 2020a, 2020b; Bucholz, Sleeper, & Newburger, 2018; Gaynor et al., 2015; Ortinau et al., 2018a; Peyvandi et al., 2018). Parent mental health and family stress factors are also a critical consideration (Kasparian et al., 2019; Sood et al., 2021). Mothers and fathers of children with CHD may experience and respond to CHD-related stress differently than one another, which is important to keep in mind when working with families (Sood et al., 2018). Timing of CHD diagnosis is also relevant in predicting outcome. Prenatal diagnosis is generally associated with lower mortality and morbidity, including better neurobehavioral outcomes (Calderon et al., 2012) and less preoperative brain injury (Peyvandi et al., 2016), than postnatal diagnosis, likely due to improved hemodynamics secondary to access to a more controlled delivery environment with immediate availability of prostaglandins, acidosis correction, and needed catheterization and open-heart surgical procedures. Of course, receiving a prenatal diagnosis of CHD is also highly stressful for expectant mothers and fathers (Rychik et al., 2012; Kasparian, 2019), and high levels of maternal stress during pregnancy may increase the risk of atypical brain development in fetuses with CHD (Wu et al., 2020). Rates of spontaneous preterm birth are twice as high for newborns with CHD than they are in the general population (Laas et al., 2012); and, both preterm (< 37 weeks' gestation) and early-term birth (37–38 weeks' gestation) have been associated with worse neurobehavioral outcomes among children with CHD (Calderon et al., 2016), as has low birthweight (Gaynor et al., 2015).

Several biological predictors have also been identified, including both genetic and medical/surgical factors. Children with CHD and a comorbid genetic condition (vs. isolated CHD) are recognized as being at a greater risk for adverse neurobehavioral and psychosocial outcomes. The *APOE* ε2 allele has also been associated with worse outcomes among younger children with CHD (Gaynor et al., 2003), but may protect against ADHD during adolescence (Schmithorst et al., 2016). With respect to medical and surgical factors, increased length of postoperative hospital stay—often a proxy for increased medical complexity (Ravishankar et al., 2016)—seems to confer increased risk for neurodevelopmental impairment. Additional factors portending worse outcomes include longer duration of cardiopulmonary bypass, higher number of surgical procedures, single-ventricle cardiac anatomy, aortic arch obstruction, increased exposure to anesthetics and potentially noxious operative and postoperative environments, need for extracorporeal life support (e.g., extracorporeal membrane oxygenation [ECMO]), and perioperative neurological complications such as seizures (Marino et al., 2012; Cassidy et al., 2018).

An understanding of neurobehavioral risk and resilience in this diverse population likely requires an appreciation of the dynamic interplay of adverse and protective forces. Figure 8.1 presents a conceptual model of a range of demographic/psychosocial, pre- and perioperative, and current physical health factors known to be associated with outcomes in CHD. In the model, adverse and protective factors are depicted in a state of theoretical

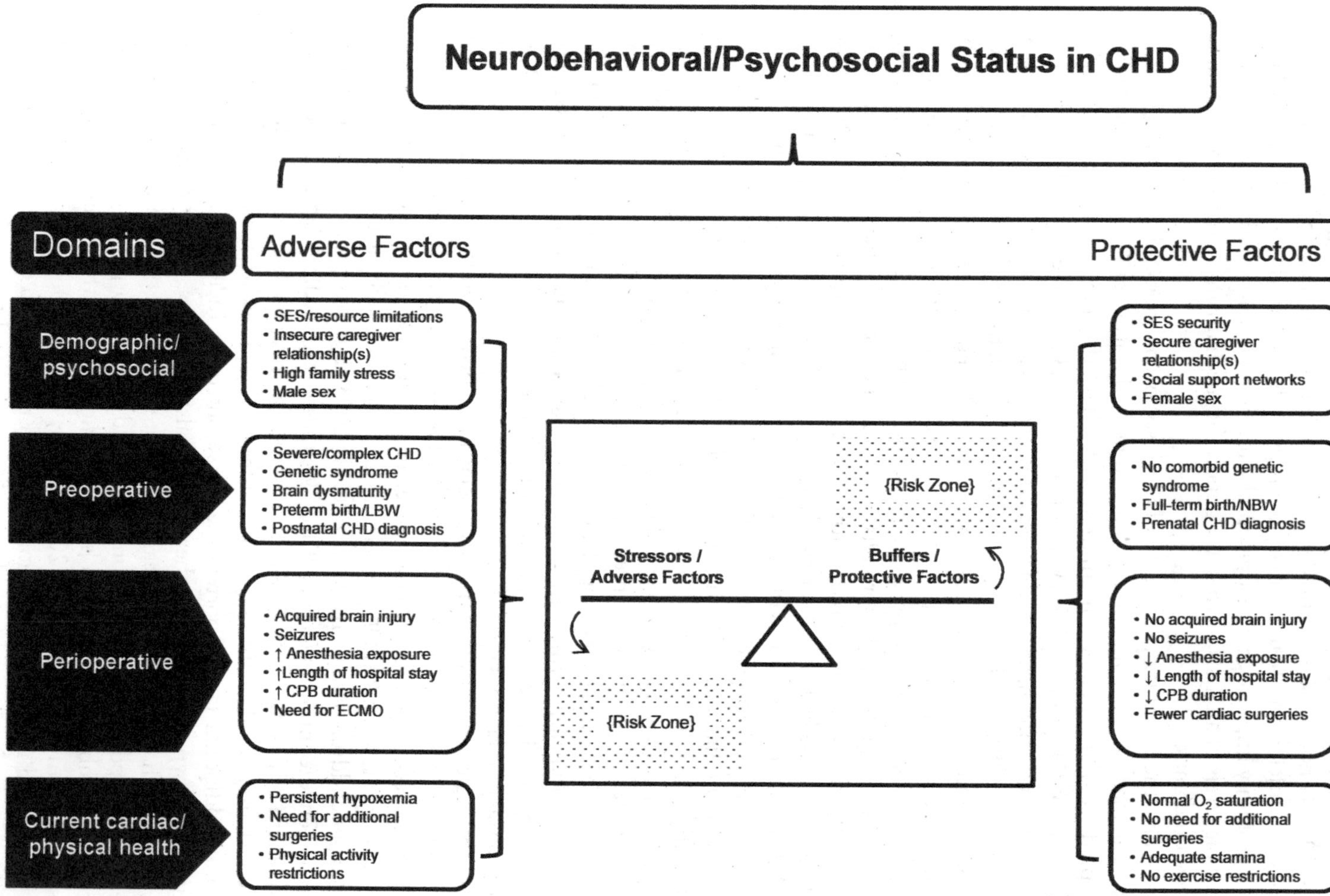

FIGURE 8.1. Conceptual model depicting a range of adverse and protective factors known to be associated with neurobehavioral and psychosocial outcomes in CHD. SES, socioeconomic status; CPB, cardiopulmonary bypass; ECMO, extracorporeal membrane oxygenation; LBW, low birthweight; NBW, normal birthweight.

equilibrium that is subject to change in response to the presence/absence (and relative weighting) of stressors and buffers. In this way, adverse outcomes become more likely as the balance shifts toward a predominance of stressors that cannot be effectively mitigated by available protective factors. Conversely, resilience is more likely to emerge when the balance tilts more toward protective factors and the fit between the child and his or her world is optimized.

TREATMENT AND INTERVENTION

Guided by a landmark scientific statement endorsed by both the American Heart Association and the American Academy of Pediatrics, systematic neurodevelopmental surveillance, screening, and evaluation are now considered the standard of care for children with severe CHD (Marino et al., 2012). The designation "high risk for developmental disorders or disabilities" was suggested for patients with CHD meeting any of the following criteria: (1) neonates or infants requiring open heart surgery; (2) children with cyanotic CHD who did not require open heart surgery during the neonatal or infant period; (3) children with CHD who were also born preterm, identified as having a developmental delay in infancy, suspected of having a genetic abnormality or syndrome, had a history of mechanical support (e.g., ECMO), underwent heart transplantation, received cardiopulmonary resuscitation, experienced prolonged hospitalization of more than 2 weeks following surgery or experienced perioperative seizures, or presented with microcephaly or significant neuroimaging abnormalities; or (4) children with other conditions who were otherwise determined to be at high risk by their medical home providers (Marino et al., 2012). As awareness of the needs of the CHD population has increased, so too has early detection and referral for specialized services. Unfortunately, evidence-based approaches for the prevention and treatment of developmental, psychosocial, and neurobehavioral challenges remain limited (Cassidy et al., 2021; Phillips & Longoria, 2019).

Some support exists for the use of psychosocial interventions in families of children with severe CHD. Parent-oriented psychoeducational interventions have proved effective in improving aspects of family functioning and maternal anxiety, and were associated with increases in Bayley Scales of Infant Development, Second Edition (BSID-II) mental (but not psychomotor) scores during infancy (McCusker et al., 2010). A similarly designed randomized controlled trial utilizing both parent- and child-oriented psychoeducation reported only small, nonsignificant improvements in child psychosocial adjustment relative to standard care. These interventions have also been associated with fewer missed days during the first year of formal schooling, although no effects were found on child behavior or academic performance (McCusker et al., 2012). Children did not receive any direct intervention in these studies, however; and a subsequent randomized controlled trial evaluating the impact of a combined child- and parent-oriented psychosocial intervention for 4- to 7-year-olds with CHD found only a small and non-significant impact on child psychosocial status (van der Mheen et al., 2019).

Data on the efficacy or effectiveness of targeted neurocognitive interventions in children or adolescents with CHD are also limited, although two phase II randomized controlled trials examining the effects of a computerized working memory training program (i.e., Cogmed) on EF and social skills are notable (Calderon et al., 2019; Calderon et al.,

2020). In addition, despite some early concerns regarding adverse effects, the prevailing consensus among experts is that psychopharmacological treatment of ADHD symptoms, including the use of stimulant and nonstimulant medications, can be implemented safely in children with CHD but should be managed in consultation with the child's cardiology team and with careful monitoring (Berger, 2016). The impact of ADHD medication on neurobehavioral and psychosocial outcomes adversely affected by CHD has not been formally evaluated in this population and deserves further investigation.

CONCLUSIONS AND FUTURE DIRECTIONS

When the first edition of this book went to print in 2000, so little was known about the neuropsychological implications of CHD that it would have been difficult to write an entire chapter about them. Since that time, it has become increasingly clear that CHD has the potential to alter brain and behavior in numerous subtle and profound ways. Atypical brain development begins *in utero*, well before cardiac surgery, and is evident across the lifespan, the product of a complex amalgam of dysmaturation and injury, and affected by a range of medical, demographic, and personal factors. Developing white matter is particularly susceptible to disruption in infants with CHD, although anomalies in gray matter, cortical thickness, gyrification, and network topology have also been reported. And against this backdrop, early self-regulatory challenges may give rise to a broad array of neurobehavioral and psychosocial difficulties that can vary considerably from person to person and cannot be accurately predicted by the child's heart condition alone.

Outcomes in CHD are indeed highly variable, and even in the most sophisticated and large-scale studies to date, risk factors often account for only a small portion of the variability in outcomes. Sociodemographic indices such as parental education and income tend to carry more weight than medical or surgical variables—a reality that, while not unique to CHD, may nonetheless imply the existence of as-yet-unidentified modifiable factors that could, at least in theory, be harnessed to promote more positive outcomes. Of course, doing so would require a more precise mechanistic understanding of risk and resilience than is currently available. It is not enough to know that children with CHD who have more educated parents or are from more affluent households fare better; we need to know *why*, so that we can figure out *how* to intervene.

Knowledge of the neuropsychology of CHD has come, with a few notable exceptions, from small, single-center, cross-sectional, observational studies. Findings from these studies provide important insight into the broad range of challenges associated with CHD, yet most have not been replicated. Furthermore, group-based findings may have limited applicability in evaluating and managing children referred for clinical neuropsychological assessment. Simply differentiating a child with CHD from the general population on some standardized metric—even one that is correlated with relevant, real-world functioning—does not necessarily provide the information needed to help that child succeed in the real world. This is particularly true when formal criteria for a specific learning disorder are not met, yet the neuropsychological profile clearly portends a high risk for failure to meet expectations at home, school, or within the community—an all-too-common scenario for children and adolescents with CHD.

Lack of specificity in the prediction of functional, ecologically relevant outcomes remains a major limitation of the field in general and of CHD research in particular, as does the dearth of empirically supported interventions for addressing specific neurobehavioral impairments (e.g., visuospatial processing deficits). Moreover, it is not enough to focus on secondary or tertiary interventions that aim to remediate or accommodate identified deficits in children with CHD; neuropsychology must also work to support primary interventions that promote positive development and prevent negative outcomes from occurring in the first place, beginning at the time of diagnosis, which for most will be during pregnancy. A focus on infancy and early childhood, when the foundations of attachment and self-regulation are just beginning to emerge and set the stage for the subsequent development of critical executive function capacities, will also be necessary for children and families affected by CHD. This developmental period can be one of profound stress and instability for the families of children with CHD, who may understandably struggle to adapt to the unique and harder-to-meet needs of the child, while at the same time having to manage the worry, isolation, and financial burdens that so often accompany CHD. Individualized developmental care interventions have shown promise in other patient populations within noncardiac intensive care settings, and their safety and feasibility should be examined in cardiac intensive care units as well (Butler, Huyler, Kaza, & Rachwal, 2017). The transition to adolescence and onset of puberty should also be recognized as potential "windows of opportunity" for individuals with CHD during which interventions may be able to harness inherent brain plasticity to maintain development on more adaptive trajectories (Dorn & Susman, 2019). As experts in both clinical psychology and development, pediatric neuropsychologists are well-poised to contribute to these important intervention-oriented goals.

Focusing even earlier in the disease course, there is a strong interest among cardiac researchers in neuroprotective interventions that preempt the brain dysmaturation and injury associated with CHD. One particularly compelling area of study is maternal hyperoxygenation during pregnancy. A clinical trial is currently underway to determine whether continuous inhaled supplemental oxygen is safe and feasible in pregnancies affected by CHD (*https://clinicaltrials.gov/ct2/show/NCT03136835*), with assessment of infant/child neurodevelopmental outcomes likely to follow thereafter. Yet another avenue of innovative ongoing research involves regenerative medicine and the use of pluripotent stem cells to reengineer native cardiac muscle to improve clinical outcomes (Nelson & Catero Peral, 2016; Peral, Burkhart, & Nelson, 2014; Vincenti et al., 2020). Studies of potential biomarkers of brain injury are being conducted and in one recent study of infants with CHD, higher levels of glial fibrillary acidic protein—an astrocyte intermediate filament protein that is detectable in the blood following injury to astrocytes—at the time of cardiac surgery predicted worse neurodevelopmental outcomes at 12 months of age (Graham et al., 2019). Innovative nonhuman models of CHD have also been created in sheep (Lawrence et al., 2019) and pigs (Stinnett et al., 2017), and have reported early evidence that inhaled hydrogen during circulatory arrest may mitigate some of the risk for ischemic injury associated with cardiac surgery and extracorporeal life support (Cole et al., 2019). These models allow for a greater degree of scientific control, as well as the experimental manipulation of surgical and other parameters, that will hopefully identify novel ways of protecting brain health against the risks imposed by CHD.

Among the most exciting advances in CHD in recent years has been the establishment of the Cardiac Neurodevelopmental Outcome Collaborative (CNOC; *www.cardiacneuro.*

org), a multisite, multinational, multidisciplinary organization whose overarching mission is to determine and implement best practices to promote optimal neurodevelopmental outcomes for individuals with CHD (Marino et al., 2020a, 2020b; Sood, Jacobs, & Marino, 2020). Toward this end, in 2019, CNOC launched a clinical registry that will database neurodevelopmental, neurobehavioral, psychosocial, and other pertinent clinical information collected from children and adolescents with CHD using standard recommended protocols (Ilardi et al., 2020; Ware et al., 2020), and permit linkage of those data with existing, high-quality cardiology and cardiac surgery registries under the auspices of Cardiac Networks United (Gaies et al., 2019). In a short time, the CNOC clinical registry will comprise the largest and most comprehensive source of information about how children with CHD develop, and will generate new insights into how better to support children and families affected by CHD.

ACKNOWLEDGMENTS

I would like to thank Johanna Calderon, Megan Cassidy, Dawn Ilardi, and Jacquie Sanz for their thoughtful comments on earlier versions of this chapter.

REFERENCES

Abda, A., Bolduc, M.-E., Tsimicalis, A., Rennick, J., Vatcher, D., & Brossard-Racine, M. (2019). Psychosocial outcomes of children and adolescents with severe congenital heart defect: A systematic review and meta-analysis. *Journal of Pediatric Psychology, 44*, 463–477.

Alton, G. Y., Taghados, S., Joffe, A. R., Robertson, C. M. T., Dinu, I., Blakely, P., . . . Synnes, A. (2015). Prediction of preschool functional abilities after early complex cardiac surgery. *Cardiology in the Young, 25*(4), 655–662.

Andropoulos, D. B., Ahmad, H. B., Haq, T., Brady, K., Stephen, A., Meador, M. R., . . . Blaine, R. (2014). The association between brain injury, perioperative anesthetic exposure, and 12-month neurodevelopmental outcomes after neonatal cardiac surgery: A retrospective cohort study. *Paediatric Anaesthesia, 24*(3), 266–274.

Andropoulos, D. B., Hunter, J. V., Nelson, D. P., Stayer, S. A., Stark, A. R., McKenzie, E. D., . . . Fraser, C. D. (2010). Brain immaturity is associated with brain injury before and after neonatal cardiac surgery with high-flow bypass and cerebral oxygenation monitoring. *Journal of Thoracic and Cardiovascular Surgery, 139*(3), 543–556.

Bagge, C. N., Henderson, V. W., Laursen, H. B., Adelborg, K., Olsen, M., & Madsen, N. L. (2018). Risk of dementia in adults with congenital heart disease: Population-based cohort study. *Circulation, 137*(18), 1912–1920.

Bean Jaworski, J. L., White, M. T., DeMaso, D. R., Newburger, J. W., Bellinger, D. C., & Cassidy, A. R. (2018). Visuospatial processing in adolescents with critical congenital heart disease: Organization, integration, and implications for academic achievement. *Child Neuropsychology, 24*, 451–468.

Beca, J., Gunn, J. K., Coleman, L., Hope, A., Reed, P. W., Hunt, R. W., . . . Shekerdemian, L. S. (2013). New white matter brain injury after infant heart surgery is associated with diagnostic group and the use of circulatory arrest. *Circulation, 127*(9), 971–979.

Bellinger, D. C. (2008). Are children with congenital cardiac malformations at increased risk of deficits in social cognition? *Cardiology in the Young, 18*(1), 3–9.

Bellinger, D. C., Bernstein, J. H., Kirkwood, M. W., Rappaport, L. A., & Newburger, J. W. (2003a). Visual-spatial skills in children after open-heart surgery. *Journal of Developmental and Behavioral Pediatrics, 24*(3), 169–179.

Bellinger, D. C., Rivkin, M. J., Demaso, D., Robertson, R. L., Stopp, C., Dunbar-Masterson, C., . . . Newburger, J. W. (2015a). Adolescents with tetralogy of Fallot: Neuropsychological assessment and structural brain imaging. *Cardiology in the Young, 25*(02), 338–347.

Bellinger, D. C., Watson, C. G., Rivkin, M. J., Robertson, R. L., Roberts, A. E., Stopp, C., . . . Newburger, J. W. (2015b). Neuropsychological status and structural brain imaging in adolescents with single ventricle who underwent the Fontan Procedure. *Journal of the American Heart Association, 4*(12), e002302.

Bellinger, D. C., Wypij, D., DuPlessis, A. J., Rappaport, L. A., Jonas, R. A., Wernovsky, G., & Newburger, J. W. (2003b). Neurodevelopmental status at eight years in children with dextro-transposition of the great arteries: The Boston Circulatory Arrest Trial. *Journal of Thoracic and Cardiovascular Surgery, 126*(5), 1385–1396.

Bellinger, D. C., Wypij, D., Kuban, K. C. K., Rappaport, L. A., Hickey, P. R., Wernovsky, G., . . . Newburger, J. W. (1999). Developmental and neurological status of children at 4 years of age after heart surgery with hypothermic circulatory arrest or low-flow cardiopulmonary bypass. *Circulation, 100*(5), 526–532.

Bellinger, D. C., Wypij, D., Rivkin, M. J., DeMaso, D. R., Robertson, R. L., Dunbar-Masterson, C., . . . Newburger, J. W. (2011). Adolescents with d-transposition of the great arteries corrected with the arterial switch procedure: neuropsychological assessment and structural brain imaging. *Circulation, 124*(12), 1361–1369.

Berger, S. (2016). Attention deficit hyperactivity disorder medications in children with heart disease. *Current Opinion in Pediatrics, 28*(5), 607–612.

Bernstein, J. H., & Waber, D. P. (1996). *Developmental Scoring System for the Rey–Osterrieth Complex Figure (DSS-ROCF)*. Odessa, FL: Psychological Assessment Resources.

Bolduc, M.-E. E., Lambert, H., Ganeshamoorthy, S., & Brossard-Racine, M. (2018). Structural brain abnormalities in adolescents and young adults with congenital heart defect: A systematic review. *Developmental Medicine and Child Neurology, 60*, 1209–1224.

Brosig, C. L., Mussatto, K. A., Kuhn, E. M., & Tweddell, J. S. (2007). Neurodevelopmental outcome in preschool survivors of complex congenital heart disease: Implications for clinical practice. *Journal of Pediatric Health Care, 21*(1), 3–12.

Brosig, C. L., Mussatto, K., Hoffman, G., Hoffmann, R. G., Dasgupta, M., Tweddell, J., & Ghanayem, N. (2013). Neurodevelopmental outcomes for children with hypoplastic left heart syndrome at the age of 5 years. *Pediatric Cardiology, 34*(7), 1597–1604.

Bucholz, E. M., Sleeper, L. A., Goldberg, C. S., Pasquali, S. K., Anderson, B. R., Gaynor, J. W., . . . Newburger, J. W. (2020a). Socioeconomic status and long-term outcomes in single ventricle heart disease. *Pediatrics, 146*(4), e202001240.

Bucholz, E. M., Sleeper, L. A., & Newburger, J. W. (2018). Neighborhood socioeconomic status and outcomes following the Norwood procedure: An analysis of the Pediatric Heart Network Single Ventricle Reconstruction Trial public data set Emily. *Journal of the American Heart Association, 7*, 1–9.

Bucholz, E. M., Sleeper, L. A., Sananes, R., Brosig, C. L., Goldberg, C. S., Pasquali, S. K., & Newburger, J. W. (2020b). Trajectories in neurodevelopmental, health-related quality of life, and functional status outcomes by socioeconomic status and maternal education in children with single ventricle heart disease. *The Journal of Pediatrics, 229*, 289–293.

Butler, S. C., Huyler, K., Kaza, A., & Rachwal, C. (2017). Filling a significant gap in the cardiac ICU: Implementation of individualised developmental care. *Cardiology in the Young, 27*, 1797–1806.

Butler, S. C., Sadhwani, A., Stopp, C., Singer, J., Wypij, D., Dunbar-Masterson, C., . . . Newburger, J. W. (2019). Neurodevelopmental assessment of infants with congenital heart disease in the early postoperative period. *Congenital Heart Disease, 14*, 236–245.

Calderon, J., Angeard, N., Moutier, S., Plumet, M.-H., Jambaqué, I., & Bonnet, D. (2012). Impact of prenatal diagnosis on neurocognitive outcomes in children with transposition of the great arteries. *Journal of Pediatrics, 161*(1), 94–98.

Calderon, J., Angeard, N., Pinabiaux, C., Bonnet, D., & Jambaqué, I. (2014a). Facial expression recognition and emotion understanding in children after neonatal open-heart surgery for transposition of the great arteries. *Developmental Medicine and Child Neurology, 56*(6), 564–571.

Calderon, J., Bellinger, D. C., Hartigan, C., Lord, A., Stopp, C., Wypij, D., & Newburger, J. W. (2019). Improving neurodevelopmental outcomes in children with congenital heart disease: Protocol for a randomised controlled trial of working memory training. *BMJ Open, 9*, Article e023304.

Calderon, J., Bonnet, D., Courtin, C., Concordet, S., Plumet, M.-H., & Angeard, N. (2010). Executive function and theory of mind in school-aged children after neonatal corrective cardiac surgery for transposition of the great arteries. *Developmental Medicine and Child Neurology, 52*(12), 1139–1144.

Calderon, J., Jambaqué, I., & Bonnet, D. (2014b). Executive functions development in 5- to 7-year-old children with transposition of the great arteries: A longitudinal study. *Developmental Neuropsychology, 39,* 365–384.

Calderon, J., Bellinger, D. C., & Newburger, J. W. (2019). Autism and congenital heart disease: Evidence and unresolved questions. *Pediatrics, 144*(5), e20184114.

Calderon, J., Stopp, C., Wypij, D., DeMaso, D. R., Rivkin, M., Newburger, J. W., & Bellinger, D. C. (2016). Early-term birth in single-ventricle congenital heart disease after the Fontan Procedure: Neurodevelopmental and psychiatric outcomes. *Journal of Pediatrics, 179,* 96–103.

Calderon, J., Wypij, D., Rofeberg, V., Stopp, C., Roseman, A., Albers, D., . . . Bellinger, D. C. (2020). Randomized controlled trial of working memory intervention in congenital heart disease. *Journal of Pediatrics, 227,* 191–198.

Cassidy, A. R. (2020). Cognitive flexibility in critical CHD: A target for intervention. *Cardiology in the Young, 30*(8), 1061–1069.

Cassidy, A. R., Bernstein, J. H., Bellinger, D. C., Newburger, J. W., & DeMaso, D. R. (2019). Visual–spatial processing style is associated with psychopathology in adolescents with critical congenital heart disease. *Clinical Neuropsychologist, 33,* 760–778.

Cassidy, A. R., Butler, S., Briend, J., Calderon, J., Casey, F., Crosby, L., . . . Butcher, J. (2021). Neurodevelopmental and psychosocial interventions for individuals with CHD: A research agenda and recommendations from the Cardiac Neurodevelopmental Outcome Collaborative. *Cardiology in the Young, 31,* 888–899.

Cassidy, A. R., Ilardi, D., Bowen, S. R., Hampton, L. E., Heinrich, K. P., Loman, M. M., . . . Wolfe, K. R. (2018). Congenital heart disease: A primer for the pediatric neuropsychologist. *Child Neuropsychology, 24*(7), 859–902.

Cassidy, A. R., Newburger, J. W., & Bellinger, D. C. (2017). Learning and memory in adolescents with critical biventricular congenital heart disease. *Journal of the International Neuropsychological Society, 23,* 1–23.

Cassidy, A. R., White, M. T., DeMaso, D. R., Newburger, J. W., & Bellinger, D. C. (2015). Executive function in children and adolescents with critical cyanotic congenital heart disease. *Journal of the International Neuropsychological Society, 20,* 34–49.

Cassidy, A. R., White, M. T., DeMaso, D. R., Newburger, J. W., & Bellinger, D. C. (2016). Processing speed, executive function, and academic achievement in children with dextro-transposition of the great arteries: Testing a longitudinal developmental cascade model. *Neuropsychology, 30*(7), 874–885.

Chen, C. Y., Harrison, T., & Heathcock, J. (2015). Infants with complex congenital heart diseases show poor short-term memory in the mobile paradigm at 3 months of age. *Infant Behavior and Development, 40,* 12–19.

Chong, L. S. H., Fitzgerald, D. A., Craig, J. C., Manera, K. E., Hanson, C. S., Celermajer, D., . . . Hanson, C. S. (2018). Children's experiences of congenital heart disease: A systematic review of qualitative studies. *European Journal of Pediatrics, 177,* 319–336.

Claessens, N. H. P., Breur, J. M. P. J., Groenendaal, F., Asperen, R. M. W., Stegeman, R., Haas, F., . . . Benders, M. J. N. L. (2019). Brain microstructural development in neonates with critical congenital heart disease: An atlas-based diffusion tensor imaging study. *NeuroImage: Clinical, 21,* Article 101672.

Clouchoux, C., du Plessis, A. J., Bouyssi-Kobar, M., Tworetzky, W., McElhinney, D. B., Brown, D. W., . . . Limperopoulos, C. (2013). Delayed cortical development in fetuses with complex congenital heart disease. *Cerebral Cortex (New York), 23*(12), 2932–2943.

Cole, A. R., Perry, D. A., Nedder, A., Pollack, E., Regan, W. L., van den Bosch, S. J., . . . Kheir, J. N. (2019). Perioperatively inhaled hydrogen gas diminishes neurologic injury following experimental circulatory arrest in swine. *JACC: Basic to Translational Science, 4,* 176–187.

Daliento, L., Mapelli, D., Russo, G., Scarso, P., Limongi, F., Iannizzi, P., . . . Volpe, B. (2005). Health related quality of life in adults with repaired tetralogy of Fallot: Psychosocial and cognitive outcomes. *Heart, 91*(2), 213–218.

DeMaso, D. R., Calderon, J., Taylor, G. A., Holland, J. E., Stopp, C., White, M. T., . . . Newburger, J. W. (2017). Psychiatric disorders in adolescents with single ventricle congenital heart disease. *Pediatrics, 139*(3), Article e20162241.

DeMaso, D. R., Labella, M., Taylor, G. A., Forbes, P. W., Stopp, C., Bellinger, D. C., . . . Newburger, J. W. (2014). Psychiatric Disorders and function in adolescents with d-transposition of the great arteries. *Journal of Pediatrics, 165*(4), 760–766.

Dimitropoulos, A., McQuillen, P. S., Sethi, V., Moosa, A., Chau, V., Xu, D., . . . Miller, S. P. (2013). Brain injury and development in newborns with critical congenital heart disease. *Neurology, 81*(3), 241–248.

Distefano, R., Galinsky, E., McClelland, M. M., Zelazo, P. D., & Carlson, S. M. (2018). Autonomy-supportive parenting and associations with child and parent executive function. *Journal of Applied Developmental Psychology, 58,* 77–85.

Dorn, L. D., & Susman, E. J. (2019). Conceptualizing puberty as a window of opportunity for impacting health and well-being across the life span. *Journal of Research on Adolescence, 29*(1), 155–176.

Fasano-McCarron, M. E., Bernstein, J. H., Waber, D. P., Bellinger, D. C., & Cassidy, A. R. (2021). Performance on the ROCF at 8 years predicts academic achievement at 16 years in individuals with dextro-transposition of the great arteries. *Journal of the International Neuropsychological Society*, 1–8.

Feldmann, M., Bataillard, C., Ehrler, M., Ullrich, C., Knirsch, W., Gosteli-Peter, M., . . . Latal, B. (2021). Cognitive and executive function in congenital heart disease: A meta-analysis. *Pediatrics, 148*(4), e2021050875.

Fontes, K., Rohlicek, C. V., Saint-Martin, C., Gilbert, G., Easson, K., Majnemer, A., . . . Brossard-Racine, M. (2019). Hippocampal alterations and functional correlates in adolescents and young adults with congenital heart disease. *Human Brain Mapping, 40*, 3548–3560.

Gaies, M., Anderson, J., Kipps, A., Lorts, A., Madsen, N., Marino, B., . . . Pasquali, S. (2019). Cardiac networks united: An integrated paediatric and congenital cardiovascular research and improvement network. *Cardiology in the Young, 29*(2), 111–118.

Gao, S., Wu, Q., Zhang, T., Shen, Z., Liu, C., Xu, X., . . . Zhao, H. (2017). Fluoxetine and congenital malformations: A systematic review and meta-analysis of cohort studies. *British Journal of Clinical Pharmacology, 83*, 2134–2147.

Gaynor, J. W., Gerdes, M., Nord, A. S., Bernbaum, J., Zackai, E. l, Wernovsky, G., . . . Jarvik, G. P. (2010). Is cardiac diagnosis a predictor of neurodevelopmental outcome after cardiac surgery in infancy? *Journal of Thoracic and Cardiovascular Surgery, 140*(6), 1230–1237.

Gaynor, J. W., Gerdes, M., Zackai, E. H., Bernbaum, J., Wernovsky, G., Clancy, R. R., . . . Jarvik, G. P. (2003). Apolipoprotein E genotype and neurodevelopmental sequelae of infant cardiac surgery. *Journal of Thoracic and Cardiovascular Surgery, 126*(6), 1736–1745.

Gaynor, J. W., Stopp, C., Wypij, D., Andropoulos, D. B., Atallah, J., Atz, A. M., . . . Newburger, J. W. (2015). Neurodevelopmental outcomes after cardiac surgery in infancy. *Pediatrics, 135*(5), 816–825.

Gerstle, M., Beebe, D. W., Drotar, D., Cassedy, A., & Marino, B. S. (2016). Executive functioning and school performance among pediatric survivors of complex congenital heart disease. *Journal of Pediatrics, 173*, 1–6.

Graham, E. M., Martin, R. H., Atz, A. M., Hamlin-Smith, K., Kavarana, M. N., Bradley, S. M., . . . Everett, A. D. (2019). Association of intraoperative circulating-brain injury biomarker and neurodevelopmental outcomes at 1 year among neonates undergoing cardiac surgery. *Journal of Thoracic and Cardiovascular Surgery, 57*, 1996–2002.

Grasty, M. A., Ittenbach, R. F., Knightly, C., Solot, C. B., Gerdes, M., Bernbaum, J. C., . . . Burnham, N. B. (2018). Hearing loss after cardiac surgery in infancy: An unintended consequence of life-saving care. *Journal of Pediatrics, 192*, 144–151.

Guo, T., Chau, V., Peyvandi, S., Latal, B., McQuillen, P. S., Knirsch, W., . . . Miller, S. P. (2018). White matter injury in term neonates with congenital heart diseases: Topology and comparison with preterm newborns. *NeuroImage, 185*, 742–749.

Hoang, T. T., Marengo, L. K., Mitchell, L. E., Can, M. A., & Agopian, A. J. (2017). Systematic reviews and meta- and pooled analyses original findings and updated meta-analysis for the association between maternal diabetes and risk for congenital heart disease phenotypes. *American Journal of Epidemiology, 186*(1), 118–128.

Hoffman, J. I. E., & Kaplan, S. (2002). The incidence of congenital heart disease. *Journal of the American College of Cardiology, 39*(12), 1890–1900.

Holland, J. E., Cassidy, A. R., Stopp, C., White, M. T., Bellinger, D. C., Rivkin, M. J., . . . DeMaso, D. R. (2017). Psychiatric disorders and function in adolescents with tetralogy of Fallot. *Journal of Pediatrics, 187*, 165–173.

Homsy, J., Zaidi, S., Shen, Y., Ware, J. S., Samocha, K. E., Karczewski, K. J., . . . Chung, W. K. (2015). De novo mutations in congenital heart disease with neurodevelopmental and other congenital anomalies. *Science, 350*(6265), 1262–1266.

Hövels-Gürich, H., Konrad, K., Skorzenski, D., Herpertz-Dahlmann, B., Messmer, B., & Seghaye, M. (2007). Attentional dysfunction in children after corrective cardiac surgery in infancy. *Annals of Thoracic Surgery, 83*(4), 1425–1430.

Ilardi, D., Ono, K. E., McCartney, R., Book, W., & Stringer, A. Y. (2017). Neurocognitive functioning in adults with congenital heart disease. *Congenital Heart Disease, 12*, 166–173.

Ilardi, D., Sanz, J., Cassidy, A. R., Sananes, R., Rollins, C., Ullman Shade, C., & Bellinger, D. (2020). Neurodevelopmental evaluation for school-age children with congenital heart disease: Recommendations from the cardiac neurodevelopmental outcome collaborative. *Cardiology in the Young, 30*(11), 1623–1636.

Jackson, W., David, N., Calderon, J., Lee, J., Feirsen, N., Bellinger, D. C., & Sun, L. (2021). Executive functions in children and adolescents with heart disease: A systematic review and meta-analysis. *Cardiology in the Young*, 1–9.

Jakab, A., Meuwly, E., Feldmann, M., von Rhein, M., & Kottke, R. (2019). Left temporal plane growth predicts language development in newborns with congenital heart disease. *Brain, 142*, 1270–1281.

Jenkins, K. J., Correa, A., Feinstein, J. A., Botto, L., Britt, A. E., Daniels, S. R., . . . Webb, C. L. (2007). Noninherited risk factors and congenital cardiovascular defects: Current knowledge: A scientific statement from the American Heart Association Council on Cardiovascular Disease in the Young. *Circulation, 115*, 2995–3014.

Karsdorp, P. A., Everaerd, W., Kindt, M., & Mulder, B. J. M. (2007). Psychological and cognitive functioning in children and adolescents with congenital heart disease: A meta-analysis. *Journal of Pediatric Psychology, 32*(5), 527–541.

Kasparian, N. A. (2019). Heart care before birth: A psychobiological perspective on fetal cardiac diagnosis. *Progress in Pediatric Cardiology*, 101142.

Kasparian, N. A., Kan, J. M., Sood, E., Wray, J., Pincus, H. A., & Newburger, J. W. (2019). Mental health care for parents of babies with congenital heart disease during intensive care unit admission: Systematic review and statement of best practice. *Early Human Development, 139*, 104837.

Kelly, C. J., Christiaens, D., Batalle, D., Makropoulos, A., Cordero-Grande, L., Steinweg, J. K., . . . Counsell, S. J. (2019). Abnormal microstructural development of the cerebral cortex in neonates with congenital heart disease is associated with impaired cerebral oxygen delivery. *Journal of the American Heart Association, 8*, Article e009893.

Kirshbom, P. M., Flynn, T. B., Clancy, R. R., Ittenbach, R. F., Hartman, D. M., Paridon, S. M., . . . Gaynor, J. W. (2005). Late neurodevelopmental outcome after repair of total anomalous pulmonary venous connection. *Journal of Thoracic and Cardiovascular Surgery, 129*(5), 1091–1097.

Kovacs, A. H., Saidi, A. S., Kuhl, E. A., Sears, S. F., Silversides, C., Harrison, J. L., . . . Nolan, R. P. (2009). Depression and anxiety in adult congenital heart disease: Predictors and prevalence. *International Journal of Cardiology, 137*(2), 158–164.

Laas, E., Lelong, N., Thieulin, A.-C., Houyel, L., Bonnet, D., Ancel, P.-Y., . . . Khoshnood, B. (2012). Preterm birth and congenital heart defects: A population-based study. *Pediatrics, 130*(4), e829–e837.

Lage, K., Greenway, S. C., Rosenfeld, J. A., Wakimoto, H., Gorham, J. M., Segre, A. V, . . . Larsen, L. A. (2012). Genetic and environmental risk factors in congenital heart disease functionally converge in protein networks driving heart development. *Proceedings of the National Academy of Sciences USA, 109*(35), 14035–14040.

Laraja, K., Sadhwani, A., Tworetzky, W., Marshall, A. C., Gauvreau, K., Freud, L., . . . Newburger, J. W. (2017). Neurodevelopmental outcome in children after fetal cardiac intervention for aortic stenosis with evolving hypoplastic left heart syndrome. *Journal of Pediatrics, 184*, 130–136.

Lawrence, K. M., McGovern, P. E., Mejaddam, A., Rossidis, A. C., Baumgarten, H., Kim, A., . . . Gaynor, J. W. (2019). Chronic intrauterine hypoxia alters neurodevelopment in fetal sheep. *Journal of Thoracic and Cardiovascular Surgery, 157*, 1982–1991.

Licht, D. J., Shera, D. M., Clancy, R. R., Wernovsky, G., Montenegro, L. M., Nicolson, S. C., . . . Vossough, A. (2009). Brain maturation is delayed in infants with complex congenital heart defects. *Journal of Thoracic and Cardiovascular Surgery, 137*(3), 529–536; discussion 536–537.

Limperopoulos, C., Tworetzky, W., McElhinney, D. B., Newburger, J. W., Brown, D. W., Robertson, R. L., . . . du Plessis, A. J. (2010). Brain volume and metabolism in fetuses with congenital heart disease: Evaluation with quantitative magnetic resonance imaging and spectroscopy. *Circulation, 121*(1), 26–33.

Mahle, W. T., Clancy, R. R., Moss, E. M., Gerdes, M., Jobes, D. R., & Wernovsky, G. (2000). Neurodevelopmental outcome and lifestyle assessment in school-aged and adolescent children with hypoplastic left heart syndrome. *Pediatrics, 105*(5), 1082–1089.

Mahle, W. T., Tavani, F., Zimmerman, R. A., Nicolson, S. C., Galli, K. K., Gaynor, J. W., . . . Kurth, C. D. (2002). An MRI study of neurological injury before and after congenital heart surgery. *Circulation, 106*(12, Suppl. 1), 109–114.

Marelli, A., Miller, S. P., Marino, B. S., Jefferson, A. L., & Newburger, J. W. (2016). Brain in congenital heart disease across the lifespan. *Circulation, 133*(20), 1951–1962.

Marino, B. S., Lipkin, P. H., Newburger, J. W., Peacock, G., Gerdes, M., Gaynor, J. W., . . . Mahle, W. T. (2012). Neurodevelopmental outcomes in children with congenital heart disease: evaluation and management: A scientific statement from the American Heart Association. *Circulation, 126*(9), 1143–1172.

Marino, B. S., Sood, E., Cassidy, A. R., Miller, T. A., Sanz, J. H., Bellinger, D., . . . Goldberg, C. S. (2020a). The origins and development of the cardiac neurodevelopment outcome collaborative: Creating innovative clinical, quality improvement, and research opportunities. *Cardiology in the Young, 31*(1), 175.

Marino, B. S., Sood, E., Cassidy, A. R., Miller, T. A., Sanz, J. H., Bellinger, D., . . . Goldberg, C. S. (2020b). The origins and development of the cardiac neurodevelopmental outcome collaborative: Creating innovative clinical, quality improvement, and research opportunities—Corrigendum. *Cardiology in the Young, 30*(11), 1597–1602.

McCusker, C. G., Armstrong, M., Mullen, M., Doherty, N., & Casey, F. (2013). A sibling-controlled, prospective study of outcomes at home and school in children with severe congenital heart disease. *Cardiology in the Young, 23*(4), 507–516.

McCusker, C. G., Doherty, N. N., Molloy, B., Rooney, N., Mulholland, C., Sands, A., . . . Casey, F. (2010). A controlled trial of early interventions to promote maternal adjustment and development in infants born with severe congenital heart disease. *Child: Care, Health and Development, 36*(1), 110–117.

McCusker, C. G., Doherty, N. N., Molloy, B., Rooney, N., Mulholland, C., Sands, A., . . . Casey, F. (2012). A randomized controlled trial of interventions to promote adjustment in children with congenital heart disease entering school and their families. *Journal of Pediatric Psychology, 37*(10), 1089–1103.

McQuillen, P. S., & Miller, S. P. (2010). Congenital heart disease and brain development. *Annals of the New York Academy of Sciences, 1184*, 68–86.

Miatton, M., De Wolf, D., François, K., Thiery, E., & Vingerhoets, G. (2007a). Behavior and self-perception in children with a surgically corrected congenital heart disease. *Journal of Developmental and Behavioral Pediatrics, 28*(4), 294–301.

Miatton, M., De Wolf, D., François, K., Thiery, E., & Vingerhoets, G. (2007b). Intellectual, neuropsychological, and behavioral functioning in children with tetralogy of Fallot. *Journal of Thoracic and Cardiovascular Surgery, 133*(2), 449–455.

Miatton, M., De Wolf, D., François, K., Thiery, E., & Vingerhoets, G. (2007c). Neuropsychological performance in school-aged children with surgically corrected congenital heart disease. *Journal of Pediatrics, 151*(1), 73–78.

Miller, A., Riehle-Colarusso, T., Siffel, C., Frías, J. L., & Correa, A. (2011). Maternal age and prevalence of isolated congenital heart defects in an urban area of the United States. *American Journal of Medical Genetics: A, 155*(9), 2137–2145.

Miller, S. P., McQuillen, P. S., Hamrick, S., Xu, D., Glidden, D. V, Charlton, N., . . . Vigneron, D. B. (2007). Abnormal brain development in newborns with congenital heart disease. *New England Journal of Medicine, 357*(19), 1928–1938.

Mills, R., McCusker, C. G., Tennyson, C., & Hanna, D. (2018). Neuropsychological outcomes in CHD beyond childhood: A meta-analysis. *Cardiology in the Young, 28*, 421–431.

Morton, S. U., Maleyeff, L., Wypij, D., Yun, H. J., Newburger, J. W., Bellinger, D. C., . . . Im, K. (2020). Abnormal left-hemispheric sulcal patterns correlate with neurodevelopmental outcomes in subjects with single ventricular congenital heart disease. *Cerebral Cortex, 30*, 476–4872.

Morton, S. U., Quiat, D., Seidman, J. G., & Seidman, C. E. (2021). Genomic frontiers in congenital heart disease. *Nature Reviews Cardiology*, 0123456789.

Munoz-Lopez, M., Hoskote, A., Chadwick, M. J., Dzieciol, A. M., Gadian, D. G., Chong, K., . . . Vargha-khadem, F. (2017). Hippocampal damage and memory impairment in congenital cyanotic heart disease. *Hippocampus, 27*, 417–424.

Murphy, L. K., Compas, B. E., Reeslund, K. L., Gindville, M. C., Mah, M. L., Markham, L. W., & Jordan, L. C. (2017). Cognitive and attentional functioning in adolescents and young adults with tetralogy of Fallot and d-transposition of the great arteries. *Child Neuropsychology, 23*(1), 99–110.

Mussatto, K. A., Hoffmann, R. G., Hoffman, G. M., Tweddell, J. S., Bear, L., Cao, Y., & Brosig, C. (2014). Risk and prevalence of developmental delay in young children with congenital heart disease. *Pediatrics, 133*(3), e570–e577.

National Scientific Council on the Developing Child. (2004). *Young children develop in an environment of relationships: Working Paper No. 1.* Cambridge, MA: Center of the Developing Child (Harvard).

Nelson, T. J., & Cantero Peral, S. (2016). Stem cell therapy and congenital heart disease. *Journal of Cardiovascular Development and Disease, 3*(3), 24.

Nicoll, R. (2018). Environmental contaminants and congenital heart defects: A re-evaluation of the evidence. *International Journal of Environmental Research and Public Health, 15,* 1–23.

Opić, P., Roos-Hesselink, J. W., Cuypers, J. A. A., Witsenburg, M., van den Bosch, A., van Domburg, R. T., . . . Utens, E. M. W. J. (2015). Psychosocial functioning of adults with congenital heart disease: Outcomes of a 30–43 year longitudinal follow-up. *Clinical Research in Cardiology, 104,* 388–400.

Ortinau, C. M., Alexopoulos, D., Dierker, D., Van Essen, D., Beca, J., & Inder, T. (2013). Cortical folding is altered before surgery in infants with congenital heart disease. *Journal of Pediatrics, 163*(5), 1507–1510.

Ortinau, C. M., Anadkat, J. S., Smyser, C. D., & Eghtesady, P. (2018a). Intraventricular hemorrhage in moderate to severe congenital heart disease. *Pediatric Critical Care Medicine, 19*(1), 56–63.

Ortinau, C. M., Beca, J., Lambeth, J., Ferdman, B., Alexopoulos, D., Shimony, J. S., . . . Inder, T. (2012). Regional alterations in cerebral growth exist preoperatively in infants with congenital heart disease. *Journal of Thoracic and Cardiovascular Surgery, 143*(6), 1264–1270.

Ortinau, C. M., Mangin-Heimos, K., Moen, J., Alexopoulos, D., Inder, T. E., Gholipour, A., . . . Smyser, C. D. (2018b). Prenatal to postnatal trajectory of brain growth in complex congenital heart disease. *NeuroImage: Clinical, 20,* 913–922.

Ortinau, C. M., Rollins, C., Gholipour, A., Yun, H., Marshall, M., Gagoski, B., . . . Im, K. (2019). Early emerging sulcal patterns are atypical in fetuses with congenital heart disease. *Cerebral Cortex, 29,* 3605–3616.

Oster, M. E., Watkins, S., Hill, K. D., Knight, J. H., & Meyer, R. E. (2017). Academic outcomes in children with congenital heart defects. *Circulation: Cardiovascular Quality and Outcomes, 10*(2), Article e003074.

Owen, M., Shevell, M., Donofrio, M., Majnemer, A., McCarter, R., Vezina, G., . . . Limperopoulos, C. (2013). Brain volume and neurobehavior in newborns with complex congenital heart defects. *Journal of Pediatrics, 3,* 1–8.

Panigrahy, A., Schmithorst, V. J., Wisnowski, J. L., Watson, C. G., Bellinger, D. C., Newburger, J. W., & Rivkin, M. J. (2015). Relationship of white matter network topology and cognitive outcome in adolescents with d-transposition of the great arteries. *NeuroImage: Clinical, 7,* 438–448.

Peral, S. C., Burkhart, H. M., & Nelson, T. J. (2014). Utilization of stem cells to treat congenital heart disease: Hype and hope. *Current Opinion in Pediatrics, 26*(5), 553–560.

Peyvandi, S., Baer, R. J., Moon-Grady, A. J., Oltman, S. P., Chambers, C. D., Norton, M. E., . . . Steurer, M. A. (2018). Socioeconomic mediators of racial and ethnic disparities in congenital heart disease outcomes: A population-based study in California. *Journal of the American Heart Association, 7*(20), 1–12.

Peyvandi, S., De Santiago, V., Chakkarapani, E., Chau, V., Campbell, A., Poskitt, K. J., . . . McQuillen, P. (2016). Association of prenatal diagnosis of critical congenital heart disease with postnatal brain development and the risk of brain injury. *JAMA Pediatrics, 170,* Article e154450.

Phillips, J. M., & Longoria, J. N. (2019). Addressing the neurodevelopmental needs of children and adolescents with congenital heart disease: A review of the existing intervention literature. *Child Neuropsychology, 26*(4), 433–459.

Pike, N. A., Woo, M. A., Poulsen, M. K., Evangelista, W., Faire, D., Halnon, N. J., . . . Kumar, R. (2016). Predictors of memory deficits in adolescents and young adults with congenital heart disease compared to healthy controls. *Frontiers in Pediatrics, 4,* Article 117.

Ravishankar, C., Gerstenberger, E., Sleeper, L. A., Atz, A. M., Affolter, J. T., Bradley, T. J., . . . Newburger, J. W. (2016). Factors affecting Fontan length of stay: Results from the Single Ventricle Reconstruction Trial. *Journal of Thoracic and Cardiovascular Surgery, 151*(3), 669–675.

Razzaghi, H., Oster, M., & Reefhuis, J. (2015). Long-term outcomes in children with congenital heart disease: National Health Interview Survey. *Journal of Pediatrics, 166*(1), 119–124.

Ricci, M. F., Martin, B. J., Joffe, A. R., Dinu, I. A., Alton, G. Y., Guerra, G. G., & Robertson, C. M. T. (2018). Deterioration of functional abilities in children surviving the Fontan operation. *Cardiology in the Young, 28*(6), 868–875.

Rivkin, M. J., Watson, C. G., Scoppettuolo, L. A., Wypij, D., Vajapeyam, S., Bellinger, D. C., . . . Newburger, J. W. (2013). Adolescents with D-transposition of the great arteries repaired in early infancy demonstrate reduced white matter microstructure associated with clinical risk factors. *Journal of Thoracic and Cardiovascular Surgery, 146*(3), 543–539.

Rollins, C. K., Watson, C. G., Asaro, L. A., Wypij, D., Vajapeyam, S., Bellinger, D. C., . . . Rivkin, M. J. (2014). White matter microstructure and cognition in adolescents with congenital heart disease. *Journal of Pediatrics, 165*(5), 936–944.

Russell, M. W., Chung, W. K., Kaltman, J. R., & Miller, T. A. (2018). Advances in the understanding of the genetic determinants of congenital heart disease and their impact on clinical outcomes. *Journal of the American Heart Association, 7*(6), 1–16.

Rychik, J., Donaghue, D. D., Levy, S., Fjardo, C., Combs, J., Zhang, X., . . . Diamond, G. S. (2013). Maternal psychological stress after prenatal diagnosis of congenital heart disease. *Journal of Pediatrics, 162*(2), 303–307.

Sanz, J. H., Anixt, J., Bear, L., Basken, A., Beca, J., Marino, B. S., . . . Ilardi, D. (2021). Characterization of neurodevelopmental and psychological outcomes in congenital heart disease: A research agenda and recommendations from the Cardiac Neurodevelopmental Outcome Collaborative. *Cardiology in the Young, 3*(6), 876–887.

Sanz, J. H., Berl, M. M., Armour, A. C., Wang, J., Cheng, Y. I., & Donofrio, M. T. (2017). Prevalence and pattern of executive dysfunction in school age children with congenital heart disease. *Congenital Heart Disease, 12*, 202–209.

Sanz, J. H., Wang, J., Berl, M. M., Armour, A. C., Cheng, Y. I., & Donofrio, M. T. (2018). Executive function and psychosocial quality of life in school age children with congenital heart disease. *Journal of Pediatrics, 202*, 63–69.

Sarrechia, I., Miatton, M., De Wolf, D., François, K., Gewillig, M., Meyns, B., & Vingerhoets, G. (2016). Neurocognitive development and behaviour in school-aged children after surgery for univentricular or biventricular congenital heart disease. *European Journal of Cardio-Thoracic Surgery, 49*(1), 167–174.

Sarrechia, I., Miatton, M., François, K., Gewillig, M., Meyns, B., Vingerhoets, G., & De Wolf, D. (2015). Neurodevelopmental outcome after surgery for acyanotic congenital heart disease. *Research in Developmental Disabilities, 45–46*, 58–68.

Schellen, C., Ernst, S., Gruber, G. M., Mlczoch, E., Weber, M., Brugger, P. C., . . . Kasprian, G. (2015). Fetal MRI detects early alterations of brain development in Tetralogy of Fallot. *American Journal of Obstetrics and Gynecology, 213*(3), 392e1-392e7.

Schmithorst, V. J., Panigrahy, A., Gaynor, J. W., Watson, C. G., Lee, V., Bellinger, D. C., . . . Newburger, J. W. (2016). Organizational topology of brain and its relationship to ADHD in adolescents with d-transposition of the great arteries. *Brain and Behavior, 504*, Article e00504.

Semmel, E. S., Dotson, V. M., Burns, T. G., Mahle, W. T., & King, T. Z. (2018). Posterior cerebellar volume and executive function in young adults with congenital heart disease. *Journal of the International Neuropsychological Society, 24*(9), 1–10.

Shillingford, A. J., Glanzman, M. M., Ittenbach, R. F., Clancy, R. R., Gaynor, J. W., & Wernovsky, G. (2008). Inattention, hyperactivity, and school performance in a population of school-age children with complex congenital heart disease. *Pediatrics, 121*(4), e759–e767.

Siciliano, R. E., Prussien, K. V, Lee, C. A., Patel, N. J., Murphy, L. K., Compas, B. E., & Jordan, L. C. (2019). Cognitive function in pediatric hypoplastic left heart syndrome: Systematic review and meta-analysis. *Journal of Pediatric Psychology, 44*, 937–947.

Sommariva, G., Zilli, T., Crescentini, C., Marini, A., Venchiarutti, M., Gortan, A. J., & Fabbro, F. (2020). Toward a characterization of language development in children with congenital heart disease: A pilot study. *Child Neuropsychology, 26*, 1–14.

Sood, E., Jacobs, J. P., & Marino, B. S. (2020). The Cardiac Neurodevelopmental Outcome Collaborative: A new community improving outcomes for individuals with congenital heart disease. *Cardiology in the Young, 30*(11), 1595–1596.

Sood, E., Karpyn, A., Demianczyk, A. C., Ryan, J., Delaplane, E. A., Neely, T., . . . Kazak, A. E. (2018). Mothers and fathers experience stress of congenital heart disease differently. *Pediatric Critical Care Medicine, 19*, 626–634.

Sood, E., Lisanti, A., Woolf-King, S., Wray, J., Kasparian, N., Jackson, E., . . . Brosig, C. L. (2021). Parent mental health and family functioning following diagnosis of congenital heart disease: A research agenda and recommendations from the Cardiac Neurodevelopmental Outcome Collaborative. *Cardiology in the Young, 31*(6), 900–914.

Spector, L. G., Menk, J. S., Knight, J. H., McCracken, C., Thomas, A. S., Vinocur, J. M., . . . Kochilas, L. (2018). Trends in long-term mortality after congenital heart surgery. *Journal of the American College of Cardiology, 71*(21), 2434–2446.

Spijkerboer, A. W., Utens, E. M. W. J., Bogers, A. J. J. C., Verhulst, F. C., & Helbing, W. A. (2008). Long-term behavioural and emotional problems in four cardiac diagnostic groups of children and adolescents after invasive treatment for congenital heart disease. *International Journal of Cardiology, 125*(1), 66–73.

Stinnett, G. R., Lin, S., Korotcov, A. V., Korotcova, L., Morton, P. D., Ramachandra, S. D., . . . Ishibashi, N. (2017). Microstructural alterations and oligodendrocyte dysmaturation in white matter after cardiopulmonary bypass in a juvenile porcine model. *Journal of the American Heart Association, 6*(8), 1–28.

Sun, L., Macgowan, C., Sled, J., Yoo, S., Manlhiot,

C., Porayette, P., . . . Seed, M. (2015). Reduced fetal cerebral oxygen consumption is associated with smaller brain size in fetuses with congenital heart disease. *Circulation, 131,* 1313–1323.

Tararbit, K., Lelong, N., Houyel, L., Bonnet, D., Goffinet, F., & Khoshnood, B. (2014). Assessing the role of multiple pregnancies in the association between tetralogy of Fallot and assisted reproductive techniques: A path-analysis approach. *Orphanet Journal of Rare Diseases, 9*(27), 1–11.

Tindall, S., Rothermel, R. R., Delamater, A., Pinsky, W., & Klein, M. D. (1999). Neuropsychological abilities of children with cardiac disease treated with extracorporeal membrane oxygenation. *Developmental Neuropsychology, 16*(1), 101–115.

Tsao, P.-C., Lee, Y.-S., Jeng, M.-J., Hsu, J.-W., Huang, K.-L., Tsai, S.-J., . . . Kou, Y. R. (2017). Additive effect of congenital heart disease and early developmental disorders on attention-deficit/hyperactivity disorder and autism spectrum disorder: A nationwide population-based longitudinal study. *European Child and Adolescent Psychiatry, 26,* 1351–1359.

van der Mheen, M., van Beynum, I. M., Dulfer, K., van der Ende, J., van Galen, E., Duvekot, J.,. . . . Utens, E. M. W. J. (2018). The CHIP-Family study to improve the psychosocial wellbeing of young children with congenital heart disease and their families: Design of a randomized controlled trial. *BMC Pediatrics, 18*(1), Article 230.

van der Mheen, M., Meentken, M., van Beynum, I., van der Ende, J., van Galen, E., Zirar, A., . . . Utens, E. (2019). CHIP-Family intervention to improve the psychosocial well-being of young children with congenital heart disease and their families: Results of a randomised controlled trial. *Cardiology in the Young, 29*(9), 1172–1182.

Vincenti, M., O'Leary, P. W., Qureshi, M. Y., Seisler, D. K., Burkhart, H. M., Cetta, F., & Nelson, T. J. (2020). Clinical impact of autologous cell therapy on Hypoplastic Left Heart syndrome after bidirectional cavopulmonary anastomosis. *Seminars in Thoracic and Cardiovascular Surgery, 33*(3), 791–801.

Volpe, J. J., Kinney, H. C., Jensen, F. E., & Rosenberg, P. A. (2011). The developing oligodendrocyte: Key cellular target in brain injury in the premature infant. *International Journal of Developmental Neuroscience, 29*(6), 565–582.

von Rhein, M., Buchmann, A., Hagmann, C., Dave, H., Bernet, V., Scheer, I., . . . Latal, B. (2015a). Severe congenital heart defects are associated with global reduction of neonatal brain volumes. *Journal of Pediatrics, 167*(6), 1259–1263.

von Rhein, M., Buchmann, A., Hagmann, C., Huber, R., Klaver, P., Knirsch, W., & Latal, B. (2014). Brain volumes predict neurodevelopment in adolescents after surgery for congenital heart disease. *Brain, 137*(1), 268–276.

von Rhein, M., Kugler, J., Liamlahi, R., Knirsch, W., Latal, B., & Kaufmann, L. (2015b). Persistence of visuo-constructional and executive deficits in adolescents after open-heart surgery. *Research in Developmental Disabilities, 36,* 303–310.

von Rhein, M., Scheer, I., Loenneker, T., Huber, R., Knirsch, W., & Latal, B. (2011). Structural brain lesions in adolescents with congenital heart disease. *Journal of Pediatrics, 158*(6), 984–989.

Ware, J., Butcher, J., Latal, B., Sadhwani, A., Rollins, C., Brosig, C., . . . Wernovsky, G. (2020). Neurodevelopmental evaluation strategies for children with complex congenital heart disease aged birth through five years: Recommendations from the cardiac neurodevelopmental outcome collaborative. *Cardiology in the Young, 30*(11), 1609–1622.

Warnes, C. A., Liberthson, R., Danielson, G. K., Dore, A., Harris, L., Hoffman, J. I., . . . Webb, G. D. (2001). Task Force 1: The changing profile of congenital heart disease in adult life. *Journal of the American College of Cardiology, 37*(5), 1170–1175.

Watson, C. G., Asaro, L. A., Wypij, D., Robertson, R. L., Newburger, J. W., & Rivkin, M. J. (2016). Altered gray matter in adolescents with d-transposition of the great arteries. *Journal of Pediatrics, 169,* 36–43.

Wotherspoon, J., Eagleson, K. J., Gilmore, L., Auld, B., Hirst, A., Johnson, S., . . . Justo, R. N. (2020). Neurodevelopmental and health-related quality-of-life outcomes in adolescence after surgery for congenital heart disease in infancy. *Developmental Medicine and Child Neurology, 62,* 214–220.

Wu, Y., Kapse, K., Jacobs, M., Niforatos-Andescavage, N., Donofrio, M. T., Krishnan, A., . . . Limperopoulos, C. (2020). Association of maternal psychological distress with *in utero* brain development in fetuses with congenital heart disease. *JAMA Pediatrics, 174*(3), 1–10.

Wu, Y., Lu, Y., Kapse, K., Jacobs, M., Andescavage, H., Donofrio, M. T., . . . Limperopoulos, C. (2021). In utero MRI identifies impaired second trimester subplate growth in fetuses with congenital heart disease. *Cerebral Cortex,* 1–10.

CHAPTER 9

Fetal Alcohol Spectrum Disorders

Gemma Bernes
Eileen M. Moore
Linnea Vaurio
Sarah N. Mattson

HISTORICAL OVERVIEW AND DIAGNOSTIC CRITERIA

Although historical documentation suggests that teratogenic effects of prenatal alcohol exposure have been known for centuries, fetal alcohol syndrome (FAS) was not formally recognized until 1973, when Kenneth Lyons Jones and David Smith described 11 children born to alcohol-abusing mothers (Jones, Smith, Ulleland, & Streissguth, 1973). Based on the examination of this small group of children, Jones and Smith defined FAS as consisting of prenatal growth deficiency, developmental delay, craniofacial abnormality, and limb defects (Jones & Smith, 1973). Since the original description of FAS, revised and updated diagnostic guidelines have been published (Bertrand, Floyd, & Weber, 2005; Hoyme et al., 2016; Stratton, Howe, & Battaglia, 1996). These guidelines vary slightly but are generally consistent with the original criteria and require abnormalities in three domains for a diagnosis of FAS: (1) prenatal or postnatal growth (height and/or weight) deficiency (< 10th centile after adjustment for age, sex, gestational age and race or ethnicity); (2) specific pattern of facial dysmorphia (palpebral fissures ≤ 10th centile, smooth philtrum, and thin vermillion border); and (3) evidence of central nervous system (CNS) dysfunction (e.g., abnormal structural CNS development and/or neurobehavioral impairment). Although the combination of the three criteria, including the facial features, is considered unique, several partial phenocopies (e.g., velocardiofacial, Williams, and de Lange syndromes) exist and should be ruled out prior to diagnosing FAS (Hoyme et al., 2005).

Early reports exclusively focused on children with FAS; however, it is now clear that individuals exposed to heavy amounts of alcohol, who do not have the physical markers seen in FAS have similar neurobehavioral deficits. A variety of terms have been used to describe individuals who are affected by the teratogenic effects of alcohol but may not show all physical symptoms of FAS: partial FAS (pFAS), alcohol-related neurodevelopmental disorder (ARND), and alcohol-related birth defects (ARBD). The guidelines from the Institute of Medicine (IOM) and subsequent updates (Hoyme et al., 2005, 2016; Stratton et al., 1996) provide criteria for the diagnosis of pFAS, ARND, and ARBD to facilitate identification of individuals with prenatal exposure to alcohol who may not meet all diagnostic criteria for FAS. Additionally, the American Psychiatric Association (2013) included neurobehavioral disorder associated with prenatal alcohol exposure (ND-PAE) in DSM-5 as a proposed diagnosis that needs further study. Unlike ARND, which cannot be used in the presence of diagnostic facial dysmorphia, ND-PAE can be diagnosed in affected individuals independently of physical features.

To acknowledge the continuum of deficits caused by prenatal alcohol exposure, the National Task Force on Fetal Alcohol Syndrome and Fetal Alcohol Effect adopted the term *fetal alcohol spectrum disorders* (FASD; Bertrand et al., 2004), which was originally coined by the nonprofit FASD United (formerly known as the National Organization on Fetal Alcohol Syndrome [NOFAS; *www.nofas.org*]). In the United States, FASD is not a diagnosis, but an umbrella term used to emphasize the range of deleterious physical, mental, and behavioral outcomes that can occur with exposure to alcohol. In Canada and other countries, FASD is used diagnostically (Cook et al., 2016). In this chapter we use the term FASD and focus on children with heavy prenatal alcohol exposure, including those with and without FAS. When describing research herein, the two groups are combined, unless group differences have been found, in which case differences are made explicit.

EPIDEMIOLOGY

FASD is caused by *in utero* alcohol exposure. Alcohol is recognized as toxic to the developing CNS (Stratton et al., 1996). Because alcohol freely crosses the placenta, a mother's blood alcohol content will be the same as that of the developing embryo or fetus, leading to disruption of the CNS and other body systems. Despite a proliferation of evidence demonstrating toxic effects of prenatal alcohol exposure, the rates of such exposure are relatively high. Approximately 11.5% of pregnant women in the United States report drinking alcohol during pregnancy, and 3.9% of women of childbearing age report drinking alcohol at *risk levels,* defined as consumption of five or more drinks on one occasion in the past 30 days (Denny, Acero, Naimi, & Kim, 2019). Thus, although FASD is preventable, continued efforts are needed to both delineate effects and develop intervention strategies suitable for children affected by prenatal alcohol exposure.

Estimates of incidence of FAS in the United States range between 0.2 and 1.5 cases per 1,000 live births, with current estimates suggesting that 1,000–6,000 infants are born each year with FAS (Centers for Disease Control and Prevention, 2002, 2015). Rates of FASD are as high as 11.3–50.0 per 1,000 children (May et al., 2018). Global prevalence rates of FASD are estimated to be 7.7 per 1,000 children in the general population, with South Africa having the highest estimates (111.1 per 1,000) of the countries with available prevalence data (Lange et al., 2017). In 2004, the estimated median adjusted annual expenditures for all individuals with FAS in the United States was $3.6 million (Lupton, Burd, & Harwood, 2004). This estimate included costs associated with medical services, residential services, special education services, and lost productivity. Total lifetime cost per individual with FAS was estimated to be $2.9 million. No current estimates are available for costs associated with the full spectrum of outcomes associated with alcohol exposure in the United States. However, the economic burden of FASD was estimated in Canada to be approximately CAD $1.8 billion (Popova, Lange, Burd, & Rehm, 2016a). Therefore, based on incidence estimates, we can expect that expenditures will also increase dramatically when considering the full FASD population in the United States.

NEUROPATHOLOGY AND NEURAL SUBSTRATES

The brain is particularly sensitive to the teratogenic effect of alcohol exposure. In general, the smaller brain size and regional abnormalities seen in imaging studies of individuals with FAS are also observed in individuals with FASD, but with somewhat decreased severity (Riley, McGee, & Sowell, 2004; Roebuck, Mattson, & Riley, 1998a).

Brain Volume

One of the diagnostic features of FAS is head circumference ≤ 10th centile. Not surprisingly, therefore, a consistent finding in neuroimaging investigations of FASD is that of smaller overall brain size (Moore, Migliorini, Infante, & Riley, 2014). As a result, examination of the specificity of alcohol's effects is important. Diffuse and consistent overall smaller size may be indicative of a global effect of prenatal alcohol exposure, while a specific pattern of disproportionately small brain regions would indicate that certain brain regions (and, by extension, certain types of behavior or cognition) are more sensitive to the teratogenic insult. Neuroimaging data suggest that certain brain regions and structures are differentially affected by prenatal alcohol exposure, most notably the corpus callosum, basal ganglia, and cerebellum.

Corpus Callosum

Dramatic abnormalities in the corpus callosum were observed in early brain autopsies in children with FAS (Jones & Smith, 1975) and have been confirmed in magnetic resonance imaging (MRI) investigations (Moore et al., 2014; Riley & McGee, 2005). Early studies reported cases of partial or full agenesis (absence) of the corpus callosum (ACC) in alcohol-exposed individuals (Riley & McGee, 2005). While complete or partial agenesis is rare in FASD, agenesis may be found at a higher rate in FAS than in any other developmental disorder (Jeret & Serur, 1991). In one study, the rate of ACC was conservatively estimated at 6.8% (Riley et al., 1995), which is higher than the estimate of 2.3% in the developmentally disabled population. Imaging studies have yielded a wide range of callosal outcomes in FASD, including agenesis, hypoplasia, thinning, displacement, and disproportionate regional reductions (Autti-Rämö et al., 2002; Riley et al., 1995; Sowell et al., 2001a). Alterations in the corpus callosum have been documented into adulthood (Bookstein, Sampson, Connor, & Streissguth, 2002; Bookstein, Sampson, Streissguth, & Connor, 2001; Chen, Coles, Lynch, & Hu, 2012).

While the macrostructural effects of prenatal alcohol exposure on the corpus callosum are striking, diffusion tensor imaging studies have also revealed microstructural abnormalities in individuals with FASD. Lower fractional anisotropy, higher mean diffusivity, and higher radial diffusivity have been reported (Moore et al., 2014; Wozniak & Muetzel, 2011). The observed pattern of microstructural changes suggests that myelination or axonal density/caliber may be affected in FASD (Feldman, Yeatman, Lee, Barde,

& Gaman-Bean, 2010). Similar to the reported macrostructural abnormalities, the genu and more posterior regions of the corpus callosum (isthmus–splenium) may be most sensitive to these microstructural changes (Moore et al., 2014; Wozniak & Muetzel, 2011).

Basal Ganglia

The basal ganglia appear to be particularly vulnerable to prenatal alcohol exposure. After controlling for microcephaly, individuals with FAS and nondysmorphic FASD have smaller basal ganglia volume (Inkelis, Moore, Bischoff-Grethe, & Riley, 2020; Mattson et al., 1992). Regional investigation of the basal ganglia demonstrates that the caudate nucleus accounts for most of the size discrepancy (Archibald et al., 2001; Mattson et al., 1992). One analysis of the caudate indicated that smaller volumes of this region were not only proportional to total brain size but also revealed areas of deformation dispersed across the head and tail regions of the bilateral caudate that were related to quantity of prenatal alcohol exposure (Joseph et al., 2014). While initial studies indicated that the caudate may be most affected, recent studies have also indicated disproportionately small putamen and pallidum volumes (Inkelis et al., 2020; Nardelli, Lebel, Rasmussen, Andrew, & Beaulieu, 2011; Roussotte et al., 2012).

Cerebellum

A number of researchers have reported that the cerebellum is disproportionately smaller, hypoplastic, malformed, or displaced among individuals with FASD (Inkelis et al., 2020; Lebel, Roussotte, & Sowell, 2011; Moore et al., 2014). In young adults, the volume of the cerebellum negatively relates to quantity of prenatal alcohol exposure (Chen et al., 2012). In addition to overall cerebellar reductions, the cerebellar vermis appears to be particularly sensitive to alcohol exposure. Earlier studies using manual tracing indicated that the anterior regions of the vermis were disproportionately affected, while more posterior regions were relatively spared (O'Hare et al., 2005; Sowell et al., 1996); however, more recent analyses using an automated segmentation technique indicate that both anterior (lobules I–V) and inferior posterior (lobules VIII–X) regions are disproportionately affected (Cardenas et al., 2014), as in reports from animal models (Goodlett, Marcussen, & West, 1990).

Other Subcortical Regions

Limbic structures are also affected by prenatal alcohol exposure, though the extent of this effect is not clear. For example, for both the hippocampus and the amygdala, evidence exists for both proportionate and disproportionate reductions (Donald et al., 2016a; Nardelli et al., 2011). Reductions in both structures may be dose- and diagnosis-dependent, with more severe reductions in more heavily exposed individuals (Chen et al., 2012) and those with FAS (Coles et al., 2011).

Smaller diencephalic structures have also been reported in FASD (Mattson et al., 1996c; Nardelli et al., 2011; Roussotte et al., 2012; Treit et al., 2013, 2017), including disproportionate reductions in the thalamus (Nardelli et al., 2011; Treit et al., 2013). The pituitary gland is disproportionately smaller in adolescent females with FASD, while posterior pituitary signal intensity is lower in both sexes (Moore, Infante, Migliorini, Mattson, &

Riley, 2016). Diencephalic structures have also been reported to relate to degree of facial dysmorphology (i.e., palpebral fissure length) in alcohol-exposed children (Roussotte et al., 2012).

The Cortex

Early studies investigating regional differences in cortical volume between those with FASD and controls revealed that the parietal (Archibald et al., 2001) and frontal areas (Sowell et al., 2002) were most affected. However, later studies indicated that these effects may vary by age and facial dysmorphology (Chen et al., 2012; Hendrickson et al., 2018; Lebel et al., 2011; Li et al., 2008). Other measures of cortical integrity also provide insight. Cortical thickness, surface area, and gyrification have been investigated. These are thought to be phenotypically and genetically independent measures with distinct developmental trajectories (Panizzon et al., 2009; Wierenga, Langen, Oranje, & Durston, 2014) and may detect more subtle structural differences that could potentially go undetected in volumetric analyses (Migliorini et al., 2015). Evidence exists for both increased (Fernandez-Jaen et al., 2011; Sowell et al., 2008; Yang et al., 2012) and decreased (Treit et al., 2013, 2014; Zhou et al., 2011; Zhou et al., 2018) cortical thickness across widespread regions of the cortex. A longitudinal study shows that alcohol-exposed children have differing developmental trajectories of cortical thickness in frontal, temporal, and parietal areas and of cortical gyrification across all four lobes (Hendrickson et al., 2018). Generally, alcohol-exposed children showed flatter change or more pronounced decreases with development that result in bigger group discrepancies during adolescence as compared to younger ages and suggested a more immature cortical structure. Only two studies have examined cortical surface area. One study indicated reduced surface area in the anterior cingulate (Migliorini et al., 2015), while the other suggested that regional reductions in surface area attenuated after correction for total brain volume (Rajaprakash, Chakravarty, Lerch, & Rovet, 2014). Finally, gyrification is generally attenuated in youth with histories of prenatal alcohol exposure (De Guio et al., 2014; Hendrickson et al., 2017; Infante et al., 2015).

White Matter

As described previously, the corpus callosum is particularly sensitive to prenatal alcohol exposure. However, white matter in general is also susceptible to alcohol's teratogenic effects. White matter hypoplasia in the cerebrum has been reported to be more severe than gray matter hypoplasia in children with FAS (Archibald et al., 2001), and disproportionate regional effects in white matter across the brain are apparent in children with heavy prenatal alcohol exposure (Bjorkquist, Fryer, Reiss, Mattson, & Riley, 2010; Gautam et al., 2015; Gautam, Nunez, Narr, Kan, & Sowell, 2014). Children with ARND have been shown to have smaller volumes of white matter tracts and fewer number of fibers (Malisza et al., 2012).

Diffusion tensor studies have also indicated microstructural changes throughout the brain in children with FASD. Children with prenatal alcohol exposure have poorer white matter integrity, as indicated by lower fractional anisotropy in a number of tracts, including the inferior and superior longitudinal fasciculi, anterior and superior corona radiata, and right uncinate (Fan et al., 2016; Moore et al., 2014; Wozniak & Muetzel,

2011). Sex-specific changes have also been noted, with alcohol-exposed girls having lower fractional anisotropy in inferior fronto-occipital and uncinate fasciculi, while alcohol-exposed boys have higher fractional anisotropy in the callosal body, cingulum, corticospinal tract, optic radiation, and superior longitudinal fasciculus (Uban, Herting, Wozniak, Sowell, & CIFASD, 2017). Children with FASD also have atypical developmental trajectories in several of these tracts (Treit et al., 2013, 2017). The impact of prenatal alcohol on white matter microstructure can be seen in newborns, although radial diffusivity rather than fractional anisotropy is the metric sensitive to alcohol exposure at this age (Taylor et al., 2015). Studies that have examined additional diffusion measures beyond fractional anisotropy (i.e., mean diffusivity, radial diffusivity) indicate that the pattern of changes is indicative of poorer axon packing density or myelination in FASD (Fan et al., 2016).

Functional Brain Imaging Studies

Functional magnetic resonance imaging (fMRI) studies have examined hemodynamic brain response for alcohol-exposed adults and children during a variety of tasks. Generally, such studies indicate that alcohol-exposed individuals have altered patterns of brain activation and tend to recruit different or a broader range of brain regions when completing tasks (Coles & Li, 2011; Moore et al., 2014). Often the activation patterns are more similar to those observed in younger children, perhaps indicating a less mature neural system. Additionally, differences in patterns of activation may indicate that groups utilize different strategies or that greater effort and compensatory mechanisms are required to complete the tasks.

Resting-state fMRI studies utilize a task-independent approach in which participants are scanned while looking at a fixation cross or with their eyes closed. Resting-state studies indicate that prenatal alcohol exposure disrupts neural networks in neonates and that these effects continue through at least young adulthood, although the nature of the disruption may differ depending on age. For example, atypical increases in functional connectivity are observed in somatosensory and motor control networks in neonates (Donald et al., 2016b); functional connectivity of sensorimotor networks is atypically increased in the default-mode network but atypically decreased in salience networks in children (Long, Little, Beaulieu, & Lebel, 2018); and atypical decreases in functional connectivity are noted between the hemispheres (Wozniak et al., 2011) and in several networks that are important for child cognition (Fan et al., 2017; Little, Reynolds, & Beaulieu, 2018), as well as in the default-mode network in young adults (Santhanam et al., 2011). Additionally, graph theory analyses indicate that children with heavy prenatal alcohol exposure have a local network efficiency disadvantage of 1.3–3.5% (Wozniak et al., 2013). While this may seem relatively small, it may have high clinical significance, as a 1% decrease in local network efficiency has been shown to relate to a 36-point difference in global cognitive functioning standard scores in children (Wozniak et al., 2017).

NEUROPSYCHOLOGICAL CONSEQUENCES

Delineation of a neuropsychological signature or profile associated with prenatal alcohol exposure has been the subject of much debate and research. Recent findings support the presence of a distinct neurobehavioral profile. In addition to generally diminished IQ, individuals with prenatal alcohol exposure show deficits in attentional, learning, psychomotor, verbal, executive, visual–spatial, and adaptive functioning domains.

Global Deficits

Given the spectrum of outcomes in FASD, it is not surprising that estimates of general intellectual functioning vary. In studies of children with FAS, IQ scores range from 20 to 120, averaging between 65 and 72 (Mattson & Riley, 1998). Although FAS is thought to be the leading preventable cause of intellectual disability in the United States (Williams, Smith, & Committee on Substance Abuse, 2015), most individuals with FAS are not intellectually disabled (Streissguth, Barr, Kogan, & Bookstein, 1996). Nondysmorphic alcohol-exposed individuals tend to have slightly higher IQ scores than dysmorphic alcohol-exposed individuals, although still significantly lower than nonexposed peers; nonetheless, absence of facial dysmorphology does not indicate absence of cognitive impairment in this population (Mattson & Riley, 1998). Developmental delay, learning disability and low academic achievement are outcomes related to decreased IQ (Bertrand et al., 2005). While some reports indicate that children with FAS and FASD are relatively more impaired on nonverbal intelligence measures (as indicated by Performance IQ) when compared to verbal intelligence measures (Bertrand et al., 2005; Streissguth, Barr, Sampson, & Bookstein, 1994a), these findings are not consistent (Mattson & Riley, 1998).

Attention and Hyperactivity

Attention deficits are well-documented effects of prenatal alcohol exposure (Burden, Jacobson, Sokol, & Jacobson, 2005), and children with FASD frequently have a diagnosis of attention-deficit/hyperactivity disorder (ADHD; Fryer, McGee, Matt, Riley, & Mattson, 2007; Ware et al., 2013). Although FASD is associated with several other disorders, including oppositional defiant disorder and conduct disorder, ADHD appears to be the most common, with prevalence rates ranging from 63% to as high as 95% (Mattson, Bernes, & Doyle, 2019). Attention deficits observed in heavily exposed children are worse than would be predicted by IQ scores (Mattson & Riley, 2000) and are also apparent in prospective studies of individuals with low to moderate prenatal alcohol exposure (e.g., Burden et al., 2005; Streissguth et al., 1994a). Measures of attention and attention-related behavior can discriminate between alcohol-exposed children and controls with a high degree of accuracy even after researchers control for overall IQ (Lee, Mattson, & Riley, 2004). Thus, attention deficits may be more sensitive than intellectual deficits or facial dysmorphology in detecting prenatal alcohol exposure.

Several studies have compared children with FASD to unexposed children with ADHD; these two groups can be distinguished from each other based on measures of vigilance, visual–spatial processing, executive functioning, learning and memory, and adaptive behavior (generally, FASD is more impaired than ADHD; for review, see Mattson et al., 2019). This is somewhat surprising given the high rates of ADHD in the FASD population, but it suggests that a singular model of attention deficits may not be appropriate in classifying these two populations.

Learning and Memory

Multiple studies have addressed learning and memory in children with FASD. General consensus is that deficits in this domain exist, but careful delineation of the nature and types of deficits is required. As in other areas of function, some, but not all, types of learning and memory are affected in individuals with FASD. While most studies have focused on verbal learning and memory, a small number have addressed nonverbal learning and memory, and others have made the distinction between learning and memory or recall and retention.

Verbal Learning and Memory

Several studies of FASD have used the California Verbal Learning Test—Children's Version (CVLT-C), a 15-word recall test. Children with FASD learn fewer words initially, have more difficulty recalling words after a delay, and show impaired discrimination of correct words in comparison to controls (Lewis et al., 2015; Mattson, Riley, Gramling, Delis, & Jones, 1998; Mattson & Roebuck, 2002). While they are not able to reach the level of learning shown by controls, children with FASD do benefit from repeated exposure to new material. Importantly, these deficits are present for children with and without the physical features associated with FAS (Mattson et al., 1998; Mattson & Roebuck, 2002), as well as after controlling for IQ (Lewis et al., 2015; Vaurio, Riley, & Mattson, 2011). Retention of learned verbal material is comparable between groups, suggesting that exposed children are able to retain verbal information that is encoded (Coles, Lynch, Kable, Johnson, & Goldstein, 2010; Mattson, Riley, Delis, Stern, & Jones, 1996b; Mattson et al., 1998).

Nonverbal Learning and Memory

Studies of nonverbal memory are sparse, and existing results are inconsistent. In some studies, alcohol-exposed children benefit from repeated exposure but demonstrate both encoding and retrieval deficits for nonverbal information (Mattson & Roebuck, 2002; Roebuck-Spencer & Mattson, 2004). Other research demonstrates that alcohol-exposed children have a pattern of spared long-term retention in visual learning measures, similar to that described earlier in the verbal domain (Kaemingk, Mulvaney, & Tanner Halverson, 2003).

Speech and Language

Although not as extensively studied as other domains, a number of studies have demonstrated both speech production and language processing dysfunction in heavily exposed populations (Church, Eldis, Blakley, & Bawle, 1997; Conry, 1990; Janzen, Nanson, & Block, 1995; Wyper & Rasmussen, 2011). While impairments are observed in both receptive and expressive language abilities, more pronounced impairments are found with expressive language skills (McGee, Bjorkquist, Riley, & Mattson, 2009). Individuals with FASD demonstrate a range of speech production deficiencies, including poorer simple phonemic production, an increased number of grammatical errors, and more marked deficits that result in low intelligibility of speech, possibly related to the high proportion of craniofacial and dentofacial abnormalities in this population (Church et al., 1997; Thorne, 2017). Younger alcohol-exposed children display global deficits in language, while older children present with more specific syntactic deficits (Carney & Chermak, 1991). However, these deficits may be secondary to the impaired intellectual functioning associated with prenatal alcohol exposure, as deficits are no longer significant after researchers control for IQ (McGee et al., 2009). Despite this, measures of grammatical error rates were able to better differentiate between children with FASD and typically developing children compared to measures of language productivity and grammatical complexity, highlighting the potential utility of language skill assessments as a diagnostic tool (Thorne, 2017).

Executive Functioning

Examinations of executive functioning (EF) in individuals with FASD generally document impairments; indeed, EF deficits are often considered a hallmark of this disorder. However, deficits are not uniform and may depend on underlying modality or task characteristics. In one study, performance on a measure of self-regulatory behavior yielded no significant differences compared to controls, children with prenatal alcohol exposure did display increased deficits on a task of problem solving and planning (Kodituwakku, Handmaker, Cutler, Weathersby, & Handmaker, 1995). Exposed children spend less time preplanning, use inefficient problem-solving strategies, and are more likely to violate a given rule compared to typically developing children (Green et al., 2009b; Kodituwakku et al., 1995; Mattson, Goodman, Caine, Delis, & Riley, 1999). In utilization of feedback tasks, alcohol-exposed participants are impaired on the Wisconsin Card Sorting Test, but equal to controls on a go/no-go task (Kodituwakku et al., 1995). These results suggest that individuals with FASD have a specific pattern of EF deficits rather than global deficits.

In another investigation, individuals with heavy alcohol exposure demonstrated deficits on tasks in the Delis–Kaplan Executive Functioning System, which allows for a simultaneous hierarchical investigation of perceptual/lower-order and higher-order integrative abilities (Delis, Kaplan, & Kramer, 2001). Exposed children performed significantly worse on tests tapping cognitive flexibility, response inhibition, and planning and concept formation, even after taking into account lower-order processing (Mattson et al., 1999). In examinations of verbal fluency in alcohol-exposed children, consistent impairment on letter fluency has been found, while category fluency appears to be diminished but less robustly affected (Kodituwakku et al., 1995; Mattson et al., 1999; Vaurio, Riley, & Mattson, 2008). This fluency deficit appears to be global, as children with FASD have shown similarly poor performance across verbal and nonverbal fluency tasks (Schonfeld, Mattson, Lang, Delis, & Riley, 2001), and may be related to the ability to switch cognitive set (Hayden, 2005). Deficits observed in children appear to extend throughout the lifespan, as adults with FASD have similarly impaired performance on EF tasks (Connor, Sampson, Bookstein, Barr, & Streissguth, 2000).

Results are equivocal regarding the relationship of EF deficits and IQ, which are traditionally thought to be relatively independent. One study of adults found that EF deficits were worse than predicted by IQ, suggesting that EF deficits are independent of diminished intellectual ability (Connor et al., 2000). Other studies indicate that EF ability in alcohol-exposed participants is either not significantly associated with IQ (Mattson et al., 1999) or is better than would be predicted by IQ (Mattson, Vaurio, & Riley, 2006), suggesting that at least some EF abilities may be a relative strength in this population. However, different patterns may exist for varying EF tasks, as verbally mediated tasks of EF were found to be related to IQ levels and not necessarily to prenatal alcohol exposure (Vaurio et al., 2011). Further research is necessary to better understand the relationship between EF and IQ in this population.

One domain of EF that has been surprisingly understudied in individuals with heavy prenatal alcohol exposure is working memory. In one study using a delayed matching to sample task and a self-ordered pointing task, two widely used working memory measures, no significant impairments were found in children with prenatal alcohol exposure (Kodituwakku et al., 1995). In a prospective study of low to moderate prenatal alcohol exposure, more moderately exposed children demonstrated worse performance on tasks thought to test working memory, and a dose–response relationship was observed, with a one-fifth of a standard deviation decrease in working memory for each ounce of absolute alcohol consumed during pregnancy (Burden et al., 2005). A recent study (Moore et al., 2021) that examined the relation between spatial working memory and age found that prenatal alcohol exposure was associated with slower improvement, resulting in a larger gap between groups as youth matured. However, a preliminary study found that when participants with lower-order processing deficits were excluded from analysis, performance of alcohol-exposed participants did not differ from controls (Vaurio, Repp, McGee, Riley, & Mattson, 2006). This suggests that deficits observed in working memory may be due to perceptual dysfunction rather than a specific higher-order deficit. Further systematic examination of working memory is required to determine if it is indeed a central dysfunction in alcohol-exposed individuals.

Motor Functioning

Children with prenatal alcohol exposure demonstrate motor impairments. Tremors, weak grasp, and poor hand–eye coordination are associated with FAS and FASD (Jones & Smith, 1973; Mattson & Riley, 1998). In one study, children with FASD showed impaired balance and were unable to compensate for body sway with their visual or vestibular systems when somatosensory or visual input was unreliable (Roebuck, Simmons, Mattson, & Riley, 1998b). Fine motor skills (e.g., dexterity) are more negatively affected than gross motor abilities (e.g., balance) in individuals with FASD, although impairment is found in both domains (Kalberg et al., 2006). Furthermore, children with prenatal alcohol exposure are more likely to display deficits in complex fine motor skills (e.g., visual–motor integration) than basic fine motor skills (e.g., grip strength; Doney et al., 2014). Other motor impairments associated with prenatal alcohol exposure include impaired oculomotor control (Green et al., 2009a), longer reaction times (Simmons, Thomas, Levy, & Riley, 2010), impaired hand–eye coordination (Adnams et al., 2001), impaired bimanual coordination (Roebuck-Spencer, Mattson, Marion, Brown, & Riley, 2004), and poor sensorimotor abilities (Jirikowic, Olson, & Kartin, 2008). Increased impairment in both fine and gross motor skills is associated with moderate to high prenatal alcohol exposure levels, with fewer studies finding impairment in children with lower levels (Doney et al., 2014; Lucas et al., 2014). In addition, motor deficits persist into adulthood for heavily exposed populations (Connor, Sampson, Streissguth, Bookstein, & Barr, 2006).

Visual–Spatial Ability

While visual–spatial ability is understudied in FASD, deficits have been noted in visual–spatial construction as measured by a figure copy test, the Beery–Buktenica Developmental Test of Visual–Motor Integration (Conry, 1990; Franklin, Deitz, Jirikowic, & Astley, 2008; Janzen et al., 1995; Mattson et al., 1998). However, these deficits may be secondary to motor rather than perceptual ability (Janzen et al., 1995). On a more complex visual–spatial task, children with histories of prenatal alcohol exposure were asked to recall hierarchical figures (Mattson, Gramling, Delis, Jones, & Riley, 1996a). Deficits were found in children's recall of local but not global features of the hierarchical stimuli, and these deficits were not due to the stimuli size or to memory performance. Previous research suggests that this type of performance may relate to a pattern of brain abnormality that involves the left hemisphere to a greater degree than the right hemisphere, which is supported by brain imaging studies in this population (Sowell et al., 2001b). Additional investigation is needed to determine if visual–spatial processing is affected in specific or global ways and to determine the contribution of lower-order (perceptual, motor) deficits to visual–spatial processing.

Social Skills and Secondary Disabilities

In addition to perceptual and cognitive deficits, children with prenatal alcohol exposure demonstrate deficits in interpersonal domains. Based on parent ratings, alcohol-exposed children are more likely to be classified as hyperactive, disruptive, impulsive, or delinquent (Mattson & Riley, 2000; Roebuck, Mattson, & Riley, 1999) and have significant deficits in adaptive behavior (Crocker, Vaurio, Riley, & Mattson, 2009; Jirikowic et al., 2008). These deficits persist throughout childhood and adulthood (Carr, Agnihotri, & Keightley, 2010; Panczakiewicz et al., 2016), though abilities related to communication and socialization have been found to decline further with age (Crocker et al., 2009; Whaley, O'Connor, & Gunderson, 2001). Parent-reported deficits in social skills, as measured by the Social Skills Rating System, have been shown to be significantly correlated with parent-reported EF deficits, suggesting that higher-order cognitive deficits may contribute to interpersonal difficulties (Schonfeld, Paley, Frankel, & O'Connor, 2006).

Heavy prenatal alcohol exposure also results in high levels of secondary disabilities and psychopathology, which are important to consider, because individuals affected by prenatal alcohol exposure who do not have an IQ below 70 are often disabled but do not qualify for special services. Deficits have been noted in social problem solving, including the ability to identify a problem, as well as generate and implement the best possible solution (McGee, Fryer, Bjorkquist, Mattson, & Riley, 2008), and high rates of inappropriate sexual behavior, disrupted school experience, delinquency, incarceration, and drug and alcohol problems have all been documented in children and adults with FASD (Streissguth et al., 1996, 2004). However, in a study of a low socioeconomic status, predominantly African American sample, no association was found between alcohol exposure and law-breaking behavior. Rather, delinquent acts were predicted by factors such as increased life stress, drug use, and decreased supervision (Lynch, Coles, Corley, & Falek, 2003). This finding highlights the importance of considering contextual factors when examining behavioral outcomes in alcohol-exposed individuals. In terms of psychopathology, elevated rates of ADHD, depressive disorders, oppositional defiant disorder, conduct disorder, and specific phobia have been documented (Fryer et al., 2007; Popova et al., 2016b; Weyrauch, Schwartz, Hart, Klug, & Burd, 2017) and these elevations persist even after researchers control for confounding variables (Barr et al., 2006; Fryer et al., 2007). Although identification of individuals with prenatal alcohol exposure may not always be based on physical characteristics or IQ scores, evidence of significant adaptive disability and risk for psychopathology and delinquency suggests that increased efforts to ameliorate negative outcomes are essential.

Neurobehavioral Profile

Given the array of deficits that are associated with prenatal alcohol exposure and the clinical overlap with other disorders, clinical identification of affected individuals is difficult. Adding to this difficulty is the fact that most alcohol-exposed individuals do not exhibit the physical phenotype of FAS but can still experience the associated neuropsychological impairments. Missed diagnosis rates as high as 80.1%, as well as significant misdiagnosis within the FASD spectrum (6.4%), have been reported (Chasnoff, Wells, & King, 2015). Consequently, a growing body of research is aimed at the development of a neurobehavioral profile to improve the identification of individuals with and without the physical dysmorphology (Mattson et al., 2019; Mattson & Riley, 2011).

As discussed earlier, ADHD is common in individuals with prenatal alcohol exposure (Popova et al., 2016b; Weyrauch et al., 2017). Studies comparing these two clinical groups support the presence of a distinct neurobehavioral profile for individuals with prenatal alcohol exposure. Both children with FASD and those with ADHD displayed EF deficits, but alcohol-exposed children demonstrated greater impairment on measures of planning, fluency, and set shifting (Kingdon, Cardoso, & McGrath, 2016). Similarly, both groups are impaired on measures of verbal learning and memory, but alcohol-exposed children display impairment in encoding information, whereas children with ADHD displayed poorer retrieval of learned material (Crocker, Vaurio, Riley, & Mattson, 2011). Additional differential deficits are reported in areas of social cognition and facial emotion processing, with children with FASD displaying increased deficits in these domains compared to children with ADHD (Greenbaum, Stevens, Nash, Koren, & Rovet, 2009). Differences in the pattern of adaptive functioning deficits are also apparent between both clinical groups. Children with alcohol exposure display a developmental plateau in adaptive abilities, whereas children with ADHD exhibit a delay, as scores continue to improve with age (Crocker et al., 2009). Furthermore, increased impairment in daily living skills is found for alcohol-exposed children compared to children with ADHD. A diagnosis of ADHD in children with FASD appears to be associated with worse impairments in communication skills (Ware et al., 2014) and increased risk of psychiatric disorders (Ware et al., 2013) compared to alcohol-exposed children without ADHD; however, overall neuropsychological performance is not further affected by a diagnosis of ADHD (Glass et al., 2013).

Neuropsychological performance of children with prenatal alcohol exposure has also been compared to children with low IQ scores. Children with FASD perform similarly to nonexposed children with low IQ scores on measures of visual attention and memory for verbal information (Vaurio et al., 2011), as well as speech production and processing skills (McGee et al., 2009). However, alcohol-exposed children display increased severity of impairment in areas of verbal learning (Vaurio et al., 2011), adaptive functioning (Fagerlund et al., 2012) and parent-reported problematic behaviors (Mattson & Riley, 2000; Vaurio et al., 2011) compared to IQ-matched nonexposed children. Taken together, these results demonstrate that prenatal alcohol exposure can result in severe neurobehavioral deficits that are not entirely explained by the intellectual deficits observed in this population.

Several studies have investigated whether the use of a neurobehavioral profile is successful in identifying children with prenatal alcohol exposure. Using latent profile analysis, researchers have demonstrated that a preliminary neurobehavioral profile is able to distinguish between children with FAS and typically developing children with an overall accuracy rate of 92% (Mattson et al., 2010). Additionally, children with prenatal alcohol exposure but no FAS were correctly differentiated from nonexposed children with 84.7% accuracy. A follow-up study had slightly lower but still significant overall classification accuracy rates (Mattson et al., 2013). Children with FAS were correctly distinguished from controls with 76.1% accuracy, and children with prenatal alcohol but not FAS were accurately identified from controls with 71.5% accuracy. Differences in overall classification accuracy rates between these two studies could, in part, be explained by the inclusion of a clinical contrast group of children with ADHD in the second study, as well as the use of more sites, which increased the diversity of the sample. Importantly, these accuracy rates were determined to be higher than those found when differentiating between groups using IQ alone (Mattson et al., 2010). Results from these studies highlight the importance of the use of neuropsychological assessments as a diagnostic tool. Additional research is necessary to further clarify this neurobehavioral profile.

DEVELOPMENTAL CONSIDERATIONS

Although the initial brain insult caused by prenatal alcohol exposure will be expressed differently with advancing age, very few longitudinal studies that have been conducted can be used to describe developmental trends in FASD. Most relevant results have come from prospective studies of lower levels of exposure, with limited research suggesting that disabilities (e.g., IQ deficits) seen in children with FASD persist into adulthood (Streissguth, Randels, & Smith, 1991). In addition, separate studies of children and adults with FASD document similar results, supporting the permanence of the neurobehavioral effects seen in this population. For example, such studies have indicated effects in children and adults in the following domains: psychopathology (Barr et al., 2006; Famy, Streissguth, & Unis, 1998; Fryer et al., 2007), alcohol problems (Baer, Sampson, Barr, Connor, & Streissguth, 2003), secondary disabilities (e.g., mental health issues and delinquency; Streissguth et al., 1996), attention (Connor, Streissguth, Sampson, Bookstein, & Barr, 1999; Mattson, Calarco, & Lang, 2006), adaptive functioning (Jirikowic et al., 2008), motor performance (Connor et al., 2006; Roebuck et al., 1998b), verbal learning (Mattson et al., 1996b), memory (Coles et al., 2010), and executive function (Malisza et al., 2005; Tamana, Pei, Massey, Massey, & Rasmussen, 2014). Longitudinal prospective studies that have followed cohorts of children into adulthood provide additional support for the long-term nature of alcohol's teratogenic effects (e.g., Connor et al., 2006; Streissguth et al., 1994a). When comparing young children and adolescents with FASD, greater impairments have been found for older children in areas of EF (Rasmussen & Bisanz, 2009; Tamana et al., 2014), processing of complex material (Tamana et al., 2014), basic math skills (Taylor & Enns, 2018), and adaptive behaviors (Fagerlund et al., 2012), indicating that some deficits may become more pronounced with age.

PREDICTORS AND MODERATORS

Although prenatal alcohol exposure is a necessary precursor to development of FASD, not all exposed children display similar outcomes. Several factors related to alcohol consumption (e.g., dose, timing, pattern of exposure) may influence the effects seen in offspring (Maier & West, 2001). Most relevant results in this area come from prospective cohort studies. These studies have demonstrated a dose–response relationship: Increased alcohol consumption is associated with worse outcomes in the domains of growth, head circumference, attention, memory, language, mathematical skills, and need for special education (Autti-Rämö, 2000; Day et al., 2002; Streissguth et al., 1994a). While greater exposure is generally associated with worse outcomes, studies have demonstrated adverse effects of prenatal alcohol exposure at doses as low as one to two drinks per day (Day et al., 2002; Streissguth, Barr, & Sampson, 1990). Timing and pattern of *in utero* alcohol exposure are additional moderators. Timing of exposure interacts with critical developmental periods to influence the nature of the deficits. Exposure in the first trimester interferes with migration of brain cells and facial development (Kotch & Sulik, 1992; Miller, 1996; Sulik, 2005). Third-trimester exposure is related to malformations in the cerebellum, hippocampus, and prefrontal cortex (Livy, Miller, Maier, & West, 2003; West & Pierce, 1986). In addition, maternal drinking habits may relate to outcome. Specifically, binge drinking is associated with increased severity of behavioral and cognitive impairments, as well as mental health problems and poor academic abilities compared to continuous drinking patterns (Flak, Su, Bertrand, Denny, Kesmodel, & Cogswell, 2014; Sayal et al., 2014). Therefore, an exposed individual's deficits will relate to not only to the amount but also the timing and pattern of maternal alcohol consumption over the course of gestation. A small number of studies has suggested that genetic factors are important in the expression of alcohol's teratogenesis. For example, the *ADH1B*3* allele may have a protective effect. The mechanism for this effect is unclear, however, and may relate to an effect on the efficiency with which alcohol is metabolized or more directly, through an effect on maternal alcohol drinking behavior (Dodge, Jacobson, & Jacobson, 2014). Additionally, a relatively recent meta-analysis revealed an increased risk of ADHD in individuals with prenatal alcohol exposure that exceeds the risk associated with parental alcohol dependence or other genetic factors (Wetherill, Foroud, & Goodlett, 2018).

A frequent confounding factor is use of other drugs by the mother during pregnancy. Abuse of any substance is unlikely to occur in isolation. In one prospective longitudinal study examining the use of cocaine during pregnancy, women who used cocaine were more likely than controls to have used marijuana, alcohol, other amphetamines, and barbiturates prior to and during pregnancy (Richardson, Conroy, & Day, 1996). Substances such as cocaine and nicotine can have consequences for physical and behavioral outcomes, such as growth deficiency and attention deficits that may be similar to the effects of prenatal alcohol exposure (Thompson, Levitt, & Stanwood, 2009). Polysubstance use during pregnancy can also have complex effects on neurobehavioral outcomes (Fisher et al., 2011). While alcohol exposure has been associated with poor attention and inhibitory control, one study found that when considering effects of tobacco, marijuana, and alcohol exposures on a sustained and selective attention task, both tobacco and marijuana, but not alcohol exposure, were related to deficits (Richardson et al., 1996). Therefore, screening for exposure to other substances is essential in study designs, and determining a unique neurobehavioral profile resulting from prenatal alcohol exposure, rather than focusing on isolated deficits, may be the most useful approach.

Several maternal factors are associated with an increased risk of FASD. These include increased maternal age, lower maternal body weight and height, poor nutrition, low maternal education, rural residency, and lower socioeconomic status (Chiodo et al., 2010; Esper & Furtado, 2014; May et al., 2008, 2013, 2016; Rubio, Kraemer, Farrell, & Day, 2008). Additional risk factors include late recognition of pregnancy, increased number of binge-drinking episodes prior to becoming pregnant, and previous drug use (Balachova et al., 2012; Esper & Furtado, 2014; Mallard, Connor, & Houghton, 2013). Postbirth environmental factors are also associated with outcome. Early diagnosis of FASD, a stable and enriched domestic environment, having basic needs met, and never experiencing violence are associated with improved outcomes in a heavily exposed population (Streissguth et al., 1996, 2004). Conversely, living in a home with substance-abusing individuals and experiencing violence are associated with poorer outcomes (May et al., 2008; Streissguth et al., 1996). Low paternal IQ and increased number of children present in the household also have been identified as risk factors (Streissguth et al., 1990). Identification of risk and protective environmental factors may indicate appropriate intervention strategies and improved outcomes.

TREATMENT AND INTERVENTION

Given the array of deficits observed in relation to prenatal alcohol exposure, designing effective interventions is challenging for this population. Environmental interventions are symptom-based and aimed at addressing the specific cognitive and behavioral effects of FASD, such as improving attention, self-regulation, and adaptive functioning skills (Petrenko & Alto, 2017). Within an academic setting, providing structure and routine, decreasing visual and auditory stimulation, and modifying the teaching approach to match the student's needs is associated with positive outcomes for alcohol-exposed individuals (Millar et al., 2017). Parent training and support programs concentrated on improving parenting skills have shown positive effects for the child, as well as the parent–child relationship (Paley & O'Connor, 2011; Petrenko & Alto, 2017). In a double-blind, placebo-controlled trial of 9-month choline supplementation that was provided to children with FASD between ages 2 and 5 years, immediate follow-up showed some beneficial effects of choline on a nonverbal explicit memory task in the youngest children (Wozniak et al., 2015). At the 4-year follow-up, relative to the placebo group, the choline-treated group had higher nonverbal intelligence, visual–spatial, working memory, and verbal memory scores, as well as fewer behavioral symptoms of ADHD (Wozniak et al., 2020). Research is ongoing to further translate treatments deemed successful in animal studies (Idrus & Thomas, 2011) into clinical interventions.

CRITIQUE OF EXISTING RESEARCH

Most of the research discussed herein entails retrospective study designs, which involves identification of participants any time after birth. Recruitment of participants is typically based on known exposure or by clinical referral of children with identified difficulties, usually in behavior or learning. Because heavily exposed populations and participants with known deficits will likely exhibit significant outcomes, larger effect sizes are seen in retrospectively recruited samples than in those recruited prospectively. Smaller sample sizes and overall lower costs are therefore possible with retrospective samples. However, valuable information may be lost with the use of a retrospective design. Birth mothers may be unavailable, and valuable medical and demographic history, as well as data regarding dose and timing of alcohol consumption, are difficult to obtain. Retrospective designs are strengthened by selection of groups that are well matched on important confounders to help control for nonrandomization and the relatively remote reports of maternal alcohol consumption.

Recruitment for prospective studies involves identifying participants before behavioral outcomes are observed. Generally, this is accomplished by targeting women who are likely to drink during pregnancy or identifying exposed infants at the time of birth. An advantage of prospective studies is that maternal drinking is measured closer to the time of exposure, which may yield more accurate reports on timing and dosage of alcohol, two important parameters when studying teratogenic effects (Streissguth, Sampson, Barr, Bookstein, & Olson, 1994b). In addition, when the mother is identified, more accurate information on demographic and environmental history is available. Another advantage of prospective studies is the possibility of adopting a longitudinal design. Initial brain changes resulting from prenatal alcohol exposure may not have consistent manifestations across different developmental periods, and repeated measures of an exposed individual's outcome can thus be helpful in detailing these changes over time. Prospective designs also have drawbacks. One goal of teratogenic research is to delineate a dose–response relationship. However, prospectively identified participants typically are not heavily exposed; therefore, much larger samples are required to detect effects. Additionally, longitudinal prospective studies are costly and time-consuming and therefore not always feasible. Because public policy and funding are based, at least in part, on scientific investigation, one consequence of not detecting teratogenic effects of alcohol may be less allocation of resources to a disabled population (Vorhees, 1986).

SUGGESTIONS FOR FUTURE DIRECTIONS

Although nearly 50 years of research on the teratogenic effects of alcohol has yielded an impressive amount of information, some areas have been understudied, and current research will likely lead to new lines of investigation. Increased use of longitudinal study designs will help in identifying the cognitive and behavioral manifestations of prenatal alcohol exposure over time and may help demonstrate potential environmental moderators of the effect of the initial alcohol insult. Improved sensitivity and specificity of a neurobehavioral profile of FASD will also enable identification and diagnosis of alcohol-exposed individuals, leading to more appropriate and informed care.

Neuroimaging of individuals with FASD has increased awareness of brain areas particularly vulnerable to prenatal alcohol exposure and differences in brain activation that may underlie cognitive and behavioral deficits. Recent studies have also used advanced statistical and machine learning techniques to determine whether neuroimaging markers, either alone or in combination with facial or neurobehavioral testing, can be used to improve identification of children with FASD (e.g., Little & Beaulieu, 2020; Suttie et al., 2018; Zhang et al., 2019). Such techniques hold promise for assisting health professionals in identifying children who either lack or have subtler facial dysmorphia, which can be challenging even for experienced clinicians (Suttie et al., 2018).

Continued and increased use of multidisciplinary approaches will lead to well-informed formulation and scientific investigations. Prenatal alcohol exposure leads to significant adverse outcomes in all spheres of functioning (e.g., health, neurocognitive, family, social, financial). Dissemination of current neurobehavioral and neuroimaging findings into medical and educational settings, and associated dialogue with health professionals and educators, are essential in ensuring that the questions asked and conclusions reached are ecologically valid for the population. Similarly, increased information on relative strengths and weaknesses in the population will aid in guiding intervention programs. Additionally, the identification of possible biomarkers, as well as risk and resiliency factors, will not only assist in earlier identification and more accurate diagnosis but also aid in prevention efforts. Some promising research suggests that early identification and a stable/nurturing home environment appear to be critical protective factors against the adverse life outcomes (e.g., alcohol and drug problems) associated with FASD (Streissguth et al., 2004), but additional research on resiliency factors is needed. Researchers have begun to develop school- and laboratory-based intervention programs with some success (Petrenko & Alto, 2017). Along with continued efforts to identify individuals affected by FASD, developing avenues to assist with learning, attending, and understanding contingencies and consequences will be invaluable.

CONCLUSION

In utero exposure to alcohol can cause permanent brain changes and lifelong neurobehavioral deficits. Imaging research has revealed a general pattern of overall reduction in brain size for heavily exposed individuals, as well as areas of relative alteration, after considering overall brain size. Size and cortical shape alterations have been found in parietal and frontal lobes. Specific structures of relative vulnerability include the corpus callosum, cerebellum, and caudate nucleus, which are reduced in size and altered in shape. Brain abnormalities are likely related to cognitive deficits found in this population. Significant research efforts have begun to delineate a neurobehavioral profile for individuals with prenatal alcohol exposure. Determining strengths and weaknesses will allow for better diagnostic specificity, as well as guide interventions for the many adversely affected children in this large population. Findings thus far generally show that individuals with heavy prenatal alcohol exposure have reduced overall IQ, as well as specific deficits in visual–spatial, psychomotor, attention, learning, and EF domains. In addition, individuals with a history of alcohol exposure demonstrate impairments in socialization that are worse than expected based on IQ and are at increased risk for negative life events such as incarceration, substance abuse, and psychopathology. The effects of prenatal alcohol exposure on brain structure and function can vary between individuals and some moderating factors have been identified, including timing and dose of maternal alcohol consumption, concurrent use of other substances by the mother, and other environmental factors.

Finally, the economic impact of FASD in the United States alone is staggering, as estimates of the prevalence of FASD suggest that as many as 1 in 100 individuals are affected by prenatal alcohol exposure. Recent studies of international samples have confirmed that alcohol consumption during pregnancy is a worldwide phenomenon, and further investigation into diverse samples will provide a better representation of outcomes. In summary, FASD is a widespread disorder with great public health and economic significance. Integration of new imaging techniques, continued delineation of neuropsychological profiles, and collaboration between medical, educational, and psychological disciplines are required to identify and assist this large and currently under identified population.

ACKNOWLEDGMENTS

Preparation of this chapter was supported in part by National Institute on Alcohol Abuse and Alcoholism Grant Nos. U01 AA014834, K99/R00 AA022661, and R01 AA026994. We gratefully acknowledge the assistance and support of the Center for Behavioral Teratology, San Diego State University.

REFERENCES

Adnams, C. M., Kodituwakku, P. W., Hay, A., Molteno, C. D., Viljoen, D., & May, P. A. (2001). Patterns of cognitive-motor development in children with fetal alcohol syndrome from a community in South Africa. *Alcoholism: Clinical and Experimental Research, 25*(4), 557–562.

American Psychiatric Association. (2013). *Diagnostic and statistical manual of mental disorders* (5th ed.). Arlington, VA: Author.

Archibald, S. L., Fennema-Notestine, C., Gamst, A., Riley, E. P., Mattson, S. N., & Jernigan, T. L. (2001). Brain dysmorphology in individuals with severe prenatal alcohol exposure. *Developmental Medicine and Child Neurology, 43*(3), 148–154.

Autti-Rämö, I. (2000). Twelve-year follow-up of children exposed to alcohol *in utero*. *Developmental Medicine and Child Neurology, 42*(6), 406–411.

Autti-Rämö, I., Autti, T., Korkman, M., Kettunen, S., Salonen, O., & Valanne, L. (2002). MRI findings in children with school problems who had been exposed prenatally to alcohol. *Developmental Medicine and Child Neurology, 44*(2), 98–106.

Baer, J. S., Sampson, P. D., Barr, H. M., Connor, P. D., & Streissguth, A. P. (2003). A 21-year longitudinal analysis of the effects of prenatal alcohol exposure on young adult drinking. *Archives of General Psychiatry, 60*(4), 377–385.

Balachova, T., Bonner, B., Chaffin, M., Bard, D., Isurina, G., Tsvetkova, L., & Volkova, E. (2012). Women's alcohol consumption and risk for alcohol-exposed pregnancies in Russia. *Addiction, 107*(1), 109–117.

Barr, H. M., Bookstein, F. L., O'Malley, K. D., Connor, P. D., Huggins, J. E., & Streissguth, A. P. (2006). Binge drinking during pregnancy as a predictor of psychiatric disorders on the Structured Clinical Interview for DSM-IV in young adult offspring. *American Journal of Psychiatry, 163*(6), 1061–1065.

Bertrand, J., Floyd, R. L., & Weber, M. K. (2005). Guidelines for identifying and referring persons with fetal alcohol syndrome. *Morbidity and Mortality Weekly Report Recommendations and Reports, 54*(RR-11), 1–14.

Bertrand, J., Floyd, R. L., Weber, M. K., O'Connor, M., Riley, E. P., Johnson, K. A., & Cohen, D. E. (2004). National Task Force on FAS/FAE: Guidelines for referral and diagnosis. Retrieved from *www.cdc.gov/ncbddd/fasd/documents/fas_guidelines_accessible.pdf.*

Bjorkquist, O. A., Fryer, S. L., Reiss, A. L., Mattson, S. N., & Riley, E. P. (2010). Cingulate gyrus morphology in children and adolescents with fetal alcohol spectrum disorders. *Psychiatry Research: Neuroimaging, 181*(2), 101–107.

Bookstein, F. L., Sampson, P. D., Connor, P. D., & Streissguth, A. P. (2002). Midline corpus callosum is a neuroanatomical focus of fetal alcohol damage. *Anatomical Record, 269*(3), 162–174.

Bookstein, F. L., Sampson, P. D., Streissguth, A. P., & Connor, P. D. (2001). Geometric morphometrics of corpus callosum and subcortical structures in the fetal-alcohol-affected brain. *Teratology, 64*(1), 4–32.

Burden, M. J., Jacobson, S. W., Sokol, R. J., & Jacobson, J. L. (2005). Effects of prenatal alcohol exposure on attention and working memory at 7.5 years of age. *Alcoholism: Clinical and Experimental Research, 29*(3), 443–452.

Cardenas, V. A., Price, M., Infante, M. A., Moore, E. M., Mattson, S. N., Riley, E. P., & Fein, G. (2014). Automated cerebellar segmentation: Validation and application to detect smaller volumes in children prenatally exposed to alcohol. *NeuroImage: Clinical, 4*, 295–301.

Carney, L. J., & Chermak, G. D. (1991). Performance of American Indian children with fetal alcohol syndrome on the test of language development. *Journal of Communication Disorders, 24*, 123–134.

Carr, J. L., Agnihotri, S., & Keightley, M. (2010). Sensory processing and adaptive behavior deficits of children across the fetal alcohol spectrum disorder continuum. *Alcoholism: Clinical and Experimental Research, 34*(6), 1022–1032.

Centers for Disease Control and Prevention. (2002). Fetal alcohol syndrome—Alaska, Arizona, Colorado, and New York, 1995–1997. *Morbidity and Mortality Weekly Report, 51*(20), 433–435.

Centers for Disease Control and Prevention. (2015). Fetal alcohol syndrome among children aged 7–9 years—Arizona, Colorado, and New York, 2010. *Morbidity and Mortality Weekly Report, 64*(3), 54–57.

Chasnoff, I. J., Wells, A. M., & King, L. (2015). Misdiagnosis and missed diagnoses in foster and adopted children with prenatal alcohol exposure. *Pediatrics, 135*(2), 264–270.

Chen, X., Coles, C. D., Lynch, M. E., & Hu, X. (2012). Understanding specific effects of prenatal alcohol exposure on brain structure in young adults. *Human Brain Mapping, 33*(7), 1663–1676.

Chiodo, L. M., da Costa, D. E., Hannigan, J. H., Covington, C. Y., Sokol, R. J., Janisse, J., . . . Delaney-Black, V. (2010). The impact of maternal age on the effects of prenatal alcohol exposure on attention. *Alcoholism: Clinical and Experimental Research, 34*(10), 1813–1821.

Church, M. W., Eldis, F., Blakley, B. W., & Bawle, E. V. (1997). Hearing, language, speech, vestibular, and dentofacial disorders in fetal alcohol syndrome. *Alcoholism: Clinical and Experimental Research, 21*(2), 227–237.

Coles, C. D., Goldstein, F. C., Lynch, M. E., Chen, X., Kable, J. A., Johnson, K. C., & Hu, X. (2011). Memory and brain volume in adults prenatally exposed to alcohol. *Brain and Cognition, 75*(1), 67–77.

Coles, C. D., & Li, Z. (2011). Functional neuroimaging in the examination of effects of prenatal alcohol exposure. *Neuropsychology Review, 21*(2), 119–132.

Coles, C. D., Lynch, M. E., Kable, J. A., Johnson, K. C., & Goldstein, F. C. (2010). Verbal and nonverbal memory in adults prenatally exposed to alcohol. *Alcoholism: Clinical and Experimental Research, 34*(5), 897–906.

Connor, P. D., Sampson, P. D., Bookstein, F. L., Barr, H. M., & Streissguth, A. P. (2000). Direct and indirect effects of prenatal alcohol damage on executive function. *Developmental Neuropsychology, 18*(3), 331–354.

Connor, P. D., Sampson, P. D., Streissguth, A. P., Bookstein, F. L., & Barr, H. M. (2006). Effects of prenatal alcohol exposure on fine motor coordination and balance: A study of two adult samples. *Neuropsychologia, 44*(5), 744–751.

Connor, P. D., Streissguth, A. P., Sampson, P. D., Bookstein, F. L., & Barr, H. M. (1999). Individual differences in auditory and visual attention among fetal alcohol-affected adults. *Alcoholism: Clinical and Experimental Research, 23*(8), 1395–1402.

Conry, J. (1990). Neuropsychological deficits in fetal alcohol syndrome and fetal alcohol effects. *Alcoholism: Clinical and Experimental Research, 14*(5), 650–655.

Cook, J. L., Green, C. R., Lilley, C. M., Anderson, S. M., Baldwin, M. E., Chudley, A. E., . . . Canada Fetal Alcohol Spectrum Disorder Research Network. (2016). Fetal alcohol spectrum disorder: A guideline for diagnosis across the lifespan. *Canadian Medical Associatio Journal, 188*(3), 191–197.

Crocker, N., Vaurio, L., Riley, E. P.; & Mattson, S. N. (2009). Comparison of adaptive behavior in children with heavy prenatal alcohol exposure or attention-deficit/hyperactivity disorder. *Alco-*

holism: Clinical and Experimental Research, 33(11), 2015–2023.

Crocker, N., Vaurio, L., Riley, E. P., & Mattson, S. N. (2011). Comparison of verbal learning and memory in children with heavy prenatal alcohol exposure or attention-deficit/hyperactivity disorder. *Alcoholism: Clinical and Experimental Research, 35*(6), 1114–1121.

Day, N. L., Leech, S. L., Richardson, G. A., Cornelius, M. D., Robles, N., & Larkby, C. (2002). Prenatal alcohol exposure predicts continued deficits in offspring size at 14 years of age. *Alcoholism: Clinical and Experimental Research, 26*(10), 1584–1591.

De Guio, F., Mangin, J. F., Riviere, D., Perrot, M., Molteno, C. D., Jacobson, S. W., . . . Jacobson, J. L. (2014). A study of cortical morphology in children with fetal alcohol spectrum disorders. *Human Brain Mapping, 35*(5), 2285–2296.

Delis, D. C., Kaplan, E., & Kramer, J. H. (2001). *Manual for the Delis–Kaplan Executive Function System*. San Antonio, TX: Psychological Corporation.

Denny, C. H., Acero, C. S., Naimi, T. S., & Kim, S. Y. (2019). Consumption of alcohol beverages and binge drinking among pregnant women aged 18–44 years—United States, 2015–2017. *Morbidity and Mortality Weekly Report, 68*(16), 365–368.

Dodge, N. C., Jacobson, J. L., & Jacobson, S. W. (2014). Protective effects of the alcohol dehydrogenase-ADH1B*3 allele on attention and behavior problems in adolescents exposed to alcohol during pregnancy. *Neurotoxicology and Teratology, 41*, 43–50.

Donald, K. A., Fouche, J. P., Roos, A., Koen, N., Howells, F. M., Riley, E. P., . . . Stein, D. J. (2016a). Alcohol exposure *in utero* is associated with decreased gray matter volume in neonates. *Metabolic Brain Disease, 31*(1), 81–91.

Donald, K. A., Ipser, J. C., Howells, F. M., Roos, A., Fouche, J. P., Riley, E. P., . . . Stein, D. J. (2016b). Interhemispheric functional brain connectivity in neonates with prenatal alcohol exposure: Preliminary findings. *Alcoholism: Clinical and Experimental Research, 40*(1), 113–121.

Doney, R., Lucas, B. R., Jones, T., Howat, P., Sauer, K., & Elliott, E. J. (2014). Fine motor skills in children with prenatal alcohol exposure or fetal alcohol spectrum disorder. *Journal of Developmental and Behavioral Pediatrics, 35*(9), 598–609.

Esper, L. H., & Furtado, E. F. (2014). Identifying maternal risk factors associated with fetal alcohol spectrum disorders: A systematic review. *European Child and Adolescent Psychiatry, 23*(10), 877–889.

Fagerlund, A., Autti-Rämö, I., Kalland, M., Santtila, P., Hoyme, H. E., Mattson, S. N., & Korkman, M. (2012). Adaptive behaviour in children and adolescents with foetal alcohol spectrum disorders: A comparison with specific learning disability and typical development. *European Journal of Child and Adolescent Psychiatry, 21*(4), 221–231.

Famy, C., Streissguth, A. P., & Unis, A. S. (1998). Mental illness in adults with fetal alcohol syndrome or fetal alcohol effects. *American Journal of Psychiatry, 155*(4), 552–554.

Fan, J., Jacobson, S. W., Taylor, P. A., Molteno, C. D., Dodge, N. C., Stanton, M. E., . . . Meintjes, E. M. (2016). White matter deficits mediate effects of prenatal alcohol exposure on cognitive development in childhood. *Human Brain Mapping, 37*(8), 2943–2958.

Fan, J., Taylor, P. A., Jacobson, S. W., Molteno, C. D., Gohel, S., Biswal, B. B., . . . Meintjes, E. M. (2017). Localized reductions in resting-state functional connectivity in children with prenatal alcohol exposure. *Human Brain Mapping, 38*(10), 5217–5233.

Feldman, H. M., Yeatman, J. D., Lee, E. S., Barde, L. H., & Gaman-Bean, S. (2010). Diffusion tensor imaging: A review for pediatric researchers and clinicians. *Journal of Developmental and Behavioral Pediatrics, 31*(4), 346–356.

Fernandez-Jaen, A., Fernandez-Mayoralas, D. M., Quinones Tapia, D., Calleja-Perez, B., Garcia-Segura, J. M., Arribas, S. L., & Munoz Jareno, N. (2011). Cortical thickness in fetal alcohol syndrome and attention deficit disorder. *Pediatric Neurology, 45*(6), 387–391.

Fisher, P. A., Lester, B. M., DeGarmo, D. S., Lagasse, L. L., Lin, H., Shankaran, S., . . . Higgins, R. (2011). The combined effects of prenatal drug exposure and early adversity on neurobehavioral disinhibition in childhood and adolescence. *Development and Psychopathology, 23*(3), 777–788.

Flak, A. L., Su, S., Bertrand, J., Denny, C. H., Kesmodel, U. S., & Cogswell, M. E. (2014). The association of mild, moderate, and binge prenatal alcohol exposure and child neuropsychological outcomes: A meta-analysis. *Alcoholism: Clinical and Experimental Research, 38*(1), 214–226.

Franklin, L., Deitz, J., Jirikowic, T., & Astley, S. (2008). Children with fetal alcohol spectrum disorders: Problem behaviors and sensory processing. *American Journal of Occupational Therapy, 62*(3), 265–273.

Fryer, S. L., McGee, C. L., Matt, G. E., Riley, E. P., & Mattson, S. N. (2007). Evaluation of psychopathological conditions in children with heavy prenatal alcohol exposure. *Pediatrics, 119*(3), e733–e741.

Gautam, P., Lebel, C., Narr, K. L., Mattson, S. N., May, P. A., Adnams, C. M., . . . Sowell, E. R. (2015). Volume changes and brain-behavior relationships in white matter and subcortical gray matter in children with prenatal alcohol exposure. *Human Brain Mapping, 36*(6), 2318–2329.

Gautam, P., Nunez, S. C., Narr, K. L., Kan, E. C., & Sowell, E. R. (2014). Effects of prenatal alcohol exposure on the development of white matter volume and change in executive function. *NeuroImage: Clinical, 5*, 19–27.

Glass, L., Ware, A. L., Crocker, N., Deweese, B. N., Coles, C. D., Kable, J. A., . . . Collaborative Initiative on Fetal Alcohol Spectrum Disorders. (2013). Neuropsychological deficits associated with heavy prenatal alcohol exposure are not exacerbated by comorbid ADHD. *Neuropsychology, 27*(6), 713–724.

Goodlett, C. R., Marcussen, B. L., & West, J. R. (1990). A single day of alcohol exposure during the brain growth spurt induces brain weight restriction and cerebellar Purkinje cell loss. *Alcohol, 7*(2), 107–114.

Green, C. R., Mihic, A. M., Brien, D. C., Armstrong, I. T., Nikkel, S. M., Stade, B. C., . . . Reynolds, J. N. (2009a). Oculomotor control in children with fetal alcohol spectrum disorders assessed using a mobile eye-tracking laboratory. *European Journal of Neuroscience, 29*(6), 1302–1309.

Green, C. R., Mihic, A. M., Nikkel, S. M., Stade, B. C., Rasmussen, C., Munoz, D. P., & Reynolds, J. N. (2009b). Executive function deficits in children with fetal alcohol spectrum disorders (FASD) measured using the Cambridge Neuropsychological Tests Automated Battery (CANTAB). *Journal of Child Psychology and Psychiatry, 50*(6), 688–697.

Greenbaum, R. L., Stevens, S. A., Nash, K., Koren, G., & Rovet, J. (2009). Social cognitive and emotion processing abilities of children with fetal alcohol spectrum disorders: A comparison with attention deficit hyperactivity disorder. *Alcoholism: Clinical and Experimental Research, 33*(10), 1656–1670.

Hayden, K. E. (2005). *Verbal fluency clustering and switching in children with heavy prenatal alcohol exposure.* Master's thesis, San Diego State University, San Diego, CA.

Hendrickson, T. J., Mueller, B. A., Sowell, E. R., Mattson, S. N., Coles, C. D., Kable, J. A., . . . Wozniak, J. R. (2018). Two-year cortical trajectories are abnormal in children and adolescents with prenatal alcohol exposure. *Developmental Cognitive Neuroscience, 30*, 123–133.

Hendrickson, T. J., Mueller, B. A., Sowell, E. R., Mattson, S. N., Coles, C. D., Kable, J. A., . . . Wozniak, J. R. (2017). Cortical gyrification is abnormal in children with prenatal alcohol exposure. *NeuroImage: Clinical, 15*, 391–400.

Hoyme, H. E., Kalberg, W. O., Elliott, A. J., Blankenship, J., Buckley, D., Marais, A. S., . . . May, P. A. (2016). Updated clinical guidelines for diagnosing fetal alcohol spectrum disorders. *Pediatrics, 138*(2), Article e20154256.

Hoyme, H. E., May, P. A., Kalberg, W. O., Kodituwakku, P., Gossage, J. P., Trujillo, P. M., . . . Robinson, L. K. (2005). A practical clinical approach to diagnosis of fetal alcohol spectrum disorders: Clarification of the 1996 Institute of Medicine criteria. *Pediatrics, 115*(1), 39–47.

Idrus, N. M., & Thomas, J. D. (2011). Fetal alcohol spectrum disorders: Experimental treatments and strategies for intervention. *Alcohol Research and Health, 34*(1), 76–85.

Infante, M. A., Moore, E. M., Bischoff-Grethe, A., Migliorini, R., Mattson, S. N., & Riley, E. P. (2015). Atypical cortical gyrification in adolescents with histories of heavy prenatal alcohol exposure. *Brain Research, 1624*, 446–454.

Inkelis, S. M., Moore, E. M., Bischoff-Grethe, A., & Riley, E. P. (2020). Neurodevelopment in adolescents and adults with fetal alcohol spectrum disorders (FASD): A magnetic resonance region of interest analysis. *Brain Research, 1732*, Article 146654.

Janzen, L. A., Nanson, J. L., & Block, G. W. (1995). Neuropsychological evaluation of preschoolers with fetal alcohol syndrome. *Neurotoxicology and Teratology, 17*(3), 273–279.

Jeret, J. S., & Serur, D. (1991). Fetal alcohol syndrome in adolescents and adults [Letter to the editor]. *Journal of the American Medical Association, 266*(8), 1077.

Jirikowic, T., Olson, H. C., & Kartin, D. (2008). Sensory processing, school performance, and adaptive behavior of young school-age children with fetal alcohol spectrum disorders. *Physical and Occupational Therapy in Pediatrics, 28*(2), 117–136.

Jones, K. L., & Smith, D. W. (1973). Recognition of the fetal alcohol syndrome in early infancy. *Lancet, 2*(7836), 999–1001.

Jones, K. L., & Smith, D. W. (1975). The fetal alcohol syndrome. *Teratology, 12*, 1–10.

Jones, K. L., Smith, D. W., Ulleland, C. N., & Streissguth, A. P. (1973). Pattern of malformation in offspring of chronic alcoholic mothers. *Lancet, 1*(7815), 1267–1271.

Joseph, J., Warton, C., Jacobson, S. W., Jacobson, J. L., Molteno, C. D., Eicher, A., . . . Meintjes, E. M. (2014). Three-dimensional surface deformation-based shape analysis of hippocampus and caudate nucleus in children with fetal alcohol spectrum disorders. *Human Brain Mapping, 35*(2), 659–672.

Kaemingk, K. L., Mulvaney, S., & Tanner Halverson, P. (2003). Learning following prenatal alcohol exposure: Performance on verbal and visual multitrial tasks. *Archives of Clinical Neuropsychology, 18*(1), 33–47.

Kalberg, W. O., Provost, B., Tollison, S. J., Tabachnick, B. G., Robinson, L. K., Hoyme, H. E., . . . May, P. A. (2006). Comparison of motor delays in young children with fetal alcohol syndrome to those with prenatal alcohol exposure and with no prenatal alcohol exposure. *Alcoholism: Clinical and Experimental Research, 30*(12), 2037–2045.

Kingdon, D., Cardoso, C., & McGrath, J. J. (2016). Research review: Executive function deficits in fetal alcohol spectrum disorders and attention-deficit/hyperactivity disorder—A meta-analysis. *Journal of Child Psychology and Psychiatry, 57*(2), 116–131.

Kodituwakku, P. W., Handmaker, N. S., Cutler, S. K., Weathersby, E. K., & Handmaker, S. D. (1995). Specific impairments in self-regulation in children exposed to alcohol prenatally. *Alcoholism: Clinical and Experimental Research, 19*(6), 1558–1564.

Kotch, L. E., & Sulik, K. K. (1992). Experimental fetal alcohol syndrome: Proposed pathogenic basis for a variety of associated facial and brain anomalies. *American Journal of Medical Genetics, 44*, 168–176.

Lange, S., Probst, C., Gmel, G., Rehm, J., Burd, L., & Popova, S. (2017). Global prevalence of fetal alcohol spectrum disorder among children and youth: A systematic review and meta-analysis. *JAMA Pediatrics, 171*(10), 948–956.

Lebel, C., Roussotte, F., & Sowell, E. R. (2011). Imaging the impact of prenatal alcohol exposure on the structure of the developing human brain. *Neuropsychology Review, 21*(2), 102–118.

Lee, K. T., Mattson, S. N., & Riley, E. P. (2004). Classifying children with heavy prenatal alcohol exposure using measures of attention. *Journal of the International Neuropsychological Society, 10*(2), 271–277.

Lewis, C. E., Thomas, K. G., Dodge, N. C., Molteno, C. D., Meintjes, E. M., Jacobson, J. L., & Jacobson, S. W. (2015). Verbal learning and memory impairment in children with fetal alcohol spectrum disorders. *Alcoholism: Clinical and Experimental Research, 39*(4), 724–732.

Li, Z., Ma, X., Peltier, S., Hu, X., Coles, C. D., & Lynch, M. E. (2008). Occipital–temporal reduction and sustained visual attention deficit in prenatal alcohol exposed adults. *Brain Imaging and Behavior, 2*(1), 39–48.

Little, G., & Beaulieu, C. (2020). Multivariate models of brain volume for identification of children and adolescents with fetal alcohol spectrum disorder. *Human Brain Mapping, 41*, 1181–1194.

Little, G., Reynolds, J., & Beaulieu, C. (2018). Altered functional connectivity observed at rest in children and adolescents prenatally exposed to alcohol. *Brain Connectivity, 8*(8), 503–515.

Livy, D. J., Miller, E. K., Maier, S. E., & West, J. R. (2003). Fetal alcohol exposure and temporal vulnerability: Effects of binge-like alcohol exposure on the developing rat hippocampus. *Neurotoxicology and Teratology, 25*(4), 447–458.

Long, X., Little, G., Beaulieu, C., & Lebel, C. (2018). Sensorimotor network alterations in children and youth with prenatal alcohol exposure. *Human Brain Mapping, 39*(5), 2258–2268.

Lucas, B. R., Latimer, J., Pinto, R. Z., Ferreira, M. L., Doney, R., Lau, M., . . . Elliott, E. J. (2014). Gross motor deficits in children prenatally exposed to alcohol: A meta-analysis. *Pediatrics, 134*(1), e192–e209.

Lupton, C., Burd, L., & Harwood, R. (2004). Cost of fetal alcohol spectrum disorders. *American Journal of Medical Genetics C: Seminars in Medical Genetics, 127*(1), 42–50.

Lynch, M. E., Coles, C. D., Corley, T., & Falek, A. (2003). Examining delinquency in adolescents differentially prenatally exposed to alcohol: The role of proximal and distal risk factors. *Journal of Studies on Alcohol, 64*, 678–686.

Maier, S. E., & West, J. R. (2001). Drinking patterns and alcohol-related birth defects. *Alcohol Research and Health, 25*(3), 168–174.

Malisza, K. L., Allman, A.-A., Shiloff, D., Jakobson, L., Longstaffe, S., & Chudley, A. E. (2005). Evaluation of spatial working memory function in children and adults with fetal alcohol spectrum disorders: A functional magnetic resonance imaging study. *Pediatric Research, 58*(6), 1150–1157.

Malisza, K. L., Buss, J. L., Bolster, R. B., de Gervai, P. D., Woods-Frohlich, L., Summers, R., . . . Longstaffe, S. (2012). Comparison of spatial working memory in children with prenatal alcohol exposure and those diagnosed with ADHD: A functional magnetic resonance imaging study. *Journal of Neurodevelopmental Disorders, 4*(1), 12.

Mallard, S. R., Connor, J. L., & Houghton, L. A. (2013). Maternal factors associated with heavy periconceptional alcohol intake and drinking following pregnancy recognition: A post-partum survey of New Zealand women. *Drug and Alcohol Review, 32*(4), 389–397.

Mattson, S. N., Bernes, G. A., & Doyle, L. R. (2019). Fetal alcohol spectrum disorders: A review of the neurobehavioral deficits associated with prenatal alcohol exposure. *Alcoholism: Clinical and Experimental Research, 43*(6), 1046–1062.

Mattson, S. N., Calarco, K. E., & Lang, A. R. (2006). Focused and shifting attention in children with heavy prenatal alcohol exposure. *Neuropsychology, 20*(3), 361–369.

Mattson, S. N., Goodman, A. M., Caine, C., Delis, D. C., & Riley, E. P. (1999). Executive functioning in children with heavy prenatal alcohol exposure. *Alcoholism: Clinical and Experimental Research, 23*(11), 1808–1815.

Mattson, S. N., Gramling, L., Delis, D., Jones, K. L., & Riley, E. P. (1996a). Global–local processing in children prenatally exposed to alcohol. *Child Neuropsychology, 2*(3), 165–175.

Mattson, S. N., & Riley, E. P. (1998). A review of the neurobehavioral deficits in children with fetal alcohol syndrome or prenatal exposure to alcohol. *Alcoholism: Clinical and Experimental Research, 22*(2), 279–294.

Mattson, S. N., & Riley, E. P. (2000). Parent ratings of behavior in children with heavy prenatal alcohol exposure and IQ-matched controls. *Alcoholism: Clinical and Experimental Research, 24*(2), 226–231.

Mattson, S. N., & Riley, E. P. (2011). The quest for a neurobehavioral profile of heavy prenatal alcohol exposure. *Alcohol Research and Health, 34*(1), 51–55.

Mattson, S. N., Riley, E. P., Delis, D. C., Stern, C., & Jones, K. L. (1996b). Verbal learning and memory in children with fetal alcohol syndrome. *Alcoholism: Clinical and Experimental Research, 20*(5), 810–816.

Mattson, S. N., Riley, E. P., Gramling, L., Delis, D. C., & Jones, K. L. (1998). Neuropsychological comparison of alcohol-exposed children with or without physical features of fetal alcohol syndrome. *Neuropsychology, 12*(1), 146–153.

Mattson, S. N., Riley, E. P., Jernigan, T. L., Ehlers, C. L., Delis, D. C., Jones, K. L., . . . Bellugi, U. (1992). Fetal alcohol syndrome: A case report of neuropsychological, MRI and EEG assessment of two children. *Alcoholism: Clinical and Experimental Research, 16*(5), 1001–1003.

Mattson, S. N., Riley, E. P., Sowell, E. R., Jernigan, T. L., Sobel, D. F., & Jones, K. L. (1996c). A decrease in the size of the basal ganglia in children with fetal alcohol syndrome. *Alcoholism: Clinical and Experimental Research, 20*(6), 1088–1093.

Mattson, S. N., & Roebuck, T. M. (2002). Acquisition and retention of verbal and nonverbal information in children with heavy prenatal alcohol exposure. *Alcoholism: Clinical and Experimental Research, 26*(6), 875–882.

Mattson, S. N., Roesch, S. C., Fagerlund, A., Autti-Ramo, I., Jones, K. L., May, P. A., . . . Riley, E. P. (2010). Toward a neurobehavioral profile of fetal alcohol spectrum disorders. *Alcoholism: Clinical and Experimental Research, 34*(9), 1640–1650.

Mattson, S. N., Roesch, S. C., Glass, L., Deweese, B. N., Coles, C. D., Kable, J. A., . . . CIFASD. (2013). Further development of a neurobehavioral profile of fetal alcohol spectrum disorders. *Alcoholism: Clinical and Experimental Research, 37*(3), 517–528.

Mattson, S. N., Vaurio, L., & Riley, E. P. (2006, February). *Differences in executive functioning in children with fetal alcohol spectrum disorders and/or ADHD.* Presented at the meeting of the International Neuropsychological Society, Boston, MA.

May, P. A., Chambers, C. D., Kalberg, W. O., Zellner, J., Feldman, H., Buckley, D., . . . Hoyme, H. E. (2018). Prevalence of fetal alcohol spectrum disorders in 4 US communities. *Journal of the American Medical Association, 319*(5), 474–482.

May, P. A., Gossage, J. P., Marais, A.-S., Hendricks, L. S., Snell, C. L., Tabachnick, B. G., . . . Viljoen, D. L. (2008). Maternal risk factors for fetal alcohol syndrome and partial fetal alcohol syndrome in South Africa: A third study. *Alcoholism: Clinical and Experimental Research, 32*(5), 738–753.

May, P. A., Hamrick, K. J., Corbin, K. D., Hasken, J. M., Marais, A. S., Blankenship, J., . . . Gossage, J. P. (2016). Maternal nutritional status as a contributing factor for the risk of fetal alcohol spectrum disorders. *Reproductive Toxicology, 59,* 101–108.

May, P. A., Tabachnick, B. G., Gossage, J. P., Kalberg, W. O., Marais, A. R., Robinson, L. K., . . . Adnams, C. M. (2013). Maternal factors predicting cognitive and behavioral characteristics of children with fetal alcohol spectrum disorders. *Journal of Developmental and Behavioral Pediatrics, 34*(5), 314–325.

McGee, C. L., Bjorkquist, O. A., Riley, E. P., & Mattson, S. N. (2009). Impaired language performance in young children with heavy prenatal alcohol exposure. *Neurotoxicology and Teratology, 31*(2), 71–75.

McGee, C. L., Fryer, S. L., Bjorkquist, O. A., Mattson, S. N., & Riley, E. P. (2008). Deficits in social problem solving in adolescents with prenatal exposure to alcohol. *American Journal of Drug and Alcohol Abuse, 34*(4), 423–431.

Migliorini, R., Moore, E. M., Glass, L., Infante, M. A., Tapert, S. F., Jones, K. L., . . . Riley, E. P. (2015). Anterior cingulate cortex surface area relates to behavioral inhibition in adolescents with and without heavy prenatal alcohol exposure. *Behavioural Brain Research, 292*, 26–35.

Millar, J. A., Thompson, J., Schwab, D., Hanlon-Dearman, A., Goodman, D., Koren, G., & Masotti, P. (2017). Educating students with FASD: Linking policy, research and practice. *Journal of Research in Special Educational Needs, 17*(1), 3–17.

Miller, M. W. (1996). Limited ethanol exposure selectively alters the proliferation of precursor cells in the cerebral cortex. *Alcoholism: Clinical and Experimental Research, 20*(1), 139–143.

Moore, E. M., Glass, L., Infante, M. A., Coles, C., Kable, J., Jones, K. L., . . . CIFASD [Collaborative Initiative on Fetal Alcohol Spectrum Disorders]. (2021). Cross-sectional analysis of spatial working memory development in children with heavy prenatal alcohol exposure. *Alcoholism: Clinical and Experimental Research, 45*, 215–223.

Moore, E. M., Infante, M. A., Migliorini, R., Mattson, S. N., & Riley, E. P. (2016). Pituitary lacks sexual dimorphism and displays reduced signal intensity on T1-weighted MRI in adolescents with histories of heavy prenatal alcohol exposure. *Neurotoxicology and Teratology, 57*, 106–111.

Moore, E. M., Migliorini, R., Infante, M. A., & Riley, E. P. (2014). Fetal alcohol spectrum disorders: Recent neuroimaging findings. *Current Developmental Disorders Reports, 1*(3), 161–172.

Nardelli, A., Lebel, C., Rasmussen, C., Andrew, G., & Beaulieu, C. (2011). Extensive deep gray matter volume reductions in children and adolescents with fetal alcohol spectrum disorders. *Alcoholism: Clinical and Experimental Research, 35*(8), 1404–1417.

O'Hare, E., Kan, E., Yoshii, J., Mattson, S., Riley, E., Thompson, P., . . . Sowell, E. (2005). Mapping cerebellar vermal morphology and cognitive correlates in prenatal alcohol exposure. *NeuroReport, 16*(12), 1285–1290.

Paley, B., & O'Connor, M. J. (2011). Behavioral interventions for children and adolescents with fetal alcohol spectrum disorders. *Alcohol Research and Health, 34*(1), 64–75.

Panczakiewicz, A. L., Glass, L., Coles, C. D., Kable, J. A., Sowell, E. R., Wozniak, J. R., . . . Collaborative Initiative on Fetal Alcohol Spectrum Disorders. (2016). Neurobehavioral deficits consistent across age and sex in youth with prenatal alcohol exposure. *Alcoholism: Clinical and Experimental Research, 40*(9), 1971–1981.

Panizzon, M. S., Fennema-Notestine, C., Eyler, L. T., Jernigan, T. L., Prom-Wormley, E., Neale, M., . . . Kremen, W. S. (2009). Distinct genetic influences on cortical surface area and cortical thickness. *Cerebral Cortex, 19*(11), 2728–2735.

Petrenko, C. L., & Alto, M. E. (2017). Interventions in fetal alcohol spectrum disorders: An international perspective. *European Journal of Medical Genetics, 60*(1), 79–91.

Popova, S., Lange, S., Burd, L., & Rehm, J. (2016a). The economic burden of fetal alcohol spectrum disorder in Canada in 2013. *Alcohol and Alcoholism, 51*(3), 367–375.

Popova, S., Lange, S., Shield, K., Mihic, A., Chudley, A. E., Mukherjee, R. A. S., . . . Rehm, J. (2016b). Comorbidity of fetal alcohol spectrum disorder: A systematic review and meta-analysis. *Lancet, 387*(10022), 978–987.

Rajaprakash, M., Chakravarty, M. M., Lerch, J. P., & Rovet, J. (2014). Cortical morphology in children with alcohol-related neurodevelopmental disorder. *Brain and Behavior, 4*(1), 41–50.

Rasmussen, C., & Bisanz, J. (2009). Executive functioning in children with fetal alcohol spectrum disorders: Profiles and age-related differences. *Child Neuropsychology, 15*(3), 201–215.

Richardson, G. A., Conroy, M. L., & Day, N. L. (1996). Prenatal cocaine exposure: Effects on the development of school-age children. *Neurotoxicology and Teratology, 18*(6), 627–634.

Riley, E. P., Mattson, S. N., Sowell, E. R., Jernigan, T. L., Sobel, D. F., & Jones, K. L. (1995). Abnormalities of the corpus callosum in children prenatally exposed to alcohol. *Alcoholism: Clinical and Experimental Research, 19*(5), 1198–1202.

Riley, E. P., & McGee, C. L. (2005). Fetal alcohol spectrum disorders: An overview with emphasis on changes in brain and behavior. *Experimental Biology and Medicine (Maywood), 230*(6), 357–365.

Riley, E. P., McGee, C. L., & Sowell, E. R. (2004). Teratogenic effects of alcohol: A decade of brain imaging. *American Journal of Medical Genetics C: Seminars in Medical Genetics, 127*(1), 35–41.

Roebuck, T. M., Mattson, S. N., & Riley, E. P. (1998a). A review of the neuroanatomical findings in children with fetal alcohol syndrome or prenatal exposure to alcohol. *Alcoholism: Clinical and Experimental Research, 22*(2), 339–344.

Roebuck, T. M., Mattson, S. N., & Riley, E. P. (1999). Behavioral and psychosocial profiles of alcohol-exposed children. *Alcoholism: Clinical and Experimental Research, 23*(6), 1070–1076.

Roebuck, T. M., Simmons, R. W., Mattson, S. N., & Riley, E. P. (1998b). Prenatal exposure to alcohol affects the ability to maintain postural balance. *Alcoholism: Clinical and Experimental Research, 22*(1), 252–258.

Roebuck-Spencer, T. M., & Mattson, S. N. (2004). Implicit strategy affects learning in children with heavy prenatal alcohol exposure. *Alcoholism: Clinical and Experimental Research, 28*(9), 1424–1431.

Roebuck-Spencer, T. M., Mattson, S., Marion, S., Brown, W., & Riley, E. (2004). Bimanual coordination in alcohol-exposed children: Role of the corpus callosum. *Journal of the International Neuropsychological Society, 10*(4), 536–548.

Roussotte, F. F., Sulik, K. K., Mattson, S. N., Riley, E. P., Jones, K. L., Adnams, C. M., . . . Sowell, E. R. (2012). Regional brain volume reductions relate to facial dysmorphology and neurocognitive function in fetal alcohol spectrum disorders. *Human Brain Mapping, 33*(4), 920–937.

Rubio, D. M., Kraemer, K. L., Farrell, M. H., & Day, N. L. (2008). Factors associated with alcohol use, depression, and their co-occurrence during pregnancy. *Alcoholism: Clinical and Experimental Research, 32*(9), 1543–1551.

Santhanam, P., Coles, C. D., Li, Z., Li, L., Lynch, M. E., & Hu, X. (2011). Default mode network dysfunction in adults with prenatal alcohol exposure. *Psychiatry Research, 194*(3), 354–362.

Sayal, K., Heron, J., Draper, E., Alati, R., Lewis, S. J., Fraser, R., . . . Gray, R. (2014). Prenatal exposure to binge pattern of alcohol consumption: Mental health and learning outcomes at age 11. *European Child and Adolescent Psychiatry, 23*(10), 891–899.

Schonfeld, A. M., Mattson, S. N., Lang, A. R., Delis, D. C., & Riley, E. P. (2001). Verbal and nonverbal fluency in children with heavy prenatal alcohol exposure. *Journal of Studies on Alcohol, 62*(2), 239–246.

Schonfeld, A. M., Paley, B., Frankel, F., & O'Connor, M. J. (2006). Executive functioning predicts social skills following prenatal alcohol exposure. *Child Neuropsychology, 12*(6), 439–452.

Simmons, R. W., Thomas, J. D., Levy, S. S., & Riley, E. P. (2010). Motor response programming and movement time in children with heavy prenatal alcohol exposure. *Alcohol, 44*(4), 371–378.

Sowell, E. R., Jernigan, T. L., Mattson, S. N., Riley, E. P., Sobel, D. F., & Jones, K. L. (1996). Abnormal development of the cerebellar vermis in children prenatally exposed to alcohol: Size reduction in lobules I-V. *Alcoholism: Clinical and Experimental Research, 20*(1), 31–34.

Sowell, E. R., Mattson, S. N., Kan, E., Thompson, P. M., Riley, E. P., & Toga, A. W. (2008). Abnormal cortical thickness and brain–behavior correlation patterns in individuals with heavy prenatal alcohol exposure. *Cerebral Cortex, 18*(1), 136–144.

Sowell, E. R., Mattson, S. N., Thompson, P. M., Jernigan, T. L., Riley, E. P., & Toga, A. W. (2001a). Mapping callosal morphology and cognitive correlates: Effects of heavy prenatal alcohol exposure. *Neurology, 57*(2), 235–244.

Sowell, E. R., Thompson, P. M., Mattson, S. N., Tessner, K. D., Jernigan, T. L., Riley, E. P., & Toga, A. W. (2001b). Voxel-based morphometric analyses of the brain in children and adolescents prenatally exposed to alcohol. *NeuroReport, 12*(3), 515–523.

Sowell, E. R., Thompson, P. M., Mattson, S. N., Tessner, K. D., Jernigan, T. L., Riley, E. P., & Toga, A. W. (2002). Regional brain shape abnormalities persist into adolescence after heavy prenatal alcohol exposure. *Cerebral Cortex, 12*(8), 856–865.

Stratton, K., Howe, C., & Battaglia, F. (1996). *Fetal alcohol syndrome: Diagnosis, epidemiology, prevention, and treatment.* Washington, DC: National Academy Press.

Streissguth, A. P., Barr, H. M., Kogan, J., & Bookstein, F. L. (1996). *Final Report: Understanding the occurrence of secondary disabilities in clients with fetal alcohol syndrome (FAS) and fetal alcohol effects (FAE).* Seattle, WA: University of Washington Publication Services.

Streissguth, A. P., Barr, H. M., & Sampson, P. D. (1990). Moderate prenatal alcohol exposure: Effects on child IQ and learning problems at age 7 1/2 years. *Alcoholism: Clinical and Experimental Research, 14*(5), 662–669.

Streissguth, A. P., Barr, H. M., Sampson, P. D., & Bookstein, F. L. (1994a). Prenatal alcohol and offspring development: The first fourteen years. *Drug and Alcohol Dependence, 36*, 89–99.

Streissguth, A. P., Bookstein, F. L., Barr, H. M., Sampson, P. D., O'Malley, K., & Young, J. K.

(2004). Risk factors for adverse life outcomes in fetal alcohol syndrome and fetal alcohol effects. *Journal of Developmental and Behavioral Pediatrics, 25*(4), 228–238.

Streissguth, A. P., Randels, S. P., & Smith, D. F. (1991). A test–retest study of intelligence in patients with fetal alcohol syndrome: Implications for care. *Journal of the American Academy of Child and Adolescent Psychiatry, 30*(4), 584–587.

Streissguth, A. P., Sampson, P. D., Barr, H. M., Bookstein, F. L., & Olson, H. C. (1994b). The effects of prenatal exposure to alcohol and tobacco: Contributions from the Seattle longitudinal prospective study and implications for public policy. In H. L. Needleman & D. Bellinger (Eds.), *Prenatal exposure to toxicants: Developmental consequences* (pp. 148–183). Baltimore: Johns Hopkins University Press.

Sulik, K. (2005). Genesis of alcohol-induced craniofacial dysmorphism. *Experimental Biology and Medicine, 230*(6), 366–375.

Suttie, M., Wozniak, J. R., Parnell, S. E., Wetherill, L., Mattson, S. N., Sowell, E. R., . . . Hammond, P. (2018). Combined face-brain morphology and associated neurocognitive correlates in fetal alcohol spectrum disorders. *Alcoholism: Clinical and Experimental Research, 42*(9), 1769–1782.

Tamana, S., Pei, J., Massey, D., Massey, V., & Rasmussen, C. (2014). Neuropsychological Impairments and age-related differences in children and adolescents with fetal alcohol spectrum disorders. *Journal of Population Therapeutics and Clinical Pharmacology, 21*(2), e167–e180.

Taylor, N. M., & Enns, L. N. (2018). Age-related differences in neuropsychological assessment of fetal alcohol spectrum disorder: A cross-sectional study. *Biochemistry and Cell Biology, 96*(2), 252–259.

Taylor, P. A., Jacobson, S. W., van der Kouwe, A., Molteno, C. D., Chen, G., Wintermark, P., . . . Meintjes, E. M. (2015). A DTI-based tractography study of effects on brain structure associated with prenatal alcohol exposure in newborns. *Human Brain Mapping, 36*(1), 170–186.

Thompson, B. L., Levitt, P., & Stanwood, G. D. (2009). Prenatal exposure to drugs: Effects on brain development and implications for policy and education. *Nature Reviews: Neuroscience, 10*(4), 303–312.

Thorne, J. C. (2017). Accentuate the negative: Grammatical errors during narrative production as a clinical marker of central nervous system abnormality in school-aged children with fetal alcohol spectrum disorders. *Journal of Speech, Language, and Hearing Research, 60*(12), 3523–3537.

Treit, S., Chen, Z., Zhou, D., Baugh, L., Rasmussen, C., Andrew, G., . . . Beaulieu, C. (2017). Sexual dimorphism of volume reduction but not cognitive deficit in fetal alcohol spectrum disorders: A combined diffusion tensor imaging, cortical thickness and brain volume study. *NeuroImage: Clinical, 15*, 284–297.

Treit, S., Lebel, C., Baugh, L., Rasmussen, C., Andrew, G., & Beaulieu, C. (2013). Longitudinal MRI reveals altered trajectory of brain development during childhood and adolescence in fetal alcohol spectrum disorders. *Journal of Neuroscience, 33*(24), 10098–10109.

Treit, S., Zhou, D., Lebel, C., Rasmussen, C., Andrew, G., & Beaulieu, C. (2014). Longitudinal MRI reveals impaired cortical thinning in children and adolescents prenatally exposed to alcohol. *Human Brain Mapping, 35*(9), 4892–4903.

Uban, K. A., Herting, M. M., Wozniak, J. R., Sowell, E. R., & CIFASD [Collaborative Initiative on Fetal Alcohol Spectrum Disorders]. (2017). Sex differences in associations between white matter microstructure and gonadal hormones in children and adolescents with prenatal alcohol exposure. *Psychoneuroendocrinology, 83*, 111–121.

Vaurio, L., Repp, A., McGee, C. L., Riley, E. P., & Mattson, S. N. (2006). Visual working memory deficits in children with heavy prenatal alcohol exposure are secondary to lower-order deficits. *Alcoholism: Clinical and Experimental Research, 30*(S2), 178A.

Vaurio, L., Riley, E. P., & Mattson, S. N. (2008). Differences in executive functioning in children with heavy prenatal alcohol exposure or attention-deficit/hyperactivity disorder. *Journal of the International Neuropsychological Society, 14*(1), 119–129.

Vaurio, L., Riley, E. P., & Mattson, S. N. (2011). Neuropsychological comparison of children with heavy prenatal alcohol exposure and an IQ-matched comparison group. *Journal of the International Neuropsychological Society, 17*(3), 463–473.

Vorhees, C. V. (1986). Principles of behavioral teratology. In E. P. Riley & C. V. Vorhees (Eds.), *Handbook of behavioral teratology* (pp. 23–48). New York: Plenum.

Ware, A. L., Glass, L., Crocker, N., Deweese, B. N., Coles, C. D., Kable, J. A., . . . Mattson, S. N. (2014). Effects of prenatal alcohol exposure and attention-deficit/hyperactivity disorder on adaptive functioning. *Alcoholism: Clinical and Experimental Research, 38*(5), 1439–1447.

Ware, A. L., O'Brien, J. W., Crocker, N., Deweese, B. N., Roesch, S. C., Coles, C. D., . . . Collaborative Initiative on Fetal Alcohol Spectrum Disorders. (2013). The effects of prenatal alcohol exposure and attention-deficit/hyperactivity disorder on psychopathology and behavior. *Alcoholism: Clinical and Experimental Research, 37*(3), 507–516.

West, J. R., & Pierce, D. R. (1986). Perinatal alcohol exposure and neuronal damage. In J. R. West (Ed.), *Alcohol and brain development* (pp. 120–157). New York: Oxford University Press.

Wetherill, L., Foroud, T., & Goodlett, C. (2018). Meta-analyses of externalizing disorders: Genetics or prenatal alcohol exposure? *Alcoholism: Clinical and Experimental Research, 42*(1), 162–172.

Weyrauch, D., Schwartz, M., Hart, B., Klug, M. G., & Burd, L. (2017). Comorbid mental disorders in fetal alcohol spectrum disorders: A systematic review. *Journal of Developmental and Behavioral Pediatrics, 38*(4), 283–291.

Whaley, S. E., O'Connor, M. J., & Gunderson, B. (2001). Comparison of the adaptive functioning of children prenatally exposed to alcohol to a nonexposed clinical sample. *Alcoholism: Clinical and Experimental Research, 25*(7), 1018–1024.

Wierenga, L. M., Langen, M., Oranje, B., & Durston, S. (2014). Unique developmental trajectories of cortical thickness and surface area. *NeuroImage, 87*, 120–126.

Williams, J. F., Smith, V. C., & Committee on Substance Abuse. (2015). Fetal alcohol spectrum disorders. *Pediatrics, 136*(5), e1395–e1406.

Wozniak, J. R., Fink, B. A., Fuglestad, A. J., Eckerle, J. K., Boys, C. J., Sandness, K. E., . . . Georgieff, M. K. (2020). Four-year follow-up of a randomized controlled trial of choline for neurodevelopment in fetal alcohol spectrum disorder. *Journal of Neurodevelopmental Disorders, 12*(1), Article 9.

Wozniak, J. R., Fuglestad, A. J., Eckerle, J. K., Fink, B. A., Hoecker, H. L., Boys, C. J., . . . Georgieff, M. K. (2015). Choline supplementation in children with fetal alcohol spectrum disorders: a randomized, double-blind, placebo-controlled trial. *American Journal of Clinical Nutrition, 102*(5), 1113–1125.

Wozniak, J. R., Mueller, B. A., Bell, C. J., Muetzel, R. L., Hoecker, H. L., Boys, C. J., & Lim, K. O. (2013). Global functional connectivity abnormalities in children with fetal alcohol spectrum disorders. *Alcoholism: Clinical and Experimental Research, 37*(5), 748–756.

Wozniak, J. R., Mueller, B. A., Mattson, S. N., Coles, C. D., Kable, J. A., Jones, K. L., . . . Collaborative Initiative on Fetal Alcohol Spectrum Disorders. (2017). Functional connectivity abnormalities and associated cognitive deficits in fetal alcohol spectrum disorders (FASD). *Brain Imaging and Behavior, 11*(5), 1432–1445.

Wozniak, J. R., Mueller, B. A., Muetzel, R. L., Bell, C. J., Hoecker, H. L., Nelson, M. L., . . . Lim, K. O. (2011). Inter-hemispheric functional connectivity disruption in children with prenatal alcohol exposure. *Alcoholism: Clinical and Experimental Research, 35*(5), 849–861.

Wozniak, J. R., & Muetzel, R. L. (2011). What does diffusion tensor imaging reveal about the brain and cognition in fetal alcohol spectrum disorders? *Neuropsychology Review, 21*(2), 133–147.

Wyper, K. R., & Rasmussen, C. R. (2011). Language impairments in children with fetal alcohol spectrum disorders. *Journal of Population Therapeutics and Clinical Pharmacology, 18*(2), e364–e376.

Yang, Y., Roussotte, F., Kan, E., Sulik, K. K., Mattson, S. N., Riley, E. P., . . . Sowell, E. R. (2012). Abnormal cortical thickness alterations in fetal alcohol spectrum disorders and their relationships with facial dysmorphology. *Cerebral Cortex, 22*(5), 1170–1179.

Zhang, C., Paolozza, A., Tseng, P. H., Reynolds, J. N., Munoz, D. P., & Itti, L. (2019). Detection of children/youth with fetal alcohol spectrum disorder through eye movement, psychometric, and neuroimaging data. *Frontiers in Neurology, 10*, Article 80.

Zhou, D., Lebel, C., Lepage, C., Rasmussen, C., Evans, A., Wyper, K., . . . Beaulieu, C. (2011). Developmental cortical thinning in fetal alcohol spectrum disorders. *NeuroImage, 58*(1), 16–25.

Zhou, D., Rasmussen, C., Pei, J., Andrew, G., Reynolds, J. N., & Beaulieu, C. (2018). Preserved cortical asymmetry despite thinner cortex in children and adolescents with prenatal alcohol exposure and associated conditions. *Human Brain Mapping, 39*(1), 72–88.

CHAPTER 10

Type 1 Diabetes

David D. Schwartz
Rachel M. Wasserman

HISTORICAL OVERVIEW

Diabetes, one of most common diseases of childhood, is a group of metabolic disorders "characterized by hyperglycemia resulting from defects in insulin secretion, insulin action, or both" (American Diabetes Association [ADA], 2014, p. S81). Insulin is a hormone that transports blood glucose across the cell membrane, where it is used as fuel for cellular metabolism. When the body is unable to produce enough insulin or use it effectively, glucose builds up in the bloodstream, with deleterious long-term effects on multiple organs, including the eyes, kidneys, nerves, heart, and brain.

The two most common forms of diabetes are type 1 (T1D) and type 2 (T2D). T1D is an autoimmune disorder in which the immune system attacks and destroys insulin-producing pancreatic beta cells. As a result, insulin production declines and, in most cases, eventually ceases entirely. T2D is characterized by insulin resistance and (often) an increasing deficiency in insulin production. While both T1D and T2D can occur at any age, T1D is more commonly diagnosed in children, whereas T2D is more common in adults, largely due to its association with lifestyle factors (e.g., obesity, inactivity). Other forms of diabetes (e.g., gestational; latent autoimmune diabetes of adulthood) are highly uncommon in children. In this chapter we focus on T1D, which accounts for ~90% of cases of pediatric diabetes (Mayer-Davis et al., 2018). While most of the studies we review here were completed with children and youth, we have included some studies of adults as well, as the vast majority of adults were first diagnosed in childhood. Adult studies therefore provide a window into the long-term impact of this largely pediatric-onset disease.

T1D requires daily completion of a complex treatment regimen that involves monitoring carbohydrate intake, adjusting insulin dose based on intake, administering insulin, and monitoring blood glucose throughout the day. It therefore places large demands on cognitive skills such as memory, attention, planning, and organization. The goal of treatment is to maintain blood sugars within a targeted range. Mean blood glucose levels are typically measured with the hemoglobin A1c (A1c) assay, which provides a measure of blood sugar concentrations over the past 2–3 months. A1c is the primary metric used for evaluating and managing blood sugars clinically, and for indexing glycemic levels in research studies. Current guidelines recommend an A1c target of < 7.5% (58 mmol/mol) for children and youth with T1D (ADA, 2019), though it is estimated that only 1 in 5 actually meet this goal (Wood et al., 2013). Moreover, a large number of youth have chronically high blood sugars (i.e., A1c ≥ 9.5% [≥ 80 mmol/mol]), with a prevalence of 12.3% of non-Hispanic Whites, 27.3% of Hispanics, 35.5% of African Americans, 26.0% of Asian/Pacific Islanders, and 52.2% of Native Americans (Hamman et al., 2014). The risk for complications increases dramatically as A1c values exceed 7.5%, and continues to increase with each additional percentage point.

The primary complications of diabetes include nephropathy, retinopathy, and peripheral neuropathy, all of which are related to hyperglycemia-induced microvascular damage (Brownlee, 2005). As early as the 1920s, it was recognized that T1D also has an effect on the brain and cognitive functioning (Miles & Root, 1922), but only since the 1980s and 1990s has significant scientific attention has been paid to this relation. There are limited data on the prevalence of cognitive complications of T1D. One study reported cognitive impairment in 28% of adults with childhood-onset T1D (compared to 5% of controls) (Nunley et al., 2015), and executive dysfunction has been reported in 10–18% of youth with T1D (Caruso et al., 2014; Perez et al., 2017). The increased awareness of the neurocognitive complications of T1D has highlighted a previously unrecognized role for the neuropsychologist in diabetes care (ADA, 2019; Ryan, van Duinkerken, & Rosano, 2016).

EPIDEMIOLOGY

The prevalence of T1D has been increasing worldwide, especially in children under age 5 (Hamman et al., 2014). As of 2015, 0.18% of U.S. youth younger than 18 years and 0.24% of youth younger than 20 years had diabetes of any type. Approximately 1.25 million children and adults in the United States have T1D. T1D is most prevalent among non-Hispanic Whites (~2.5 cases/1,000), followed by African Americans (1.7 cases/1,000) and Hispanics (1.3 cases/1,000) (Hamman et al., 2014). Prevalence varies throughout the world and between different ethnic populations (Mayer-Davis et al., 2018), likely due to differences in environmental and genetic factors. Onset has a bimodal distribution, with a first peak between ages 5 and 7 years and a second peak between ages 10 and 14 years, or around the onset of puberty (Harjutsalo, Sjöberg, & Tuomilehto, 2008). Almost half of all cases are diagnosed prior to age 10, and approximately 80% are diagnosed before age 16. Worldwide, T1D is equally likely in males and females, but in some populations (e.g., people of European ancestry) prevalence may be slightly higher in males (Ostman et al., 2008).

ETIOLOGY, NEUROPATHOLOGY, AND NEURAL SUBSTRATES

Etiology

The etiology of T1D likely reflects the combined effect of genetic susceptibility and environmental triggers. The risk of T1D is approximately 0.5% in the general population, 4–10% for siblings of individuals with T1D, and at least 30–35% in identical twins (Mayer-Davis et al., 2018) if not much higher (Redondo, Jeffrey, Fain, Eisenbarth, & Orban,

2008). While diabetes is clearly a polygenic disorder, polymorphisms in the major histocompatibility complex on chromosome *6p21* are currently believed to confer the highest risk genetically (Davies et al., 1994). Little is known about environmental triggers, though viruses are thought to play a primary role, perhaps by infecting pancreatic beta cells, which are then targeted by the immune system. Enteroviruses in particular have been implicated, especially when infection occurs prenatally or in early childhood. As with autism, there does not appear to be a causal link between childhood vaccines and development of T1D (Hviid, Stellfeld, Wohlfahrt, & Melbye, 2004).

Studies have shown that T1D progresses through a series of stages that can last for years before becoming symptomatic (Insel et al., 2015). Stage 1 is defined by the presence of diabetes-related islet autoantibodies with normal blood sugars. In Stage 2, there is development of glucose intolerance due to decreasing beta cells, but the individual remains asymptomatic. Stage 2 is also characterized by a decrease in C-peptide levels and increased insulin resistance, which are associated with risk for cognitive dysfunction. Stage 3 is defined by the onset of symptomatic disease (e.g., polydipsia, polyuria, weight loss), most likely after a critical mass of beta cells has been destroyed. It is unclear how long the perionset period lasts. Some authors have argued that symptomatic onset is generally rapid, occurring within 1–2 weeks (Roche, Menon, Gill, & Hoey, 2005), while others have suggested that this stage may last for months or longer (Atkinson, Eisenbarth, & Michels, 2014). During this time, the individual is exposed to a prolonged period of untreated hyperglycemia that has the potential to impact brain development (Ryan, 2006, 2008).

Neuropathology

The glycemic dysregulation that characterizes diabetes can affect brain development and functioning. The primary mechanisms of neuropathology are hypoglycemia (low blood glucose levels), hyperglycemia (high blood glucose), and diabetic ketoacidosis (DKA).

Hypoglycemia

Glucose is the brain's primary energy source, yet it cannot synthesize or store more than a few minutes' worth, so any interruption of glucose supply results in acute disturbance of neuronal function. Current guidelines classify hypoglycemia at three levels, which can be characterized as mild (glucose < 70 mg/dL [3.9 mmol/L] and ≥ 54 mg/dL [3.0 mmol/L]), moderate (glucose < 54 mg/dL [3.0 mmol/L]), and severe (ADA, 2019). Severe hypoglycemia (SH) is defined not by glucose levels, but by altered mental and/or physical status that impairs the person's function to the degree that he or she requires immediate help from someone else (e.g., administration of glucagon). SH results in a potentially devastating sequence of events that may progress from acute cognitive dysfunction to seizures and loss of consciousness. Eventually, cessation of electrical brain activity (a flat or isoelectric electroencephalogram [EEG]) may occur, resulting in neuronal death (Cryer, 2007; Languren, Montiel, Julio-Amilpas, & Massieu, 2013). Irreversible brain damage is especially likely when blood glucose falls below 20 mg/dL (i.e., profound hypoglycemia; Languren et al., 2013).

Fortunately, in most cases, hypoglycemia is interrupted before permanent injury to the brain occurs, and acute cognitive sequelae tend to resolve with a return to euglycemia.

However, SH may still have an effect on cognition, especially at younger ages. Brain regions particularly vulnerable to SH include the hippocampus (Ho et al., 2008), insular cortex, thalamus (Seaquist, 2015), frontotemporal cortex, basal ganglia (McCrimmon, Ryan, & Frier, 2012), and the default mode network (Passow et al., 2015). Neuroimaging studies have shown reduced gray matter volume in the left superior temporal gyrus (Perantie et al., 2007) and reduced gray matter density in the cerebellum (Musen et al., 2006) in response to SH. One study showed that children with greater exposure to hypoglycemia have decreased regional white matter in the occipital–parietal cortex (Perantie et al., 2011), though a later study did not find a similar effect (Barnea-Goraly et al., 2014).

Recurrent SH was long thought to be the primary factor in diabetes-related neurocognitive dysfunction, but longitudinal data from the landmark Diabetes Control and Complications Trial/Epidemiology of Diabetes Intervention and Complications (DCCT/EDIC) study, which followed a large cohort of adults with T1D over an 18-year period, showed no association between repeated episodes of SH and cognitive dysfunction (Austin & Deary, 1999; DCCT/EDIC Study Research Group, 2007; Jacobson et al., 2011). Meta-analyses of adults with T1D have produced conflicting results, with one analysis finding no effects of SH on cognition (Brands, Biessels, De Haan, Kappelle, & Kessels, 2005), and another finding specific effects on memory and executive function (Tonoli et al., 2014). Findings from children more consistently suggest an association between recurrent SH and cognitive dysfunction, specifically in memory. In a meta-analysis of eight studies, Naguib, Kulinskaya, Lomax, and Garralda (2009) found no effects of SH on cognitive functioning with the exception of short-term verbal memory. A more focused meta-analysis found associations between recurrent SH and IQ (small effect), learning (small to medium effect), memory (medium effect), and verbal fluency (small effect) (Blasetti et al., 2011), though the authors argued that differences in IQ and verbal fluency most probably reflected an underlying memory deficit. In a meta-analysis, Gaudieri, Chen, Greer, and Holmes (2008) found a small effect of hypoglycemic seizures on IQ ($d = -0.19$ to -0.21) but nominally *better* visual memory ($d = 0.13$) and learning ($d = 0.12$). They hypothesized that this discrepancy may have been "due to the opposing effects of those in relatively poorer versus better metabolic control" (p. 1896).

Hyperglycemia

Chronic hyperglycemia appears to be the primary cause of cognitive dysfunction in individuals with T1D. Hyperglycemia exacerbates cerebral ischemia and is associated with neuron-damaging acidosis and production of extracellular glutamate, which can be neurotoxic (Kawai, Keep, Betz, & Nagao, 1998). It changes the composition of metabolite concentrations in neural tissue, which can affect neuronal integrity (Arbalaez, Semenkovich, & Hershey, 2013). It also disrupts the blood–brain barrier (Kawai et al., 1998), resulting in changes that either increase or decrease neural exposure to glucose (Malone, 2016), which in turn might expose the brain to a damaging flood of glucose in the perionset period (Ryan 2006, 2008). Hyperglycemia contributes to the formation of advanced glycation end products that can affect cerebral microvasculature (Wessels, Scheltens, Barkhof, & Heine, 2008), and it induces oxidative stress in cells that cannot down-regulate transport of glucose across the cell membrane, which explains why cells in the eyes, kidneys, and peripheral nervous system are selectively damaged by diabetes (Brownlee, 2005). Oxidative stress has also been shown to cause selective damage to neurons in the hippocampus, cerebellum, substantia nigra, and ventral tegmental area (VTA) (Wang & Michaelis, 2010).

Animal studies have demonstrated that hyperglycemia impedes myelination (Malone, Hanna, & Saporta, 2006) and affects axonal integrity (Sharma et al., 2010). In humans, neuroimaging studies have shown effects of hyperglycemia on white matter volume and integrity (e.g., Wessels et al., 2007), and slower growth of white matter throughout the cortex and cerebellum (Barnea-Goraly et al., 2014; Mauras et al., 2015; Mazaika et al., 2016). Hyperglycemia-related changes in gray matter have been observed in children in the right posterior cortex (Perantie et al., 2007) and in whole-brain gray matter (Perantie et al., 2011). Findings from the DirecNet study group showed slower growth of whole brain gray matter in terms of reduced cortical volume and total surface area (Barnea-Goraly et al., 2014; Mauras et al., 2015; Mazaika et al., 2016). In adults, gray matter changes have been reported in the hippocampus, parahippocampal gyrus, and superior temporal gyrus (Musen et al., 2006), with more widespread changes noted in individuals diagnosed prior to age 7 (Ferguson et al., 2005). As discussed in more detail below, hyperglycemia has been found to be associated with reduced information processing speed, attention, executive functioning (Jacobson et al., 2011; Wessels et al., 2007) and IQ (Fox et al., 2018; Perantie et al., 2008).

Diabetic Ketoacidosis

DKA is an acute metabolic crisis that can lead to coma and death. It is evident at the time of diabetes diagnosis in 30–40% of cases (Dabelea et al., 2014), and is more likely in younger children (Iovane et al., 2018). In ~1% of cases, DKA results in frank cerebral edema (Wolfsdorf, Glaser, & Sperling, 2006; Wolfsdorf et al., 2007), though it is likely associated with subclinical edema in more than half of all cases (Glaser et al., 2006). DKA at diagnosis is associated with reduced white matter volume in frontal, temporal, and parietal regions, reduced neuronal density in frontal gray matter (Cameron et al., 2014), and abnormal growth of gray and white matter 18 months postdiagnosis, associated with reduced IQ and attention (Aye et al., 2019). It is also associated with changes in mean diffusivity in the thalamus (Antenor-Dorsey et al., 2013).

Glucose Variability

Glucose variability is defined as the degree to which an individual's blood sugars fluctuate between high and low levels. While blood sugars vary throughout the day in individuals without diabetes (e.g., they might vary from 80 to 140 mg/dL in response to carbohydrate intake or exercise), glycemic variability is heightened in people with diabetes (< 40 mg/dL to > 400 mg/dL). Studies using data from continuous glucose monitors (CGM) have shown that even children with T1D whose average blood glucose levels are in range spend on average 12 hours/day in the hyperglycemic range, and 1 hour/day in the hypoglycemic range (Mauras et al., 2012; Tansey et al., 2016). This daily variability is not captured by the A1c assay, and thus may be an unrecognized contributor to cognitive dysfunction. Glucose variability is strongly associated with oxidative stress in T2D (Monnier et al., 2006) but only weakly in T1D (Wentholt, Kulik, Michels, Hoekstra, & DeVries, 2008). Studies using CGM data have shown that greater variability is associated with abnormal growth of whole-brain gray and white matter, and reduced IQ (Barnea-Goraly et al., 2014; Mauras et al., 2015; Mazaika et al., 2016).

Functional Connectivity

One of the more intriguing findings of the past 10 years has been the recognition of T1D-related changes in the default mode network (DMN), a distributed network that includes the frontal lobes, posterior cingulate, and lateral parietal–occipital cortices. The DMN tends to be most active when a person is not involved in any overt tasks and may have a role in introspection and planning. Studies have identified gray and white matter changes in the cuneus, precuneus, and cingulate cortex in T1D (Kaufmann et al., 2011; Perantie et al., 2007) that were associated with both SH and chronic hyperglycemia (Arbelaez et al., 2013). Other functional brain differences have begun to emerge. Hosseini et al. (2016) found reduced global integration of brain networks in children with T1D and greater vulnerability of these networks to insult. A second study with the same group of children found increased resting state functional connectivity in T1D, which correlated with processing speed, executive functioning, learning and memory (Saggar et al., 2017). The authors interpreted this as most likely indicating functional reorganization of the brain as a compensatory response to abnormal gray and white matter development (e.g., Barnea-Goraly et al., 2014; Mauras et al., 2015; Mazaika et al., 2016). While their functional significance is still unclear, these studies are beginning to inform a more complete understanding of brain development and function in T1D.

Other Factors

Other diabetes-related factors can affect central nervous system (CNS) integrity and therefore *may* impact cognition in T1D. Insulin stimulates neuronal growth and differentiation, synaptic plasticity, and neurotransmission, so deficiencies in insulin have the potential to disrupt cognitive functioning (Malone, 2016). Impaired C-peptide action is associated with cognitive dysfunction and hippocampal apoptosis in rats with T1D (Sima & Li, 2005). However, research on the potential impact of these factors in humans with T1D is currently lacking (Tonoli et al., 2014). Genetic factors may also contribute to cognitive vulnerability. One study suggested that the ε4 allele of the APOE gene might affect IQ in T1D (Ferguson et al., 2003), but subsequent research did not find an association (Jacobson et al., 2011). Deletion in glutathione S-transferase is associated with retinopathy in T1D (Hovnik, Dolžan, Bratina, Podkrajšek, & Battelino, 2009), but a relation to cognitive outcomes has not been reported.

NEUROPSYCHOLOGICAL CONSEQUENCES

General Intellectual Functioning

Meta-analyses comparing children with and without T1D suggest a small effect of T1D on IQ in children, translating to a 2- to 3-point reduction in Full Scale, Verbal/crystallized, and Performance/fluid IQ (Gaudieri et al., 2008; Nauguib et al., 2009). Tonoli et al. (2014)

found a larger effect on Full Scale IQ (FSIQ) (~6 point reduction), but no effect on Verbal IQ (VIQ) or Performance IQ (PIQ).

Effects of early-onset of disease (EOD; i.e., onset in the first 5–7 years of life) are well documented. Children with EOD showed reduced crystallized intelligence compared to children with later onset of T1D ($d = -0.15$) and to healthy controls ($d = -0.28$ to -0.35) (Gaudieri et al., 2008). In adults, Brands et al. (2005) found a 12- to 14-point difference in crystallized IQ, and a 6-point difference in fluid IQ, and Tonoli et al. (2014) reported an approximate 5 point reduction in VIQ and PIQ. The larger effects in adults suggest there may be a diabetes-related decline in IQ over time, a possibility supported by longitudinal research. In a 12-year study, Northam and colleagues (1995) found no T1D-control group differences in IQ at diabetes diagnosis, but after 2 years, differences emerged in PIQ (though only in children with EOD; Northam et al., 1998), and after 6 years, changes were evident in VIQ (Northam et al., 2001). Diabetes-related declines in IQ may be secondary to white matter changes affecting attention (Cato et al., 2014) and/or to hypoglycemia-related hippocampal damage affecting memory (Blasetti et al., 2011; Northam et al., 2001).

In terms of the effect of diabetes risk factors on IQ, findings are mixed for SH (Blasetti et al., 2011; Gaudieri et al., 2008; Naguib et al., 2009; Tonoli et al., 2014), chronic hyperglycemia (Perantie et al., 2008; Schoenle, Schoenle, Molinari, & Largo, 2002; Semenkovich et al., 2016; Tonoli et al., 2014), and DKA (Aye et al., 2019; Cato et al., 2014). A possible explanation is that the effect of T1D on IQ may depend on interactions between these risk factors, and with EOD (Cato et al., 2014; Lin, Northam, Rankins, Werther, & Cameron, 2010; Lin, Northam, Werther, & Cameron, 2015).

Perceptual and Sensorimotor Skills

Slowed processing speed is one of the most common neurocognitive sequelae of T1D (Jacobson et al., 2011). Meta-analyses indicate a small effect of T1D on information processing and psychomotor efficiency in children ($d = -0.10$ to -0.22; Gaudieri et al., 2008; Naguib et al., 2009) and a medium-size effect in adults ($d = -0.6$; Brands et al., 2005). Deficits in psychomotor efficiency are especially likely in children with EOD (Gaudieri et al., 2008). Meta-analytic findings also consistently show reduced fine-motor speed in children with T1D, with effect sizes in the small ($d = -0.16$ to -0.26; Gaudieri et al., 2008; Naguib et al., 2009) to medium range ($d = -0.38$; Tonoli et al., 2014), with larger differences again evident in adults ($d = -0.5$ to -0.6; Brands et al., 2005; Tonoli et al., 2014).

Changes in processing speed also appear to be linked to hyperglycemia and its complications (Wessels et al., 2008), and there is evidence that such changes may be initiated early in the disease process, possibly due to prolonged exposure to hyperglycemia in the perionset period (Ryan, 2006, 2008). For example, deficits on the Grooved Pegboard test have been found within days of diabetes diagnosis and were predictive of glycemic levels 2 years postdiagnosis, suggesting that reduced psychomotor speed may be a leading indicator of neurocognitive dysfunction in children with T1D (Schwartz, Axelrad, & Anderson, 2014a). In contrast, simple reaction time may not be impaired at diagnosis (Semenkovich et al., 2016). Longitudinal studies indicate that psychomotor speed and mental efficiency show mild declines over time in individuals with chronically elevated A1c (DCCT/EDIC Study Research Group, 2007) and microvascular complications (Jacobson et al., 2011).

Thus, declines in processing speed may be isolated to patients with EOD, chronic hyperglycemia, and/or microvascular complications.

Deficits in visuospatial processing and visuomotor integration are also reported in T1D, with effect sizes in the small range for children (*d* = −0.18 to −0.29; Gaudieri et al., 2008; Naguib et al., 2009) and adults (*d* = −0.4; Brands et al., 2005). An earlier review (Desrocher & Rovet, 2004) found effects of SH and EOD on visuospatial and visuomotor skills in T1D, but these findings were not supported by later meta-analyses (Brands et al., 2005; Gaudeiri et al., 2008; Naguib et al., 2009).

Language

Two meta-analyses have looked at language functioning. Naguib et al. (2009) found no difference in language abilities between children with and without T1D, though in a subset of studies they found a marginal effect of hypoglycemic seizures (*d* = −0.66; *p* = .08). In adults with and without T1D, no differences in naming and comprehension were found (Brands et al., 2005). Deficits in verbal fluency were noted in children with SH (Blasetti et al., 2011), but this may reflect more basic deficits in processing speed, memory, and executive functioning. Small deficits in reading (*d* = −0.24) and writing (*d* = −0.28) have been reported (Naguib et al., 2009), with general academic difficulties appearing to be more common in EOD (Gaudieri et al., 2008). It is unclear whether these deficits might be secondary to other factors (e.g., attention, memory). In a study of Finnish children with EOD, Hannonen et al. (2010) found a deficit in phonemic perception (*d* = −0.59). Overall, it appears that diabetes has a minimal effect on language, with the possible exception of children who experience SH early in life.

Attention

Compared to healthy controls, children with T1D show mild to moderate deficits in sustained attention (*d* = −0.217; Naguib et al., 2009). Gaudieri et al. (2008) reported a smaller effect (*d* = −0.10) when looking at a combined index of attention and executive functioning. In adults, Brands et al. (2005) found effects of T1D on visual (*d* = −0.4), sustained (*d* = −0.3), and selective attention (*d* = −0.2), but not on divided attention. EOD is associated with decrements in attention compared to later disease onset (*d* = −0.27; Gaudieri et al., 2008). Microangiopathy is associated with reduced connectivity in attention networks and lower performance on tests of attention and processing speed in adults with long-standing T1D (van Duinkerken et al., 2012). Attention deficits in T1D appear most strongly linked to hyperglycemia. While some studies have found an effect of SH on attention, meta-analyses have not supported this association (Brands et al., 2005; Tonoli et al., 2014).

Memory

Meta-analyses comparing children with and without T1D generally show a small effect of T1D on verbal learning (*d* = −0.17, *p* = .07, Gaudieri et al., 2008; *d* = −0.367, *p* < .01, Naguib et al., 2009), but little to no effect on verbal and visuospatial memory. In adults, a small effect of diabetes on memory was found in Tonoli et al. (2014; *d* = −0.19) but not in Brands et al. (2005). Thus, there appears to be little support for a general effect of T1D on memory functioning.

However, the story becomes very different when examining age-of-onset effects. Compared to children with later disease onset, children with EOD show clear deficits in verbal (d = −0.25 to −0.28) and visuospatial learning and memory (d = −0.25 to −0.52) (Gaudieri et al., 2008; Tonoli et al., 2014). As noted earlier, a history of SH is also associated with poorer memory performance. Naguib et al. (2009) found a small effect of SH on verbal short-term memory (d = −0.14), whereas Blasetti et al. (2011) found a moderately larger effect on memory overall (d = −0.38). DKA has been found to be associated with reduced verbal memory performance at the time of diagnosis (Cameron et al., 2014), and with reduced visual memory 3.5 months later (Semenkovich et al., 2016). DKA history is also associated with more chronic memory dysfunction, especially in children with EOD (Antenor-Dorsey et al., 2013; Ghetti, Lee, Sims, DeMaster, & Glaser, 2010). Overall, it appears that T1D has a negligible effect on memory except for individuals with EOD, an effect that may in part be driven by the increased likelihood of SH and DKA in younger children (Guadieri et al., 2008; Ryan et al., 2016).

Executive Functions

Most research examining executive functioning (EF) in youth with T1D has focused on EF as a predictor of self-management or glycemic control (discussed in the section "Behavioral Functioning"). Fewer studies have looked at EF as an outcome. Due to the paucity of studies 10 years ago, Gaudieri et al. (2008) combined the domains of EF and attention in their meta-analysis, finding a small overall effect (d = −0.10). A more recent meta-analysis by Broadley, White, and Andrew (2017) found small to medium effects of T1D on inhibition (Hedges's g = −0.28), working memory (g = 0.34), set-shifting (g = −0.31), and overall EF (g = −0.42). Too few studies were available to conduct meta-analyses on diabetes-related risk factors, but findings from relevant studies were summarized: EOD was associated with reduced inhibition and set shifting; chronic hypoglycemia was associated with poorer working memory; SH was associated with reduced inhibition, working memory, and set shifting; and complications of hyperglycemia were possibly related to disinhibition. Findings are mixed regarding DKA and EF, though some studies have found an association (Cato et al., 2014, 2016). SH occurring before age 6 has been found to be a risk factor for worse EF in young adults (Ly, Anderson, McNamara, Davis, & Jones, 2011).

Even fewer studies have examined EF as an outcome using questionnaire-based assessments such as the BRIEF (Gioia, Isquith, Guy, & Kenworthy, 2000). This is important, as questionnaires likely do not measure the same constructs as performance-based assessments of EF (Toplak, West, & Stanovich, 2013), and questionnaire data might be more predictive of behaviors involved in diabetes self-management (Suchy et al., 2016). Studies using questionnaires have found reduced EF in youth with T1D compared to healthy controls (Berg et al., 2018). Mean scores have typically been within the average range, though the prevalence of clinically significant scores may be elevated, ranging from 10–18% in some studies (Caruso et al., 2014; Perez et al., 2017; Vloemans et al., 2019). These findings suggest that group differences in real-world EF may be limited to a subset of patients. Nonetheless, even small differences in EF are associated with poorer diabetes self-management (Duke & Harris, 2014; Wasserman, Hilliard, Schwartz, & Anderson, 2015), which in turn is associated with A1c (Hood, Peterson, Rohan, & Drotar, 2009). Thus, a bidirectional or cyclical relationship may exist between glycemic levels and EF.

Acute Cognitive Effects

While most studies have examined long-term effects of T1D on neurocognitive functioning, acute glycemic extremes are also associated with cognitive deficits, though they tend to be transient. Mental speed and efficiency are slower during hypoglycemia and hyperglycemia (Gonder-Frederick et al., 2009), and acute hypoglycemia has detrimental effects on selective attention (McAulay, Deary, Ferguson, & Frier, 2001) and vigilance (Warren & Frier, 2005). The effects of acute hyperglycemia on attention are less clear, with some studies showing an effect (Sattar, Renneboog, & Decaux, 2017) and others not (Draelos et al., 1995). Given that even children who meet recommended A1c targets experience significant glycemic variability throughout the day (Mauras et al., 2012; Tansey et al., 2016), it is likely that they also experience daily fluctuations in attention and processing speed. This has implications for activities such as driving (ADA, 2012) and school performance. In a small intervention study, Daley, Wodrich, and Hasan (2006) demonstrated that stabilization of blood glucose using an insulin pump resulted in increased on-task classroom behavior and a reduction in off-task behavior in four boys with T1D and attention problems.

Adaptive and Social Functioning

Few studies have examined adaptive functioning in youth with T1D, though evidence suggests generally age-appropriate attainment of responsibility and independence (Pacaud et al., 2007). Nonetheless, the complexities of diabetes self-management require additional skills and resources that complicate the transition into adulthood for individuals with T1D (Hilliard et al., 2014). Children and youth with T1D also tend to have typical social functioning, though social factors have a significant impact on adjustment to and management of diabetes. In general, good social support from family and friends is associated with positive outcomes, whereas poorer outcomes are associated with parental underinvolvement or overly controlling behavior, conflict, and criticism (Wiebe, Helgeson, & Berg, 2016). Conflict may have a stronger impact on outcomes than support (Palladino & Helgeson, 2012).

Emotional and Behavioral Adjustment

Emotional Functioning

The complexity and unrelenting nature of diabetes and its treatment, the disruptive effect it has on children's lives, and the stress that comes from the "high-stakes" nature of maintaining tight glycemic control mean that diabetes distress (Reynolds & Helgeson, 2011) and burnout (Polonsky, 1996) are quite common. These problems tend to be heightened in youth with chronically high blood sugars (Reynolds & Helgeson, 2011) and may in turn result in problematic self-management and an increased risk for depression. Some authors suggest a twofold increase in lifetime prevalence of depression in T1D (Cameron, Northam, Ambler, & Daneman, 2007; Ducat, Philipson, & Anderson 2014), though depressive disorders in youth with T1D may be overestimated, as it can be difficult to distinguish depressive symptoms from diabetes distress and burnout.

Eating disordered behavior, which may be triggered by the intense focus on carbohydrate intake in T1D, is associated with elevated A1c and increased risk for DKA (Goebel-Fabbri, 2013). Insulin omission to control weight is a more widespread problem that also increases risk for hyperglycemia and DKA (Weinger & Beverly, 2010). There is also an elevated risk for other mental health concerns, including adjustment disorders at diagnosis (Cameron et al., 2007), anxiety (Rechenberg, Whittemore, & Grey, 2017), and behavior problems (Cohen, Lumley, Naar-King, Partridge, & Cakan, 2004). Family conflict, which may be exacerbated by disagreements over diabetes management, can have a substantial impact on treatment-related behaviors and glycemic levels (Anderson, 2004).

Behavioral Functioning

Problematic diabetes management is perhaps the main behavioral concern for which psychologists are consulted when working with children and youth with T1D. As noted earlier, many of the challenges to optimal management reflect the socioemotional burden of diabetes and its treatment. Cognitive factors also play an important role, especially beginning in adolescence, when youth take on more responsibility for diabetes self-care. Much of the research in this area has focused on EF given the importance of skills such as planning, organization, and working memory for managing daily tasks. Duke and Harris (2014) summarized the literature to date and found small to medium effects of EF on self-management, though only one study (of six) identified a relationship between EF and glycemic levels. More recent studies have shown that poorer performance on the Iowa Gambling Task predicts a larger increase in A1c during the year after high school (Suchy et al., 2017), whereas better performance on EF tasks predicts a slower increase in A1c across the same transition period (Berg et al., 2018). Consistent with these findings, youth with attention-deficit/hyperactivity disorder (ADHD) are at greater risk for problems with diabetes management, chronically high blood sugars, DKA, and SH (Hilgard et al., 2017; Lin, Lin, Hsu, Lin, & Fu, 2019; Nylander, Lindström, Khalifa, & Fernell, 2018; Yazar et al., 2019). Other cognitive factors that likely affect self-management behaviors include IQ (Gottfredson & Deary, 2004; Suchy et al., 2016); problem solving (Cook, Herold, Edidin, & Briars, 2002; Hill-Briggs, 2003); verbal memory, which predicts daily blood glucose monitoring (Holmes et al., 2006); and math skills, which are needed for correct calculation of carbohydrate consumption and insulin-dose adjustments (Soutor, Chen, Streisand, Kaplowitz, & Holmes, 2004).

DEVELOPMENTAL CONSIDERATIONS

Brain areas that are still developing (Rice & Barone, 2000) or that undergo prolonged development (Pechtel & Pizzagalli, 2011) are more vulnerable to insult than areas that have matured. In T1D, there is strong support for the effects of EOD on neurodevelopment (Schwartz, Wasserman, Powell, & Axelrad, 2014b), likely due in part to the exceptionally high glucose requirements of the developing brain, which reach adult rates by age 2 years and double the adult rate by ages 4–5, when neuronal and synaptic proliferation peak (Kuzawa et al., 2014). T1D-related disruption of cerebral glucose supply can therefore have particularly deleterious effects on brain development at these ages (Arbelaez et al., 2013; Cato & Hershey, 2016). Ryan (2006, 2008) applied a diathesis–stress model to understanding EOD effects, arguing that unidentified hyperglycemia leading up to symptomatic onset might create a vulnerability to later effects of dysglycemia. In addition, the impact of these initial insults may not immediately be evident in later-developing abilities such as EF (i.e., they may represent cognitive late-effects; Schwartz et al., 2014b). As discussed earlier, meta-analyses show small effects of EOD on cognition compared to children with later onset, and medium effects compared to healthy controls (Gaudieri et al., 2008). Consistent memory deficits are *only* found in individuals with EOD, though it difficult to tease out the effects of EOD alone from increased incidence of SH and DKA in younger children. Also of note, effects of EOD on later EF have been reported (Tonoli et al., 2014), potentially consistent with a cognitive late-effects account.

The cognitive impact of T1D has additional ramifications in adolescence. The nervous system goes though substantial reorganization at this time, especially in areas related to EF and social-emotional processing (Colver & Longwell, 2013; Sisk & Zehr, 2005), potentially making development in these areas more vulnerable to diabetes-related disruption (Schwartz et al., 2014b). As a result of these changes, adolescents are less likely to plan ahead and defer immediate reward (McClure, Laibson, Lowenstein, & Cohen, 2004), and more likely to act without thinking and take risks (Steinberg, 2010). This is a recipe for problematic diabetes control, and it occurs at just the time that responsibility for illness management typically shifts from parent to child (Anderson & Schwartz, 2014). Not surprisingly, management tends to decline and A1c to increase in adolescence.

These developmental findings led to the suggestion that some suboptimal self-management may be the result of adolescent risk taking (Schwartz & Axelrad, 2015). Specifically, when faced with completing diabetes management tasks, adolescents may engage in a reasoned decision-making process that overvalues immediate benefits and downplays long-term risks or costs (Gerrard, Gibbons, Houlihan, Stock, & Pomery, 2008; McClure et al., 2004). For example, when socializing with friends, an adolescent with T1D may defer taking insulin until later, resulting in acutely high blood sugars and increased risk for DKA if he or she subsequently forgets to take it. Wasserman, Anderson, and Schwartz (2017) developed these ideas into a model of diabetes-specific risk taking that is currently under investigation. Preliminary findings suggest that diabetes-specific risk taking is correlated to general executive dysfunction, poorer diabetes self-management, and report of SH (but not DKA) over the past year (Wasserman et al., 2018).

Adulthood has been described as a period of relative cognitive stability in T1D (Biessels, Deary, & Ryan, 2008), although cognitive dysfunction may increase slowly over the course of the disease in individuals with chronically out-of-range blood sugars, especially in processing speed and cognitive efficiency (DCCT/EDIC Study Research Group 2007; Jacobson et al., 2011). Studies have demonstrated accelerated cognitive aging and increased rates of dementia in older adults with T2D, but it is not known whether similar problems are evident in T1D. Given that a large number of adults are living into old age, widespread cognitive decline in the T1D population would have significant public health implications (Moheet, Mangia, & Seaquist 2015).

Predictors and Moderators

Biological Factors

The primary known biological risk factors for neurocognitive dysfunction in T1D are the glycemic extremes discussed earlier and microvascular complications. Microvascular complications outside the brain (retinopathy and neuropathy) are associated with changes in cerebral white matter (Ferguson et al., 2003; Musen et al., 2006; Wessels et al., 2007) and decreased gray matter density in the interior frontal gyrus and occipital lobe (Wessels et al., 2006), and thus appear to be markers for microvascular disease inside the brain (Wessels et al., 2008).

Psychological Factors

Emotional and behavioral factors have a significant impact on diabetes management (Datye, Moore, Russell, & Jaser, 2015; Helgeson, Siminerio, Escobar, & Becker, 2009), which in turn affects glycemic control (Hood et al., 2009).

Social and Cultural Factors

Minority youth experience significant disparities in diabetes care (Naranjo, Schwartz, & Delamater, 2015) and have higher rates of chronic hyperglycemia (Hamman et al., 2014), placing them at heightened risk for cognitive dysfunction. Poor and minority youth are also exposed to greater levels of chronic stress (Pechtel & Pizzagall, 2011), which has deleterious effects on the CNS (Bos, Fox, Zeanah, & Nelson, 2009) and contributes directly to hyperglycemia (Brand, Johnson, & Johnson, 1986). However, research on cognitive outcomes in different racial and socioeconomic groups with T1D is currently lacking. There are also few studies examining gender differences, though Naguib et al. (2009) found no gender effects on cognition in youth with T1D.

Treatment and Intervention

The primary treatment of T1D involves administration of insulin multiple times a day, either through subcutaneous injection or via an insulin pump, with the goal of maintaining glucose homeostasis in much the same way a functioning pancreas would. This also requires frequent monitoring of carbohydrate intake and blood sugars (ADA, 2019). Traditionally, blood glucose monitoring has been accomplished with a hand-held glucometer, but within the past several years, CGMs have come under increasingly wide use. Apart from maintaining tight glycemic control (i.e., A1c < 7.5%), no other treatments have been shown to prevent complications in T1D (Wessels et al., 2008).

Current treatment guidelines also recommend psychosocial care for all people with diabetes, with the goal of "achieving satisfactory medical outcomes and psychological well-being"; such care should include "assessment for symptoms of diabetes distress, depression, anxiety, disordered eating, and cognitive capacities," and "referral to a mental health specialist familiar with diabetes management" when indicated (ADA, 2019, pp. S54–S55). While it is beyond the scope of this chapter to review interventions to improve self-management, multicomponent interventions that target some combination of behavioral, emotional, social, and family processes have small but positive effects (Hood et al., 2009).

There is also an important role for the neuropsychologist in helping patients with diabetes. This includes screening for cognitive and executive deficits in youth with T1D (Wasserman, Anderson, & Schwartz, 2016) and their parents (Goethals et al., 2018), consideration of EF skills in formulating diabetes care plans (Duke & Harris, 2014), and providing clinically informed recommendations for family management or environmental accommodations to support EF (Wasserman et al., 2015).

CONCLUSIONS AND FUTURE DIRECTIONS

T1D diabetes is a life-changing disease that places a substantial burden on children and their families in the form of a highly complex medical regimen that must be followed closely every day to prevent significant long-term complications. Problems with self-management, stress, and other psychological difficulties are well-known correlates of the disease and its treatment. While we have known of the neurological impact and cognitive sequelae of T1D for some time, the impact of these additional morbidities is really only now coming into focus.

Multiple meta-analyses support the conclusion that the effects of T1D on cognition are relatively small, typically on the order of a 2- to 4-point decrement on tests of IQ, attention, EF, and psychomotor speed and efficiency, with somewhat larger effects evident in children with onset of diabetes in the first 5–7 years of life. These subtle cognitive deficits have to be understood in the broader context of living with diabetes, as even small problems in reasoning, attention, memory, and EF can complicate diabetes management, reduce glycemic control, and contribute even more to the daily stress of this chronic condition.

Glycemic extremes appear to be at the root of these decrements, with effects that appear to begin at or even before diabetes onset, and may increase over time in response to chronic hyperglycemia and its complications. A number of relationships emerge from the data that have been reviewed in this chapter:

1. A general effect of early-onset diabetes across most cognitive domains.
2. An effect of chronic hyperglycemia on white matter tracts throughout the brain, resulting in reduced speed of processing and attention.
3. An effect of severe hypoglycemia and DKA on the hippocampus and other medial-temporal structures, especially during the sensitive period between birth and 7 years, resulting in decrements in learning and memory.
4. An effect of severe hyperglycemia, hypoglycemia, and DKA on the brain at or even before symptomatic onset of T1D.
5. "Downstream" developmental effects of the above deficits on IQ, and possibly also on academic achievement.

An important caveat is that glycemic extremes tend to co-occur, such that children with chronic hyperglycemia also tend to have more episodes of SH (Ryan et al., 2016) and may be more vulnerable to its effects (McNeilly & McCrimmon, 2015), so there are likely synergistic effects that have proved difficult to measure. Also, events such as DKA and SH are more likely in younger children, and thus occur more often in children with EOD. Diabetes duration is also conflated with chronic hyperglycemia and number of episodes of SH and DKA. These interrelationships complicate research trying to tease apart risk factors for different cognitive deficits, though well-designed studies can help minimize their effects.

There are other limitations to the studies reviewed in this chapter. We have relied on meta-analyses to best understand overall effects of diabetes on cognition, but the analyses had somewhat differing definitions of cognitive domains and included different neuropsychological tests within domains. Definitions of SH and DKA also vary among studies. These differences limit the strength of conclusions that can be made at this time. Other limitations include use of SH or hypoglycemic seizures as a proxy for hypoglycemic exposure, which may obscure cumulative effects of moderate hypoglycemia (McNeilly & McCrimmon, 2015), and use of A1c as a proxy measure of hyperglycemic exposure, which as an average can obscure clinically relevant variations in blood glucose throughout the day (Siegelaar, Holleman, Hoekstra, & DeVries, 2010), including hypoglycemic lows (Ryan et al., 2016).

Some of these problems can be mitigated by use of CGMs, which are increasingly being used in research. This is a very important development, as a CGM can give accurate measurements of mean blood glucose, glycemic variability, and exposure to hypoglycemia over any time period, providing more fine-grained data for comparisons. It can also be used to measure acute effects of high or low blood sugars without resorting to insulin clamps, which for ethical reasons cannot be used with children, and to provide a better understanding of the effects of acute glycemic dysregulation on "in-the-moment" functioning.

More longitudinal research is needed to examine changes over time in cognitive function and the CNS. It will be especially important to follow children from diagnosis forward to better understand the impact of diabetes on neurodevelopment. If screening for prediabetes or presymptomatic T1D becomes more common, prospective studies could start even earlier in the disease course. Study designs will be enhanced by newly available technologies such as the CGM and neuroimaging techniques that can even be used with very young children (e.g., Aye et al., 2011).

As noted earlier, little is known about the effect of moderating and mediating variables on cognitive outcomes in T1D. Genetic polymorphisms have been identified that confer increased neurodevelopmental risk in other conditions (e.g., pediatric cancer; Krull et al., 2013); whether there are genetic contributors to cognitive dysfunction in T1D is unknown. Equally important will be research looking to identify possible neuroprotective genes (e.g., Malik, Motamedi, Royo, LeBold, & Watson, 2011) and neuroprotective therapies (Vajda, 2002).

Another promising area for future research is in investigating the impact of stress on cognitive outcomes in T1D. We know little about how stress and diabetes might interact in their effects on brain development, and whether environmental stressors and adverse childhood experiences (Anda et al., 2006) might predispose some children to greater vulnerability to the cognitive effects of T1D. We also know little about whether there are differences in cognitive vulnerability to diabetes based on race, ethnicity, or gender.

Large-scale research with more diverse samples of children and youth with T1D will be crucial in the coming years.

REFERENCES

American Diabetes Association. (2014). Diagnosis and classification of diabetes mellitus. *Diabetes Care, 32*(Suppl. 1), S81–S90.

American Diabetes Association. (2012). Diabetes and driving. *Diabetes Care, 35*(Suppl. 1), S81–S86.

American Diabetes Association. (2019). Standards of Medical Care in Diabetes—2019. *Diabetes Care, 42*(Suppl. 1), S1–S2.

Anda, R. F., Felitti, V. J., Bremner, J. D., Walker, J. D., Whitfield, C., Perry, B. D., . . . Giles, W. H. (2006). The enduring effects of abuse and related adverse experiences in childhood: A convergence of evidence from neurobiology and epidemiology. *European Archives of Psychiatry and Clinical Neuroscience, 256*(3), 174–186.

Anderson, B. J. (2004). Family conflict and diabetes management in youth: Clinical lessons from child development and diabetes research. *Diabetes Spectrum, 17*(1), 22–26.

Anderson, B. J., & Schwartz, D. D. (2014). Psychosocial and family issues in children with type 1 diabetes. In G. Umpierrez (Ed.), *Therapy for diabetes mellitus and related disorders* (6th ed., pp. 134–155). Alexandria, VA: American Diabetes Association.

Antenor-Dorsey, J. A., Meyer, E., Rutlin, J., Perantie, D. C., White, N. H., Arbalaez, A. M., . . . Hershey, T. (2013). White matter microstructural integrity in youth with type 1 diabetes. *Diabetes, 62*, 581–589.

Arbelaez, A. M., Semenkovich, K., & Hershey, T. (2013). Glycemic extremes in youth with T1DM: The structural and functional integrity of the developing brain. *Pediatric Diabetes, 14*, 541–553.

Atkinson, M. A., Eisenbarth, G. S., & Michels, A. W. (2014). Type 1 diabetes. *Lancet, 383*, 69–82.

Austin, E., & Deary, I. (1999). Effects of repeated hypoglycemia on cognitive function: A psychometrically validated reanalysis of the Diabetes Control and Complications Trial data. *Diabetes Care, 22*, 1273–1277.

Aye, T., Mazaika, P. K., Mauras, N., Marzelli, M. J., Shen, H., Hershey, T., . . . Diabetes Research in Children Network (DirecNet) Study Group. (2019). Impact of early diabetic ketoacidosis on the developing brain. *Diabetes Care, 42*, 443–449.

Aye, T., Reiss, A. L., Kesler, S., Hoang, S., Drobney, J., Park, Y. . . . Buckingham, B. A. (2011). The feasibility of detecting neuropsychologic and neuroanatomic effects of type 1 diabetes in young children. *Diabetes Care, 34*, 1458–1462.

Barnea-Goraly, N., Raman, M., Mazaika, P., Marzelli, M., Hershey, T., Weinzimer, S. A. . . . Diabetes Research in Children Network (DirecNet). (2014). Alterations in white matter structure in young children with type 1 diabetes. *Diabetes Care, 37*, 332–340.

Berg, C. A., Wiebe, D. J., Suchy, Y., Turner, S. L., Butner, J., Munion, A., . . . Murray, M. (2018). Executive function predicting longitudinal change in type 1 diabetes management during the transition to emerging adulthood. *Diabetes Care, 41*(11), 2281–2288.

Biessels, G. J., Deary, I. J., & Ryan, C. M. (2008). Cognition and diabetes: A lifespan perspective. *Lancet Neurology, 7*, 184–190.

Blasetti, A., Chiuri, R. M., Tocco, A. M., Di Giulio, C., Mattei, P. A., Ballone, E., . . . Verroti, A. (2011). The effect of recurrent severe hypoglycemia on cognitive performance in children with type 1 diabetes: A meta-analysis. *Journal of Child Neurology, 26*, 1383–1391.

Bos, K. J., Fox, N., Zeanah, C. H., & Nelson, C. A., III. (2009). Effects of early psychosocial deprivation on the development of memory and executive function. *Frontiers in Behavioral Neuroscience, 3*, Article 16.

Brand, A. H., Johnson, J. H., & Johnson, S. B. (1986). Life stress and diabetic control in children and adolescents with insulin-dependent diabetes. *Journal of Pediatric Psychology, 11*(4), 481–495.

Brands, A. M., Biessels, G. J., De Haan, E. H., Kappelle, L. J., & Kessels, R. P. (2005). The effects of type 1 diabetes on cognitive performance: A meta-analysis. *Diabetes Care, 28*(3), 726–735.

Broadley, M. M., White, M. J., & Andrew, B. (2017). A systematic review and meta-analysis of executive function performance in type 1 diabetes mellitus. *Psychosomatic Medicine, 79*(6), 684–696.

Brownlee, M. (2005). The pathobiology of diabetic complications: A unifying mechanism. *Diabetes, 54*, 1615–1625.

Cameron, F. J., Northam, E. A., Ambler, G. R., & Daneman, D. (2007). Routine psychological screening in youth with type 1 diabetes and their parents: A notion whose time has come? *Diabetes Care, 30,* 2716–2724.

Cameron, F. J., Scratch, S. E., Nadebaum, C., Northam, E. A., Koves, I., Jennings, J., . . . DKA Brain Injury Study Group. (2014). Neurological consequences of diabetic ketoacidosis at initial presentation of type 1 diabetes in a prospective cohort study of children. *Diabetes Care, 37*(6), 1554–1562.

Caruso, N. C., Radovanovic, B., Kennedy, J. D., Couper, J., Kohler, M., Kavanagh, P. S., . . . Lushington, K. (2014). Sleep, executive functioning and behaviour in children and adolescents with type 1 diabetes. *Sleep Medicine, 15*(12), 1490–1499.

Cato, A., & Hershey, T. (2016). Cognition and type 1 diabetes in children and adolescents. *Diabetes Spectrum, 29,* 197–202.

Cato, M. A., Mauras, N., Ambrosino, J., Bondurant, A., Conrad, A. L., Kollman, C., . . . Reiss, A. L. (2014). Cognitive functioning in young children with type 1 diabetes. *Journal of the International Neuropsychological Society, 20*(2), 238–247.

Cato, M. A., Mauras, N., Mazaika, P., Kollman, C., Cheng, P., Aye, T., . . . Tansey, M. (2016). Longitudinal evaluation of cognitive functioning in young children with type 1 diabetes over 18 months. *Journal of the International Neuropsychological Society, 22*(3), 293–302.

Cohen, D. M., Lumley, M. A., Naar-King, S., Partridge, T., & Cakan, N. (2004). Child behavior problems and family functioning as predictors of adherence and glycemic control in economically disadvantaged children with type 1 diabetes: A prospective study. *Journal of Pediatric Psychology, 29,* 171–284.

Colver, A., & Longwell, S. (2013). New understanding of adolescent brain development: Relevance to transitional healthcare for young people with long term conditions. *Archives of Disease in Childhood, 98,* 902–907.

Cook, S., Herold, K., Edidin, D. V., & Briars, R. (2002). Increasing problem solving in adolescents with type 1 diabetes: The choices diabetes program. *Diabetes Educator, 28,* 115–124.

Cryer, P. E. (2007). Hypoglycemia, functional brain failure, and brain death. *Journal of Clinical Investigation, 117,* 868–870.

Dabelea, D., Rewers, A., Stafford, J. M., Standiford, D. A., Lawrence, J. M., Saydah, S, . . . SEARCH for Diabetes in Youth Study Group. (2014). Trends in the prevalence of ketoacidosis at diabetes diagnosis: The SEARCH for Diabetes in Youth Study. *Pediatrics, 133,* e938–e945.

Daley, K. B., Wodrich, D. L., & Hasan, K. (2006). Classroom attention in children with type 1 diabetes mellitus: The effect of stabilizing serum glucose. *Journal of Pediatrics, 148,* 201–206.

Datye, K. A., Moore, D. J., Russell, W. E., & Jaser, S. S. (2015). A review of adolescent adherence in type 1 diabetes and the untapped potential of diabetes providers to improve outcomes. *Current Diabetes Reports, 15,* 51–59.

Davies, J. L., Kawaguchi, Y., Bennett, S. T., Copeman, J. B., Cordell, H. J., Pritchard, L. E., . . . Palmer, S. M. (1994). A genome-wide search for human type 1 diabetes susceptibility genes. *Nature, 371*(6493), 130–136.

Desrocher, M., & Rovet, J. (2004) Neurocognitive correlates of type 1 diabetes mellitus in childhood. *Child Neuropsychology, 10,* 36–52.

Diabetes Control and Complications Trial/Epidemiology of Diabetes Interventions and Complications (DCCT/EDIC) Study Research Group. (2007). Long-term effect of diabetes and its treatment on cognitive function. *New England Journal of Medicine, 356,* 1842–1852.

Draelos, M. T., Jacobson, A. M., Weinger, K., Widom, B., Ryan, C. M., Finkelstein, D. M., & Simonson, D. C. (1995). Cognitive function in patients with insulin-dependent diabetes mellitus during hyperglycemia and hypoglycemia. *American Journal of Medicine, 98,* 135–144.

Ducat, L., Philipson, L. H., & Anderson, B. J. (2014). The mental health comorbidities of diabetes. *Journal of the American Medical Society, 312,* 691–692.

Duke, D. C., & Harris, M. A. (2014). Executive function, adherence, and glycemic control in adolescents with type 1 diabetes: A literature review. *Current Diabetes Reports, 14*(10), 532.

Ferguson, S. C., Blane, A., Wardlaw, J., Frier, B. M., Perros, P., McCrimmon, R. J., & Deary, I. J. (2005). Influence of an early-onset age of type 1 diabetes on cerebral structure and cognitive function. *Diabetes Care, 28,* 1431–1437.

Ferguson, S. C., Deary, I. J., Evans, J. C., Ellard, S., Hattersley, A. T., & Frier, B. M. (2003). Apolipoprotein-E influences aspects of intellectual ability in type 1 diabetes. *Diabetes, 52,* 145–148.

Fox, L. A., Hershey, T., Mauras, N., Arbelaez, A. M., Tamborlane, W. V., Buckingham, B., . . . Diabetes Research in Children Network. (2018).

Persistence of abnormalities in white matter in children with type 1 diabetes. *Diabetologia, 61*(7), 1538–1547.

Gaudieri, P. A., Chen, R., Greer, T. F., & Holmes, C. S. (2008). Cognitive function in children with type 1 diabetes: A meta-analysis. *Diabetes Care, 31*(9), 1892–1897.

Gerrard, M., Gibbons, F. X., Houlihan, A. E., Stock, M. L., & Pomery, E. A. (2008). A dual-process approach to health risk decision-making: The prototype-willingness model. *Developmental Review, 28*, 29–61.

Ghetti, S., Lee, J. K., Sims, C., DeMaster, D. M., & Glaser, N. S. (2010). Diabetic ketoacidosis and memory dysfunction in children with type 1 diabetes. *Journal of Pediatrics, 156*, 109–114.

Gioia, G., Isquith, P., Guy, S., & Kenworthy, L. (2000). *Behavior rating inventory of executive functions.* Lutz, FL: Psychological Assessment Resources.

Glaser, N. S., Wooton-Gorges, S., Buonocore, M., Marcin, J. P., Rewers, A., Strain, J., . . . Kupperman, N. (2006). Frequency of sub-clinical cerebral edema in children with diabetic ketoacidosis. *Pediatric Diabetes, 7*, 75–80.

Goebel-Fabbri, A. E. (2013). Eating disorders. In A. Peters & L. Laffel (Eds.), *Type 1 diabetes sourcebook* (pp. 180–186). Alexandria, VA: American Diabetes Association.

Goethals, E. R., de Wit, M., Van Broeck, N., Lemiere, J., Van Liefferinge, D., Böhler, S., . . . Van Impe, S. (2018). Child and parental executive functioning in type 1 diabetes: Their unique and interactive role toward treatment adherence and glycemic control. *Pediatric Diabetes, 19*(3), 520–526.

Gonder-Frederick, L. A., Zrebiec, J. F., Bauchowitz, A. U., Ritterband, L. M., Magee, J. C., Cox, D. J., & Clarke, W. L. (2009). Cognitive function is disrupted by both hypo- and hyperglycemia in school aged children with type 1 diabetes: A field study. *Diabetes Care, 32*, 1001–1006.

Gottfredson, L. S., & Deary, I. J. (2004). Intelligence predicts health and longevity, but why? *Current Directions in Psychological Science, 13*, 1–4.

Hamman, R. F., Bell, R. A., Dabelea, D., D'Agostino, R. B., Dolan, L., Imperatore, G., . . . SEARCH for Diabetes in Youth Study Group. (2014). The SEARCH for Diabetes in Youth study: Rationale, findings, and future directions. *Diabetes Care, 37*, 3336–3344.

Hannonen, R., Komulainen, J., Eklund, K., Tolvanen, A., Riikonen, R., & Ahonen, T. (2010). Verbal and academic skills in children with early-onset type 1 diabetes. *Developmental Medicine and Child Neurology, 52*, e143–e147.

Harjutsalo, V., Sjöberg, L., & Tuomilehto, J. (2008). Time trends in the incidence of type 1 diabetes in Finnish children: A cohort study. *Lancet, 371*(9626), 1777–1782.

Helgeson, V. S., Siminerio, L., Escobar, O., & Becker, D. (2009). Predictors of metabolic control among adolescents with diabetes: A 4-year longitudinal study. *Journal of Pediatric Psychology, 34*(3), 254–270.

Hilgard, D., Konrad, K., Meusers, M., Bartus, B., Otto, K. P., Lepler, R., . . . German/Austrian DPV Study Group, the Working Group on Psychiatric, Psychotherapeutic Psychological Aspects of Paediatric Diabetology (PPAG eV) and the BMBF Competence Network Diabetes, Germany. (2017). Comorbidity of attention deficit hyperactivity disorder and type 1 diabetes in children and adolescents: Analysis based on the multicentre DPV registry. *Pediatric Diabetes, 18*(8), 706–713.

Hill-Briggs, F. (2003). Problem solving in diabetes self-management: A model of chronic illness self-management behavior. *Annals of Behavioral Medicine, 25*, 182–193.

Hilliard, M. E., Perlus, J. G., Clark, L. M., Haynie, D. L., Plotnick, L. P., Guttman-Bauman, I., & Iannotti, R. J. (2014). Perspectives from before and after the pediatric to adult care transition: A mixed-methods study in type 1 diabetes. *Diabetes Care, 37*, 346–354.

Ho, M., Weller, N. J., Ives, F., Carne, C. L., Murray, K., Vanden Driessen, R., . . . Jones, T. W. (2008). Prevalence of structural central nervous system abnormalities in early-onset type 1 diabetes mellitus. *Journal of Pediatrics, 153*, 385–390.

Holmes, C. S., Chen, R., Streisand, R., Marschall, D. E., Souter, S., Swift, E. E., & Peterson, C. C. (2006). Predictors of youth diabetes care behaviors and metabolic control: A structural equation modeling approach. *Journal of Pediatric Psychology, 31*, 770–784.

Hood, K. K., Peterson, C. M., Rohan, J. M., & Drotar, D. (2009). Association between adherence and glycemic control in pediatric type 1 diabetes: A meta-analysis. *Pediatrics, 124*(6), e1171–e1179.

Hosseini, S. M., Mazaika, P., Mauras, N., Buckingham, B., Weinzimer, S. A., Tsalikian, E., . . . Diabetes Research in Children Network (DirecNet). (2016). Altered integration of structural covariance networks in young children with type 1 diabetes. *Human Brain Mapping, 37,* 4034–4046.

Hovnik, T., Dolžan, V., Bratina, N. U., Podkrajšek, K. T., & Battelino, T. (2009). Genetic polymorphisms in genes encoding antioxidant enzymes are associated with diabetic retinopathy in type 1 diabetes. *Diabetes Care, 32*(12), 2258–2262.

Hviid, A., Stellfeld, M., Wohlfahrt, J., & Melbye, M. (2004). Childhood vaccination and type 1 diabetes. *New England Journal of Medicine, 350*(14), 1398–1404.

Insel, R. A., Dunne, J. L., Atkinson, M. A., Chiang, J. L., Dabalea, D., Gottlieb, P. A. . . . Ziegler, A.-G. (2015). Staging presymptomatic type 1 diabetes: A scientific statement of JDRF, the Endocrine Society, and the American Diabetes Association. *Diabetes Care, 38,* 1964–1974.

Iovane, B., Cangelosi, A. M., Bonaccini, I., Di Mauro, D., Scarabello, C., Panigari, A., . . . Vanelli, M. (2018). Diabetic ketoacidosis at the onset of type 1 diabetes in young children: Is it time to launch a tailored campaign for DKA prevention in children < 5 years? *Acta Biomedica, 89,* 67–71.

Jacobson, A. M., Ryan, C. M., Cleary, P. A., Waberski, B. H., Weinger, K., Musen, G., . . . DCCT/EDIC Research Group. (2011). Biomedical risk factors for decreased cognitive functioning in type 1 diabetes: An 18 year follow-up of the Diabetes Control and Complications Trial (DCCT) cohort. *Diabetologia, 54,* 245–255.

Kaufmann, L., Pixner, S., Starke, M., Zotter, S., Kohle, J., Dagmar, M., . . . Hofer, S. (2011). Neurocognition and brain structure in pediatric patients with type 1 diabetes. *Journal of Pediatric Neuroradiology, 1*(1), 25–35.

Kawai, N., Keep, R. F., Betz, A. L., & Nagao, S. (1998). Hyperglycemia induces progressive changes in the cerebral microvasculature and blood–brain barrier transport during focal cerebral ischemia. In A. Marmarou et al. (Eds.), Intracranial Pressure and Neuromonitoring in Brain Injury (Vol. 71, pp. 25–29). *Acta Neurochirurgica Supplements.* Vienna: Springer.

Krull, K. R., Bhojwani, D., Conklin, H. M., Pei, D., Cheng, C., Reddick, W. E., . . . Pui, C. (2013). Genetic mediators of neurocognitive outcomes in survivors of childhood acute lymphoblastic leukemia. *Journal of Clinical Oncology, 31,* 2182–2188.

Kuzawa, C. W., Chugani, H. T., Grossman, L. I., Lipovich, L., Muzik, O., Hof, P. R. . . . Lange, N. (2014). Metabolic costs an evolutionary implications of human brain development. *Proceedings of the National Academy of Sciences USA, 111,* 13010–13015.

Languren, G., Montiel, T., Julio-Amilpas, A., & Massieu, L. (2013). Neuronal damage and cognitive impairment associated with hypoglycemia: An integrated view. *Neurochemistry International, 63*(4), 331–343.

Lin, A., Northam, E. A., Rankins, D., Werther, G. A., & Cameron, F. J. (2010). Neuropsychological profiles of young people with type 1 diabetes 12 yr after disease onset. *Pediatric Diabetes, 11*(4), 235–243.

Lin, A., Northam, E. A., Werther, G. A., & Cameron, F. J. (2015). Risk factors for decline in IQ in youth with type 1 diabetes over the 12 years from diagnosis/illness onset. *Diabetes Care, 38,* 236–242.

Lin, S. Y., Lin, C. L., Hsu, W. H., Lin, C. C., & Fu, Y. C. (2019). Association of attention deficit hyperactivity disorder with recurrent hypoglycemia in type 1 diabetes mellitus. *Pediatric Diabetes, 20*(2), 189–196.

Ly, T. T., Anderson, M., McNamara, K. A., Davis, E. A., & Jones, T. W. (2011). Neurocognitive outcomes in young adults with early-onset type 1 diabetes: a prospective follow-up study. *Diabetes Care, 34*(10), 2192–2197.

Malik, S. Z., Motamedi, S., Royo, N. C., LeBold, D., & Watson, D. J. (2011). Identification of potentially neuroprotective genes upregulated by neurotrophin treatment of CA3 neurons in the injured brain. *Journal of Neurotrauma, 28,* 415–430.

Malone, J. I. (2016). Diabetic central neuropathy: CNS damage related to hyperglycemia. *Diabetes, 65*(2), 355–357.

Malone, J. I., Hanna, S. K., & Saporta, S. (2006). Hyperglycemic brain injury in the rat. *Brain Research, 1076,* 9–15.

Mauras, N., Beck, R., Xing, D., Ruedy, K., Buckingham, B., Tansey, M., . . . Diabetes Research in Children Network (DirecNet) Study Group. (2012). A randomized clinical trial to assess the efficacy and safety of realtime continuous glucose monitoring in the management of type 1 diabetes in young children aged 4 to < 10 years. *Diabetes Care, 35,* 204–210.

Mauras, N., Mazaika, P., Buckingham, B., Weinzimer, S., White, N. H., Tsalikian, E., . . . Diabetes Research in Children Network (DirecNet). (2015). Longitudinal assessment of neuroanatomical and cognitive differences in young children with type 1 diabetes: Association with hyperglycemia. *Diabetes, 64,* 1770–1779.

Mayer-Davis, E. J., Kahkoska, A. R., Jefferies, C., Dabelea, D., Balde, N., Gon, C. X., . . . Craig, M. E. (2018). ISPAD clinical practice consensus guidelines 2018: Definition, epidemiology and classification of diabetes in children and adolescents. *Pediatric Diabetes, 19*(Suppl. 27), 7–19.

Mazaika, P. K., Weinzimer, S. A., Mauras, N., Buckingham, B., White, N. H., Tsalikian, E., . . . Diabetes Research in Children Network (DirecNet). (2016). Variations in brain volume and growth in young children with type 1 diabetes. *Diabetes, 65*(2), 476–485.

McAulay, V., Deary, I. J., Ferguson, S. C., & Frier, B. M. (2001). Acute hypoglycemia in humans causes attentional dysfunction while nonverbal intelligence is preserved. *Diabetes Care, 24,* 1745–1750.

McClure, S. M., Laibson, D. I., Lowenstein, G., & Cohen, J. D. (2004). Separate neural systems value immediate and delayed monetary rewards. *Science, 306,* 503–507.

McCrimmon, R. J., Ryan, C. M., & Frier, B. M. (2012). Diabetes and cognitive dysfunction. *Lancet, 379,* 2291–2299.

McNeilly, A. D., & McCrimmon, R. J. (2015). The Scylla and Charybdis of glucose control in childhood type 1 diabetes? *Pediatric Diabetes, 16,* 235–241.

Miles, W. R., & Root, H. F. (1922). Psychologic tests applied to diabetic patients. *Archives of Internal Medicine, 30,* 767–777.

Moheet, A., Mangia, S., & Seaquist, E. R. (2015). Impact of diabetes on cognitive function and brain structure. *Annals of the New York Academy of Sciences, 1353,* 60–71.

Monnier, L., Mas, E., Ginet, C., Michel, F., Villon, L., Cristol, J. P., & Colette, C. (2006). Activation of oxidative stress by acute glucose fluctuations compared with sustained chronic hyperglycemia in patients with type 2 diabetes. *Journal of the American Medical Association, 295,* 1681–1687.

Musen, G., Lyoo, I. K., Sparks, C. R., Weinger, K., Hwang, J., Ryan, C. M., . . . Jacobson, A. M. (2006). Effects of type 1 diabetes on gray matter density as measured by voxel-based morphometry. *Diabetes, 55,* 326–333.

Naguib, J. M., Kulinskaya, E., Lomax, C. L., & Garralda, M. E. (2009). Neuro-cognitive performance in children with type 1 diabetes—a meta-analysis. *Journal of Pediatric Psychology, 34*(3), 271–282.

Naranjo, D., Schwartz, D. D., & Delamater, A. M. (2015). Diabetes in ethnic minority youth: Disparate burden and intervention approaches. *Current Diabetes Reviews, 11*(4), 251–260.

Northam, E., Anderson, P., Werther, G., Adler, R., & Andrewes, D. (1995). Neuropsychological complications of insulin dependent diabetes in children. *Child Neuropsychology, 1,* 884–890.

Northam, E. A., Anderson, P. J., Werther, G. A., Warne, G. L., Adler, R. G., & Andrewes, D. (1998). Neuropsychological complications of IDDM in children 2 years after disease onset. *Diabetes Care, 21,* 379–384.

Northam, E. A., Rankins, D., Lin, A., Wellard, R. M., Pell, G. S., Finch, S. J., . . . Cameron, F. J. (2009). Central nervous system function in youth with type 1 diabetes 12 years after disease onset. *Diabetes Care, 32,* 445–450.

Northam, E. A., Anderson, P. J., Jacobs, R., Hughes, M., Warne, G. L., & Werther, G. A. (2001). Neuropsychological profiles of children with type 1 diabetes 6 years after disease onset. *Diabetes Care, 24*(9), 1541–1546.

Nunley, K. A., Rosano, C., Ryan, C. M., Jennings, J. R., Aizenstein, H. J., Zgibor, J. C., . . . Saxton, J. A. (2015). Clinically relevant cognitive impairment in middle-aged adults with childhood-onset type 1 diabetes. *Diabetes Care, 38,* 1768–1776.

Nylander, C., Lindström, K., Khalifa, N., & Fernell, E. (2018). Previously undiagnosed attention-deficit/hyperactivity disorder associated with poor metabolic control in adolescents with type 1 diabetes. *Pediatric Diabetes, 19*(4), 816–822.

Ostman, J., Lönnberg, G., Arnqvist, H. J., Blohmé, G., Bolinder, J., Ekbom, S. A. . . . Nyström, L. (2008). Gender differences and temporal variation in the incidence of type 1 diabetes: Results of 8012 cases in the nationwide Diabetes Incidence Study in Sweden 1983–2002. *Journal of Internal Medicine, 263*(4), 386–394.

Pacaud, D., Crawford, S., Stephure, D. K., Dean, H. J., Couch, R., & Dewey, D. (2007). Effect of type 1 diabetes on psychosocial maturation in young adults. *Journal of Adolescent Health, 40,* 29–35.

Palladino, D. K., & Helgeson, V. S. (2012). Friends or foes?: A review of peer influence on self-care and glycemic control in adolescents with type 1 diabetes. *Journal of Pediatric Psychology, 37,* 591–603.

Passow, S., Specht, K., Adamsen, T. C., Biermann, M., Brekke, N., Craven, A. R., . . . Hugdahl, K. (2015). Default-mode network functional connectivity is closely related to metabolic activity. *Human Brain Mapping, 36,* 2027–2038.

Pechtel, P., & Pizzagalli, D. A. (2011). Effects of early life stress on cognitive and affective function: An integrated review of human literature. *Psychopharmacology (Berlin), 214*(1), 55–70.

Perantie, D. C., Koller, J. M., Weaver, P. M., Lugar, H. M., Black, K. J., White, N. H., & Hershey, T. (2011). Prospectively determined impact of type 1 diabetes on brain volume during development. *Diabetes, 60*, 3006–3014.

Perantie, D. C., Lim, A., Wu, J., Weaver, P., Warren, S. L., Sadler, M., . . . Hershey, T. (2008). Effects of prior hypoglycemia and hyperglycemia on cognition in children with type 1 diabetes mellitus. *Pediatric Diabetes, 9*, 87–95.

Perantie, D. C., Wu, J., Koller, J. M., Lim, A., Warren, S. L., Black, K . J., . . . Hershey, T. (2007). Regional brain volume differences associated with hyperglycemia and severe hypoglycemia in youth with type 1 diabetes. *Diabetes Care, 30*, 2331–2337.

Perez, K. M., Patel, N. J., Lord, J. H., Savin, K. L., Monzon, A. D., Whittemore, R., & Jaser, S. S. (2017). Executive function in adolescents with type 1 diabetes: Relationship to adherence, glycemic control, and psychosocial outcomes. *Journal of Pediatric Psychology, 42*(6), 636–646.

Polonsky, W. H. (1996). Understanding and treating patients with diabetes burnout. In B. J. Anderson & R. R. Rubin (Eds.), *Practical psychology for diabetes clinicians* (pp. 183–191). Alexandria, VA: American Diabetes Association.

Rechenberg K., Whittemore, R., & Grey, M. (2017). Anxiety in youth with type 1 diabetes. *Journal of Pediatric Nursing, 32*, 64–71.

Redondo, M. J., Jeffrey, J., Fain, P. R., Eisenbarth, G. S., & Orban, T. (2008). Concordance for islet autoimmunity among monozygotic twins. *New England Journal of Medicine, 359*, 2849–2850.

Reynolds, K. A., & Helgeson, V. S. (2011). Children with diabetes compared to peers: Depressed? Distressed? A meta-analytic review. *Annals of Behavioral Medicine, 42*, 29–41.

Roche, E. F., Menon, A., Gill, D., & Hoey, H. (2005). Clinical presentation of type 1 diabetes. *Pediatric Diabetes, 6*, 75–78.

Ryan, C. (2006). Why is cognitive dysfunction associated with the development of diabetes early in life?: The diathesis hypothesis. *Pediatric Diabetes, 7*, 289–297.

Ryan, C. (2008). Searching for the origin of brain dysfunction in diabetic children: Going back to the beginning. *Pediatric Diabetes, 9*, 527–530.

Ryan, C. M., van Duinkerken, E., & Rosano, C. (2016). Neurocognitive consequences of diabetes. *American Psychologist, 71*, 563–576.

Saggar, M., Tsalikian, E., Mauras, N., Mazaika, P., White, N. H., Weinzimer, S., . . . Diabetes Research in Children Network (DirecNet). (2017). Compensatory hyper-connectivity in developing brains of young children with type 1 diabetes. *Diabetes, 66*(3), 754–762.

Sattar, L., Renneboog, B., & Decaux, G. (2017). Hyperglycemia induces attention and gait deficits in diabetic mellitus patients. *Acta Diabetologica, 54*, 953–959.

Schoenle, E . J., Schoenle, D., Molinari, L., & Largo, R. H. (2002). Impaired intellectual development in children with type1 diabetes: Association with HBA(1c), age at diagnosis and sex. *Diabetologia, 45*, 108–114.

Schwartz, D. D., & Axelrad, M. E. (2015). *Healthcare partnerships for pediatric adherence: Promoting collaborative management for pediatric chronic illness care*. Cham, Switzerland: Springer International.

Schwartz, D. D., Axelrad, M. E., & Anderson, B. J. (2014a). Neurocognitive functioning in children and adolescents at the time of type 1 diabetes diagnosis: Associations with glycemic control one year after diagnosis. *Diabetes Care, 37*(9), 2475–2482.

Schwartz, D. D., Wasserman, R., Powell, P. W., & Axelrad, M. E. (2014b). Neurocognitive outcomes in pediatric diabetes: A developmental perspective. *Current Diabetes Reports, 10*, Article 533.

Seaquist, E. R. (2015). The impact of diabetes on cerebral structure and function. *Psychosomatic Medicine, 77*, 616–621.

Semenkovich, K., Bischoff, A., Doty, T., Nelson, S., Siller, A. F., Hershey, T., & Arbeláez, A. M. (2016). Clinical presentation and memory function in youth with type 1 diabetes. *Pediatric Diabetes, 17*(7), 492–499.

Sharma, R., Buras, E., Terashima, T., Serrano, F., Massaad, C. A., Hu, L., . . . Pautler, R. G. (2010). Hyperglycemia induces oxidative stress and impairs axonal transport rates in mice. *PLoS ONE*, 5(10), Article e13463.

Siegelaar, S. E., Holleman, F., Hoekstra, J. B., & DeVries, J. H. (2010). Glucose variability: Does it matter? *Endocrine Reviews, 31*(2), 171–182.

Sima, A. A., & Li, Z. G. (2005). The effect of C-peptide on cognitive dysfunction and hippocampal apoptosis in type 1 diabetic rats. *Diabetes, 54*, 1497–1505.

Sisk, C., & Zehr, J. (2005). Pubertal hormones organize the adolescent brain and behavior. *Frontiers of Neuroendocrinology, 26*, 163–174.

Soutor, S. A., Chen, R., Streisand, R., Kaplowitz, P., & Holmes, C. S. (2004). Memory matters: Developmental differences in predictors of diabetes care behaviors. *Journal of Pediatric Psychology, 29*, 493–505.

Steinberg, L. (2010). A dual systems model of adolescent risk-taking. *Developmental Psychobiology, 52*(3), 216–224.

Suchy, Y., Queen, T. L., Huntbach, B., Wiebe, D. J., Turner, S. L., Butner, J., . . . Berg, C. A. (2017). Iowa gambling task performance prospectively predicts changes in glycemic control among adolescents with type 1 diabetes. *Journal of the International Neuropsychological Society, 23*(3), 204–213.

Suchy, Y., Turner, S. L., Queen, T. L., Durracio, K., Wiebe, D. J., Butner, J., . . . Berg, C. A. (2016, May 12). The relation of questionnaire and performance-based measures of executive functioning with type 1 diabetes outcomes among late adolescents. *Health Psychology*.

Tansey, M., Beck, R., Ruedy, K., Tamborlane, W., Cheng, P., Kollman, C., . . . Diabetes Research in Children Network (DirecNet). (2016). Persistently high glucose levels in young children with type 1 diabetes. *Pediatric Diabetes, 17*, 93–100.

Tonoli, C., Heyman, E., Roelands, B., Pattyn, N., Buyse, L., Piacentini, M. F., . . . Meeusen, R. (2014). Type 1 diabetes-associated cognitive decline: A meta-analysis and update of the current literature. *Journal of Diabetes, 6*, 499–513.

Toplak, M. E., West, R. F., & Stanovich, K. E. (2013). Practitioner review: Do performance-based measures and ratings of executive function assess the same construct? *Journal of Child Psychology and Psychiatry, 54*, 131–143.

Vajda, F. J. (2002). Neuroprotection and neurodegenerative disease. *Journal of Clinical Neuroscience, 9*, 4–8.

van Duinkerken, E., Schoonheim, M. M., Sanz-Arigita, E. J., IJzerman, R. G., Moll, A. C., Snoek, F. J., . . . Barkhof, F. (2012). Resting-state brain networks in type 1 diabetic patients with and without microangiopathy and their relation to cognitive functions and disease variables. *Diabetes, 61*(7), 1814–1821.

Vloemans, A. F., Eilander, M. M., Rotteveel, J., Bakker-van Waarde, W. M., Houdijk, E. C., Nuboer, R., . . . De Wit, M. (2019). Youth with type 1 diabetes taking responsibility for self-management: The importance of executive functioning in achieving glycemic control: Results from the longitudinal DINO study. *Diabetes Care, 42*(2), 225–231.

Wang, X., & Michaelis, E. K. (2010). Selective neuronal vulnerability to oxidative stress in the brain. *Frontiers in Aging Neuroscience, 2*, Article 12.

Warren, R. E., & Frier, B. M. (2005). Hypoglycaemia and cognitive function. *Diabetes, Obesity and Metabolism, 7*(5), 493–503.

Wasserman, R., Anderson, B. J., & Schwartz, D. D. (2017). Illness-specific risk-taking in adolescence: A missing piece of the nonadherence puzzle for youth with type 1 diabetes? *Diabetes Spectrum, 30*(1), 3–10.

Wasserman, R. M., Anderson, B. J., & Schwartz, D. D. (2016). Screening of neurocognitive and executive functioning in children, adolescents, and young adults with type 1 diabetes. *Diabetes Spectrum, 29*(4), 202–210.

Wasserman, R. M., Hilliard, M. E., Schwartz, D. D., & Anderson, B. J. (2015). Practical strategies to enhance executive functioning and strengthen diabetes management across the lifespan. *Current Diabetes Reports, 15*(8), Article 52.

Wasserman, R. M., Patton, S. R., Clements, M. A., Finch, J. H., Boschert, K. N., Schwartz, D. D., & Anderson, B. J. (2018). Diabetes-specific risk-taking: Psychometric properties of a measure for adolescents with type 1 diabetes. *Diabetes, 67*(Suppl. 1).

Weinger, K., & Beverly, E. A. (2010). Barriers to achieving glycemic targets: Who omits insulin and why? *Diabetes Care, 33*, 450–452.

Wentholt, I., Kulik, W., Michels, R., Hoekstra, J., & DeVries, J. (2008). Glucose fluctuations and activation of oxidative stress in patients with type 1 diabetes. *Diabetologia, 51*, 183–190.

Wessels, A. M., Rombouts, S. A., Remijnse, P. L., Boom, Y., Scheltens, P., Barkhof, F., . . . Snoek, F. J. (2007). Cognitive performance in type 1 diabetes patients is associated with cerebral white matter volume. *Diabetologia, 50*, 1763–1769.

Wessels, A. M., Scheltens, P., Barkhof, F., & Heine, R. J. (2008). Hyperglycaemia as a determinant of cognitive decline in patients with type 1 diabetes. *European Journal of Pharmacology, 585*, 88–96.

Wessels, A. M., Simsek, S., Remijnse, P. L., Veltman, D. J., Biessels, G. J., Barkhof, F., . . . Rombouts, S. A. (2006). Voxel-based morphometry demonstrates reduced gray matter density on brain MRI in patients with diabetic retinopathy. *Diabetologia, 49*, 2474–2480.

Wiebe, D. J., Helgeson, V., & Berg, C. A. (2016). The social context of managing diabetes across the life span. *American Psychologist, 71,* 526–538.

Wolfsdorf, J., Craig, M. E., Daneman, D., Dunger, D., Edge, J., Lee, W. R., . . . International Society for Pediatric and Adolescent Diabetes. (2007). Diabetic ketoacidosis. *Pediatric Diabetes, 8,* 28–43.

Wolfsdorf, J., Glaser, N., & Sperling, M. A. (2006). Diabetic ketoacidosis in infants, children, and adolescents: A consensus statement from the American Diabetes Association. *Diabetes Care, 29,* 1150–1159.

Wood, J. R., Miller, K. M., Maahs, D. M., Beck, R. W., DiMeglio, L. A., Libman, I. M., . . . T1D Exchange Clinic Network. (2013). Most youth with type 1 diabetes in the T1D Exchange Clinic Registry do not meet American Diabetes Association or International Society for Pediatric and Adolescent Diabetes clinical guidelines. *Diabetes Care, 36*(7), 2035–2037.

Yazar, A., Akın, F., Akça, Ö. F., Eklioğlu, B. S., Türe, E., Coşkun, F., & Atabek, M. E. (2019). The effect of attention deficit/hyperactivity disorder and other psychiatric disorders on the treatment of pediatric diabetes mellitus. *Pediatric Diabetes, 20*(3), 345–352.

PART III
NEURODEVELOPMENTAL DISORDERS

CHAPTER 11

Attention-Deficit/Hyperactivity Disorder

Erik G. Willcutt

HISTORICAL OVERVIEW

Although the cluster of behaviors now known as attention-deficit/hyperactivity disorder (ADHD) was described in the medical literature at least a century ago (Still, 1902; see review by Barkley, 2015), it was not formally defined as a diagnosis until the second edition of the *Diagnostic and Statistical Manual of Mental Disorders* (DSM-II) included a syndrome named *hyperkinetic reaction of childhood or adolescence* (American Psychiatric Association, 1968). The name of the syndrome was then changed to *attention deficit disorder* (ADD) in the third edition of the DSM (DSM-III; American Psychiatric Association, 1980) before being renamed as ADHD in the revised edition of DSM-III (DSM-III-R; American Psychiatric Association, 1987) and subsequent versions of the DSM.

The diagnostic criteria for ADHD in DSM-IV incorporated separate dimensions of nine symptoms of inattention and disorganization, and nine symptoms of hyperactivity and impulsivity. Definitions of three diagnostic subtypes were based on differential elevations on these symptom dimensions. The combined type (ADHD-C) was defined by six or more symptoms of inattention and six or more symptoms of hyperactivity–impulsivity. The predominantly inattentive type (ADHD-I) was defined by six or more inattention symptoms and fewer than six hyperactive–impulsive symptoms, whereas the predominantly hyperactive–impulsive type (ADHD-H) was defined by six or more hyperactive–impulsive symptoms and fewer than six inattention symptoms.

After the publication of DSM-IV, concerns were raised about the longitudinal stability of the DSM-IV subtypes (e.g., Lahey, Pelham, Loney, Lee, & Willcutt, 2005; Lahey & Willcutt, 2010; Todd et al., 2008), the validity of ADHD-H in older children (e.g., Willcutt, Chhabildas, & Pennington, 2001), and the extent to which the criteria for ADHD-I effectively capture a hypothesized inattentive group without hyperactivity (e.g., Milich, Balentine, & Lynam, 2001). Therefore, to aid decision making during the development of the criteria for ADHD in DSM-5 and other future diagnostic systems, we completed a comprehensive literature review and meta-analysis of 546 studies of the DSM-IV model of ADHD (Willcutt et al., 2012). Results of the review provided strong support for the DSM-IV model that includes separate dimensions of inattention symptoms (e.g., careless mistakes, forgetfulness, difficulty organizing tasks) and hyperactive–impulsive symptoms (e.g., excessive activity, interrupting or intruding on conversations), and recommended that these two symptom dimensions be retained in DSM-5. The review also provided strong support for the overall validity of ADHD as a diagnosis, but several findings called into question the validity of ADHD subtypes, at least as defined by DSM-IV. Most importantly, results of the meta-analysis indicated that the DSM-IV subtype classifications were unstable, with children often shifting between subtypes across development in both systematic and unpredictable ways.

In part due to the longitudinal instability of the DSM-IV subtypes, DSM-5 reconceptualized the subtypes as diagnostic specifiers that indicate *current* levels of inattention versus hyperactivity–impulsivity symptoms during the 6 months prior to the assessment. The predominantly inattentive presentation describes individuals with maladaptive levels of inattention but not hyperactivity–impulsivity, the predominantly hyperactive–impulsive presentation is characterized by maladaptive levels of hyperactivity–impulsivity but not inattention, and the combined presentation describes individuals who exhibit significant current symptoms of both inattention and hyperactivity–impulsivity. Additional DSM-5 criteria specify that ADHD symptoms must have an onset during childhood and must lead to significant impairment that is present in multiple settings, must have been present for at least 6 months, and are not better explained by another mental disorder (psychosis, mood disorder, anxiety disorder, dissociative disorder, personality disorder, or substance intoxication or withdrawal).

EPIDEMIOLOGY

Several systematic reviews have estimated the prevalence of ADHD based on over 150 population-based studies from around the United States and most regions of the world (e.g., Polanczyk, de Lima, Horta, Biederman, & Rohde, 2007; Willcutt, 2012). Although estimates vary across studies, pooled results indicate that approximately 5% of children, adolescents, and adults meet full diagnostic criteria for ADHD. The remainder of this section summarizes studies that tested whether the prevalence of ADHD differs as a function of gender, race/ethnicity, country, or socioeconomic status.

Gender Differences

Results of our meta-analysis indicated that males are approximately twice as likely than females to meet criteria for ADHD in epidemiological samples (Willcutt, 2012). This gender difference is even more pronounced in clinic samples (male:female ratio of 4:1 or higher), indicating that males are also more likely than females to be referred for clinical services (Willcutt et al., 2012). We recently found that gender differences in cognitive predictors of ADHD such as response speed and executive functions account for a small proportion (14%) of the higher prevalence of ADHD in males (Arnett, Pennington, Willcutt, DeFries, & Olson, 2015), but the remainder of the gender difference in the prevalence of ADHD remains unexplained.

Comparisons between Countries

Although a handful of studies have reported prevalence differences between countries in specific comparisons (e.g., MacDonald et al., 2019), the overall results of the meta-analyses indicate no significant differences in the prevalence of ADHD when results are stratified by region of the United States, country, or region of the world (Polanczyk et al., 2007; Willcutt et al., 2012). These results provide important evidence that ADHD occurs across cultures and is not a unique cultural construct that is restricted to the United States or any other specific culture or region.

Socioeconomic Status

Only a handful of epidemiological studies have stratified their results by socioeconomic status (SES). Studies in Colombia (Pineda et al., 1999), Germany (Dopfner, Breuer, Wille, Erhart, & Ravens-Sieberer, 2008), Australia (Graetz, Sawyer, Hazell, Arney, & Baghurst, 2001), and the United States (Costello, Keeler, & Angold, 2001; Froehlich et al., 2007) indicate that individuals from low SES environments are 1.5 to 4.0 times more likely to meet criteria for ADHD than individuals from families with high SES. However, other studies do not find a significant relation between SES and prevalence of ADHD (e.g., Canino et al., 2004; Nolan, Gadow, & Sprafkin, 2001; Waschbusch, King, & Gregus, 2007; Zwirs et al., 2007), suggesting that additional research is needed to test more conclusively whether low SES is a risk factor for ADHD in at least some populations.

Race/Ethnicity

Some initial studies in the United States that defined ADHD based on parent and teacher ratings suggested that African American children exhibit more symptoms of ADHD than non-Hispanic White or Hispanic children (e.g., DuPaul, Power, Anastopoulos, & Reid, 1998; Nolan et al., 2001; Reid et al., 1998). Similarly, a later study that measured ADHD with a structured interview in a sample of 4-year-old children reported higher rates of ADHD in African American and Hispanic children than in White, non-Hispanic children, but these differences were no longer significant after differences in SES were controlled (Lavigne, LeBailly, Hopkins, Gouze, & Binns, 2009). In contrast, two other studies in the United States that used structured interviews to diagnose ADHD based on full DSM-IV criteria found no difference in the overall prevalence of DSM-IV ADHD in samples of African American and non-Hispanic White children (Angold et al., 2002; Froehlich et al., 2007). In fact, one of these studies (Froehlich et al., 2007) found that non-Hispanic White children were *more* likely to meet criteria for ADHD than Hispanic children. Few studies outside the United States have tested for differences in the prevalence of ADHD as a function of race or ethnicity.

Overall, existing studies clearly indicate that ADHD occurs across social classes, racial/ethnic groups, and countries. Differences in prevalence as a function of race or ethnicity may be most likely to emerge when ADHD is defined by rating scales only, rather than full diagnostic criteria, but the small number of available studies underscores the critical need for additional research in this area. Additional research is also needed to determine the etiology of the higher prevalence of ADHD in males than in females and to clarify the extent to which the prevalence of ADHD may vary as a function of SES or other demographic variables.

ETIOLOGY, NEUROPATHOLOGY, AND NEURAL SUBSTRATES

Etiology

Family Studies

Previous studies demonstrate clearly that ADHD is familial (e.g., Faraone, Biederman, & Friedman, 2000; Friedman, Chhabildas, Budhiraja, Willcutt, & Pennington, 2003). Approximately 30–35% of the full siblings of ADHD probands also meet criteria for ADHD, indicating that the relative risk for ADHD is six to eight times higher among first-degree relatives of individuals with ADHD than the base rate of ADHD in the population (Willcutt et al., 2010b). However, because biological relatives living in the same home share both their home environment and some of their genes, family studies cannot be used to test whether these familial influences are genetic or environmental. Instead, other methods, such as twin studies, are needed to disentangle the relative contributions of genetic and family environmental influences on ADHD.

Twin Studies

By comparing the similarity of pairs of identical versus fraternal twins, twin studies provide an estimate of the extent to which ADHD is due to genetic or environmental influences. Nearly all twin studies of ADHD report a higher concordance (i.e., both twins met criteria for ADHD) in identical twin pairs (60–80% of pairs) than fraternal twin pairs (25–35% of pairs), and subsequent analyses indicate that approximately 70% of the risk for ADHD is due to genetic influences (see systematic reviews by Faraone & Larsson, 2019; Willcutt et al., 2010b). The variance in ADHD symptoms that is not accounted for by genetic influences is primarily explained by nonshared environmental influences that specifically affect one twin in a pair and not the other, whereas shared environmental influences are not significant in most studies. Based on these results, subsequent studies have attempted to identify the specific environmental or genetic factors that increase the likelihood that a child will develop ADHD.

Molecular Genetic Studies

The high heritability observed in twin studies led to initial optimism that specific genes would be identified that explain a large proportion of the risk for ADHD, but results of molecular genetic studies have turned out to be much more complicated than anticipated. Initial studies used a "candidate gene" approach that investigates the role of a specific gene identified because it is part of a biological system that is associated with a disorder. For example, because psychostimulant medication increases dopamine availability by blocking reuptake at the synapse, many early molecular genetic studies of ADHD examined polymorphisms in genes that influence the dopamine pathway (for an early meta-analytic review, see Faraone et al., 2005). Although results of candidate gene studies were inconsistent and frequently contradictory, a meta-analytic review reported small but significant effects for polymorphisms in three genes in the dopamine system, two genes that play a role in serotonin transmission, and a gene coding for a synaptic vesicle regulating protein (Gizer, Ficks, & Waldman, 2009). However, small effect sizes indicated that each of these risk factors accounted for a very small proportion of the total genetic risk for ADHD.

Genomewide Analyses

Because most of the genetic variance in ADHD symptoms was not explained by the polymorphisms included in initial candidate gene studies, the next generation of molecular genetic studies took advantage of advances in DNA technology that make it possible to screen the entire human genome for chromosomal regions that may contain genes that increase risk for ADHD. This systematic approach tests for associations between ADHD and millions of DNA markers spaced relatively evenly across the genome. Because each marker is tested individually, the large number of statistical tests required for this approach is a key limitation, and very large samples are required to obtain adequate statistical power to detect effects after controlling for multiple testing. One recent study identified several locations in the genome that were significantly associated with ADHD but once again the effects of these individual risk factors are very small (Demontis et al., 2019).

Specific Environmental Risk Factors

In addition to the SES studies described earlier, studies of other environmental variables suggest that ADHD may also have small but significant associations with environmental risk factors that include prenatal or perinatal complications, specific prenatal exposure to nicotine or other substances, and potentially exposure to lead or other environmental toxins (reviewed by Froehlich et al., 2012). However, much like the results of molecular genetic studies, effects are small and often inconsistent across studies. Furthermore, interpretation of these results is complicated by important methodological issues such as psychometric weaknesses in measures of environmental risk and potential biases due to retrospective reports of environmental factors.

Conclusions from Etiologically Informative Studies

Despite the high heritability of ADHD, each individual genetic and environmental risk factor explains a very small proportion of the risk for ADHD. This pattern of results suggests that dozens or even hundreds of genes act in combination with a range of environmental risk factors to lead to the development of ADHD. Future studies that incorporate neuropsychological measures may provide a useful approach to begin to disentangle the complex etiological structure of ADHD.

Neural Substrates

Executive Functions

As described in more detail in the overview of neuropsychological studies of ADHD in the subsequent section, initial theoretical models of ADHD focused on the possibility that ADHD may be due to dysfunction in prefrontal cortices and related networks that result in deficits in executive functions (EF), cognitive processes that facilitate the maintenance of an optimal problem-solving set to attain a future goal (e.g., Barkley, 1997; Pennington & Ozonoff, 1996). In a simplified model of cognitive control and decision-making processes, EF represent "top-down" cognitive inputs that facilitate decision making by maintaining information about possible choices in working memory, suppressing irrelevant information, and inhibiting responses that are maladaptive or simply off-task, then integrating this knowledge with information about reinforcement probabilities to select the optimal action for the situation.

Although executive control processes involve several distributed brain networks, studies of primates and neuropsychological, neuroimaging, and lesion studies of humans suggest that the primary neural circuit includes the thalamus, basal ganglia, and dorsolateral and ventrolateral regions of the prefrontal cortex (for a review, see Pennington, McGrath, & Peterson, 2019). Initial functional neuroimaging studies of ADHD reported reduced activation in the frontostriatal networks that play an important role in overall executive functions and motor response inhibition (e.g., Rubia et al., 1999; Vaidya et al., 1998), and these results have been replicated consistently in later individual studies and systematic meta-analyses (e.g., Hart, Radua, Nakao, Mataix-Cols, & Rubia, 2013; McCarthy, Skokauskas, & Frodl, 2014; Rubia, 2018). These functional results are also consistent with earlier structural neuroimaging studies that showed reduced volumes in prefrontal cortex and related structures such as the basal ganglia were associated with both the diagnosis of ADHD and weaker performance on specific EF tasks (e.g., Casey et al., 1997; Castellanos et al., 1996; Filipek et al., 1997).

Results of meta-analyses also suggest that underactivation in the anterior cingulate cortex (ACC) is associated with ADHD and with specific weaknesses in other aspects of executive control, such as error monitoring and interference control (Hart, Radua, Nakao, Mataix-Cols, & Rubia, 2013). Interestingly, results of this review also suggest that ADHD may be associated with dysfunction in right-hemispheric frontostriatal networks, whereas ADHD is most often associated with dysfunction in left ACC.

Other Neural Substrates

Although data from multiple levels of analysis suggest that EF deficits are an important component of an overall neurocognitive model of ADHD, the results of the neuropsychological studies summarized in the next section also indicate that EF weaknesses are neither necessary nor sufficient to cause ADHD in isolation (e.g., Willcutt, Doyle, Nigg, Faraone, & Pennington, 2005b). Alternative theoretical models have suggested that symptoms of ADHD may result from dysfunctional responses to reward and/or punishment contingencies (e.g., Luman, Oosterlaan, & Sergeant, 2005), pronounced aversion to the experience of delay (e.g., Sonuga-Barke, Taylor, Sembi, & Smith, 1992), inconsistent cognitive responses due to attentional fluctuations (e.g., Sergeant, Geurts, Huijbregts, Scheres, & Oosterlaan, 2003; Sonuga-Barke & Castellanos, 2007), or overall slow and variable cognitive processing speed (e.g., McGrath et al., 2011; Shanahan et al., 2006).

Neuroimaging studies provide initial support for several of these theories. Results of several meta-analyses of functional magnetic resonance imaging (fMRI) studies indicate that ADHD is associated with underactivation in frontoparietal networks that are active during tasks that require selective and sustained attention, along with frontocerebellar networks that are involved in a range of timing tasks (e.g., Hart et al., 2012, 2013; for a comprehensive review, see Rubia, 2018). Furthermore, a number of recent studies suggest that ADHD may be associated with increased activation in the default mode network (DMN; Castellanos, Kelly, & Milham, 2009; Rubia, 2018). The DMN includes connections between a number of regions of the prefrontal cortex, cingulate cortex, and parietal cortex, and it is most active when an individual is at rest and not actively engaged in a cognitive task (e.g., Buckner, Andrews-Hanna, & Schacter, 2008). While the DMN typically becomes less active when other regions are activated to perform a cognitive task, meta-analyses suggest that individuals with ADHD exhibit enhanced activation of the DMN during cognitive tasks (Cortese et al., 2012). This pattern may potentially reflect poor regulation of connectivity between the regions involved in key networks, an inefficiency that may then manifest as behavioral distractibility or slow and inconsistent responses.

Neuropsychological Studies

The neuropsychological literature on ADHD is immense. As of the end of 2018, over 750 studies had examined some aspect of the neuropsychological correlates of ADHD. This rapid accumulation of new knowledge has provided a key resource to facilitate continued refinement of theoretical models of ADHD, but it has also underscored the complexity of the neuropsychological dysfunction that is associated with ADHD.

Over the past 15 years, our group and several others have completed a series of meta-analyses of different aspects of the neuropsychology of ADHD (e.g., Frazier, Demaree, & Youngstrom, 2004; Hervey, Epstein, & Curry, 2004; Huang-Pollock, Karalunas, Tam, & Moore, 2012; Lansbergen, Kenemans, & Van, 2007; Lijffijt, Kenemans, Verbaten, & Van Engeland, 2005; Martinussen, Hayden, Hogg-Johnson, & Tannock, 2005; Pauli-Pott & Becker, 2011; Schoechlin & Engel, 2005; Sonuga-Barke, Sergeant, Nigg, & Willcutt, 2008; van Mourik, Oosterlaan, & Sergeant, 2005; Willcutt & Bidwell, 2011; Willcutt et al., 2005a, 2005b, 2012; Willcutt, Sonuga-Barke, Nigg, & Sergeant, 2008; Woods, Lovejoy, & Ball, 2002). Meta-analysis is a statistical procedure that is used to combine effect sizes from multiple studies to compute a single, pooled estimate of the overall effect size in the population. For the purposes of this section of the chapter, all effect sizes have been converted to Cohen's *d*, a widely used measure that reflects the mean difference between groups with and without ADHD divided by the pooled standard deviation (Cohen, 1988). Therefore, an effect size of 0.50 would indicate that the means of the ADHD group and control group differ by half of one standard deviation.

To remain consistent with the structure of the other chapters in this volume, this section first summarizes the latest results regarding the association between ADHD and specific domains of neuropsychological functioning. The section then concludes with a discussion of important constraints that are provided by these results for current and future theoretical models of ADHD, and examines the strengths and weaknesses of a recent shift toward theoretical models that explicitly hypothesize that ADHD may be associated with weaknesses in two or more domains.

General Intellectual Functioning

Meta-analyses of studies of both children and adults indicate that groups with ADHD score lower than groups without ADHD on measures of general intellectual functioning (e.g., Frazier et al., 2004; Willcutt, 2015; Willcutt et al., 2012). The overall pooled effect size across studies suggests that this effect is medium in magnitude for measures of Full Scale IQ (d = approximately 0.50, or 6–8 IQ points). However, it is important to underscore that most children and adults with ADHD score in the average range on measures of general cognitive ability.

Processing Speed

In comparison to the results for Full Scale IQ, recent evidence from our laboratory and others indicates that groups with ADHD may exhibit even larger deficits on measures of specific aspects of intelligence such as processing speed (e.g., McGrath et al., 2011; Rucklidge & Tannock, 2002; Shanahan et al., 2006). Meta-analyses indicate that overall pooled effect sizes are medium to large for both children and adults with ADHD (d = 0.60–0.80; Willcutt et al., 2012). Furthermore, these weaknesses remain significant when group differences in general intelligence are controlled (e.g., McGrath et al., 2011; Rucklidge & Tannock, 2002; Shanahan et al., 2006), indicating that these effects do not simply reflect lower global intelligence. While no theoretical models have proposed that slow processing speed is a necessary and sufficient cause of ADHD, these robust and consistent effects indicate that a comprehensive cognitive model of ADHD must account for specific weakness in processing speed.

Perceptual and Sensorimotor Skills

Far fewer studies have tested for associations between ADHD and perceptual or motor skills. A handful of studies have suggested that ADHD may be associated with weaknesses in both gross-motor and fine-motor difficulties (e.g., Hinshaw, Carte, Sami, Treuting, & Zupan, 2002; Piek, Pitcher, & Hay, 1999), but effects have not been significant in other samples (e.g., Loo et al., 2007; Semrud-Clikeman, Walkowiak, Wilkinson, & Christopher, 2010), and overall effect sizes are small (Willcutt et al., 2012). Future research is also needed to clarify whether these weaknesses remain significant when potential confounding variables such as global cognitive ability are controlled.

Language

Groups with ADHD tend to perform worse than groups without ADHD on measures of a range of different aspects of receptive and expressive language (pooled d = 0.90–1.20; Korrel, Miller, Silk, Anderson, & Sciberras, 2017). Additional research is needed to clarify whether any of these weaknesses may be limited to the subgroup of 25–40% of individuals with ADHD who also meet criteria for reading disability. However, initial results suggest that most effects are reduced but remain significant even after researchers control for reading achievement and other potential confounding variables (Helland, Posserud, Helland, Heimann, & Lundervold, 2016; Willcutt, Pennington, Olson, Chhabildas, & Hulslander, 2005c).

Attention

Previous studies of ADHD have examined multiple constructs that fall under the broad umbrella of attention. The majority of this literature focuses on measures of attentional vigilance or sustained attention, typically operationalized by the successful detection of infrequent targets during a lengthy task. Studies of both children and adults with ADHD have found significant differences between groups with and without ADHD, with a medium overall pooled effect size (*d* = 0.50–0.70; e.g., Chhabildas, Pennington, & Willcutt, 2001; Egeland, Johansen, & Ueland, 2009; for a review, see Willcutt et al., 2012). Once again, several individual studies have demonstrated that these effects remain significant after controlling for group differences in general cognitive ability and other potential confounding variables (e.g., Willcutt et al., 2005a).

Memory

Some evidence suggests that ADHD is associated with small but significant weaknesses in short-term memory span and long-term memory storage (e.g., Hinshaw, Carte, Fan, Jassy, & Owens, 2007; see review by Willcutt et al., 2012). However, impairments on basic memory span tasks such as digit span forward are typically smaller than the effects observed on measures that require both storage and manipulation of information in working memory (e.g., digits backward), suggesting that any memory weaknesses are most pronounced on tasks that include an executive component.

Executive Functions

As noted earlier, a majority of the neuropsychological research on ADHD has focused on EF. Some theories proposed that ADHD may be due to a general EF weakness (Pennington & Ozonoff, 1996), whereas others suggested that ADHD is associated with a more focused weakness in a specific aspect of EF such as motor response inhibition (Barkley, 1997). Although initial studies often described EF as a single, unitary construct, subsequent exploratory and confirmatory factor analyses and more recent functional neuroimaging studies suggest that EFs are more accurately characterized as a collection of related but separable processes (e.g., Collette et al., 2005; Friedman et al., 2008; Miyake et al., 2000; Willcutt et al., 2005c). Specific dimensions of EF include response inhibition, verbal and spatial working memory, set shifting, planning, and interference control.

Meta-analyses of over 250 studies of children and adults indicate that ADHD is associated with significant weaknesses on measures of most EF domains (Willcutt et al., 2005b, 2012), and results of individual studies indicate that these group differences remain significant after researchers control for group differences in intelligence, reading ability, and symptoms of frequently comorbid disorders such as conduct disorder (e.g., Barkley, Murphy, & Bush, 2001; Nigg, Hinshaw, Carte, & Treuting, 1998; Willcutt et al., 2010a, 2005c). Pooled effect sizes are largest for measures of response inhibition and working memory (*d* = 0.60–0.80), whereas substantially smaller effects were reported for measures of set shifting and interference control such as a Stroop task (van Mourik et al., 2005; Willcutt et al., 2005b).

Overall, these results provide strong support for the theory that ADHD is due at least in part to weaknesses in inhibitory control and other aspects of EF. However, the overall effect sizes from meta-analyses of children and adults also indicAate that each specific EF weakness accounts for no more than 10% of the variance in ADHD symptoms, suggesting that none of these weaknesses is necessary or sufficient to cause ADHD in isolation.

Studies of Other Functional Domains

As part of the development of the criteria for DSM-5, we completed a systematic meta-analysis of studies that tested whether ADHD is associated with significant impairment in important domains of adaptive, academic, social, behavioral, or emotional functioning (Willcutt et al., 2012). Although these constructs are not typically included in classic definitions of neuropsychological constructs, they are reviewed here to maintain consistency with other chapters and to facilitate a complete understanding of the difficulties associated with ADHD.

ADAPTIVE AND ACADEMIC FUNCTIONING

ADHD is associated with weaknesses in nearly every domain of adaptive or academic functioning that has been assessed (Willcutt et al., 2012), including performance on academic achievement tests (d = 0.8–1.0), daily academic functioning in school (d = 1.0–1.2), and overall global or adaptive functioning (d = 1.4–1.6). Furthermore, these results remained significant in individual studies that controlled for confounding variables such as general cognitive ability, learning disabilities, and other frequently comorbid disorders, providing strong support for the external validity of ADHD (e.g., Lahey et al., 1998; Willcutt et al., 2005c).

SOCIAL FUNCTIONING

The meta-analysis revealed similar results for measures of social functioning (Willcutt et al., 2012). Children and adults with ADHD exhibited significant social impairment, with large effect sizes on nearly all social skills measures (d = 1.1–1.5) (e.g., Mikami, Huang-Pollock, Pfiffner, McBurnett, & Hangai, 2007; Shipp, Burns, & Desmul, 2010; Willcutt et al., 2011), prosocial behaviors (e.g., Carlson, Booth, Shin, & Canu, 2002; Lahey et al., 1998), social assertiveness (e.g., Bauermeister et al., 2005), and stability of social relationships in adulthood (e.g., Sobanski et al., 2008).

EMOTIONAL AND BEHAVIORAL ADJUSTMENT

As described in more detail earlier, the core symptoms of ADHD include two dimensions of behavioral symptoms characterized by inattention and hyperactivity–impulsivity. In addition to these deficits in behavioral functioning, increasing evidence suggests that ADHD may also be characterized by specific difficulties with the regulation of negative emotions (e.g., Barkley, 2015). Specific areas of weakness often include impatience, difficulty inhibiting frustration, hostility and emotional reactivity, and overall emotional lability. These difficulties with emotion regulation uniquely predict important impairment in social functioning after researchers control for level of ADHD symptoms, and may be especially pronounced in individuals with both ADHD and oppositional defiant disorder (see review by Barkley, 2015). Additional research is needed to better understand the neuropsychological correlates and consequences of these specific difficulties and their behavioral and neuropsychological relationship with the DSM-5 symptom dimensions of ADHD.

Implications of Neuropsychological Studies: A Paradigm Shift to Multiple-Deficit Models

The results summarized in this chapter indicate that ADHD is associated with a range of neuropsychological weaknesses, with medium to large effect sizes on measures of EFs and multiple other cognitive domains. However, all of these effects are far smaller than the effect size of the difference between groups on measures of ADHD symptoms (d = 3.0–4.0), and each individual weakness accounts for a maximum of approximately 10–15% of the variance in ADHD symptoms.

To understand the clinical implications of the relatively modest amount of variance explained by the most well-replicated neuropsychological weaknesses in ADHD, we tested how well measures of each of the most prominent theoretical models of ADHD predicted ADHD status (Willcutt, 2015; Willcutt et al., 2005b). We used a cutoff score at the 10th percentile on each measure to create a categorical measure of impairment in each neuropsychological domain (e.g., response inhibition, working memory, processing speed, response variability, and vigilance), then calculated the proportion of individuals with ADHD who exhibited each neuropsychological weakness. Between 20 and 45% of individuals with ADHD exhibited a weakness in each specific domain, a rate that is two to four times higher than the 10% that would be expected by chance. However, these results also indicate that fewer than half of all individuals with ADHD exhibit a significant deficit in any specific domain.

These results clearly indicate that no neuropsychological weakness is necessary or sufficient to cause all cases of ADHD, which has precipitated a significant reconceptualization of theoretical models of the disorder. Rather than attempting to identify a single neuropsychological weakness that is necessary and sufficient to cause ADHD, several theoretical models explicitly hypothesize that ADHD is a complex and heterogeneous disorder that is associated with weaknesses in multiple cognitive domains (Nigg, 2006; Pennington, 2006; Sonuga-Barke, 2005; Sonuga-Barke, Dalen, & Remington, 2003; Willcutt, 2015; Willcutt et al., 2008).

Two broad types of theoretical models have been proposed to incorporate multiple neurocognitive deficits. *Independent pathway models* suggest that dysfunction in any of two or more pathophysiological substrates may independently lead to the same final behavioral manifestation of a disorder. In other words, these models propose that there are distinct neuropsychological subtypes of ADHD (e.g., Nigg, Willcutt, Doyle, & Sonuga-Barke, 2005). For example, Sonuga-Barke (2002, 2003) and his colleagues proposed an influential example of a dual-pathway model in which some individuals exhibit ADHD symptoms due to significant aversion to delay, whereas others have ADHD due to weak inhibitory control. This model received important support from studies indicating that delay aversion and response inhibition predict ADHD symptoms independently (e.g., Solanto et al., 2001; Sonuga-Barke et al., 2003). However, other researchers found that a significant subset of individuals with ADHD exhibit weaknesses in both domains, suggesting that these pathways may not be entirely independent (Sonuga-Barke et al., 2008).

In contrast to the distinct neuropsychological subtypes proposed by independent pathway models, *multiple-deficit models* suggest that ADHD symptoms arise from the additive and interactive combination of multiple neuropsychological weaknesses, none of which is necessary or sufficient to cause the disorder when it occurs in isolation (e.g., Pennington, 2006; Willcutt et al., 2010a). Consistent with this possibility, results in our samples indicate that over 50% of individuals with ADHD exhibit significant impairment in at least two neuropsychological domains, and over 25% exhibit three or more weaknesses (e.g., Willcutt, 2015). The profile of specific weaknesses is likely to vary across individuals, helping to explain the striking clinical heterogeneity observed in groups with ADHD. For example, individuals with weaknesses in executive control and processing speed might be most likely to exhibit significant inattention and comorbid learning difficulties, whereas EF weaknesses coupled with aversion to delay or disruption in other motivational processes might be more strongly associated with hyperactive and impulsive behaviors and comorbidity with disorders such as conduct disorder.

Summary

In summary, a growing literature suggests that a comprehensive neurocognitive model of ADHD is likely to involve dysfunction in multiple cognitive processes that are mediated by neural networks distributed across many locations in the brain. Components of this multiple-deficit model are likely to include independent weaknesses in EFs, processing speed, attentional vigilance, and emotion regulation. Further research is needed to test whether dysfunction in these different domains leads to distinct neuropsychological subtypes within the overall population of individuals with ADHD, or whether multiple dysfunctional processes act in combination to increase susceptibility to ADHD in each individual. Perhaps the most likely scenario is a hybrid of these two models, in which some cases of ADHD are attributable to a primary deficit in a relatively specific neurocognitive process, whereas other cases may be caused by the combined effects of dysfunction in multiple neural substrates.

DEVELOPMENTAL CONSIDERATIONS

Age of Onset

ADHD is a developmental disorder with onset in early childhood, and most children are first referred for an evaluation by the end of elementary school (American Psychiatric Association, 2013). However, while the majority of cases of ADHD are identified during childhood, a subset of individuals with significant ADHD symptoms early in development may not receive a clinical evaluation and diagnosis until adolescence or adulthood. This may occur for a range of reasons, including lack of access to clinical services, parental concerns about the potential implications of a diagnosis or subsequent pharmacological treatment, or initially mild impairment that becomes more severe when an individual is confronted with the dramatic increase in attentional and organizational demands in adolescence and adulthood. Therefore, the age-of-onset criterion in DSM-5 specifies that the onset of symptoms and impairment must occur during childhood (i.e., before age 12 years), but this criterion can be fulfilled if it can be confirmed through retrospective reports that the individual exhibited significant symptoms and impairment during childhood, even if a clinical assessment was not sought at that time.

Developmental Course

Longitudinal studies have clearly demonstrated that the symptoms of ADHD and associated functional impairment continue into adolescence and adulthood for most individuals who are first diagnosed in childhood (Barkley, Fischer, Smallish, & Fletcher, 2002; Lahey et al., 2005; Willcutt et al., 2007). However, while the overall diagnosis of ADHD is highly stable over time, longitudinal studies of both unselected samples and samples of children with ADHD suggest that levels of hyperactivity–impulsivity symptoms decline significantly from early childhood through adolescence, whereas inattention symptoms decline minimally with age (e.g., Hinshaw, Owens, Sami, & Fargeon, 2006; Lahey et al., 2005; Lahey & Willcutt, 2010; Larsson, Lichtenstein, & Larsson, 2006; Leopold, Christopher, Olson, Petrill, & Willcutt, 2019).

The different developmental trajectories of the two symptom dimensions also lead to changes in ADHD subtype classifications over time. In addition to unpredictable shifts between subtypes due to random fluctuations in levels of symptoms and measurement error, a subset of individuals with ADHD shift systematically between subtypes across development in a pattern that is consistent with the developmental trajectories of the symptom dimensions (Willcutt et al., 2012). Specifically, individuals who meet criteria for the DSM-IV hyperactive–impulsive type in preschool often shift to the combined type early in elementary school as increased attentional demands in school make their symptoms of inattention more noticeable and impairing. Then, because inattention symptoms remain relatively stable across later development, whereas hyperactivity–impulsivity symptoms decline with age, individuals who initially meet criteria for the combined type in childhood often meet criteria for the predominantly inattentive presentation as they get older and their hyperactivity–impulsivity symptoms decline below the diagnostic threshold. This pattern is also reflected in prevalence studies of ADHD in adults, which consistently find that the majority of adults with ADHD meet criteria for the predominantly inattentive type (Willcutt, 2012).

PREDICTORS AND MODERATORS

The extensive literature summarized in this chapter clearly indicates that ADHD is associated with impairment on a range of concurrent and long-term functional outcomes. However, it is also clear that the severity of this impairment varies across individuals with ADHD. This section and the subsequent section on treatment and intervention summarize results for several potential moderators that have been studied most extensively.

ADHD Subtype

Although this chapter focuses on the overall diagnosis of ADHD, ADHD is clearly heterogeneous at the level of behavioral symptoms. Results of our meta-analysis of studies of DSM-IV ADHD indicated that nearly all neuropsychological measures were more highly correlated with symptoms of inattention than with symptoms of hyperactivity–impulsivity (Willcutt et al., 2012). Consistent with the findings for symptom dimensions, the two subtypes that are characterized by significant inattention (combined type and predominantly inattentive type) performed significantly worse than comparison groups without ADHD on measures of response inhibition, planning, vigilance, processing and naming speed, but there were very few differences between the combined and inattentive types on these measures. In contrast, effect sizes were much smaller and often nonsignificant when the hyperactive–impulsive type was compared to a group without ADHD, and the hyperactive–impulsive type performed significantly better than the inattentive and combined types on most neuropsychological measures. These results suggest that the inattentive and combined presentations share a common neuropsychological etiology that is driven primarily by symptoms of inattention. In contrast, the minimal evidence of neuropsychological dysfunction underscores ongoing questions regarding the diagnostic validity of the hyperactive–impulsive type, and suggest that additional research is needed to clarify whether this subtype should be retained in future diagnostic systems.

Comorbid Disorders

Over 80% of individuals with ADHD also meet criteria for another disorder, and many meet criteria for multiple additional diagnoses (e.g., Faraone, Biederman, Weber, & Russell, 1998; Hinshaw, 2002; Willcutt et al., 2010a; Willcutt, Pennington, Chhabildas, Friedman, & Alexander, 1999). In our 2012 meta-analysis, the most common comorbidities included oppositional defiant disorder (pooled estimate = 50%), conduct disorder (pooled estimate = 25%), learning disabilities (20–30%), and mood or anxiety disorders (20–30%).

The nearly ubiquitous comorbidity exhibited by individuals with ADHD initially called into question whether the significant neurocognitive weaknesses observed in groups with ADHD might be associated with one of these comorbid disorders rather than ADHD per se. However, subsequent studies showed that differences between ADHD and control groups on measures of response inhibition, working memory, delay aversion, response variability, and processing speed all remained significant when symptoms of most comorbid disorders were controlled (e.g., Rucklidge & Tannock, 2002; Solanto et al., 2007; Willcutt et al., 2010a). These results provide important evidence that each of these neuropsychological weaknesses is independently associated with ADHD and not simply a consequence of a comorbid disorder.

On the other hand, the presence of comorbidity may be an important moderator of neuropsychological and other functional outcomes for individuals with ADHD. For example, individuals with ADHD with comorbid externalizing disorders are at elevated risk for later conduct problems, criminal behavior, and intimate partner aggression (e.g., Mannuzza, Klein, & Moulton, 2008; Satterfield & Schell, 1997; Wymbs et al., 2012). Similarly, individuals with ADHD and depression exhibit greater social difficulties than do individuals with ADHD alone (e.g., Daviss, 2008), and individuals with comorbid learning disabilities exhibit greater academic, neuropsychological, social, and behavioral difficulties (e.g., Willcutt et al., 2007).

Genetic and Environmental Risk Factors

Despite high estimates of heritability, molecular genetic studies indicate that the genetic etiology of ADHD is extremely complex. Because each genetic risk factor confers only a small increase in susceptibility to ADHD, it is difficult to detect a moderating effect of any specific genetic risk factor on measures of neuropsychological functioning or other functional outcomes. Similarly, few studies have tested whether specific environmental risk factors moderate the neuropsychological outcomes of individuals with ADHD.

While analyses of individual risk factors may not be fruitful, it may eventually be possible to develop probabilistic risk profiles that combine information from all genetic and environmental risk factors to provide a measure of overall risk that could then be used to identify individuals who are at higher risk for ADHD. If this approach is successful, it could then facilitate primary prevention or early intervention to reduce the probability that an individual will eventually develop ADHD.

TREATMENT AND INTERVENTION

Medication and Behavioral Modification

The National Institute of Mental Health (NIMH) collaborative Multimodal Treatment of Attention Deficit Hyperactivity Disorder (MTA) study was one of the largest treatment studies of a childhood disorder that has been completed to date (MTA Cooperative Group, 1999). This study compared the effectiveness of psychopharmacological and behavior modification interventions, the two most widely studied intervention approaches for ADHD. Children between ages 7 and 10 years were randomized into one of four treatment groups: (1) medication alone, (2) intensive behavior modification alone, (3) combined medication and behavior modification, or (4) a community comparison group in which children received whatever treatment they received from community providers (if any).

Symptoms were reduced during the intervention in all four groups. Both groups that received medication improved more than the groups that did not receive medication, with large effect sizes for reductions in ADHD symptoms and associated social, academic, and adaptive impairment. In most cases, the primary medication was a psychostimulant such as methylphenidate, dextroamphetamine, or pemoline that increases levels of dopamine and norepinephrine in brain regions that are often underactive in ADHD. Approximately 80–90% of individuals with ADHD respond to one of the stimulants, and these medications are considered the first-line treatment for ADHD (see review by Connor, 2015). Alternatively, some individuals may respond better to atomoxetine, a norepinephrine reuptake inhibitor that has also been shown to be effective for ADHD (Tanaka, Rohde, Jin, Feldman, & Upadhyaya, 2013).

In contrast to the effect of medication alone, the behavioral modification condition had a relatively small initial effect on ADHD symptoms. However, the combination of medication and behavioral modification led to greater improvement on a range of important measures of functioning beyond ADHD symptoms, including an overall composite measure of functional outcomes (Conners et al., 2001). The combined treatment was also most effective for children with anxiety disorders and children from families with lower SES. Overall, results of the MTA study and subsequent intervention studies suggest that the optimal treatment approach for most individuals should incorporate both well-managed medication and empirically supported behavior modification strategies (for a recent review, see Caye, Swanson, Coghill, & Rohde, 2019).

Other Interventions

In addition to long-standing work on pharmacological and behavioral interventions, recent studies have tested a number of other approaches (for detailed reviews, see several chapters in Barkley, 2015; Caye et al., 2019). These include social skills training (Mikami, 2015), self-regulation interventions (Pfiffner & DuPaul, 2015), and specific programs that attempt to improve EFs, working memory, or attention (Rapport, Orban, Kofler, Friedman, & Bolden, 2015). Although these approaches have been shown to improve performance on some measures of targeted constructs administered in the laboratory, these effects typically fail to generalize beyond the laboratory setting. A number of ongoing studies continue to test whether it may be possible to refine these approaches to achieve generalizable improvements in symptoms or impairment in the future, but for now, their utility appears to be limited.

CONCLUSIONS AND FUTURE DIRECTIONS

The overarching long-term objective of all neuropsychological research is to improve the validity of clinical diagnostic procedures and the effectiveness of interventions for individuals with ADHD. In contrast to earlier theories proposing that a single neuropsychological weakness is necessary and sufficient to cause ADHD, the field has shifted toward more complex models that suggest that multiple neuropsychological weaknesses act in combination to lead to the development of ADHD. Because only a minority of individuals with ADHD exhibit a significant weakness on any of the measures of competing theoretical models that have been proposed to date, no neuropsychological measures that are currently available have sufficient predictive power to be useful for clinical diagnosis. Furthermore, the neuropsychological and behavioral heterogeneity among individuals with ADHD suggest that it is likely to remain difficult or impossible to develop an objective test with adequate positive and negative predictive power for diagnostic purposes.

Even if it is not possible to use neuropsychological measures for diagnostic purposes, results of neuropsychological studies are still likely to have important clinical utility in several ways. For example, it may eventually be possible to combine neuropsychological data with information about an individual's genetic background, family history, environmental circumstances, and other etiological factors to create a probabilistic measure of overall risk for ADHD. This profile could then be used to supplement parent and teacher ratings to identify individuals who are at high risk for ADHD, facilitating primary prevention or early intervention.

Basic neuropsychological research may also facilitate the identification of specific areas of weakness that can then be targeted by interventions. This might involve pharmacological interventions that target dysfunction in a specific neural substrate or environmental interventions designed to remediate or accommodate the specific pattern of weaknesses exhibited by an individual. For example, an individual with significant EF difficulties might benefit from a structured behavioral and organizational system that provides consistent reminders about appointments and tasks that must be completed, whereas individuals with severe processing speed difficulties might benefit from increased time to complete tests and assignments, so that slow processing speed does not compromise their ability to demonstrate mastery of the material.

FINAL SUMMARY

Overall, the studies reviewed in this chapter underscore that the neuropsychology of ADHD is complex and multifactorial, with no single deficit that is necessary or sufficient to explain all cases of ADHD. A comprehensive theoretical model of ADHD must account for weaknesses in response inhibition and other aspects of executive control, increased aversion to delay, and slower and more variable response speed. Additional research is needed to clarify the relations among these complex cognitive processes and to continue to refine the best approach to describe the behavioral and neuropsychological heterogeneity that characterizes ADHD.

REFERENCES

American Psychiatric Association. (1968). *Diagnostic and statistical manual of mental disorders* (2nd ed.). Washington, DC: Author.

American Psychiatric Association. (1980). *Diagnostic and statistical manual of mental disorders* (3rd ed.). Washington, DC: Author.

American Psychiatric Association. (1987). *Diagnostic and statistical manual of mental disorders* (3rd ed., rev.). Washington, DC: Author.

American Psychiatric Association. (2013). *Diagnostic and statistical manual of mental disorders* (5th ed.). Arlington, VA: Author.

Angold, A., Erkanli, A., Farmer, E. M. Z., Fairbank, J. A., Burns, B. J., Keeler, G., & Costello, E. J. (2002). Psychiatric disorder, impairment, and service use in rural African American and White youth. *Archives of General Psychiatry, 59*, 893-901.

Arnett, A. B., Pennington, B. F., Willcutt, E. G., DeFries, J. C., & Olson, R. K. (2015). Sex differences in ADHD symptom severity. *Journal of Child Psychology and Psychiatry, 56*, 632–639.

Barkley, R. A. (1997). Behavioral inhibition, sustained attention, and executive functions: Constructing a unifying theory of ADHD. *Psychological Bulletin, 121*, 65–94.

Barkley, R. A. (2015). *Attention-deficit hyperactivity disorder* (4th ed.). New York: Guilford Press.

Barkley, R. A., Fischer, M., Smallish, L., & Fletcher, K. (2002). The persistence of attention-deficit/hyperactivity disorder into young adulthood as a function of reporting source and definition of disorder. *Journal of Abnormal Psychology, 111*, 279–289.

Barkley, R. A., Murphy, K. R., & Bush, T. (2001). Time perception and reproduction in young adults with attention deficit hyperactivity disorder. *Neuropsychology, 15*, 351-360.

Bauermeister, J. J., Matos, M., Reina, G., Salas, C. C., Martinez, J. V., Cumba, E., & Barkley, R. A. (2005). Comparison of the DSM-IV combined and inattentive types of ADHD in a school-based sample of Latino/Hispanic children. *Journal of Child Psychology and Psychiatry, 46*, 166–179.

Buckner, R. L., Andrews-Hanna, J. R., & Schacter, D. L. (2008). The brain's default network: Anatomy, function, and relevance to disease. *Annals of the New York Academy of Sciences, 1124*, 1–38.

Canino, G., Shrout, P. E., Rubio-Stipec, M., Bird, H. R., Bravo, M., Ramirez, R., . . . Martinez-Taboas, A. (2004). The DSM-IV rates of child and adolescent disorders in Puerto Rico: Prevalence, correlates, service use, and the effects of impairment. *Archives of General Psychiatry, 61*, 85–93.

Carlson, C. L., Booth, J. E., Shin, M., & Canu, W. H. (2002). Parent-, teacher-, and self-rated motivational styles in ADHD subtypes. *Journal of Learning Disabilities, 35*, 104–113.

Casey, B. J., Castellanos, F. X., Giedd, J. N., Marsh, W. L., Hamburger, S. D., Schubert, A. B., . . . Rapoport, J. L. (1997). Implication of right frontostriatal circuitry in response inhibition and attention-deficit/hyperactivity disorder. *Journal of the American Academy of Child and Adolescent Psychiatry, 36*, 374–383.

Castellanos, F. X., Giedd, J. N., Marsh, W. L., Hamburger, S. D., Vaituzis, A. C., Dickstein, D. P., . . . Rapoport, J. L. (1996). Quantitative brain magnetic resonance imaging in attention-deficit hyperactivity disorder. *Archives of General Psychiatry, 53*, 607–616.

Castellanos, F. X., Kelly, C., & Milham, M. P. (2009). The restless brain: Attention-deficit hyperactivity disorder, resting-state functional connectivity, and intrasubject variability. *Canadian Journal of Psychiatry, 54*, 665–672.

Caye, A., Swanson, J. M., Coghill, D., & Rohde, L. A. (2019). Treatment strategies for ADHD: An evidence-based guide to select optimal treatment. *Molecular Psychiatry, 24,* 390–408.

Chhabildas, N., Pennington, B. F., & Willcutt, E. G. (2001). A comparison of the neuropsychological profiles of the DSM-IV subtypes of ADHD. *Journal of Abnormal Child Psychology, 29,* 529–540.

Cohen, J. (1988). *Statistical power analyses for the behavioral sciences.* Hillsdale, NJ: Erlbaum.

Collette, F., Van der Linden, M., Laureys, S., Delfiore, G., Degueldre, C., Luxen, A., & Salmon, E. (2005). Exploring the unity and diversity of the neural substrates of executive functioning. *Human Brain Mapping, 25,* 409–423.

Conners, C. K., Epstein, J. N., March, J. S., Angold, A., Wells, K. C., Klaric, J., . . . Wigal, T. (2001). Multimodal treatment of ADHD in the MTA: An alternative outcome analysis. *Journal of the American Academy of Child and Adolescent Psychiatry, 40,* 159–167.

Connor, D. F. (2015). Stimulant and nonstimulant medications for childhood ADHD. In R. A. Barkley (Ed.), *Attention deficit hyperactivity disorder* (4th ed., pp. 666–685). New York: Guilford Press.

Cortese, S., Kelly, C., Chabernaud, C., Proal, E., Di Martino, A., Milham, M. P., & Castellanos, F. X. (2012). Toward systems neuroscience of ADHD: A meta-analysis of 55 fMRI studies. *American Journal of Psychiatry, 169,* 1038–1055.

Costello, E. J., Keeler, G. P., & Angold, A. (2001). Poverty, race/ethnicity, and psychiatric disorder: A study of rural children. *American Journal of Public Health, 91,* 1494–1498.

Daviss, W. B. (2008). A review of co-morbid depression in pediatric ADHD: Etiology, phenomenology, and treatment. *Journal of Child and Adolescent Psychopharmacology, 18,* 565–571.

Demontis, D., Walters, R. K., Martin, J., Mattheisen, M., Als, T. D., Agerbo, E., . . . Neale, B. M. (2019). Discovery of the first genome-wide significant risk loci for attention deficit/hyperactivity disorder. *Nature Genetics, 51,* 63–75.

Dopfner, M., Breuer, D., Wille, N., Erhart, M., & Ravens-Sieberer, U. (2008). How often do children meet ICD-10/DSM-IV criteria of attention deficit-/hyperactivity disorder and hyperkinetic disorder?: Parent-based prevalence rates in a national sample—results of the BELLA study. *European Child and Adolescent Psychiatry, 17*(Suppl. 1), 59–70.

DuPaul, G. J., Power, T. P., Anastopoulos, A. D., & Reid, R. (1998). *ADHD Rating Scale–IV.* New York: Guilford Press.

Egeland, J., Johansen, S. N., & Ueland, T. (2009). Differentiating between ADHD sub-types on CCPT measures of sustained attention and vigilance. *Scandinavian Journal of Psychology, 50,* 347–354.

Faraone, S. V., Biederman, J., & Friedman, D. (2000). Validity of DSM-IV subtypes of attention-deficit/hyperactivity disorder: A family study perspective. *Journal of the American Academy of Child and Adolescent Psychiatry, 39,* 300–307.

Faraone, S. V., Biederman, J., Weber, W., & Russell, R. L. (1998). Psychiatric, neuropsychological, and psychosocial features of DSM-IV subtypes of attention-deficit/hyperactivity disorder: Results from a clinically referred sample. *Journal of the American Academy of Child and Adolescent Psychiatry, 37,* 185–193.

Faraone, S. V., & Larsson, H. (2019). Genetics of attention deficit hyperactivity disorder. *Molecular Psychiatry, 24,* 562–575.

Faraone, S. V., Perlis, R. H., Doyle, A. E., Smoller, J. W., Goralnick, J. J., Holmgren, M. A., & Sklar, P. (2005). Molecular genetics of attention-deficit/hyperactivity disorder. *Biological Psychiatry, 57,* 1313–1323.

Filipek, P. A., Semrud-Clikeman, M., Steingard, R. J., Renshaw, P. F., Kennedy, D. N., & Biederman, J. (1997). Volumetric MRI analysis comparing subjects having attention-deficit hyperactivity disorder with normal controls. *Neurology, 48,* 589–601.

Frazier, T. W., Demaree, H. A., & Youngstrom, E. A. (2004). Meta-analysis of intellectual and neuropsychological test performance in attention-deficit/hyperactivity disorder. *Neuropsychology, 18,* 543–555.

Friedman, M. C., Chhabildas, N., Budhiraja, N., Willcutt, E. G., & Pennington, B. F. (2003). Etiology of the comorbidity between RD and ADHD: Exploration of the non-random mating hypothesis. *American Journal of Medical Genetics B: Neuropsychiatric Genetics, 120,* 109–115.

Friedman, N. P., Miyake, A., Young, S. E., DeFries, J. C., Corley, R. P., & Hewitt, J. K. (2008). Individual differences in executive functions are almost entirely genetic in origin. *Journal of Experimental Psychology: General, 137,* 201–225.

Froehlich, T. E., Anixt, J. S., Loe, I. M., Chirdkiatgumchai, V., Kuan, L., & Gilman, R. C. (2012). Update on environmental risk factors for attention-deficit/hyperactivity disorder. *Current Psychiatry Reports, 13,* 333–344.

Froehlich, T. E., Lanphear, B. P., Epstein, J. N., Barbaresi, W. J., Katusic, S. K., & Kahn, R. S. (2007). Prevalence, recognition, and treatment of attention-deficit/hyperactivity disorder in a national sample of US children. *Archives of Pediatric and Adolescent Medicine, 161*, 857–864.

Gizer, I. R., Ficks, C., & Waldman, I. D. (2009). Candidate gene studies of ADHD: A meta-analytic review. *Human Genetics, 126*, 51–90.

Graetz, B. W., Sawyer, M. G., Hazell, P. L., Arney, F., & Baghurst, P. (2001). Validity of DSM-IVADHD subtypes in a nationally representative sample of Australian children and adolescents. *Journal of the American Academy of Child and Adolescent Psychiatry, 40*, 1410–1417.

Hart, H., Radua, J., Mataix-Cols, D., & Rubia, K. (2012). Meta-analysis of fMRI studies of timing in attention-deficit hyperactivity disorder (ADHD). *Neuroscience and Biobehavioral Reviews, 36*, 2248–2256.

Hart, H., Radua, J., Nakao, T., Mataix-Cols, D., & Rubia, K. (2013). Meta-analysis of functional magnetic resonance imaging studies of inhibition and attention in attention-deficit/hyperactivity disorder: Exploring task-specific, stimulant medication, and age effects. *JAMA Psychiatry, 70*, 185–198.

Helland, W. A., Posserud, M.-B., Helland, T., Heimann, M., & Lundervold, A. J. (2016). Language impairments in children with ADHD and in children with reading disorder. *Journal of Attention Disorders, 20*, 581–589.

Hervey, A. S., Epstein, J. N., & Curry, J. F. (2004). Neuropsychology of adults with attention-deficit/hyperactivity disorder: A meta-analytic review. *Neuropsychology, 18*, 485–503.

Hinshaw, S. P. (2002). Preadolescent girls with attention-deficit/hyperactivity disorder: I. Background characteristics, comorbidity, cognitive and social functioning, and parenting practices. *Journal of Consulting and Clinical Psychology, 70*, 1086–1098.

Hinshaw, S. P., Carte, E. T., Fan, C., Jassy, J. S., & Owens, E. B. (2007). Neuropsychological functioning of girls with attention-deficit/hyperactivity disorder followed prospectively into adolescence: Evidence for continuing deficits? *Neuropsychology, 21*, 263–273.

Hinshaw, S. P., Carte, E. T., Sami, N., Treuting, J. J., & Zupan, B. A. (2002). Preadolescent girls with attention-deficit/hyperactivity disorder: II. Neuropsychological performance in relation to subtypes and individual classification. *Journal of Consulting and Clinical Psychology, 70*, 1099–1111.

Hinshaw, S. P., Owens, E. B., Sami, N., & Fargeon, S. (2006). Prospective follow-up of girls with attention-deficit/hyperactivity disorder into adolescence: Evidence for continuing cross-domain impairment. *Journal of Consulting and Clinical Psychology, 74*, 489–499.

Huang-Pollock, C. L., Karalunas, S. L., Tam, H., & Moore, A. N. (2012). Evaluating vigilance deficits in ADHD: A meta-analysis of CPT performance. *Journal of Abnormal Psychology, 121*, 360–371.

Korrel, H., Miller, K. L., Silk, T., Anderson, V., & Sciberras, E. (2017). Research Review: Language problems in children with attention-deficit hyperactivity disorder—a systematic meta-analytic review. *Journal of Child Psychology and Psychiatry, 58*, 640–654.

Lahey, B. B., Pelham, W. E., Loney, J., Lee, S. S., & Willcutt, E. (2005). Instability of the DSM-IV Subtypes of ADHD from preschool through elementary school. *Archives of General Psychiatry, 62*, 896–902.

Lahey, B. B., Pelham, W. E., Stein, M. A., Loney, J., Trapani, C., Nugent, K., . . . Baumann, B. (1998). Validity of DSM-IV attention-deficit/hyperactivity disorder for younger children. *Journal of the American Academy of Child and Adolescent Psychiatry, 37*, 695–702.

Lahey, B. B., & Willcutt, E. G. (2010). Predictive validity of a continuous alternative to nominal subtypes of attention-deficit hyperactivity disorder in DSM-IV. *Journal of Clinical Child and Adolescent Psychology, 39*, 761–775.

Lansbergen, M. M., Kenemans, J. L., & Van, E. H. (2007). Stroop interference and attention-deficit/hyperactivity disorder: A review and meta-analysis. *Neuropsychology, 21*, 251–262.

Larsson, H., Lichtenstein, P., & Larsson, J. O. (2006). Genetic contributions to the development of ADHD subtypes from childhood to adolescence. *Journal of the American Academy of Child and Adolescent Psychiatry, 45*, 973–981.

Lavigne, J. V., LeBailly, S. A., Hopkins, J., Gouze, K. R., & Binns, H. J. (2009). The prevalence of ADHD, ODD, depression, and anxiety in a community sample of 4-year-olds. *Journal of Clinical Child and Adolescent Psychology, 38*, 315–328.

Leopold, D. R., Christopher, M. E., Olson, R. K., Petrill, S. A., & Willcutt, E. G. (2019). Invariance of ADHD symptoms across sex and age: A latent analysis of ADHD and impairment ratings from early childhood into adolescence. *Journal of Abnormal Child Psychology, 47*, 21–34.

Lijffijt, M., Kenemans, J. L., Verbaten, M. N., & Van Engeland, H. (2005). A meta-analytic review of stopping performance in attention-deficit/hyperactivity disorder: Deficient inhibitory motor control? *Journal of Abnormal Psychology, 114,* 216–222.

Loo, S. K., Humphrey, L. A., Tapio, T., Moilanen, I. K., McGough, J. J., McCracken, J. T., . . . Smalley, S. L. (2007). Executive functioning among Finnish adolescents with attention-deficit/hyperactivity disorder. *Journal of the American Academy of Child and Adolescent Psychiatry, 46,* 1594–1604.

Luman, M., Oosterlaan, J., & Sergeant, J. A. (2005). The impact of reinforcement contingencies on AD/HD: A review and theoretical appraisal. *Clinical Psychology Review, 25,* 183–213.

MacDonald, B., Pennington, B. F., Willcutt, E. G., Dmitrieva, J., Samuelsson, S., Byrne, B., & Olson, R. K. (2019). Cross-country differences in parental reporting of symptoms of ADHD. *Journal of Crosscultural Psychology, 50,* 806–824.

Mannuzza, S., Klein, R. G., & Moulton, J. L., III. (2008). Lifetime criminality among boys with attention deficit hyperactivity disorder: A prospective follow-up study into adulthood using official arrest records. *Psychiatry Research, 160,* 237–246.

Martinussen, R., Hayden, J., Hogg-Johnson, S., & Tannock, R. (2005). A meta-analysis of working memory impairments in children with attention-deficit/hyperactivity disorder. *Journal of the American Academy of Child and Adolescent Psychiatry, 44,* 377–384.

McCarthy, H., Skokauskas, N., & Frodl, T. (2014). Identifying a consistent pattern of neural function in attention deficit hyperactivity disorder: A meta-analysis. *Psychological Medicine, 44,* 869–880.

McGrath, L. M., Pennington, B. F., Shanahan, M. A., Santerre-Lemmon, L. E., Barnard, H. D., Willcutt, E. G., . . . Olson, R. K. (2011). A multiple deficit model of reading disability and attention-deficit/hyperactivity disorder: Searching for shared cognitive deficits. *Journal of Child Psychology and Psychiatry, 52,* 547–557.

Mikami, A. Y. (2015). Social skills training for youth with ADHD. In R. A. Barkley (Ed.), *Attention deficit hyperactivity disorder* (4th ed., pp. 569–595). New York: Guilford Press.

Mikami, A. Y., Huang-Pollock, C. L., Pfiffner, L. J., McBurnett, K., & Hangai, D. (2007). Social skills differences among attention-deficit/hyperactivity disorder types in a chat room assessment task. *Journal of Abnormal Child Psychology, 35,* 509–521.

Milich, R., Balentine, A. C., & Lynam, D. R. (2001). ADHD combined type and ADHD predominantly inattentive type are distinct and unrelated disorders. *Clinical Psychology: Science and Practice, 8,* 463–488.

Miyake, A., Friedman, N. P., Emerson, M. J., Witzki, A. H., Howerter, A., & Wager, T. D. (2000). The unity and diversity of executive functions and their contributions to complex "Frontal Lobe" tasks: A latent variable analysis. *Cognitive Psychology, 41,* 49–100.

MTA Cooperative Group. (1999). A 14-month randomized clinical trial of treatment strategies for attention-deficit/hyperactivity disorder: The Multimodal Treatment Study of Children with ADHD. *Archives of General Psychiatry, 56,* 1073–1086.

Nigg, J. T. (2006). *What causes ADHD?: Understanding what goes wrong and why.* New York: Guilford Press.

Nigg, J. T., Hinshaw, S. P., Carte, E. T., & Treuting, J. J. (1998). Neuropsychological correlates of childhood attention-deficit/hyperactivity disorder: Explainable by comorbid disruptive behavior or reading problems? *Journal of Abnormal Psychology, 107,* 468–480.

Nigg, J. T., Willcutt, E. G., Doyle, A. E., & Sonuga-Barke, E. J. (2005). Causal heterogeneity in attention-deficit/hyperactivity disorder: Do we need neuropsychologically impaired subtypes? *Biological Psychiatry, 57,* 1224–1230.

Nolan, E. E., Gadow, K. D., & Sprafkin, J. (2001). Teacher reports of DSM-IV ADHD, ODD, and CD symptoms in schoolchildren. *Journal of the American Academy of Child and Adolescent Psychiatry, 40,* 241–249.

Pauli-Pott, U., & Becker, K. (2011). Neuropsychological basic deficits in preschoolers at risk for ADHD: A meta-analysis. *Clinical Psychology Review, 31,* 626–637.

Pennington, B. F. (2006). From single to multiple deficit models of developmental disorders. *Cognition, 101,* 385–413.

Pennington, B. F., McGrath, L. M., & Peterson, R. L. (2019). *Diagnosing learning disorders* (3rd ed.). New York: Guilford Press.

Pennington, B. F., & Ozonoff, S. (1996). Executive functions and developmental psychopathology. *Journal of Child Psychology and Psychiatry, 37,* 51–87.

Pfiffner, L. J., & DuPaul, G. J. (2015). Treatment of ADHD in school settings. In R. A. Barkley (Ed.), *Attention deficit hyperactivity disorder* (4th ed., pp. 596–629). New York: Guilford Press.

Piek, J. P., Pitcher, T. M., & Hay, D. A. (1999).

Motor coordination and kinaesthesis in boys with attention deficit-hyperactivity disorder. *Developmental Medicine and Child Neurology, 41*, 159–165.

Pineda, D. A., Ardila, A., Rosselli, M., Arias, B. E., Henao, G. C., Gomez, L. F., . . . Miranda, M. L. (1999). Prevalence of attention-deficit/hyperactivity disorder symptoms in 4- to 17-year-old children in the general population. *Journal of Abnormal Child Psychology, 27*, 455–462.

Polanczyk, G., de Lima, M. S., Horta, B. L., Biederman, J., & Rohde, L. A. (2007). The worldwide prevalence of ADHD: A systematic review and metaregression analysis. *American Journal of Psychiatry, 164*, 942–948.

Rapport, M. D., Orban, S. A., Kofler, M. J., Friedman, L. M., & Bolden, J. (2015). Executive function training for children with ADHD. In R. A. Barkley (Ed.), *Attention deficit hyperactivity disorder* (4th ed., pp. 641–665). New York: Guilford Press.

Reid, R., DuPaul, G. J., Power, T. J., Anastopoulos, A. D., Rogers-Adkinson, D., Noll, M. B., & Riccio, C. (1998). Assessing culturally different students for attention deficit hyperactivity disorder using behavior rating scales. *Journal of Abnormal Child Psychology, 26*, 187–198.

Rubia, K. (2018). Cognitive neuroscience of attention deficit hyperactivity disorder and its clinical translation. *Frontiers in Human Neuroscience, 12*, 1–23.

Rubia, K., Overmeyer, S., Taylor, E., Brammer, M., Williams, S. C., Simmons, A., & Bullmore, E. T. (1999). Hypofrontality in attention deficit hyperactivity disorder during higher-order motor control: A study with functional MRI. *American Journal of Psychiatry, 156*, 891–896.

Rucklidge, J. J., & Tannock, R. (2002). Neuropsychological profiles of adolescents with ADHD: Effects of reading difficulties and gender. *Journal of Child Psychology and Psychiatry, 43*, 988–1003.

Satterfield, J. H., & Schell, A. (1997). A prospective study of hyperactive boys with conduct problems and normal boys: Adolescent and adult criminality. *Journal of the American Academy of Child and Adolescent Psychiatry, 36*, 1726–1735.

Schoechlin, C., & Engel, R. (2005). Neuropsychological performance in adult attention-deficit hyperactivity disorder: Meta-analysis of empirical data. *Archives of Clinical Neuropsychology, 20*, 727–744.

Semrud-Clikeman, M., Walkowiak, J., Wilkinson, A., & Christopher, G. (2010). Neuropsychological differences among children with Asperger syndrome, nonverbal learning disabilities, attention deficit disorder, and controls. *Developmental Neuropsychology, 35*, 582–600.

Sergeant, J. A., Geurts, H., Huijbregts, S., Scheres, A., & Oosterlaan, J. (2003). The top and the bottom of ADHD: A neuropsychological perspective. *Neuroscience and Biobehavioral Reviews, 27*, 583–592.

Shanahan, M. A., Pennington, B. F., Yerys, B. E., Scott, A., Boada, R., Willcutt, E. G., . . . DeFries, J. C. (2006). Processing speed deficits in attention deficit/hyperactivity disorder and reading disability. *Journal of Abnormal Child Psychology, 34*, 585–602.

Shipp, F., Burns, G. L., & Desmul, C. (2010). Construct validity of ADHD-IN, ADHD-HI, ODD toward adults, academic and social competence dimensions with teacher ratings of Thai adolescents: Additional validity for the Child and Adolescent Disruptive Behavior Inventory. *Journal of Psychopathology and Behavioral Assessment, 32*, 557–564.

Sobanski, E., Bruggemann, D., Alm, B., Kern, S., Philipsen, A., Schmalzried, H., . . . Rietschel, M. (2008). Subtype differences in adults with attention-deficit/hyperactivity disorder (ADHD) with regard to ADHD-symptoms, psychiatric comorbidity and psychosocial adjustment. *European Psychiatry, 23*, 142–149.

Solanto, M. V., Abikoff, H., Sonuga-Barke, E., Schachar, R., Logan, G. D., Wigal, T., . . . Turkel, E. (2001). The ecological validity of delay aversion and response inhibition as measures of impulsivity in AD/HD: A supplement to the NIMH multimodal treatment study of AD/HD. *Journal of Abnormal Child Psychology, 29*, 215–228.

Solanto, M. V., Gilbert, S. N., Raj, A., Zhu, J., Pope-Boyd, S., Stepak, B., . . . Newcorn, J. H. (2007). Neurocognitive functioning in AD/HD, predominantly inattentive and combined subtypes. *Journal of Abnormal Child Psychology, 35*, 729–744.

Sonuga-Barke, E. J. (2002). Psychological heterogeneity in AD/HD—a dual pathway model of behaviour and cognition. *Behavioural Brain Research, 130*, 29–36.

Sonuga-Barke, E. J. (2003). The dual pathway model of AD/HD: An elaboration of neurodevelopmental characteristics. *Neuroscience and Biobehavioral Reviews, 27*, 593–604.

Sonuga-Barke, E. J. (2005). Causal models of attention-deficit/hyperactivity disorder: From common simple deficits to multiple developmental pathways. *Biological Psychiatry, 57*, 1231–1238.

Sonuga-Barke, E. J., & Castellanos, F. X. (2007).

Spontaneous attentional fluctuations in impaired states and pathological conditions: A neurobiological hypothesis. *Neuroscience and Biobehavioral Reviews, 31,* 977–986.

Sonuga-Barke, E. J., Dalen, L., & Remington, B. (2003). Do executive deficits and delay aversion make independent contributions to preschool attention-deficit/hyperactivity disorder symptoms? *Journal of the American Academy of Child and Adolescent Psychiatry, 42,* 1335–1342.

Sonuga-Barke, E. J., Sergeant, J. A., Nigg, J., & Willcutt, E. (2008). Executive dysfunction and delay aversion in attention deficit hyperactivity disorder: Nosologic and diagnostic implications. *Child and Adolescent Psychiatric Clinics of North America, 17,* 367–384.

Sonuga-Barke, E. J., Taylor, E., Sembi, S., & Smith, J. (1992). Hyperactivity and delay aversion—I: The effect of delay on choice. *Journal of Child Psychology and Psychiatry, 33,* 387–398.

Still, G. F. (1902). Some abnormal psychical conditions in children. *Lancet, 1,* 1008–1012, 1077–1082, 1163–1168.

Tanaka, Y., Rohde, L. A., Jin, L., Feldman, P. D., & Upadhyaya, H. P. (2013). A meta-analysis of the consistency of atomoxetine treatment effects in pediatric patients with attention-deficit/hyperactivity disorder from 15 clinical trials across four geographic regions. *Journal of Child and Adolescent Psychopharmacology, 23,* 262–270.

Todd, R. D., Huang, H., Todorov, A. A., Neuman, R. J., Reiersen, A. M., Henderson, C. A., & Reich, W. C. (2008). Predictors of stability of attention-deficit/hyperactivity disorder subtypes from childhood to young adulthood. *Journal of the American Academy of Child and Adolescent Psychiatry, 47,* 76–85.

Vaidya, C. J., Austin, G., Kirkorian, G., Ridlehuber, H. W., Desmond, J. E., Glover, G. H., & Gabrieli, J. D. (1998). Selective effects of methylphenidate in attention deficit hyperactivity disorder: A functional magnetic resonance study. *Proceedings of the National Academy of Sciences USA, 95,* 14494–14499.

van Mourik, R., Oosterlaan, J., & Sergeant, J. A. (2005). The Stroop revisited: A meta-analysis of interference control in AD/HD. *Journal of Child Psychology and Psychiatry, 46,* 150–165.

Waschbusch, D. A., King, S., & Gregus, A. (2007). Age of onset of ADHD in a sample of elementary school students. *Journal of Psychopathology and Behavioral Assessment, 29,* 9–16.

Willcutt, E. G. (2012). The prevalence of DSM-IV attention-deficit/hyperactivity disorder: A meta-analytic review. *Neurotherapeutics, 9,* 490–499.

Willcutt, E. G. (2015). Theories of ADHD. In R. Barkley (Ed.), *Attention deficit hyperactivity disorder: A clinical handbook* (4th ed., pp. 391–404). New York: Guilford Press.

Willcutt, E. G., Betjemann, R. S., McGrath, L. M., Chhabildas, N. A., Olson, R. K., DeFries, J. C., & Pennington, B. F. (2010a). Etiology and neuropsychology of comorbidity between RD and ADHD: The case for multiple-deficit models. *Cortex, 46,* 1345–1361.

Willcutt, E. G., Betjemann, R. S., Pennington, B. F., Olson, R. K., DeFries, J. C., & Wadsworth, S. J. (2007). Longitudinal study of reading disability and attention-deficit/hyperactivity disorder: Implications for education. *Mind, Brain, and Education, 4,* 181–192.

Willcutt, E. G., & Bidwell, L. C. (2011). Etiology of ADHD: Implications for assessment and treatment. In B. Hoza & S. W. Evans (Eds.), *Treating attention deficit hyperactivity disorder* (pp. 6-2–6-18). Kingston, NJ: Civic Research Institute.

Willcutt, E. G., Boada, R., Riddle, M. W., Chhabildas, N., DeFries, J. C., & Pennington, B. F. (2011). Colorado Learning Difficulties Questionnaire: Validation of a parent-report screening measure. *Psychological Assessment, 23,* 778–791.

Willcutt, E. G., Brodsky, K., Chhabildas, N. A., Shanahan, M., Yerys, B. E., Scott, A., & Pennington, B. F. (2005a). The neuropsychology of ADHD: Validity of the executive function hypothesis. In D. Gozal & D. L. Molfese (Eds.), *Attention deficit hyperactivity disorder: From genes to patients* (pp. 185–213). Totowa, NJ: Humana Press.

Willcutt, E. G., Chhabildas, N. A., & Pennington, B. F. (2001). Validity of the DSM-IV subtypes of ADHD. *The ADHD Report, 9,* 2–5.

Willcutt, E. G., Doyle, A. E., Nigg, J. T., Faraone, S. V., & Pennington, B. F. (2005b). Validity of the executive function theory of attention-deficit/hyperactivity disorder: A meta-analytic review. *Biological Psychiatry, 57,* 1336–1346.

Willcutt, E. G., Nigg, J. T., Pennington, B. F., Solanto, M. V., Rohde, L. A., Tannock, R., . . . Lahey, B. B. (2012). Validity of DSM-IV attention-deficit/hyperactivity disorder dimensions and subtypes. *Journal of Abnormal Psychology, 121,* 991–1010.

Willcutt, E. G., Pennington, B. F., Chhabildas, N. A., Friedman, M. C., & Alexander, J. (1999).

Psychiatric comorbidity associated with DSM-IV ADHD in a nonreferred sample of twins. *Journal of the American Academy of Child and Adolescent Psychiatry, 38,* 1355–1362.

Willcutt, E. G., Pennington, B. F., Duncan, L., Smith, S. D., Keenan, J. M., Wadsworth, S. J., & DeFries, J. C. (2010b). Understanding the complex etiology of developmental disorders: Behavioral and molecular genetic approaches. *Journal of Developmental and Behavioral Pediatrics, 31,* 533–544.

Willcutt, E. G., Pennington, B. F., Olson, R. K., Chhabildas, N., & Hulslander, J. (2005c). Neuropsychological analyses of comorbidity between reading disability and attention deficit hyperactivity disorder: In search of the common deficit. *Developmental Neuropsychology, 27,* 35–78.

Willcutt, E. G., Sonuga-Barke, E. J. S., Nigg, J. T., & Sergeant, J. A. (2008). Recent developments in neuropsychological models of childhood disorders. *Advances in Biological Psychiatry, 24,* 195–226.

Woods, S. P., Lovejoy, D. W., & Ball, J. D. (2002). Neuropsychological characteristics of adults with ADHD: A comprehensive review of initial studies. *Clinical Neuropsychologist, 16,* 12–34.

Wymbs, B., Molina, B., Pelham, W., Cheong, J., Gnagy, E., Belendiuk, K., . . . Waschbusch, D. (2012). Risk of intimate partner violence among young adult males with childhood ADHD. *Journal of Attention Disorders, 16,* 373–383.

Zwirs, B. W., Burger, H., Schulpen, T. W., Wiznitzer, M., Fedder, H., & Buitelaar, J. K. (2007). Prevalence of psychiatric disorders among children of different ethnic origin. *Journal of Abnormal Child Psychology, 35,* 556–566.

CHAPTER 12

Speech, Language, and Reading Disabilities

Robin L. Peterson
Bruce F. Pennington

HISTORICAL OVERVIEW

In this chapter, we review the common and related neurodevelopmental disorders of speech sound disorder, language disorder, and reading disability. Speech and language are the oldest topics in the history of neuropsychology, going back to classic case reports by Gall, Dax, Broca, Wernicke, and others in the 19th century. Although initial work focused on previously healthy adults who lost speech–language skills due to acquired neurological insults, parallel developmental conditions were noted not long after. The first case report of a child with limited speech output was published in 1825 (Gall, 1825) and many more followed, spurred in part by advances in understanding acquired aphasia. The children in these reports had extremely limited speech output despite normal hearing and apparently normal language comprehension and nonverbal intelligence. These early cases did not distinguish speech production from language. Early labels for these children included "hearing mutism" and "congenital aphasia," and later "developmental aphasia" and "developmental dysphasia." Eventually, this neurological terminology was dropped in favor of terms such as "developmental language disorder" or "specific language impairment." In addition, a clearer distinction was drawn between problems with speech and language development, and subtypes in each domain were proposed.

The first case reports of developmental reading disability were published in the late 19th century by Pringle-Morgan (1896) and Kerr (1897). These reports described children with normal vision and apparently normal intelligence who could not learn to read despite access to education. Early terms for this condition included "congenital word blindness" and "developmental alexia."

Thus, for both language and reading disorders, the earliest identified cases described children whose difficulties were both severe (near total inability to speak or read) and specific (evidence of typical or near-typical functioning in other domains). It is not surprising that such children would come to clinical and scholarly attention first, because their difficulties were so striking and puzzling. Early definitions were shaped by sociocultural context. For example, for reading disabilities, initial reports described middle- or upper-class boys, since most other segments of the population had limited educational opportunity and thus would not be expected to learn to read in any case (Kirby, 2020). These historical facts highlight three issues that have been the subject of debate in the field for decades. Although there has been progress toward consensus, some controversy about all three questions remains (For further discussion of these issues, see Elliott & Greigorenko, 2014; Fletcher, Lyon, Fuchs, & Barnes, 2018; Kirby, Nation, Snowling, & Whyte, 2020; Peterson et al., 2021; Stanovich, 2005; Washington, Terry, & Seidenberg, 2013):

1. How severe do speech, language, or reading difficulties need to be to qualify as a disorder?
2. How specific must those difficulties be? Does a child with language problems in the context of low nonverbal IQ have a language disorder? Similarly, does a child with widespread cognitive and academic challenges have a reading disability?
3. How do we distinguish lack of environmental and educational opportunity from a neurodevelopmental disorder?

DEFINITIONS

This chapter focuses on the most prevalent and best understood neurodevelopmental disorders impacting speech, language, and reading. These include (1) *speech sound disorder*, which (as the name implies) is characterized by difficulties producing speech sounds; (2) *language disorder*, which is characterized by problems in structural language, including semantics and syntax (see Table 12.1); and (3) *reading disability* or *dyslexia*, which is characterized by difficulties with accurate and fluent word reading and spelling. Other speech–language disabilities, such as childhood apraxia of speech and pragmatic language impairment, are not addressed (see Pennington et al., 2019, for discussion of those disorders).

For reading development, basic skills (decoding, word reading accuracy, fluency) can be distinguished from the complex skill of reading comprehension. According to the simple view of reading, which was proposed by Gough and Tunmer (1986) and has since accrued substantial empirical support (García & Cain, 2014), reading comprehension is the product of word reading accuracy and oral language comprehension. Because word reading and oral language are correlated, many individuals with reading comprehension problems also have dyslexia (Spencer, Quinn, & Wagner, 2014). However, some individuals have reading comprehension problems in the absence of dyslexia, with recently increasing attention to "specific reading comprehension disability" (Spencer & Wagner, 2018). As predicted by the simple view, the vast majority of these individuals have underlying weaknesses in oral language (Nation, Cocksey, Taylor, & Bishop, 2010; Spencer at al., 2014). We believe that "specific" reading comprehension disability is best understood as a form of language disorder and so do not treat it as a separate entity.

Current definitions of all three of the disorders that are the focus of this chapter have two parts. First, the index skill (speech articulation, structural language, or reading) must be substantially below age expectations and cause functional impairment. Second, the problem must not be better accounted for by a list of exclusionary conditions such

TABLE 12.1. Components of a Sound-Based Language

Structural language	
Phonemes	The individual sound units whose concatenations, in a particular order, produce morphemes.
Morphemes	The smallest meaningful units of a word, whose combination creates a word.
Syntax	The rules governing how words in phrases and sentences can be combined (called *grammar* in popular usage).
Lexicon	The collection of all words in a given language. Each lexical entry includes all information with morphological or syntactic ramifications but does not include conceptual knowledge.
Semantics	Meanings of words and sentences.
Pragmatic language	
Discourse	The linking of sentences such that they constitute a narrative.
Prosody	The vocal intonation that can modify the literal meaning of words and sentences.

as extreme environmental deprivation, more severe neurodevelopmental disorder (e.g., intellectual disability), or a sensory or motor disability. Many different terms have been used to describe these conditions over the years, some of which emphasize similarities to acquired neurological disorders and others of which make assumptions about specificity (e.g., specific language impairment, specific reading disability) or underlying neuropsychology (e.g., phonological disorder). In line with expert consensus recommendations (Bishop, Snowling, Thompson, Greenhalgh, & the CATALISE-2 Consortium, 2017), we generally prefer descriptive terms that avoid such assumptions and thus use *speech sound disorder* and *language disorder* throughout this chapter. Because the term *dyslexia* remains in widespread common usage, including in important advocacy organizations, we use it interchangeably with *reading disability*.

EPIDEMIOLOGY

Prevalence estimates depend on definition, including questions related to severity, specificity, and sociocultural context discussed earlier. Speech articulation, oral language, and word reading skills are all continuous traits, so applying a categorical diagnosis inevitably requires a somewhat arbitrary cutoff. The cutoffs are not completely arbitrary, because the diagnostic threshold can affect the longitudinal stability of the diagnosis. Lenient diagnostic cutoffs identify many children who will grow out of their speech or language delay, with the resulting low longitudinal stability undermining the important requirement of functional impairment. Approximately 75% of children who receive a diagnosis of speech sound disorder at age 3 have clinically normal speech by age 6 (Shriberg, Tomblin, &

McSweeny, 1999). Similarly, not every late talker goes on to have a persisting language disorder, although the recovery rate is lower than is the case for speech sound disorder.

Commonly used definitions for language and reading disabilities require objective test performance on the index skill that falls at least 1.5 standard deviations below the mean, which identifies approximately 7% of the population. More stringent cutoffs identify fewer individuals, and more lenient cutoffs identify more individuals. A wide range of prevalence estimates for speech sound disorder have been reported, with the variability relating to factors including age (a greater percentage of children identified in younger samples) and method of diagnosis (speech sample analysis vs. parent and/or teacher report vs. standardized speech production test). Population-based studies of school-age children using individually administered speech tasks have reported prevalence rates around 3–4% (Shriberg et al., 1999; Wren, Miller, Peters, Emond, & Roulstone, 2016). All three disorders have a small but significant male predominance in population samples (Rutter et al., 2004; Shriberg et al., 1999; Tomblin et al., 1997). The male predominance is higher in referred samples, meaning that many girls with these disorders are not referred for services, at least partly because they have lower rates of comorbid behavior problems (e.g., hyperactivity) than boys do (Willcutt & Pennington, 2000).

The question of specificity also influences prevalence. Historical definitions of reading and language disorders required not only that reading or language skill fall below age expectations, but also that problems be greater than expected for intelligence (nonverbal IQ in the case of language disorder). However, decades of research have revealed serious problems with requiring such a discrepancy. The distinction between specific (i.e., IQ-discrepant) and "garden-variety" (i.e., broad-based) language or learning problems is not valid in terms of neuropsychological profiles or helpful treatments (Stanovich, 2005). Thus, for example, children with reading difficulties tend to have notable weaknesses in phonological processing and respond best to intensive, phonics-based reading instruction regardless of whether their IQ is significantly higher than their reading skill (Vellutino, Scanlon, & Lyon, 2000). Furthermore, children meeting criteria for language disorder show similar functioning across measures of social, emotional, behavioral, and academic impairment whether or not their nonverbal IQ is below the average range (Norbury et al., 2016). Since reading and language are both correlated with measures of intelligence, older diagnostic definitions that required both age and IQ discrepancy identified fewer children than current definitions, which are less specific and only require age discrepancy. Some have argued that this broadening of diagnostic criteria leads to confusion and risks overpathologizing children who fall somewhere on a normal spectrum of functioning. However, access to appropriate resources is often contingent on diagnosis. It seems both illogical and unethical to deny children access to intervention on the basis of the fact that they have more widespread difficulties than children who do qualify for services.

To turn to the third question, there are many complex issues related to the intersection of sociocultural context with the disorders considered here. A thorough examination of these issues is beyond the scope of this chapter, but we briefly highlight a few considerations. Historically, most research on speech, language, and reading disorders has been conducted in English. Mounting attention to these disorders in other languages indicates that they occur across languages and orthographies, with some contextual variations in how disorders manifest across different cultures and linguistic groups (Leonard, 2014; Verhoeven, Perfetti, & Pugh, 2019). This cross-cultural work has sometimes led to overturning of assumptions that grew out of an Anglocentric perspective. For example, one account of language disorder held that it arose from difficulties acquiring particular aspects of grammar, most notably the past tense. While this is the case in English, it is not so for languages that mark the past tense in a more salient manner. Instead, across cultures, language disorders are characterized by particular difficulties acquiring whichever linguistic forms are initially challenging for all learners (Leonard, 2014). Notably, major cross-cultural differences exist in awareness of speech and language disorders, availability of validated instruments for assessment, and access to treatment resources (Pham et al., 2019), which clearly impact both research and clinical practice. Ultimately, a universal theory of speech and language disorders will need to account for speakers of all the world's languages.

Dyslexia exists across every written system studied, including alphabetic languages (which represent speech sounds with letters) and logographic languages (in which symbols represent meaningful components of words rather than individual sounds). Within alphabetic systems, much research has investigated the impact of *orthographic transparency*, or the consistency with which individual speech sounds are represented by particular letters. Relatively transparent orthographies (e.g., Spanish, Finnish, Italian, or Slovakian) are easier to learn to decode than more opaque orthographies such as English (Ziegler & Goswami, 2005). Seminal research demonstrated that the rate of clinically impairing reading problems was lower in transparent orthographies than in English. However, even in the absence of major educational impairment, subtle reading problems are linked to the same underlying neurobiology in transparent orthographies as in English (Paulesu et al., 2001). Subsequent research has documented impressive universality in the neuropsychological predictors of reading skill and reading difficulties across countries and written systems (Caravolas et al., 2012).

Another important consideration relates to the manifestation of these neurodevelopmental disorders across groups within countries, such as children of varying socioeconomic backgrounds, children whose home language differs from their language of instruction, and children from historically oppressed racial or ethnic groups. This variation is exemplified by the inverse relationship of socioeconomic status (SES) to language and reading skills (Hussar et al., 2020; Tomblin et al., 1997), most likely because of the association of lower SES with a wide range of risk factors that can impact neurodevelopment. Interestingly, speech sound disorder appears not to be related to SES (e.g., Dodd, Holm, Hua, & Crosbie, 2003), suggesting that individual differences in early speech development are less related to variability in environmental input than are individual differences in early language and literacy development. Thus, if language and reading disorders are defined by scores on performance-based tests, their prevalence will increase as SES decreases. However, among children with language difficulties, those from lower SES families are *less* likely to receive speech–language interventions than children from higher SES families (Wittke & Spaulding, 2018). Current diagnostic systems exclude individuals whose difficulties are thought to owe to environmental disadvantage, though, in practice, the risk factors that have led to developmental difficulties for any individual child are largely unknown. Furthermore, there is not strong evidence that interventions for reading or language difficulties should vary as a function of their etiology. Thus, deferring diagnosis on the basis of environmental disadvantage could have the unintended consequence of further limiting access to helpful resources.

A second example draws from the work of Julie Washington and colleagues, who have studied language and literacy development in African American children in the United States. Many of these children speak African American English, a rule-governed, major dialect of American English. It is used throughout the United States and in parts of Canada, with significant regional variations. It developed as an oral language without a written counterpart. Compared to mainstream American English, African American English primarily impacts morphosyntactic and phonological structures (Washington et al., 2013). It turns out there is overlap between features of African American English and the profile of difficulties that characterize language disorder in mainstream American English (including morpheme deletion or "zero-marking"—e.g., "She walk home" in place of "She walks home"). This phenomenon can make it challenging to distinguish linguistic differences from a language disorder in African American children, especially with existing standardized instruments that emphasize morphosyntax (Craig & Washington, 2006).

Turning to the impact of dialect use on literacy development, longitudinal studies and computational modeling have demonstrated that a mismatch between spoken and written dialects significantly complicates the task of learning to read for speakers of African American English (Washington, Branum-Martin, Sun, & Lee-James, 2018; Brown et al., 2015). This mismatch may contribute to the long-standing "achievement gap" for African American children in the United States. Although this achievement gap is well recognized, African American children are *less* likely to be referred for special education services than their otherwise similar, white, mainstream American, English-speaking peers, echoing the pattern for SES and language intervention discussed earlier (Morgan et al., 2015). Finally, there are individual differences in how quickly children who speak African American English learn to "code-switch" and acquire mainstream American English for the school setting, with slow acquisition of mainstream American English features contributing significant risk for persistent reading difficulties (Washington et al., 2018). These examples illustrate the complexities of comparing prevalence rates of language and reading disorders across groups and the related risks of both over- and underidentification.

ETIOLOGY

Speech sound disorder, language disorder, and reading disability are comorbid, and this comorbidity is linked to shared underlying etiological risk factors. All three disorders are familial and heritable. The heritability of speech sound disorder is the highest of the three, approaching 1.0 in some studies (e.g., Lewis & Thompson, 1992), while the heritability of language disorder is lower (Rice, Taylor, Zubrick, Hoffman, & Earnest, 2020).

The overall heritability of reading disability is moderate, with the caveat that the heritability of reading difficulties changes with age. For instance, Logan et al. (2013) demonstrated that the heritability of individual differences in reading skill steadily increases from .22 at 6 years to .82 at 12 years. This increase in heritability likely reflects (1) a narrowing of environmental influences on reading produced by a fairly standard reading curriculum once children enter formal education, and (2) an increasing correlation between genotype and environment as children increasingly are able to pick niches that fit their level of reading skills (e.g., good readers read more on their own and become even better readers, while poor readers avoid reading).

The etiological overlap between early speech and later reading appears primarily due to shared genetic influences. In contrast (but consistent with the evidence for a greater environmental etiology for language than speech problems) the etiological overlap between early language and later reading is due to a mix of more substantial shared environmental and modest shared genetic influences (Hayiou-Thomas, 2008). Interestingly, there is a substantial genetic covariance between speech sound disorder and motor problems (Bishop, 2002).

Identifying which specific genes and environments contribute to speech, language, and reading difficulties remains an active area of research. Several candidate genes for dyslexia have now been identified in at least two independent samples, many of which are known to play a role in brain development (reviewed in Mascheretti et al., 2017). However, not every study has replicated these results (e.g., Scerri et al., 2017), nor have these candidates reached significance in existing genomewide association studies of dyslexia (e.g., Eicher et al., 2013). Even if the most promising current candidate genes are ultimately confirmed to play a role in the etiology of dyslexia, each one will likely explain only a small portion of the variance in eventual reading outcome. Most of the heritability of all three of these disorders remains unaccounted for and much important work remains.

Consistent with the behavioral genetics work discussed previously, the molecular genetics work also provides more evidence for a genetic link between speech sound disorder and reading disability than between language impairment and reading disability. Speech sound disorder has shown linkage to known dyslexia risk loci, including some of the regions that include dyslexia candidate genes (e.g., Smith, Pennington, Boada, & Shriberg, 2005). However, there has not been consistent overlap in the molecular genetics findings for language and reading disorders.

In terms of specific environmental risk factors, the strongest evidence supports associations of language skills with the quantity and quality of linguistic input provided to children (e.g., Hart & Risley, 1992). Some of this variation is related to various demographic factors (e.g., higher SES families provide more verbal stimulation to their children than lower SES families on average). However, there is also considerable overlap across groups and significant variability even among families that are demographically similar. What accounts for these striking within-group differences remains largely unknown (Weisleder & Fernald, 2013) and could ultimately become important prevention/intervention targets.

NEURAL SUBSTRATES

Language Disorder and Speech Sound Disorder

The classic Wernicke–Lichtheim–Geschwind model mapped adult language processing onto a connected set of left-hemisphere perisylvian structures, including the left superior temporal gyrus (Wernicke's area), left inferior frontal gyrus (Broca's area), and the white matter tract between these two areas (the arcuate fasciculus). Despite its considerable influence and longevity, empirical findings eventually demonstrated that this model does not account for the highly distributed and interactive neural systems supporting mature human language (Kolb & Whishaw, 2009; Poeppel, Emmorey, Hickok, & Pylkkanen, 2012).

The classic model also did not account for development. Consistent with an interactive specialization view (Johnson & de Haan, 2011), the left-hemisphere specialization for language is not present at birth. Instead, early language processing is bilateral and becomes more left lateralized over the first few years of life (Redcay, Haist, & Courchesne, 2008). Based on the classic model, one would anticipate congenital left-perisylvian lesions to cause a severe language disorder. However, multiple case studies of children with such insults (Bates & Roe, 2001) found that (1) *either* left- *or* right-hemisphere lesions disrupt early language development, but not permanently, as would occur after left-hemisphere-acquired lesions in adults, and (2) early right-hemisphere lesions impair comprehension more than do early left-hemisphere lesions, again in contrast to what is seen in adults.

Hickok and Poeppel's (2007) dual-stream model of speech perception and production provides an updated framework for understanding the limited body of neuroimaging findings for children with language disorder and speech sound disorder. Similar to the well-established dual-stream model of visual processing (i.e., the "what" ventral visual pathway and the "how" dorsal visual pathway), Hickok and Poeppel propose a ventral "what" speech stream for mapping speech to objects and a dorsal "how" speech stream for planning how to produce new words. Their model also assumes more widely distributed and bilateral neural systems for speech than the classic model.

Mayes, Reilly, and Morgan (2015) conducted a systematic review of 18 neuroimaging studies of language disorder. The brain abnormalities found in these studies were variable. The most consistent results in structural neuroimaging studies were abnormalities in the volumes of the caudate nucleus and posterior superior temporal gyrus bilaterally (both smaller in the language disorder groups compared to controls) and left inferior frontal gyrus (where the direction of findings varied across studies). A smaller number of functional magnetic resonance imaging (fMRI) studies found reduced activity in the language disorder groups in these three structures. Since the systematic review, a structural brain imaging study (Lee, Dick, & Tomblin, 2020) tested the dual-stream model account of language disorder in adolescents and young adults with language disorder compared to age-matched controls. Findings included gray matter increases in both the dorsal stream (left transverse temporal gyrus, which includes primary auditory cortex) and ventral stream (right inferior frontal gyrus and bilateral temporal poles) compared to the control group. Consistent with other work (e.g., Verly et al., 2019), the group with language disorder showed reduced white matter integrity and lack of expected age-related white matter development in both the dorsal and ventral streams compared to controls.

One fMRI study (Preston et al., 2012) reported greater dorsal and bilateral activation during visual and auditory presentation of words and pseudowords for the group of school-age children with a history of speech sound disorder compared to a typically developing group. The researchers interpreted this pattern as consistent with a developmental delay. Structural MRI in the same sample (Preston et al., 2014) found results that were consistent with this hypothesis. Compared to age-matched controls, the speech sound disorder group had more gray matter bilaterally in the superior temporal gyrus and more white matter in the anterior corpus callosum, which connects frontal articulatory areas of the two cerebral hemispheres. The authors interpreted the gray matter difference as stemming from a developmental delay in pruning. The increase in anterior corpus callosum white matter could be consistent with more bilateral processing of speech.

A few other relatively recent studies also reported atypical white matter development in children with speech sound disorder (e.g., Luders et al., 2017; Morgan et al., 2018), with variability in findings across studies again being notable. For example, Luders and colleagues (2017) reported reduced volume in the anterior corpus callosum in 18 children with speech sound disorder, whereas Preston et al. (2014) reported increased volumes in this regions in their sample. The field will benefit from more studies with larger sample sizes and eventual meta-analytic approaches. More generally, establishing tight links between specific behavioral diagnoses and neural phenotypes has been challenging in research on children with neurodevelopmental disorders. As some disorders may not have a specific gray or white matter "signature," focusing on interactive networks that change with development, comorbidity, and more complex relationships, such as equifinality (different brain changes leading to the same language/reading phenotypes) and multifinality (the same brain changes leading to different language/reading phenotypes), may be more productive (Siugzdaite, Bathelt, Holmes, & Astle, 2020).

Reading Disability

Of the three disorders considered in this chapter, the neural substrates of reading disability are best understood and have now been summarized in several systematic reviews and meta-analyses (e.g., Richlan, Kronbichler, & Wimmer, 2011, 2013; Paulesu, Danelli, & Burlingeri, 2014). The neural correlates of reading disability include abnormalities in the structure and function of a left-hemisphere network that encompasses language processing regions, as well as in structures associated with visual–object processing and establishment of visual–linguistic mappings. Functional neuroimaging reveals underactivations in two posterior left-hemisphere regions: a temporoparietal region believed to be crucial for phonological processing and phoneme–grapheme conversion, and an occipitotemporal region, including the so-called "visual word form area," which is thought to participate in whole-word recognition (Richlan et al., 2011). Abnormal activation of the left inferior frontal gyrus is also commonly reported. Structural imaging studies have revealed gray matter decreases in this same network (Richlan et al., 2013). Reduced white matter integrity in tracts connecting the left temporoparietal regions to the left interior frontal gyrus (i.e., arcuate fasciculus and the superior longitudinal fasciculus) have also been consistently reported in both children and adults with reading disability (Vandermosten, Boets, Wouters, & Ghesquière, 2012). Family risk studies have demonstrated that structural and functional differences predate literacy instruction and are therefore not merely a consequence of reading failure (Raschle, Chang, & Gaab, 2011; Raschle, Zuk, & Gaab, 2012; Vandermosten et al., 2015).

NEUROPSYCHOLOGICAL CORRELATES

There is a long history of neuropsychological theories of developmental disorders, most of which have posited a single, core neuropsychological deficit as necessary and sufficient to produce the behavioral phenotype. These theories failed for at least three related reasons. First, any single cause is inconsistent with what is known about these disorders at the etiological and neural levels. Consistent with the complex disease model in medicine, the disorders considered here are more accurately attributed to multiple interacting risk and protective factors. Second, single-deficit theories generally assumed more specificity than has been evident in research on these disorders. Consistent with one theme of this chapter, most developmental disorders arise of a mix of substantial general and more modest specific influences (Pennington, McGrath, & Peterson, 2019). Third, among neurodevelopmental disorders, comorbidity is the rule rather than the exception, and single-deficit models do not account for comorbidity. Thus, the field has gradually shifted from the single-deficit view to a multiple neuropsychological deficit framework (Pennington, 2006; McGrath, Peterson, & Pennington, 2020). A multiple-deficit framework is consistent with what is known about the causes of developmental disorders at the etiological and neural levels, and allows for modeling of a combination of general and specific neuropsychological influences. In addition, the multiple-deficit framework accounts for comorbidity, because it posits that some neuropsychological problems are shared across disorders (thus explaining their overlap) while others are unique (which explains why the disorders are not identical). In the sections that follow, we discuss the neuropsychological profiles of speech sound disorder, language disorder, and reading disability within the context of a multiple-deficit framework.

General Intellectual Functioning

As discussed previously, language, speech, and reading skill are all correlated with measures of IQ, even nonverbal IQ. The extent of the relationship between general intellectual functioning and the disorders considered here varies by definition. Older definitions that required an IQ discrepancy yielded smaller associations than do current definitions. A meta-analysis (Gallinat & Spaulding, 2014) found an effect size of 0.69 for the association between language disorder and nonverbal IQ, which translates to approximately 10 standard score points, meaning that about half of children with a language disorder can be expected to have a nonverbal IQ that falls below the average range. A population cohort study comparing children with speech sound disorder to typically developing children reported group differences with effect sizes of around 0.35 for both verbal and nonverbal IQ measures (Wren et al., 2016), which translates to about 5 standard score points. The correlation of reading disability with verbal IQ is approximately 0.5 (Snowling & Melby-Lervåg, 2016), while the correlation with nonverbal IQ is relatively smaller but significant. Consistent with its robust association with language disorder, nonverbal IQ has a stronger relationship with reading comprehension than with the basic reading skills implicated in dyslexia (Peng, Wang, Wang, & Lin, 2019).

To address the issue of the distinctiveness of different learning disabilities, we explored the links among reading, other academic skills, and IQ (Peterson et al., 2021). Using bifactor modeling, we found strong evidence for a general factor related to basic literacy skills (word reading, spelling, and reading fluency), reading comprehension, math calculation and problem solving, and written expression. Analogous to cognitive *g*, we and other authors referred to this general factor as "academic *g*." Consistent with previous research (Kaufmann, Reynolds, Liu, Kaufman, & McGrew, 2012), academic *g* was strongly but not perfectly correlated with Full Scale IQ (in our study, $r = .72$). On the other hand, even while accounting for general academic and intellectual skills, we identified reliable distinct variance in basic literacy, as well as in math. We did not identify reliable variance in written expression that was distinct from general academic skills, and evidence for reliable distinct variance in reading comprehension was mixed. While supporting a degree of specificity in basic literacy and math, results highlighted the general nature of learning challenges for many children with learning disorders.

Perceptual and Sensorimotor Skills

A limitation of sensorimotor accounts of language and reading disabilities is their failure to fully account for most individuals with these disorders. For language disorder, the best-known sensory account is the auditory hypothesis, which was developed in the 1970s by Tallal and colleagues. Early studies demonstrated that children with language disorder had specific difficulty discriminating rapidly presented nonspeech sounds (Tallal & Piercy, 1973), which was postulated to lead to downstream problems processing speech and ultimately in language development. Later studies cast doubt on whether these auditory deficits were causal, because many children with language disorder do not have auditory deficits, while many typically developing children do (Bishop, Carlyon, Deeks, & Bishop, 1999b). Consistent with a multiple-deficit view, auditory deficits may complicate language development in children with other underlying risk factors (Bishop et al., 1999a) and/or may play a more substantial role in a minority of individuals with language disorder (Bishop & MacArthur, 2005).

The earliest neuropsychological theories of reading disability posited a visual deficit to explain observed letter reversals in reading and writing (Orton, 1925). A straightforward visual account of dyslexia has long been discredited (Vellutino, 1979), but interest in linking reading difficulties to low-level sensory or motor processing problems has persisted into this century (Richardson, Thomson, Scott, & Goswami, 2004). Similar to the auditory account of language disorder, the relationship between these processing deficits and reading outcomes is variable across individuals and the deficits are thus unlikely to be causal in most cases.

In contrast to these largely debunked sensory–motor accounts of reading disability and language disorder, a more promising account of speech sound disorder holds that the difficulties producing speech sounds arises from a problem in speech motor representations (Terband, Maassen, Guenther, & Brumberg, 2014a). In typical speech development, there is a tight coupling between speech perception and production, with infant babbling providing a mechanism for auditory feedback and subsequent tuning of speech motor representations (Guenther, 1995). Babbling is delayed and atypical in speech sound disorder. A computational model (Terband et al., 2014a) simulated babbling and speech imitation in speech sound disorder by adding noise to the model's motor representations. These results align with behavioral studies showing that children with speech sound disorder perform worse than controls on a range of oral motor tasks (Lewis et al., 2011; Raitano, Pennington, Tunick, Boada, & Shriberg, 2004) and compensate less well for experimental perturbations in auditory feedback (Terband, van Brenk, & van Doornik-van der Zee, 2014b).

Language

Speech sound disorder and language disorder are both defined by language problems. Awareness of the components of oral language (Table 12.1) is helpful in understanding the neuropsychology of these disorders. The structure of language is hierarchical: Speech sounds (phonemes) are combined into units of meaning (morphemes) that alone or in combination form words in the lexicon, which are combined into phrases and sentences in a lawful way (syntax), and in turn have meaning (semantics). These five components (phonemes, morphemes, lexicon, syntax, and semantics) make up structural language, which is distinguished from the social use of language, or *pragmatics* (discourse and prosody). As mentioned previously, language disorder involves deficits in structural language, mainly in syntax and the lexicon, whereas the chief problem in speech sound disorder and reading disability is at the phonological level of language.

Language Disorder

The many competing single-deficit accounts of language disorder (Leonard, 2014) posit either a deficit in an aspect of linguistic *knowledge* or a specific *processing* deficit that interferes with language development. An example of a well-known knowledge deficit hypothesis is the *extended optional infinitive hypothesis* (Rice, Wexler, & Cleave, 1995). According to this hypothesis, the core deficit in language disorder is difficulty in acquiring a particular aspect of syntax. In English, children with language disorder most notably have difficulties with the past tense, often substituting an unmarked form for a marked one (e.g., "He walk there" in place of "He walked there"). Such "zero-marking" errors are made by typically developing children early in language acquisition, but children with language disorder tend to use unmarked (or infinitive) forms much longer than even younger typically developing children matched for overall language skill. The extended optional infinitive hypothesis was developed to account for findings in English-speaking children but does not adequately account for the linguistic phenotype of language disorder in some other languages (Leonard, 2014). This account also fails to explain why most children with language disorder have difficulty with tasks that do not require syntactic competence, including vocabulary knowledge.

The *phonological memory hypothesis*, an example of a processing deficit theory of language disorder, holds that the core deficit lies in the ability to hold phonological forms in working memory (Gathercole & Baddeley, 1990). This hypothesis has been supported by convergent evidence from adults with brain damage, second-language learners, typically developing children, and computational models highlighting a key role for phonological memory in structural language learning (Baddeley, Gathercole, & Papagno, 1998; Joanisse & Seidenberg, 2003). Also, phonological memory deficits are a robust endophenotype for language disorder. They have strong genetic and behavioral correlations with language disorder, and they persist even in individuals whose broader language problems have resolved (Bishop et al., 1999a). For these reasons, a deficit in phonological memory appears to be important in most cases of language disorder.

Speech Sound Disorder

Speech sound disorder is associated with phonological processing weaknesses, including in phonological awareness and phonological memory (Bird, Bishop, & Freeman, 1995; Raitano et al., 2004). Because phonological processing has been strongly linked to basic literacy development, these findings help explain the comorbidity between speech sound disorder and reading disability. However, research has consistently reported that most of the risk for reading disability in speech sound disorder is carried by a co-occurring language disorder, while the association between an isolated speech sound disorder (i.e., without comorbid language disorder) and later literacy problems is much smaller (Hayiou-Thomas, Carrol, Leavett, Hulme, & Snowling, 2017; Lewis et al., 2015; Peterson, Pennington, Shriberg, & Boada, 2009). Somewhat surprisingly, a history of speech sound disorder is associated with phonological processing weaknesses in the school years even for children with age-appropriate literacy skills (Peterson et al., 2009), suggesting that other factors are protective against dyslexia in this group. This pattern is consistent with a multiple-deficit framework in which phonological awareness is a shared risk factor for speech sound disorder and reading disability but is not necessary and sufficient for either disorder.

Reading Disability

The dominant explanation of reading disability for many years was that the disorder is caused by a single core deficit in phonological processing (Vellutino, Fletcher, Snowling, & Scanlon, 2004). According to the phonological theory of dyslexia, the ability to attend to and manipulate linguistic sounds is crucial for the establishment and automatization of letter–sound correspondences, which in turn underlie accurate and fluent word recognition through the process of phonological coding. Although this theory has received wide support, it fails to account for the fact that some children with phonological processing deficits have normal-range reading skills (Peterson et al., 2009), whereas others with dyslexia have normal-range phonological processing (Pennington et al., 2012).

Findings from longitudinal family risk studies also challenge the notion that phonological processing is the single core deficit underlying reading disability. This work has shown that a variety of oral language skills differentiate children who develop dyslexia from those who do not, and that the best oral language predictors change with developmental level. Children who will later go on to develop dyslexia show aberrant neural response to speech stimuli in infancy (Lyytinen et al., 2005) followed by delayed speech and language development as toddlers (Scarborough, Catts, & Kamhi, 2005). By preschool, differences begin to emerge on various phonological and reading-related tasks, including those tapping phonological awareness, phonological and short-term memory, and letter knowledge (Scarborough et al., 2005). By school age, phonological processing problems and vocabulary weaknesses remain evident, but the earlier, broader oral language difficulties have otherwise largely resolved for most individuals (Snowling & Melby-Lervåg, 2016). Reading disability is thus best conceptualized as a type of subtle language learning disorder with origins early in development.

Memory

Weaknesses in phonological and verbal short-term memory have been linked to all three of the disorders considered here and may help explain their comorbidity. Although long-term declarative memory is not strongly implicated in speech, language, or reading disorders, the *procedural memory hypothesis* is another processing account of language disorder that has received some research support (Ullman & Pierpont, 2005). Much of what a typical adult knows about phonology or grammar relies on implicit rather than declarative knowledge. Infants apply statistical learning, a form of procedural learning, to parse patterns within the speech stream (Saffran, Aslin, & Newport, 1996). A deficit in this process provides a plausible explanation for language disorder and potentially even reading disability. In support of this hypothesis, individuals with language disorder show procedural learning deficits on multiple tasks (Leonard, 2014). A meta-analysis of differences between children with and without language disorder revealed evidence for only a weak average effect size of 0.33 (Lum, Conti-Ramsden, Morgan, & Ullman, 2014). Thus, deficits in procedural learning may contribute to language disorder within the multiple-deficit framework but do not suffice as a single-deficit explanation for the disorder.

Attention/Executive Functions/Processing Speed

Reading disability and language disorder are both comorbid with attention- deficit/hyperactivity disorder (ADHD). Because these comorbidities occur across a continuum of severity, individuals with reading disability or language disorder are at elevated risk for difficulties in everyday attention and executive functioning skills, even if they do not meet full symptom criteria for ADHD (Mueller & Tomblin, 2012; Willcutt & Pennington, 2000). Language disorder and reading disability are also associated with performance-based measures of attention and related skills.

Processing speed is a general risk factor for many neurodevelopmental disorders and likely contributes to comorbidities. Weaknesses in processing speed help explain the overlap of basic literacy and math skill with ADHD symptomatology (McGrath et al., 2011; Peterson et al., 2017). Research has demonstrated associations of both reading disability and language disorder to a range of speeded tasks (Norton & Wolf, 2012; Ebert & Pham, 2019). As noted earlier, speeded tasks have not been strongly linked to speech sound disorder, providing an example of a potential neuropsychological protective factor for this group.

Although visual accounts of dyslexia have been discredited, the possibility of a role of visual attentional deficits in reading difficulties has received renewed attention (Facoetti, Corradi, Ruffino, Gori, & Zorzi, 2010; Fu, Zhao, Ding, & Wang, 2019). Performance on visual attention tasks in children of preschool age significantly predicted reading ability 2 years later, after researchers accounted for the influence of reading-related phonological processing skills (Franceschini, Gori, Ruffino, Pedroll, & Facoetti, 2012). While deficits in visual attention fail to provide a convincing explanation for the early speech–language phenotype in predyslexic children, weaknesses in this area may combine with language problems as contributors to later reading disability.

Social, Emotional, and Behavioral Functioning

Language disorder is associated with a wide range of adjustment difficulties, including externalizing and internalizing symptoms, as well as problems in peer relationships (Mok, Pickles, Durkin, & Conti-Ramsden, 2014; Norbury et al., 2016). Longitudinal studies examining the developmental trajectories of social, emotional, and behavioral functioning in youth with language disorder have yielded mixed results (Conti-Ramsden et al., 2019). Some adjustment difficulties are likely a consequence of having a communication disorder, while others may be due to common etiological factors that convey risk for both language disorder and psychiatric difficulties.

Reading disability is also associated with both emotional and behavioral difficulties. The link between reading problems and externalizing disorders is primarily accounted for by their shared comorbidity with ADHD. In contrast, internalizing symptoms appear to be at least partly a response to the experience of having learning difficulties, especially in girls (Willcutt & Pennington, 2000).

Relatively little work has investigated social, emotional, and behavioral functioning in speech sound disorder. Overall, it appears that the risk for adjustment difficulties in children with a history of isolated speech difficulties (i.e., without a co-occurring language impairment) is low (Lewis et al., 2016; Snowling et al., 2006).

DEVELOPMENTAL CONSIDERATIONS

Oral language development in reading disability provides a powerful example of heterotypic continuity, in which the manifestation of an underlying impairment changes with development. As discussed in the section on neuropsychological correlates, children who will later develop dyslexia demonstrate early differences in speech processing, followed by delays in speech production, vocabulary, and syntax, and eventually by difficulties in phonological processing. The literacy profile of individuals with dyslexia also changes over time. Early problems with reading accuracy may remit, while problems with spelling and reading fluency are more likely to persist into adulthood (Bruck, 1992, 1993). The underlying vulnerability in reading disability may interfere with the acquisition of whatever linguistic task is most relevant at a particular developmental stage (Scarborough et al., 2005). Heterotypic continuity is also illustrated by speech sound disorder. As a group, individuals with a history of this disorder continue to demonstrate weaknesses in phonological processing and literacy into adulthood, even if frank speech difficulties have resolved (Peterson et al., 2009; Lewis & Freebairn, 1992).

The experience of having a learning disability can lead to the development of difficulties in other areas, as described earlier for the development of internalizing symptoms in girls with dyslexia. In addition, there is a well-documented reciprocal relationship between vocabulary and reading skill: Strong vocabulary supports strong word-level reading and comprehension skills. At the same time, because reading is itself an important contributor to vocabulary learning in older children and adolescents, weak readers are at risk for more limited vocabulary development over time (the so-called "Matthew effect"; Stanovich, 2009).

Several researchers have investigated long-term developmental trajectories in children with language disorder, from preschool age through adolescence or adulthood. Although there have been some differences in the pattern of results across studies, considerable evidence supports a relative slowing in growth over time in age-adjusted scores across several ability domains, including vocabulary knowledge, academic skills, and nonverbal IQ (Conti-Ramsden, St Clair, Pickles, & Durkin, 2012; Stothard, Snowling, Bishop, Chipchase, & Kaplan, 1998). Given the critical role of language skills in children's development (Nelson, 1998), it is not surprising that a persisting language impairment would exact a greater and greater cost.

PREDICTORS AND MODERATORS

In some ways, the three disorders considered here can be thought of as falling along a continuum of severity. Isolated speech sound disorder is the mildest of these disorders, as it is most likely to resolve in childhood and is associated with the lowest level of neuropsychological morbidity, psychiatric comorbidity, and long-term adaptive impairment. Language disorder is at the other end of the spectrum and is linked to the most widespread disruptions in neural, cognitive, and psychosocial functioning, as well as the greatest long-term adaptive impairment (Johnson, Beitchman, & Brownlie, 2010). Consistent with this view, the presence of broader oral language difficulties is a well-documented risk factor in both speech sound disorder and reading disability (Lewis et al., 2015, 2016; Peterson et al., 2009; Snowling et al., 2006; Snowling, Gallagher, & Frith, 2003). More generally, comorbidity is a child-level factor that conveys risk for poorer outcomes across neurodevelopmental disorders (Willcutt et al., 2013). Thus, it is important for clinicians working with children with speech, language, or reading disabilities to screen for co-occurring communication, learning, and emotional–behavioral disorders.

At the family level, better maternal health and well-being is a protective factor for children otherwise at risk for communication impairments (Harrison & McLeod, 2010), an association that is likely mediated in part by home language environment. Some of the variance in communication skills related to family "environmental" factors can be attributed to shared genetic influences (Scarborough, 1991). However, genetically sensitive designs and experimental intervention studies indicate independent associations of early linguistic input with later language development (Rutter, Thorpe, Greewood, Northstone, & Golding, 2003; Weber, Fernald, & Diop, 2017).

As discussed previously, various demographic factors are associated with reduced likelihood of a child coming to clinical attention and participating in language or reading intervention. These factors include female gender, lower SES, and membership in a historically oppressed racial or ethnic group, although some of these same factors convey *increased* risk for difficulties in language or academic development. Individual differences are also evident in how well children with speech, language, or reading disabilities respond to intervention. A Cochrane meta-analysis of speech–language therapy interventions (Law, Garrett, & Nye, 2003) found that the most reliable treatment effects are for children with speech and expressive vocabulary problems, while receptive language problems are more difficult to remediate. For reading disability, evidence supports the importance of early identification and intervention, as treatments for word-level reading difficulties show larger effects sizes for younger than older readers (Vaughn, Denton, & Fletcher, 2010).

TREATMENT

Speech Sound Disorder and Language Disorder

Approaches to treating speech and language disorders include imitation and modeling, as well as focused stimulation (i.e., the therapist repeatedly uses a target word or phrase while interacting with the child), conversational recasts (i.e., the therapist repeats all or part of what the child has said and builds on it), and milieu teaching (i.e., the therapist sets up an environment with preferred toys or other items about which the child will be motivated to communicate). All of these provide targeted exposure to, and practice with, the linguistic forms with which the child is struggling. These therapies provide a more intensive and focused "dose" of activities in which parents and other adults naturally engage to stimulate language development. Evaluation of these approaches documents gains relative to both untreated controls and untreated linguistic forms in the child's repertoire, as well as increased rates of language development and transfer to spontaneous speech (Law et al., 2003).

Current treatment approaches are also subject to several limitations. First, although many different forms of speech and language therapy are similarly effective (Nye, Foster, & Seaman, 1987; Baker & McCleod, 2011), the "active ingredients" common to these approaches remains unclear. Second, evidence regarding the effectiveness of therapies delivered by trained parents versus clinicians is lacking (Law et al., 2003). Third, existing interventions have not been established as effective in treating receptive language problems. Finally, milder initial speech or language difficulties are associated with better outcomes, but treatment duration is not (Bishop & Edmundson, 1987). In summary, a variety of speech–language therapy-based approaches appear helpful in treating language disorder and speech sound disorder, but these interventions do not yet meet all standards for well-established empirically supported treatments.

Reading Disability

Research on treatments for reading difficulties in the early grades indicates that (1) intervention is most effective when provided in a one-to-one or small-group setting; (2) successful interventions heavily emphasize phonics instruction; and (3) useful additional treatment elements include training in phonological awareness, supported reading of increasingly difficult connected text, writing exercises, and comprehension strategies (Scammacca, Vaughn, Roberts, Wanzek, & Torgesen, 2007). The most effective reading treatments for older children emphasize language and cognitive skills such as vocabulary and comprehension strategies. However, even adolescents can benefit from phonics and fluency training to a degree, so a combined approach may be most appropriate for older students with dyslexia (Scammacca, Roberts, Vaughn, & Stuebing, 2015). About half of successfully treated children maintain reading gains for at least 1 to 2 years. As for children with speech and language disorders, youth with milder reading difficulties respond better to treatment, although some individual children with severe reading problems also respond favorably to reading intervention (Stuebing et al., 2015).

CONCLUSIONS AND FUTURE DIRECTIONS

What does the science of speech, language, and reading disorders tell us about the questions of severity, specificity, and sociocultural context raised at the beginning of the chapter? On the issue of severity, a key point is that each of these disorders is defined by setting a partially arbitrary cutoff on a continuous distribution. Thus, along with all other behaviorally defined conditions, the three language-related disorders considered here are best conceptualized as falling on a spectrum. No matter where we set the cutoff for identifying the disorder on a given measure, there will always be individuals who fall just above or below it, or who would not meet the same cutoff on a different day or based on a different measure. For individual diagnostic decision making, this difficulty can be reduced by administering multiple correlated measures and considering other information, including history and behavioral observations, but it can never be avoided entirely. Thus, clinicians need not make a hard "yes or no" diagnostic decision in every case. From a research perspective, we know that speech, language, and academic skills are normally distributed due to their multifactorial causes, and that the same etiological, neural, and neuropsychological risk factors that influence membership in the low tail of the distribution also affect these skills across the full range of individual differences (Haworth et al., 2009; Kauffmann et al., 2011; Niogi & McCandliss, 2006; Snowling et al., 2003). These findings have led to calls for research that moves away from discrete categories and focuses instead on a dimensional approach (Casey, Oliveri, & Insel, 2014; Kovas & Plomin, 2006; Peters & Ansari, 2019).

The historical emphasis on "specific" language and learning disabilities continues to influence public perception of these disorders, as well as aspects of clinical practice and scholarship. For language disorder, expert consensus has been to remove the term *specific* from diagnostic terminology (Bishop et al., 2017), but most current nosologies retain this verbiage for reading disability (e.g., specific learning disorder). Although a degree of specificity is evident for each of the disorders considered here, substantial general influences require consideration at the etiological ("generalist" genes and environments; Kovas & Plomin, 2006), neural (distributed, bilateral networks), neuropsychological (cross-disorder links to general intelligence, processing speed, and broad oral language skill), and symptom levels (comorbidity not only with one another but also with other learning and psychiatric disorders). Thus, widespread difficulties need not exclude children from access to services for language-based disorders.

Some scientific questions concern more specific subgroups of a disorder. For example, the etiology of reading disability reflects a stronger contribution of genetic influences in individuals who meet both age- and IQ-discrepancy criteria compared to individuals who meet age-discrepancy criteria alone (Wadsworth, Olson, Pennington, & DeFries, 2000). A continued focus of some genetic investigations on the more specific phenotype of reading disability in the context of relatively high IQ is warranted. At the same time, many important scientific questions about general language and learning difficulties remain understudied. For example, neuroimaging studies have tended to exclude individuals with comorbid disorders because of the interpretive complexity and need for larger sample sizes in research on comorbidity. Systematic study of individuals with comorbid disorders is needed to better describe the brain bases of the general versus specific aspects of language and learning disorders. A recent functional neuroimaging study took this approach by comparing children with reading disability alone, math disability alone, comorbid reading and math disabilities, and no learning disability (Peters, Bulthé, Daniels, de Beeck, & De Smedt, 2018). Patterns of brain activation were similar for the three learning disability groups but differed from the patterns displayed by the control group. We need more research examining etiology, brain bases, neuropsychological correlates, and response to intervention in language and learning disorders that systematically accounts for comorbidities.

Turning to the question of sociocultural context, early case reports reflected children from advantaged backgrounds, while children from historically oppressed groups remain at risk for underidentification even today. Clinicians face a diagnostic dilemma when it appears that environmental disadvantage has contributed significantly to the development of communication or academic difficulties. In such cases, it may be useful to bear in mind that the environment plays an important role in neurodevelopment and contributes to individual differences in language and reading, and that diagnoses serve the important functions of guiding treatment and "buying" access to services regardless of etiology. Thus, in most cases, the presence of environmental risk factors need not preclude diagnosis. We need more rigorous work to develop culturally and linguistically appropriate test batteries and norms for historically understudied groups around the world. As illustrated by cross-linguistic studies of language disorder that have helped to correct the errors of an early Anglocentric perspective, such efforts would benefit both research and clinical practice.

ACKNOWLEDGMENT

This work was supported by a grant from NICHD (Grant No. HD027802).

REFERENCES

Baddeley, A., Gathercole, S., & Papagno, C. (1998). The phonological loop as a language learning device. *Psychological Review, 105*(1), 158–173.

Baker, E., & McLeod, S. (2011). Evidence-based practice for children with speech sound disorders: Part 1. Narrative review. *Language, Speech, and Hearing Services in Schools, 42*(2), 102–139.

Bates, E. A., & Roe, K. (2001). Language development in children with unilateral brain injury. In C. A. Nelson & M. Luciana (Eds.), *Handbook of developmental cognitive neuroscience* (pp. 281–307). Cambridge, MA: MIT Press.

Bird, J., Bishop, D. V., & Freeman, N. H. (1995). Phonological awareness and literacy development in children with expressive phonological impairments. *Journal of Speech, Language, and Hearing Research, 38*(2), 446–462.

Bishop, D. V. (2002). Motor immaturity and specific speech and language impairment: Evidence for a common genetic basis. *American Journal of Medical Genetics, 114*(1), 56–63.

Bishop, D. V. M., Bishop, S. J., Bright, P., James, C., Delaney, T., & Tallal, P. (1999a). Different origin of auditory and phonological processing problems in children with language impairment: Evidence from a twin study. *Journal of Speech, Language, and Hearing Research, 42*(1), 155–168.

Bishop, D. V. M., Carlyon, R. P., Deeks, J. M., & Bishop, S. J. (1999b). Auditory temporal processing impairment: Neither necessary nor sufficient for causing language impairment in children. *Journal of Speech, Language, and Hearing Research, 42*(6), 1295–1310.

Bishop, D. V. M., & Edmundson, A. (1987). Language-impaired 4-year-olds: Distinguishing transient from persistent impairment. *Journal of Speech and Hearing Disorders, 52*(2), 156–173.

Bishop, D. V. M., & Hayiou-Thomas, M. E. (2008). Heritability of specific language impairment depends on diagnostic criteria. *Genes, Brain and Behavior, 7*(3), 365–372.

Bishop, D. V., & McArthur, G. M. (2005). Individual differences in auditory processing in specific language impairment: A follow-up study using event-related potentials and behavioural thresholds. *Cortex, 41*(3), 327–341.

Bishop, D. V., Snowling, M. J., Thompson, P. A., Greenhalgh, T., & the CATALISE-2 Consortium. (2017). Phase 2 of CATALISE: A multinational and multidisciplinary Delphi consensus study of problems with language development: Terminology. *Journal of Child Psychology and Psychiatry, 58*(10), 1068–1080.

Brown, M. C., Sibley, D. E., Washington, J. A., Rogers, T. T., Edwards, J. R., MacDonald, M. C., & Seidenberg, M. S. (2015). Impact of dialect use on a basic component of learning to read. *Frontiers in Psychology, 6*, Article 196.

Bruck, M. (1992). Persistence of dyslexics' phonological awareness deficits. *Developmental Psychology, 28*(5), 874–886.

Bruck, M. (1993). Component spelling skills of

college students with childhood diagnoses of dyslexia. *Learning Disability Quarterly, 16*(3), 171–184.

Caravolas, M., Lervåg, A., Mousikou, P., Efrim, C., Litavský, M., Onochie-Quintanilla, E., . . . Seidlová-Málková, G. (2012). Common patterns of prediction of literacy development in different alphabetic orthographies. *Psychological Science, 23*(6), 678–686.

Casey, B. J., Oliveri, M. E., & Insel, T. (2014). A neurodevelopmental perspective on the research domain criteria (RDoC) framework. *Biological Psychiatry, 76*(5), 350–353.

Conti-Ramsden, G., Mok, P., Durkin, K., Pickles, A., Toseeb, U., & Botting, N. (2019). Do emotional difficulties and peer problems occur together from childhood to adolescence?: The case of children with a history of developmental language disorder (DLD). *European Child and Adolescent Psychiatry, 28*(7), 993–1004.

Conti-Ramsden, G., St Clair, M. C., Pickles, A., & Durkin, K. (2012). Developmental trajectories of verbal and nonverbal skills in individuals with a history of specific language impairment: From childhood to adolescence. *Journal of Speech, Language, and Hearing Research, 55*, 1716–1735.

Conti-Ramsden, G., Ullman, M. T., & Lum, J. A. (2015). The relation between receptive grammar and procedural, declarative, and working memory in specific language impairment. *Frontiers in Psychology, 6*, Article 1090.

Craig, H. K., & Washington, J. A. (2006). *Malik goes to school: Examining the language skills of African American students from preschool–5th grade*. Mahwah, NJ: Erlbaum.

Dodd, B., Holm, A., Hua, Z., & Crosbie, S. (2003). A normative study of British-speaking children. *Clinical Linguistic Phonology, 17*(8), 617–643.

Ebert, K. D., & Pham, G. (2019). Including nonlinguistic processing tasks in the identification of developmental language disorder. *American Journal of Speech–Language Pathology, 28*(3), 932–944.

Eicher, J. D., Powers, N. R., Miller, L. L., Akshoomoff, N., Amaral, D. G., Bloss, C. S., . . . Chang, L. (2013). Genome-wide association study of shared components of reading disability and language impairment. *Genes, Brain and Behavior, 12*(8), 792–801.

Elliott, J. G., & Grigorenko, E. L. (2014). *The dyslexia debate*. New York: Cambridge University Press.

Facoetti, A., Corradi, N., Ruffino, M., Gori, S., & Zorzi, M. (2010). Visual spatial attention and speech segmentation are both impaired in preschoolers at familial risk for developmental dyslexia. *Dyslexia, 16*, 226–239.

Fletcher, J. M., Lyon, G. R., Fuchs, L. S., & Barnes, M. A. (2018). *Learning disabilities: From identification to intervention*. New York: Guilford Press.

Franceschini, S., Gori, S., Ruffino, M., Pedroll, K., & Facoetti, A. (2012). A causal link between spatial attention and reading acquisition. *Current Biology, 22*(9), 814–819.

Fu, W., Zhao, J., Ding, Y., & Wang, Z. (2019). Dyslexic children are sluggish in disengaging spatial attention. *Dyslexia, 25*(2), 158–172.

Gall, F. J. (1825). *Sur les fonctions de cerveau et sur celles de chacune de ses parties* [*On the functions of the brain and those of each of its parts*.]. Paris: Chez J.-B. Bailliere Libraire.

Gallinat, E., & Spaulding, T. J. (2014). Differences in the performance of children with specific language impairment and their typically developing peers on nonverbal cognitive tests: A meta-analysis. *Journal of Speech, Language, and Hearing Research, 57*(4), 1363–1382.

García, J. R., & Cain, K. (2014). Decoding and reading comprehension: A meta-analysis to identify which reader and assessment characteristics influence the strength of the relationship in English. *Review of Educational Research, 84*(1), 74–111.

Gathercole, S. E., & Baddeley, A. D. (1990). Phonological memory deficits in language disordered children: Is there a causal connection? *Journal of Memory and Language, 29*(3), 336–360.

Gough, P. B., & Tunmer, W. E. (1986). Decoding, reading, and reading disability. *Remedial and Special Education, 7*(1), 6–10.

Guenther, F. H. (1995). Speech sound acquisition, coarticulation, and rate effects in a neural network model of speech production. *Psychology Review, 102*(3), 594–621.

Harrison, L. J., & McLeod, S. (2010). Risk and protective factors associated with speech and language impairment in a nationally representative sample of 4- to 5-year-old children. *Journal of Speech, Language, and Hearing Research, 53*, 508–529.

Hart, B., & Risley, T. R. (1992). American parenting of language-learning children: Persisting differences in family–child interactions observed in natural home environments. *Developmental Psychology, 28*(6), 1096–1105.

Haworth, C. M., Kovas, Y., Harlaar, N., Hayiou-Thomas, M. E., Petrill, S. A., Dale, P. S., & Plomin, R. (2009). Generalist genes and learning disabilities: A multivariate genetic analysis of low performance in reading, mathematics, language and general cognitive ability in a sample of 8000 12-year-old twins. *Journal of Child Psychology and Psychiatry, 50*(10), 1318–1325.

Hayiou-Thomas, M. E. (2008). Genetic and environmental influences on early speech, language and literacy development. *Journal of Communication Disorders, 41*(5), 397–408.

Hayiou-Thomas, M. E., Carroll, J. M., Leavett, R., Hulme, C., & Snowling, M. J. (2017). When does speech sound disorder matter for literacy?: The role of disordered speech errors, co-occurring language impairment and family risk of dyslexia. *Journal of Child Psychology and Psychiatry, 58*(2), 197–205.

Hensler, B. S., Schatschneider, C., Taylor, J., & Wagner, R. K. (2010). Behavioral genetic approach to the study of dyslexia. *Journal of Developmental and Behavioral Pediatrics, 31,* 525–532.

Hickok, G., & Poeppel, D. (2007). The cortical organization of speech processing. *Nature Reviews Neuroscience, 8*(5), 393–402.

Hussar, B., Zhang, J., Hein, S., Wang, K., Roberts, A., Cui, J., . . . Dilig, R. (2020). *The condition of education* (Publication No. 2020144). Washington, DC: National Center for Education Statistics.

Joanisse, M. F., & Seidenberg, M. S. (2003). Phonology and syntax in specific language impairment: Evidence from a connectionist model. *Brain and Language, 86*(1), 40–56.

Johnson, C. J., Beitchman, J. H., & Brownlie, E. B. (2010). Twenty-year follow-up of children with and without speech–language impairments: Family, educational, occupational, and quality of life outcomes. *American Journal of Speech–Language Pathology, 19,* 51–65.

Johnson, M. H., & de Haan, M. (2011). *Developmental cognitive neuroscience.* Oxford, UK: Blackwell.

Kaufman, S. B., Reynolds, M. R., Liu, X., Kaufman, A. S., & McGrew, K. S. (2012). Are cognitive g and academic achievement g one and the same g? An exploration on the Woodcock–Johnson and Kaufman tests. *Intelligence, 40*(2), 123–138.

Kerr, J. (1897). School hygiene, in its mental, moral, and physical aspects (Howard Medical Prize Essay). *Journal of the Royal Statistical Society, 60,* 613–680.

Kirby, P. (2020). Dyslexia debated, then and now: A historical perspective on the dyslexia debate. *Oxford Review of Education, 46*(4), 472–486.

Kirby, P., Nation, K., Snowling, M., & Whyte, W. (2020). The problem of dyslexia: Historical perspectives. *Oxford Review of Education, 46*(4), 409–413.

Kolb, B., & Whishaw, I. Q. (2009). *Fundamentals of human neuropsychology* (6th ed.). New York: Freeman.

Kovas, Y., & Plomin, R. (2006). Generalist genes: Implications for the cognitive sciences. *Trends in Cognitive Sciences, 10*(5), 198–203.

Kurth, F., Luders, E., Pigdon, L., Conti-Ramsden, G., Reilly, S., & Morgan, A. T. (2018). Altered gray matter volumes in language-associated regions in children with developmental language disorder and speech sound disorder. *Developmental Psychobiology, 60*(7), 814–824.

Law, J., Garrett, Z., & Nye, C. (2003). Speech and language therapy interventions for children with primary speech and language delay or disorder. *Cochrane Database of Systematic Reviews, 3,* CD004110.

Lee, J. C., Dick, A. S., & Tomblin, J. B. (2020). Altered brain structures in the dorsal and ventral language pathways in individuals with and without developmental language disorder (DLD). *Brain Imaging and Behavior, 14,* 2569–2586.

Lee, J. C., Nopoulos, P. C., & Tomblin, J. B. (2020). Procedural and declarative memory brain systems in developmental language disorder (DLD). *Brain and Language, 205,* Article 104789.

Leonard, L. B. (2014). *Children with specific language impairment* (2nd ed.). Cambridge, MA: MIT Press.

Lewis, B. A., & Freebairn, L. (1992). Residual effects of preschool phonology disorders in grade school, adolescence, and adulthood. *Journal of Speech and Hearing Research, 35*(4), 819–831.

Lewis, B. A., Avrich, A. A., Freebairn, L. A., Hansen, A. J., Sucheston, L. E., Kuo, I., . . . Stein, C. M. (2011). Literacy outcomes of children with early childhood speech sound disorders: Impact of endophenotypes. *Journal of Speech, Language, and Hearing Research, 54,* 1628–1643.

Lewis, B. A., Freebairn, L., Tag, J., Ciesla, A. A., Iyengar, S. K., Stein, C. M., & Taylor, H. G. (2015). Adolescent outcomes of children with early speech sound disorders with and without language impairment. *American Journal of Speech–Language Pathology, 24*(2), 150–163.

Lewis, B. A., Patton, E., Freebairn, L., Tag, J., Iyengar, S. K., Stein, C. M., & Taylor, H. G. (2016). Psychosocial co-morbidities in adolescents and adults with histories of communication disorders. *Journal of Communication Disorders, 61,* 60–70.

Lewis, B. A., & Thompson, L. A. (1992). A study of developmental speech and language disorders in twins. *Journal of Speech and Hearing Research, 35*(5), 1086–1094.

Logan, J. A. R., Cutting, L., Schatschneider, C., Hart, S. A., Deater-Deckard, K., & Peterill, S. (2013). Reading development in young children: Genetic and environmental influence *Child Development, 84,* 2131-2144.

Luders, E., Kurth, F., Pigdon, L., Conti-Ramsden, G., Reilly, S., & Morgan, A. T. (2017). Atypical callosal morphology in children with speech sound disorder. *Neuroscience, 367,* 211–218.

Lum, J. A. G., Conti-Ramsden, G., Morgan, A. T., & Ullman, M. T. (2014). Procedural learning deficits in specific language impairment (SLI): A meta-analysis of serial reaction time task performance. *Cortex, 51,* 1–10.

Lyytinen, H., Guttorm, T. K., Huttunen, T., Hämäläinen, J., Leppänen, P. H., & Vesterinen, M. (2005). Psychophysiology of developmental dyslexia: A review of findings including studies of children at risk for dyslexia. *Journal of Neurolinguistics, 18*(2), 167–195.

Mascheretti, S., Trezzi, V., Giorda, R., Boivin, M., Plourde, V., Vitaro, F., . . . Marino, C. (2017). Complex effects of dyslexia risk factors account for ADHD traits: Evidence from two independent samples. *Journal of Child Psychology and Psychiatry, 58*(1), 75–82.

Mayes, A. K., Reilly, S., & Morgan, A. T. (2015). Neural correlates of childhood language disorder: A systematic review. *Developmental Medicine and Child Neurology, 57*(8), 706–717.

McGrath, L. M., Pennington, B. F., Shanahan, M. A., Santerre-Lemmon, L. E., Barnard, H. D., Willcutt, E. G., . . . Olson, R. K. (2011). A multiple deficit model of reading disability and attention-deficit/hyperactivity disorder: Searching for shared cognitive deficits. *Journal of Child Psychology and Psychiatry, 52*(5), 547–557.

McGrath, L. M., Peterson, R. L., & Pennington, B. F. (2020). The multiple deficit model: Progress, problems, and prospects. *Scientific Studies of Reading, 24*(1), 7–13.

Mok, P. L., Pickles, A., Durkin, K., & Conti-Ramsden, G. (2014). Longitudinal trajectories of peer relations in children with specific language impairment. *Journal of Child Psychology and Psychiatry, 55*(5), 516–527.

Morgan, P. L., Farkas, G., Hillemeier, M. M., Mattison, R., Maczuga, S., Li, H., & Cook, M. (2015). Minorities are disproportionately underrepresented in special education: Longitudinal evidence across five disability conditions. *Educational Researcher, 44*(5), 278–292.

Morgan, A. T., Su, M., Reilly, S., Conti-Ramsden, G., Connelly, A., & Liégeois, F. J. (2018). A brain marker for developmental speech disorders. *Journal of Pediatrics, 198,* 234–239.

Mueller, K. L., & Tomblin, J. B. (2012). Examining the comorbidity of language disorders and ADHD. *Topics in Language Disorders, 32*(3), 228–246.

Nation, K., Cocksey, J., Taylor, J. S., & Bishop, D. V. (2010). A longitudinal investigation of early reading and language skills in children with poor reading comprehension. *Journal of Child Psychology and Psychiatry, 51*(9), 1031–1039.

Nelson, K. (1998). *Language in cognitive development: The emergence of the mediated mind.* New York: Cambridge University Press.

Niogi, S. N., & McCandliss, B. D. (2006). Left lateralized white matter microstructure accounts for individual differences in reading ability and disability. *Neuropsychologia, 44*(11), 2178–2188.

Norbury, C. F., Gooch, D., Wray, C., Baird, G., Charman, T., Simonoff, E., . . . Pickles, A. (2016). The impact of nonverbal ability on prevalence and clinical presentation of language disorder: Evidence from a population study. *Journal of Child Psychology and Psychiatry, 57*(11), 1247–1257.

Norton, E. S., & Wolf, M. (2012). Rapid automatized naming (RAN) and reading fluency: Implications for understanding and treatment of reading disabilities. *Annual Review of Psychology, 63,* 427–452.

Nye, C., Foster, S. H., & Seaman, D. (1987). Effectiveness of language intervention with the language/learning disabled. *Journal of Speech and Hearing Disorders, 52*(4), 348–357.

Orton, S. T. (1925). "Word-blindness" in school children. *Archives of Neurology and Psychiatry, 14,* 582–615.

Paulesu, E., Danelli, L., & Berlingeri, M. (2014). Reading the dyslexic brain: Multiple dysfunctional routes revealed by a new meta-analysis of PET and fMRI activation studies. *Frontiers in Human Neuroscience, 8,* Article 830.

Paulesu, E., Demonet, J. F., Fazio, F., McCrory, E., Chanoine, V., Brunswick, N., . . . Frith, U. (2001). Dyslexia: Cultural diversity and biological unity. *Science, 291,* 2165–2167.

Peng, P., Wang, T., Wang, C., & Lin, X. (2019). A meta-analysis on the relation between fluid intelligence and reading/mathematics: Effects of tasks, age, and social economics status. *Psychological Bulletin, 145*(2), 189–236.

Pennington, B. F. (2006). From single to multiple deficit models of developmental disorders. *Cognition, 101*(2), 385–413.

Pennington, B. F., McGrath, L. M., & Peterson, R.

L. (2019). *Diagnosing learning disorders: From science to practice*. New York: Guilford Press.

Pennington, B. F., Santerre-Lemmon, L., Rosenberg, J., MacDonald, B., Boada, R., Friend, A., . . . Olson, R. K. (2012). Individual prediction of dyslexia by single versus multiple deficit models. *Journal of Abnormal Psychology, 121*, 212–224.

Peters, L., & Ansari, D. (2019). Are specific learning disorders truly specific, and are they disorders? *Trends in Neuroscience and Education, 17*, Article 100115.

Peters, L., Bulthé, J., Daniels, N., de Beeck, H. O., & De Smedt, B. (2018). Dyscalculia and dyslexia: Different behavioral, yet similar brain activity profiles during arithmetic. *NeuroImage: Clinical, 18*, 663–674.

Peterson, R. L., Boada, R., McGrath, L. M., Willcutt, E. G., Olson, R. K., & Pennington, B. F. (2017). Cognitive prediction of reading, math, and attention: Shared and unique influences. *Journal of Learning Disabilities, 50*(4), 408–421.

Peterson, R. L., McGrath, L. M., Willcutt, E. G., Keenan, J. M., Olson, R. K., and Pennington, B. F. (2021). How specific are learning disabilities? *Journal of Learning Disabilities, 54*(6).

Peterson, R. L., Pennington, B. F., Shriberg, L. D., & Boada, R. (2009). What influences literacy outcome in children with speech sound disorder? *Journal of Speech, Language, and Hearing Research, 52*, 1175–1188.

Pham, G. T., Pruitt-Lord, S., Snow, C. E., Nguyen, Y. H. T., Phạm, B., Dao, T. B. T., . . . Dam, Q. D. (2019). Identifying developmental language disorder in Vietnamese children. *Journal of Speech, Language, and Hearing Research, 62*(5), 1452–1467.

Poeppel, D., Emmorey, K., Hickok, G., & Pylkkanen, L. (2012). Towards a new neurobiology of language. *Journal of Neuroscience, 32*(41), 14125–14131.

Preston, J. L., Felsenfeld, S., Frost, S. J., Mencl, W. E., Fulbright, R. K., Grigorenko, E. L., . . . Pugh, K. R. (2012). Functional brain activation differences in school-age children with speech sound errors: Speech and print processing. *Journal of Speech, Language, and Hearing Research, 55*(4), 1068–1082.

Preston, J. L., Molfese, P. J., Mencl, W. E., Frost, S. J., Hoeft, F., Fulbright, R. K., . . . Pugh, K. R. (2014). Structural brain differences in school-age children with residual speech sound errors. *Brain and Language, 128*(1), 25–33.

Pringle-Morgan, W. (1896). A case of congenital word blindness. *British Medical Journal, 2*(1871), Article 1378.

Raitano, N. A., Pennington, B. F., Tunick, R. A., Boada, R., & Shriberg, L. D. (2004). Pre-literacy skills of subgroups of children with speech sound disorders. *Journal of Child Psychology and Psychiatry, 45*(4), 821–835.

Raschle, N. M., Chang, M., & Gaab, N. (2011). Structural brain alterations associated with dyslexia predate reading onset. *NeuroImage, 57*(3), 742–749.

Raschle, N. M., Zuk, J., & Gaab, N. (2012). Functional characteristics of developmental dyslexia in left-hemispheric posterior brain regions predate reading onset. *Proceedings of the National Academy of Sciences USA, 109*(6), 2156–2161.

Redcay, E., Haist, F., & Courchesne, E. (2008). Functional neuroimaging of speech perception during a pivotal period in language acquisition. *Developmental Science, 11*(2), 237–252.

Rice, M. L., Taylor, C. L., Zubrick, S. R., Hoffman, L., & Earnest, K. K. (2020). Heritability of specific language impairment and nonspecific language impairment at ages 4 and 6 years across phenotypes of speech, language, and nonverbal cognition. *Journal of Speech, Language, and Hearing Research, 63*(3), 793–813.

Rice, M. L., Wexler, K., & Cleave, P. L. (1995). Specific language impairment as a period of extended optional infinitive. *Journal of Speech and Hearing Research, 38*(4), 850–863.

Richardson, U., Thomson, J. M., Scott, S. K., & Goswami, U. (2004). Auditory processing skills and phonological representation in dyslexic children. *Dyslexia, 10*(3), 215–233.

Richlan, F., Kronbichler, M., & Wimmer, H. (2011). Meta-analyzing brain dysfunctions in dyslexic children and adults. *NeuroImage, 56*(3), 1735–1742.

Richlan, F., Kronbichler, M., & Wimmer, H. (2013). Structural abnormalities in the dyslexic brain: A meta-analysis of voxel-based morphometry studies. *Human Brain Mapping, 34*(11), 3055–3065.

Rutter, M., Caspi, A., Fergusson, D., Horwood, L. J., Goodman, R., Maughan, B., . . . Carroll, J. (2004). Sex differences in developmental reading disability: New findings from 4 epidemiological studies. *Journal of the American Medical Association, 291*(16), 2007–2012.

Rutter, M., Thorpe, K., Greenwood, R., Northstone, K., & Golding, J. (2003). Twins as a natural experiment to study the causes of mild language delay: I: Design; twin-singleton differences in language, and obstetric risks. *Journal of Child Psychology and Psychiatry, 44*(3), 326–341.

Saffran, J. R., Aslin, R. N., & Newport, E. L. (1996).

Statistical learning by 8-month-old infants. *Science, 274*(5294), 1926–1928.

Savage, R. (2004). Motor skills, automaticity and developmental dyslexia: A review of the research literature. *Reading and Writing, 17*(3), 301–324.

Scammacca, N., Roberts, G., Vaughn, S., & Stuebing, K. K. (2015). A meta-analysis of interventions for struggling readers in grades 4–12: 1980–2011. *Journal of Learning Disabilities, 48*(4), 369–390.

Scammacca, N., Vaughn, S., Roberts, G., Wanzek, J., & Torgesen, J. K. (2007). *Extensive reading intervention in grades K–3: From research to practice.* Portsmouth, NH: Research Corporation, Center on Instruction.

Scarborough, H. S. (1991). Antecedents to reading disability: Preschool language development and literacy experiences of children from dyslexic families. *Reading and Writing, 3*(3), 219–233.

Scarborough, H. S., Catts, H. W., & Kamhi, A. G. (2005). Developmental relationships between language and reading: Reconciling a beautiful hypothesis with some ugly facts. In H. W. Catts & A. G. Kamhi (Eds.), *The connections between language and reading disabilities* (pp. 3–24). Mahwah, NJ: Erlbaum.

Scerri, T. S., Macpherson, E., Martinelli, A., Wa, W. C., Monaco, A. P., Stein, J., . . . Snowling, M. J. (2017). The DCDC2 deletion is not a risk factor for dyslexia. *Translational Psychiatry, 7*(7), Article e1182.

Shriberg, L. D., Tomblin, J. B., & McSweeny, J. L. (1999). Prevalence of speech delay in 6-year-old children and comorbidity with language impairment. *Journal of Speech, Language, and Hearing Research, 42*(6), 1461–1481.

Siugzdaite, R., Bathelt, J., Holmes, J., & Astle, D. E. (2020). Transdiagnostic brain mapping in developmental disorders. *Current Biology, 30*, 1245–1257.

Smith, S. D., Pennington, B. F., Boada, R., & Shriberg, L. D. (2005). Linkage of speech sound disorder to reading disability loci. *Journal of Child Psychology and Psychiatry, 46*(10), 1057–1066.

Snowling, M. J., Bishop, D. V. M., Stothard, S. E., Chipchase, B., & Kaplan, C. (2006). Psychosocial outcomes at 15 years of children with a preschool history of speech–language impairment. *Journal of Child Psychology and Psychiatry, 47*(8), 759–765.

Snowling, M. J., Gallagher, A., & Frith, U. (2003). Family risk of dyslexia is continuous: Individual differences in the precursors of reading skill. *Child Development, 74*(2), 358–373.

Snowling, M. J., & Melby-Lervåg, M. (2016). Oral language deficits in familial dyslexia: A meta-analysis and review. *Psychological Bulletin, 142*(5), 498–545.

Spencer, M., Quinn, J. M., & Wagner, R. K. (2014). Specific reading comprehension disability: Major problem, myth, or misnomer?. *Learning Disabilities Research and Practice, 29*(1), 3–9.

Spencer, M., & Wagner, R. K. (2018). The comprehension problems of children with poor reading comprehension despite adequate decoding: A meta-analysis. *Review of Educational Research, 88*(3), 366–400.

Stanovich, K. E. (2005). The future of a mistake: Will discrepancy measurement continue to make the learning disabilities field a pseudoscience? *Learning Disability Quarterly, 28*(2), 103–106.

Stanovich, K. E. (2009). Matthew effects in reading: Some consequences of individual differences in the acquisition of literacy. *Journal of Education, 189*(1–2), 23–55.

Stothard, S. E., Snowling, M. J., Bishop, D. V. M., Chipchase, B. B., & Kaplan, C. A. (1998). Language-impaired preschoolers: A follow-up into adolescence. *Journal of Speech, Language, and Hearing Research, 41*(2), 407–418.

Stuebing, K. K., Barth, A. E., Trahan, L. H., Reddy, R. R., Miciak, J., & Fletcher, J. M. (2015). Are child cognitive characteristics strong predictors of responses to intervention?: A meta-analysis. *Review of Educational Research, 85*(3), 395–429.

Tallal, P., & Piercy, M. (1973). Developmental aphasia: Impaired rate of nonverbal processing as a function of sensory modality. *Neuropsychologia, 11*, 389-398.

Terband, H., Maassen, B., Guenther, F. H., & Brumberg, J. (2014a). Auditory–motor interactions in pediatric motor speech disorders: Neurocomputational modeling of disordered development. *Journal of Communication Disorders, 47*, 17–33.

Terband, H., van Brenk, F., & van Doornik-van der Zee, A. (2014b). Auditory feedback perturbation in children with developmental speech sound disorders. *Journal of Communication Disorders, 51*, 64–77.

Tomblin, J. B., Records, N. L., Buckwalter, P., Zhang, X., Smith, E., & O'Brien, M. (1997). Prevalence of specific language impairment in kindergarten children. *Journal of Speech, Language, and Hearing Research, 40*(6), 1245–1260.

Ullman, M. T., & Pierpont, E. I. (2005). Specific language impairment is not specific to language: The procedural deficit hypothesis. *Cortex, 41*(3), 399–433.

Vandermosten, M., Boets, B., Wouters, J., & Ghesquière, P. (2012). A qualitative and quantitative review of diffusion tensor imaging studies in reading and dyslexia. *Neuroscience and Biobehavioral Reviews, 36*(6), 1532–1552.

Vandermosten, M., Vanderauwera, J., Theys, C., De Vos, A., Vanvooren, S., Sunaert, S., . . . Ghesquière, P. (2015). A DTI tractography study in pre-readers at risk for dyslexia. *Developmental Cognitive Neuroscience, 14,* 8–15.

Vaughn, S., Denton, C. A., & Fletcher, J. M. (2010). Why intensive interventions are necessary for students with severe reading difficulties. *Psychology in the Schools, 47*(5), 432–444.

Vellutino, F. R. (1979). The validity of perceptual deficit explanations of reading disability: A reply to Fletcher and Satz. *Journal of Learning Disabilities, 12*(3), 160–167.

Vellutino, F. R., Fletcher, J. M., Snowling, M. J., & Scanlon, D. M. (2004). Specific reading disability (dyslexia): What have we learned in the past four decades? *Journal of Child Psychology and Psychiatry, 45*(1), 2–40.

Vellutino, F. R., Scanlon, D. M., & Lyon, G. R. (2000). Differentiating between difficult-to-remediate and readily remediated poor readers: More evidence against the IQ–achievement discrepancy definition of reading disability. *Journal of Learning Disabilities, 33*(3), 223–238.

Verhoeven, L., Perfetti, C., & Pugh, K. (Eds.). (2019). *Developmental dyslexia across languages and writing systems.* New York: Cambridge University Press.

Verly, M., Gerrits, R., Sleurs, C., Lagae, L., Sunaert, S., Zink, I., & Rommel, N. (2019). The miswired language network in children with developmental language disorder: Insights from DTI tractography. *Brain Imaging and Behavior, 13*(4), 973–984.

Wadsworth, S. J., Olson, R. K., Pennington, B. F., & DeFries, J. C. (2000). Differential genetic etiology of reading disability as a function of IQ. *Journal of Learning Disabilities, 33*(2), 192–199.

Washington, J. A., Branum-Martin, L., Sun, C., & Lee-James, R. (2018). The impact of dialect density on the growth of language and reading in African American children. *Language, Speech, and Hearing Services in Schools, 49*(2), 232–247.

Washington, J. A., Terry, N. P., & Seidenberg, M. S. (2013). Language variation and literacy learning: The case of African American English. In C. A. Stone, E. R. Silliman, B. J. Ehren, & G. P. Wallach (Eds.), *Handbook of language and literacy: Development and disorders* (2nd ed., pp. 204–221). New York: Guilford Press.

Weber, A., Fernald, A., & Diop, Y. (2017). When cultural norms discourage talking to babies: Effectiveness of a parenting program in rural Senegal. *Child Development, 88*(5), 1513–1526.

Weisleder, A., & Fernald, A. (2013). Talking to children matters: Early language experience strengthens processing and builds vocabulary. *Psychological Science, 24*(11), 2143–2152.

Willcutt, E. G., & Pennington, B. F. (2000). Psychiatric comorbidity in children and adolescents with reading disability. *Journal of Child Psychology and Psychiatry, 41*(8), 1039–1048.

Willcutt, E. G., Petrill, S. A., Wu, S., Boada, R., DeFries, J. C., Olson, R. K., & Pennington, B. F. (2013). Comorbidity between reading disability and math disability: Concurrent psychopathology, functional impairment, and neuropsychological functioning. *Journal of Learning Disabilities, 46*(6), 500–516.

Wittke, K., & Spaulding, T. J. (2018). Which preschool children with specific language impairment receive language intervention? *Language, Speech, and Hearing Services in Schools, 49*(1), 59–71.

Wren, Y., Miller, L. L., Peters, T. J., Emond, A., & Roulstone, S. (2016). Prevalence and predictors of persistent speech sound disorder at eight years old: Findings from a population cohort study. *Journal of Speech, Language, and Hearing Research, 59*(4), 647–673.

Ziegler, J. C., & Goswami, U. (2005). Reading acquisition, developmental dyslexia, and skilled reading across languages: A psycholinguistic grain size theory. *Psychological Bulletin, 131*(1), 3–29.

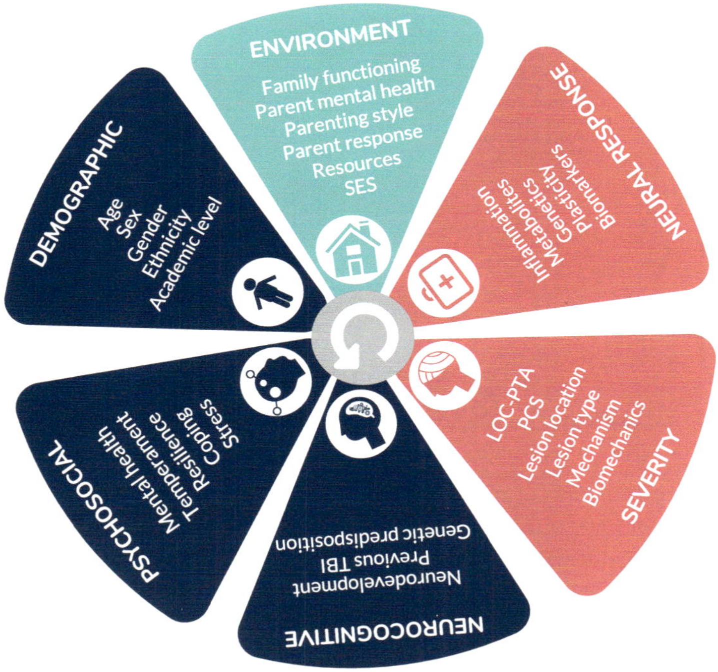

PLATE 5.1. A conceptual model of the range of factors that contribute to outcome (represented by center circle) after pediatric TBI. Child factors (dark green) represent premorbid and postinjury characteristics of the child that moderate injury consequences. These are divided into three categories, including *demographic factors* (e.g., age, sex, ethnicity, and education or academic level); historical *neurocognitive factors* (e.g., history of previous TBI, premorbid neurodevelopmental conditions, genetic predispositions); and pre- and postinjury *psychosocial factors* (e.g., child's temperament or personality, stress and mental health, and individual traits such as resilience or coping mechanisms). Environmental factors (turquoise) refer to the environment in which the child is developing (e.g., family socioeconomic status (SES), access to resources, and parent responses to the injury, and effects of family relations and parenting factors on the child's response to injury). Injury factors (pink) include both injury severity (e.g., duration of loss of consciousness [LOC] and posttraumatic amnesia [PTA], presence and duration of postconcussive symptoms [PCS], presence and location of intracranial lesions, and biomechanical aspects of injury) and indications of neural responses to injury (e.g., biomarkers, plasticity, genetic factors, and metabolic and inflammatory processes).

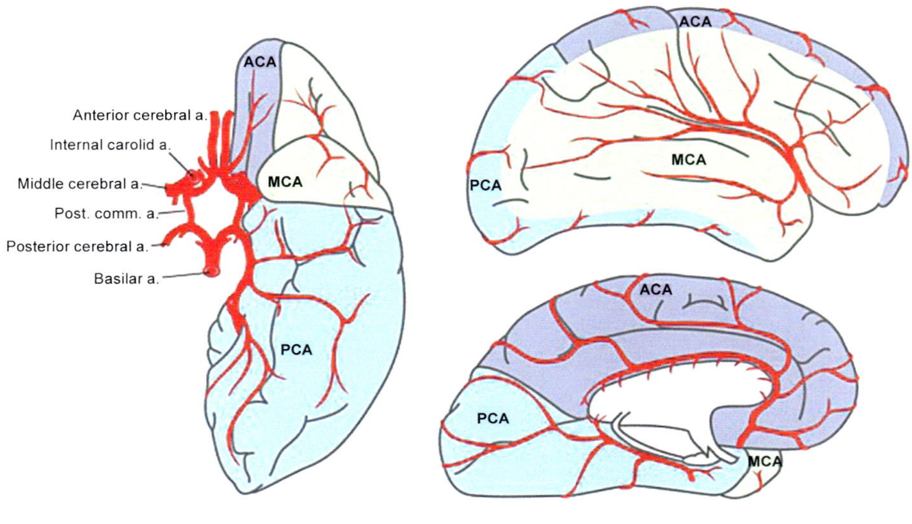

PLATE 6.1. Arterial supply of the cerebral cortex.

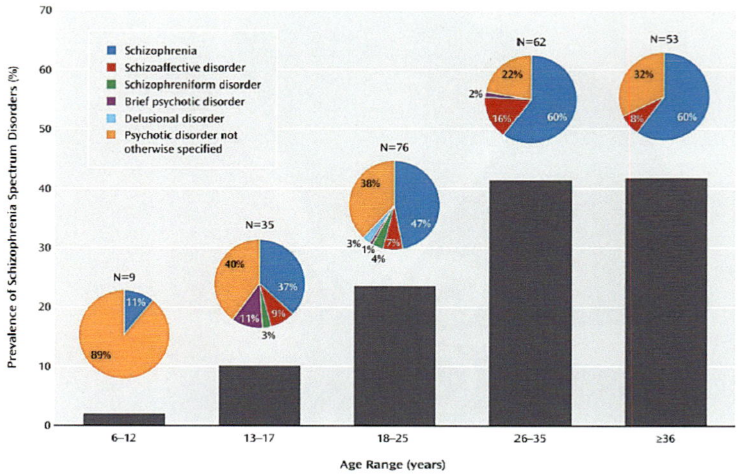

PLATE 18.1. Prevalence of schizophrenia spectrum disorders and distribution of specific disorders by age in participants with 22q11.2 deletion syndrome. From an original 1,402 participants diagnosed with 22q11.2 deletion syndrome assessed for psychiatric disorders, 235 were diagnosed with schizophrenia spectrum disorders. The prevalence of schizophrenia increased significantly with age ($\chi^2 = 12.54$, $df = 4$, $p = .01$), whereas the diagnosis of psychotic disorder not otherwise specified decreased ($\chi^2 = 17.17$, $df = 4$, $p = .002$). Reprinted from Schneider et al. (2014) with permission from American Psychiatric Association Publishing.

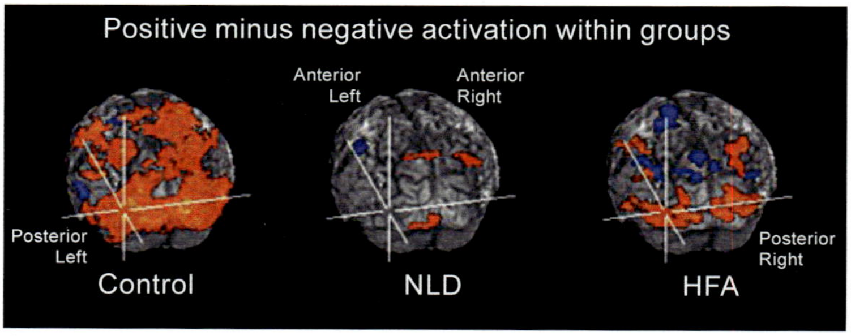

PLATE 20.1. fMRI findings indicating patterns of associated brain activity when viewing positive social interaction videos across control, NVLD, and HFA groups. The results indicate increased activity in children without social processing difficulty, as shown by the orange color, in response to positive social interactions throughout the brain, while those with HFA show more processing in the occipital lobe and those with NVLD show less activity overall (unpublished manuscript). Used with permission of Margaret Semrud-Clikeman.

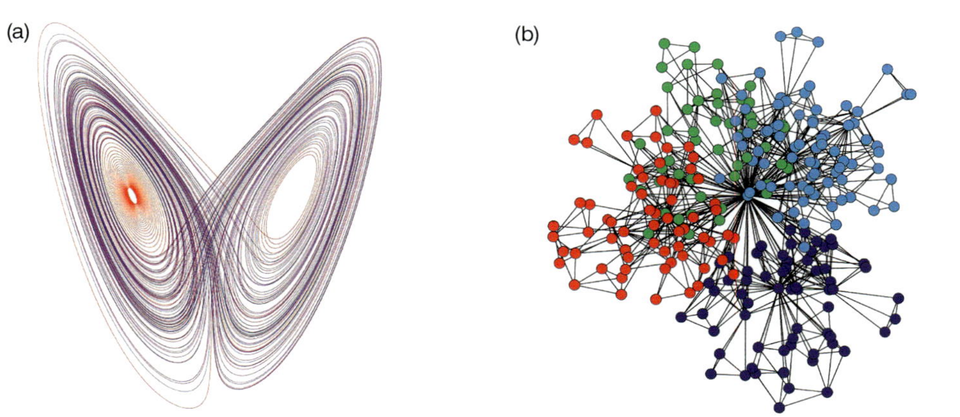

PLATE 24.1. Network metaphors: (a) Attractor in a dynamical system; (b) dynamic network image. Plate 24.1a is reprinted with permission under a Creative Commons license (*http://creativecommons.org/licenses/by-sa/3.0/deed.en*).

CHAPTER 13

Math Disability

Paul T. Cirino

HISTORICAL OVERVIEW

Background

Many of neuropsychology's classic cases involve adults with unusual and dramatic acquired symptomatology (e.g., Phineas Gage). Even among pediatric conditions, disorders in Parts II and IV of this volume are defined predominantly biologically, whereas learning disabilities and some other disorders of Part III are not. Learning disabilities do not have a sudden "onset," nor are they obvious perinatally; rather they involve a failure to acquire taught skills and so in this sense are "normative" or "distributional" disorders.

Math disability has received less attention than reading disability (RD), though this landscape has become more equitable since Geary's (1993) landmark review. Only a fraction of the literature on math disability appears in the most common neuropsychological journals; rather, it is found in educational, developmental, or cognitive outlets given that learning disorders are defined largely along a continuum (Branum-Martin, Fletcher, & Stuebing, 2013). A corollary is that knowledge of math *dis*ability is intricately connected to a broader understanding of math *a*bility from a developmental or educational or cognitive perspective. The terms *math learning disability* or *math disability* (MD), *math difficulties*, *developmental dyscalculia*, and *low achievement in math* can be seen as interchangeable, as there is not true consensus on their differentiation (except for acquired difficulties); in this chapter, the term MD is used for convenience.

Early descriptions of MD focused on adults who lost prior mathematical skills following brain insult. For example, Singer and Low (1933) were among the first to systematically parse a variety of differentiable mathematical functions in their patient. Gerstmann (1940) associated acalculia with angular gyrus lesions and recognized the overlap with other conditions (agraphia, finger agnosia, right-left disorientation). Later, Hécaen, Angelerges, and Houiller (1961) distinguished between acalculia subtypes (spatial, with alexia, and anarithmetria). This early work highlighted several key aspects of MD, namely, the debate about the relative importance of verbal and spatial contributions, the recognition that MD co-occurs with other disorders (and the extent to which it is isolatable), and the need to understand the wide array of math subskills.

Classification/Definition/Identification

MD as a diagnosis, and its precise meaning as it emerges outside of specific lesions, is often debated. Taking the United States as an example case, federal law maintains a *definition* of specific learning disability that has been constant for over 50 years (U.S. Office of Education, 1968) and is applied to any academic skill. What has changed are the *procedures/regulations* that determine how to identify such individuals. For example, the most recent of these was the Individuals with Disabilities Education Act (2004), and the most recent amendment was the Every Student Succeeds Act (2015). Current iterations indicate that states must not require the use of a severe discrepancy between intellectual ability and achievement but must permit a process based on response to intervention and may permit other research-based procedures. The most recent *Diagnostic and Statistical Manual of Mental Disorders* (DSM-5; American Psychiatric Association, 2013) recognizes that specific learning disorders occur in a variety of achievement domains, specifies that the relevant academic skill must be well below the average range, and that diagnosis includes history, test scores, observations, and response to intervention. The most common math measures in the MD literature are broadband computational measures, though such measures tap a wide range of competencies taught at different times and with different emphases (addition, subtraction, multiplication, division, fractions/decimals, algebra), each of which can be further subdivided (single digit vs. multidigit, with or without carrying/borrowing).

Although the identification of learning disabilities has evolved, clinical practice and the research literature still include a variety of classification schemes. First, *discrepancy* definitions (i.e., a difference between IQ performance and achievement) continue to be used but are increasingly rare in current research literature given strong evidence against these (e.g., Fletcher et al., 1994; Francis, Shaywitz, Stuebing, Shaywitz, & Fletcher, 1996; Stuebing et al., 2002). Second, *low achievement* definitions are also common, although the referent for *low* is debatable—common demarcations include the 5th, 7th, 10th, 15th, and 25th percentiles. Some authors have suggested a more fundamental distinction between low achievement and MD, reserving the latter term for only the most severe cases (usually below the 10th percentile) (Mazzocco & Myers, 2003; Murphy, Mazzocco, Hanich, & Early, 2007), though empirical evidence for qualitative differences among such groups is thin. A third type of definition can be labeled *persistence* (Geary, Hoard, & Hamson, 1999), meaning that a student demonstrates low achievement consistently over time (usually 1 year) to promote diagnostic reliability. A fourth approach is *cognitive strengths and weaknesses,* which suggest that differences between processing skills and with regard to achievement are diagnostic of learning disability (e.g., Flanagan, Ortiz, & Alfonso, 2013), though at least in the reading literature, the empirical evidence for this approach is weak (see debate: Fletcher & Miciak, 2017; Schneider & Kaufman, 2017). A final approach, *response to intervention* (RTI) has as a central tenet that delivery of additional services occurs according to need (performance in the classroom) rather than to a diagnostic label, although it can also lead to the conclusion that the term *learning disability* might best be reserved for students who do not improve when provided scientifically based remediation (i.e., "nonresponders"). Diagnostic approaches can be combined, such that initial weak performance for age/grade (low achievement) prompts tracking over time (persistence), meanwhile providing graded support to help students improve (RTI).

Summary

The previous discussion highlights a number of key issues regarding the historical context of MD. First, difficulties in math may occur as a result of brain injury (in adults or children), but MD is more commonly a developmental phenomenon. Therefore, the understanding of MD is to some extent not separable from the broader literature on mathematical development. Second, generalizations about MD must consider the procedures used for identification of the disorder, with most current research work deemphasizing discrepancies (among cognitive, or between cognitive and achievement domains), and instead focusing on low achievement and response to intervention. As will become more apparent throughout this chapter, it is also important to note that knowledge of MD has strong "gradient" effects, in terms of time (most work in the area is recent), in terms of age (most work is with young children), and in terms of math content (most work is focused on basic arithmetic and skills early in the math hierarchy).

EPIDEMIOLOGY

The epidemiology of MD is confounded with whatever classification approach is adopted. For example, discrepancy approaches identify fewer children than do low achievement approaches, because IQ and achievement are correlated. Within any individual classification approach, parameters may also vary (e.g., discrepancies of 2 *SD* are rarer than those of 1 *SD*; low achievement at the 10th percentile is rarer than at the 25th percentile). Epidemiology can also be confounded with the *measures* used for identification, which is often further confounded with *content*. For example, many measures (of computations, or math fact fluency, or math reasoning) are well-normed/standardized, but others (of math cognition, of fractions) are often experimental, with varying psychometric properties, which in turn affects who is identified with MD.

With such caveats in mind, work by Barbaresi, Katusic, Colligan, Weaver, and Jacobsen (2005) is an example of an *incidence* study (a followed birth cohort) in the U.S. Midwest. Cumulative incidence rates were 5.2–9.3% for discrepancy definitions, and 13% for low achievement. But most large-scale studies of MD are *prevalence* studies, denoting the proportion of the population with MD at any given time, and these estimates approximate 6% across countries (Badian, 1999; Morsanyi, van Bers, McCormack, & McGourty, 2018).

Where low achievement is used as a criterion, results will approximate the cut point. For example, Morgan, Farkas, and Wu (2009), using a 10th percentile cutoff point, found that 791 out of 7,892 (10%) students met this criterion. But when additional criteria were implemented (persistent low achievement across fall and spring of kindergarten), the rate was 5.9%. Shalev, Manor, Auerbach, and Gross-Tsur (1998) found that only half of those with MD met the same (low achievement) criteria 3 years later, but 95% remained in the bottom quartile of their school. In a later study using two large representative databases, Morgan, Farkas, Hillemeier, and Maczuga (2016), found that with a 25th percentile criterion, 16% met a *persistence* definition that spanned 1 to 5 years. Thus, even though earlier math is strongly related to later math, any given dichotomous designation (MD vs. not) will vary over time (Martin et al., 2013).

ETIOLOGY, NEUROPATHOLOGY, AND NEURAL SUBSTRATES

Genetic and Environmental Etiology

Some genetically defined disorders are associated with risk for MD (including several of those in Part IV of this volume), but there is no single or even major cause of most cases of MD. Genetic factors specific to math are not well understood, but current hints come from quantitative genetic studies, including behavioral genetic/genetically sensitive design studies (e.g., relative risk, twin studies, multivariate studies), or from molecular studies (e.g., microarrays, whole genome sequencing). On the behavioral genetics side, heritability estimates for MD are moderate (.47), and the same genetic factors appear to be relevant for RD as well (Kovas et al., 2007), supporting the generalist genes hypothesis (Plomin & Kovas, 2005). Estimates of heritability have been found to decrease from ages 7–12 (Kovas et al., 2013), and may be higher (and shared environmental influences lower) in countries with a national curriculum that reduces environmental range (e.g., in the United Kingdom vs. the United States; Petrill & Kovas, 2016). Petrill et al. (2012) found that math fluency showed a distinct heritability pattern from untimed math measures and from reading fluency, which is relevant given the strong role that math fact retrieval plays in studies of MD (Geary, 1993). On the molecular genetics side, attempts have been made to identify relevant single-nucleotide polymorphisms (SNPs) and gene × environment interactions (Docherty et al., 2010; Docherty, Kovas, & Plomin, 2011). However, more studies are needed, and existing effect sizes are small and in need of replication.

Turning to other factors, it is not hard to imagine how environmental issues (e.g., limited exposure, obstacles to learning, poor instruction, low socioeconomic status) may negatively impact math learning. For example, young children with poor math exposure may fail to gain experience with informal math learning. Similarly, instability within the family, or financial, emotional, dietary, or housing domains can negatively impact learning. And, certainly, poor math instruction can lead to weak learning, particularly if a curriculum is not systematic, explicit, based in research, or implemented with fidelity. However, such "lack of opportunity" issues are not the *etiology* of MD by definition (they are "exclusionary" criteria; American Psychiatric Association, 2013). In practice, though, it is difficult to determine how much the source of a child's math difficulty is due to environmental versus nonenvironmental issues.

Neuropathology and Neural Substrates

Neuroimaging in MD (and in math in general) has increased greatly over the past 15 years in ways that support and expand upon theoretical models (Dehaene & Cohen, 1995; von Aster & Shalev, 2007). On the structural side, children with MD show decreased gray matter (GM) across several areas of the left hemisphere (LH; superior and inferior temporal gyri), right hemisphere (RH; inferior frontal, intraparietal sulcus [IPS]), and bilaterally (medial temporal lobe, superior parietal lobule) (Ashkenazi, Black, Abrams, Hoeft, & Menon, 2013; Rykhlevskaia, Uddin, Kondos, & Menon, 2009). White matter (WM) differences have also been identified, such as reduced WM volume in children with MD relative to controls in the inferior parietal lobule and temporal lobes (Ranpura et al., 2013; Rykhlevskaia et al., 2009). Ranpura et al. (2013) also evaluated group-by-age interactions, demonstrating differences over time in GM for left supramarginal gyrus (MD gained less), and in WM for LH superior temporal, and bilateral superior frontal areas (MD stable or decrease, and controls gained).

There are more functional than structural math studies, most of which focus on typical development. Rivera, Reiss, Eckert, and Menon (2005) found that activity in some LH areas (supramarginal and inferior temporal) was greater at increased age, while several (predominantly LH) frontal areas had less activity at increased age; this anterior-to-posterior shift has been observed by others as well (Ansari & Dhital, 2006; Kucian, von Aster, Loenneker, Dietrich, & Martin, 2008). In addition, other work has found that hippocampal activity tracks with retrieval (activity is correlated during learning), which is in turn associated with a decreased reliance on prefrontal areas; finally, the relation of hippocampal activity with retrieval decreases with mastery (Cho et al., 2012; Qin et al., 2014; Menon, 2016). The few functional studies specific to MD (Kaufmann, Wood, Rubinsten, & Henik, 2011) do note group differences predominantly in frontal and parietal areas, which were supported in a subsequent study (Ashkenazi, Rosenberg-Lee, Tenison, & Menon, 2012) that also showed that children with MD (unlike typically developing children) did not show the expected increase in neural responses in key areas as problem complexity increased.

These data, together with excellent summaries of this literature (Fias, Menon, & Szücs, 2013; Peters & DeSmedt, 2018; Menon, 2016), paint a picture of a broad-based neural network that is used to complete most any arithmetic problem. Initial number identification (visual cortex and then lingual/fusiform gyri) precedes quantity processing (IPS/superior parietal), and concurrently, working memory (basal ganglia, dorsolateral prefrontal) maintains short-term memory representations/manipulations, as the long-term memory formation system (anterior and medial temporal lobe, angular gyrus) activates. All the while, a salience system (ventrolateral prefrontal, insula) helps maintain attention for problem solving.

This brief overview of the neural underpinnings of MD highlights extremely interesting developments that further understanding of MD, but with two caveats. First, most work is focused on simple arithmetic processing, with an additional branch of work focused on quantity and the role of the IPS over development, specifically with increased LH activity for symbolic stimuli (Emerson & Cantlon, 2015; Vogel, Grabner, Schneider, Siegler, & Ansari, 2013). There is less work in areas such as rational numbers or algebra. Second, neuroimaging has not progressed to the point where it can be used diagnostically or at an individual clinical level. However, it can be used as external validation in testing classification hypotheses or theorizing areas of activity for a given math cognitive function or areas that coincide with behavioral changes as a result of intervention. For example, Supekar et al. (2013) found that improvement in a math facts intervention was predicted by hippocampal volume and connectivity with basal ganglia and prefrontal areas. As noted by Bugden and Ansari (2015), knowledge of these structural and functional imaging results demonstrate that cognitive neuroscience can constrain our models of mathematics.

NEUROPSYCHOLOGICAL CORRELATES

General Intellectual Functioning

Individuals with MD have lower IQ scores on average than those without MD for multiple reasons. IQ scores and math scores are correlated (~.50–.60), so if low achievement (simple cutoff point) criteria are used, IQ scores will trend lower. The relationship between math achievement and IQ probably arises at least partly because IQ tests tend to include measures of a range of specific neurocognitive functions that are theoretically and empirically related to math (vocabulary, processing speed, working memory, spatial processing). Furthermore, MD is commonly comorbid with other neurodevelopmental disorders (e.g., reading disorder, attentional disorders, spina bifida), many of which are also associated with lower IQ scores on average.

Visuospatial, Perceptual, and Sensorimotor Skills

Visuospatial and perceptual factors have been related to mathematics at both theoretical and empirical levels (Hartje, 1987). Theoretically, the idea is that we represent magnitudes along a mental number line; therefore, in order to perceive these, we need visuospatial skills to enable this representation (Mix & Cheng, 2012; Sella, Berteletti, Lucangeli, & Zorzi, 2017). Geary (1993) reviewed visuospatial aspects as one of three manifest issues with MD, based primarily on the neuropsychological literature of acquired disorders. Supported by both cognitive and neuroimaging work, models like those of Dehaene, Piazza, Pinel, and Cohen (2003) focus on parietally mediated functions. The empirical evidence that visuospatial skills relate to mathematics is, however, decidedly mixed, likely moderated by age and by type of math outcome considered (Casey, Pezaris, & Nuttall, 1992; Cirino, Morris, & Morris, 2002, 2007; Tolar, Lederberg, & Fletcher, 2009). An important consideration is that many visuospatial tasks share variance with other cognitive domains, notably executive function (Miyake, Friedman, Rettinger, Shah, & Hegarty, 2001).

The most prominent sensorimotor skill related to mathematics concerns finger representations and use—that is, finger gnosis and fine motor skills. There is neural proximity of parietal areas important for both math and finger gnosis (the localizationist view; e.g., Dehaene et al., 2003). It is also the case that functionally, finger usage is critical to the mastery of small sums arithmetic developmentally, which proceeds from deliberate finger counting to verbal counting to automatic retrieval (Butterworth, 1999; Geary & Hoard, 2002). Finally, Penner-Wilger and Anderson (2013) describe a redeployment view, wherein shared neural circuitry supports some basic function that can be utilized in multiple ways (in this case, for both finger gnosis and number representation). Fine motor skills more generally (manipulating pegs, copying complex visual figures) are empirically related to mathematics in both typically developing individuals (Carlson, Rowe, & Curby, 2013; Pitchford, Papini, Outhwaite, & Gulliford, 2016) and neurodevelopmental populations such as spina bifida (Barnes et al., 2011; Raghubar et al., 2015).

Language

Language has long been implicated in math. For example, Geary (1993) emphasized semantic (math fact) retrieval as a key manifest deficit in MD. With mastery of math facts, neuroimaging evidence shows an increasing reliance on LH areas traditionally associated with reading (e.g., angular gyrus). There are also developmental parallels for what it takes to represent and recognize both letters and numbers, and these early symbolic skills are strongly related to early math skills (Cirino, 2011), more so than the nonsymbolic magnitude comparison skills thought by some to represent the core deficit in MD (Schneider et al., 2016; Vanbinst, Ansari, Ghesquière, & De Smedt, 2016). There is ample evidence (both theoretical and empirical) for the relation of several specific language skills, including phonological awareness (Cirino, Child, & Macdonald, 2018; Robinson, Menchetti, & Torgesen, 2002), rapid naming skills (Koponen, Georgiou, Salmi, Leskinen, & Aro, 2017), and broader language skills such as vocabulary and listening comprehension (Cirino, Tolar, & Fuchs, 2022; Fuchs et al., 2010a; Vukovic & Lesaux, 2013), to math, although some of these relationships may be indirect (Fuchs et al., 2012). For complex math skills that directly involve language, such as word problems, text comprehension plays a strong role (Fuchs, Fuchs, Compton, Hamlett, & Wang, 2015). Although colloquially it is common to associate visuospatial skills with math in contrast to the association of language with reading, this is a false dichotomy; even if the link of language is stronger for reading than math, it is still quite strong for math, and language may be more relevant for math than are visuospatial skills. Future work will no doubt continue to refine (1) which language skills are relevant for (2) which math skills, (3) when in the developmental trajectory, and (4) whether such relations are direct versus indirect, and how such relations vary depending on which other neurocognitive systems are considered.

Processing Speed

Processing speed is important for math because it may increase efficiency and/or limit decay in working memory (Andersson & Lyxell, 2007; Geary, 1993). Processing speed can also be measured along a simple-complex continuum (Chiaravalloti, Cristodoulou, Demaree, & DeLuca, 2003; Gerst et al., 2021), and may have differential relations with MD and/or RD depending on whether it is measured linguistically versus nonlinguistically (Moll, Göbel, Gooch, Landerl, & Snowling, 2016). In the case of rapid naming skills (discussed earlier as a language predictor), it is necessary to differentiate its processing speed component from its symbolic identification component. This is particularly relevant given that math fact mastery is a key milestone in the developmental math hierarchy and requires both skills. Processing speed has also been proposed as one key differentiator between computational versus problem-solving MD (Fuchs et al., 2008b), and has been implicated as a shared cognitive predictor across neurodevelopmental disorders including RD, MD, and attention-deficit/hyperactivity disorder (ADHD) (McGrath et al., 2011; Peterson et al., 2017).

Attention

A broad distinction can be made between cognitive and behavioral attention. In the math literature broadly, there are many more studies of the latter than the former. Behavioral attention is often operationalized with symptomatology related to ADHD, and comorbidity of ADHD with MD is also higher than expected given epidemiological base rates. Behavioral attention is consistently moderately ($r \sim .45$) related to various math outcomes; in most cases, it is also a unique predictor even with strong competing predictors (Hansen, Jordan, & Rodrigues, 2017; Fuchs et al., 2016); in some cases, though, with younger children, behavioral attention is not a significant predictor (Fuchs et al., 2010a; Martin, Cirino, Sharp, & Barnes, 2014), or its effect is indirect via more proximal math outcomes (Fuchs et al., 2012). In contrast, there is very little work that focuses on *cognitive* attention and its relation to achievement. Gold et al. (2013), in an MD sample, found that a teacher rating scale of attention related to math performance, but a performance-based measure of attention did not. On the other hand, Richard, Hodges, and Heinrich (2018), with a small sample of children with acute lymphoblastic leukemia, found that both sustained attention and teacher ratings of behavioral attention related to math performance. Raghubar et al. (2015) found significant zero-order correlations of their performance based-measure of attention with math in their sample of youth with spina bifida and typical development, but this measure was weakly related to group and did not mediate the relation of group and math outcomes.

Executive Function

The aspect of executive function (EF) that is most closely related to mathematics is working memory (see reviews and syntheses by Friso-van den Bos, van der Ven, Kroesbergen, & van Luit, 2013; Raghubar, Barnes, & Hecht, 2010). In a review, Peng, Namkung, Barnes, and Sun (2016) found a medium overall relation ($r = .35$), and different working memory content (numeric, verbal, visual) showed similar relations. Among math outcomes, effects were weakest for geometry compared to word problems; among populations, relations were strongest for individuals with MD comorbid with a variety of neurodevelopmental disorders, compared to individuals with MD alone or typical students. Other aspects of EF have been less investigated, and also with mixed results (St Clair-Thompson & Gathercole, 2006; Van der Ven, Kroesbergen, Boom, & Leseman, 2012). A meta-analytic study of shifting in relation to math (Yeniad, Malda, Mesman, van IJzendooren, & Pieper, 2013) showed a modest relation ($r = .26$). Fuhs et al. (2015) and Gerst, Cirino, Fletcher, and Yoshida (2017) both compared cognitive and behavioral measures of EF in relation to math and reading outcomes. In a large sample of preschoolers, Fuhs, Farran, and Nesbitt (2015) found strong relations between the two types of measures, and both types uniquely related to mathematics (though with stronger effects for cognitive than for behavioral measures of EF). In a smaller and older sample of children, Gerst et al. (2017) found much weaker relations between these EF measure types, but also showed stronger relations of cognitive measures (median $r = .50$) than behavioral ones (median $r = .38$) to math (though in regressions, only cognitive measures of EF were uniquely related). As such, this poses an interesting contrast to the attention literature, where behavioral ratings appear more strongly related to mathematics than are cognitive ones.

Memory

There is a rich literature base regarding working memory (often also including short-term memory) and mathematics, and the role of semantic retrieval is heavily emphasized in developmental studies of math. However, there is almost no work that systematically evaluates declarative or nondeclarative memory with traditional neuropsychological tasks (list learning, story memory, reproduction of visual objects over time; Blankenship, Keith, Calkins, & Bell, 2018) in typical math development or individuals with MD. As seen in another section of this chapter, however, hippocampal circuitry (including its parietal and frontal connections) appears to be very important in helping to establish math fact mastery. Given the extant literature, it might be expected that the ability to make associations and encode these into long-term memory would be highly relevant for math development. A key question is whether any potential deficit in MD is specific to alphanumeric stimuli, or whether more pure visual memory is also relevant. It would also be important to determine whether these memory functions are relevant beyond math fact retrieval per se.

Social Cognition, Adaptive and Social Functioning, and Emotional and Behavioral Adjustment

Beyond neurocognitive domains, the dominant socioemotional factor discussed specifically with regard to math is math anxiety, which has modest relations with math performance in general, $r \sim .30$ (Ma, 1999), and therefore is more prevalent in MD, even though math anxiety is not specific to MD (Devine, Hill, Carey, & Szücs, 2018). These relations appear to be reciprocal (Carey, Hill, Devine, & Szücs, 2016), and are impacted by a wide variety of variables including age, gender, sociocultural, and instructional factors (Dowker, Sarkar, & Looi, 2016); math anxiety is also related to a host of other cognitive and noncognitive variables as well. Beyond math anxiety (and behavioral attention, discussed earlier), few data focus on the relation of social, adaptive, emotional, and behavioral variables in MD, and what data there are generally do not find robust relations. For example, Claessens and Dowsett (2014) found that the effects of disruptive behavior were much weaker than were the effects of inattention. Duncan et al. (2007) analyzed several large-scale national (U.S.) studies and found meta-analytic correlations with achievement for internalizing, externalizing, or social skills that were weak (r's = –.14, –.10, and .21, respectively), none of which were significant in regression analyses (even when early achievement was removed as a control variable).

DEVELOPMENTAL CONSIDERATIONS

MD does not have an *age of onset* given that it is rarely acquired. Of more relevance is *age of diagnosis/identification*. For example, earlier diagnosis is associated with the comorbidity of MD with other neurodevelopmental disorders such as attentional or reading difficulties is high (up to two-thirds of cases; American Psychiatric Association, 2013; Barbaresi et al., 2005). This provides additional presentation targets for a child to come to the attention of teachers or neuropsychologists, in part because comorbidity often implies greater severity. Students with MD and comorbid RD perform more poorly on mathematical and neurocognitive domains than do students with only MD (Cirino, Fuchs, Elias, Powell, & Schumacher, 2015; Peng, Wang, & Namkung, 2018). Early diagnosis may also occur if parents and/or teachers of young children are otherwise sensitive to early signs of struggle (e.g., if there is a family history, or if the academic context is demanding). In contrast, later diagnosis may be associated with classification approach; for example, discrepancy-based definitions might happen at later ages (in waiting for there to be a gap between IQ and math scores). Later diagnosis may also be associated with a mismatch of educational expectations and performance, especially if these change (e.g., the student moves to a more demanding academic environment). Students have multiple opportunities for such change given natural transitions (elementary to middle school, middle to high school, beyond high school).

An important note is that because MD is defined psychometrically, the educational context is highly relevant, because the curricula themselves, and the level of demand across school, vary quite widely. For example, average performance on a nationally normed measure can appear below average if the school, district, or state as a whole is high-performing; conversely, the same score may appear above average in a low-performing context. Math is hierarchical, and this is expressed in curricula that change systematically with development and education. For example, informal exposure and naming yield to counting, then to math facts, to broader arithmetic, to word problems, to rational numbers, to algebra, and even to more complex skills (e.g., calculus) in high school and beyond, and finally to functional, "everyday" math skills (e.g., financial, health, and general mathematical "literacy"). Relatedly, *age at testing* can also very much impact the assessment of MD because of (1) which skills are expected to have been mastered at the time of assessment; (2) which skills are most recently or currently being learned, and (3) to which skills the student has not yet been exposed; of course, a loss of previously acquired skill might also occur, albeit more rarely. At school ages, widely used educational measures vary widely in the number of items that address any given skill, and so coverage may be sporadic, particularly as it corresponds to a given student's learning environment/expectations (see earlier rationale for *persistence* definitions of MD). It may also be the case that the items required to obtain "average" performance differ from school expectations for that age/grade, or from components that contribute to a student's letter grade. Because math curricula are broad, it is possible for a young student to have difficulty with the geometric, measurement, or statistical concepts covered in their school, but these are less likely to be reflected on a standardized computational measure. As students move through later elementary, middle, and high school, the focus of mathematical instruction becomes even more separate from what is measured by most standardized normative measures. For example, both fractions and algebra are key curricular foci, but they do not have widely used and available normed instruments to assess them.

Transition Issues

Transitions across development are quite important for MD, but for perhaps different reasons than some other disorders considered in this volume. For example, physicians are not usually the primary manager of care for MD, so the medical transitioning that is highly salient for some other neuropsychological disorders (from child to adult neurologist, or from developmental pediatrician to internist) is less relevant. Rather, the prominent transitions for MD are those associated with formal schooling changes (which coincide with important developmental epochs).

These transitions differ in the extent to which they are more quantitative versus qualitative. For example, the transition into early formal education (kindergarten and grade 1) is primarily qualitative, in that written arithmetic is introduced systematically for the first time. Throughout most of the remainder of elementary to middle school, there are quantitative changes involving mastery of basic facts and procedural operations that increase in difficulty. There is also some qualitative change, such as the application of calculation principles into word reasoning, and the introduction of rational numbers (e.g., fractions), where knowledge of whole numbers can interfere with understanding (van Hoof, Vamvakoussi, Van Dooren, & Verschaffel, 2017). The next shift, around the transition to secondary school and involving algebra and upper-level math, also involves qualitative shifts in understanding; this particular transition is relevant because, in the United States, for example, the timing of the first dedicated course in algebra is in part determined by prior mathematical performance, and this timing often "sets" the mathematical trajectory for students (Cirino et al., 2022). Next, for students attending postsecondary institutions, the transition is quantitative, in that many majors (outside of core science–technology–engineering–mathematics, or STEM majors) do not require extensive mathematics beyond algebra. For students with MD, however, this is potentially a large stumbling block. For example, again in the case of the United States, half of all postsecondary enrollment occurs at 2 year colleges, where up to 60% of students are required to take developmental (remedial) coursework, and only a fraction of these proceed to college-level math and earn a degree (Bailey, Jeong, & Cho, 2010; Ma & Baum, 2016). Furthermore, there are few studies of MD at the postsecondary level, and those that do exist vary tremendously in definition, application, sample size, and focus. Finally, the transition to independent adulthood (whether this occurs directly after high school or after postsecondary education) introduces both quantitative and qualitative change, where the emphasis shifts to the use of mathematical principles in health, financial, and other functional realms (Organisation for Economic Cooperation and Development, 2009) necessary to function in a technological society (Lusardi, 2015). In fact, in an international study, the range of adults who performed at or below the most basic level was 8–30% across countries; the United States, at 19%, was 11th out of 13 countries) (Organisation for Economic Cooperation and Development, 2013).

PREDICTORS AND MODERATORS

Beyond the neurocognitive and emotional–affective–behavioral factors discussed earlier, additional psychological factors are relevant for math. In the educational literature, these are often considered "noncognitive" variables (Duckworth & Yeager, 2015; Richardson, Abraham, & Bond, 2012). The term *noncognitive* is a misnomer, in that cognitive processes are involved, but the distinction made is between psychometric (task-based or performance or problem-solving tasks) and all other measures (e.g., self-report measures). For MD (and mathematics development more generally), key constructs include motivation, affect, and self-regulation (specifically, self-regulated learning). These are factors that are not diagnostic of MD but may alter its course, often in bidirectional fashion. With somewhat different terminology, Stankov (2013; Stankov & Lee, 2014) refers to a "predictability gradient hypothesis" and considers self-concept, anxiety, self-efficacy, and self-confidence as "self-beliefs," which are typically assessed in relation to a specific domain (e.g., self-efficacy of math), and which vary (in the above ascending order) in their prediction of math performance. Such variables were found to be more predictive than more distal factors such as personality, depression, well-being, learning strategies, and achievement goal orientation (performance vs. mastery).

TREATMENT AND INTERVENTION

Information regarding effective and empirically validated treatments for MD has expanded greatly in the past 20 years, including a number of reviews and meta-analyses that consolidate this information (e.g., Dennis et al., 2016; Hughes, Witzel, Riccomini, Fries, & Kanyongo, 2014; Stevens, Rodgers, & Powell, 2018). But to set the stage for this section, it is illustrative to consider examples of efficacious interventions for students with MD that target different math content and roughly track the developmental progression of math knowledge. First, *numerosity* interventions are most common at the preschool and kindergarten stage, with content focused on understanding relations between magnitudes, and between magnitudes and their symbolic value. Next, *math facts* interventions are in part premised on the idea that knowledge of basic math facts (typically taken to be single-digit addition and subtraction, and sometimes multiplication, in oral or written format) is a "bottleneck" or rate-limiting step to enable more complex mathematical performance. Fuchs et al. (2010b), who conducted a series of number combination studies, found that the bottleneck hypothesis is only partially supported—deliberate practice is key to improving these skills, but this practice can be contextualized within other math training, such as *word problems* interventions. For example, Fuchs et al. (2014a) compared a word problems intervention to a computational intervention for at-risk students, and found that computations intervention was specific to math facts and procedural computation outcomes, whereas word problems intervention improved computational, word problem, and algebraic outcomes. Fractions represent a fundamental shift from whole to rational numbers, and *fractions* interventions for struggling students have recently appeared. For example, Fuchs et al. (2013) found that an approach focused on measurement (opposed to the more common part–whole method) was effective in promoting fractions competence. Beyond fractions, and in particular beyond middle school, there are fewer systematic data for students with MD, and this remains an area ripe for investigation.

Turning to more amalgamated intervention results and their effect sizes (ESs) reported in a Cohen's *d*, Hedges's *g*, or similar metric, an earlier meta-analytic study (Kroesbergen & Van Luit, 2003) evaluated 61 studies focused on students with math difficulties and found strong overall effects that were affected by four factors: (1) duration (longer interventions showed more improvement); (2) design (single-subject studies showed more improvement than groups); (3) topic (with the largest effects for math facts, ES = 1.14); and (4) type of instruction (direct instruction yielded higher ESs than mediated/assisted or reform-based mathematics instruction, ES = 0.91 vs. 0.34). Similarly, Baker, Gersten, and Lee (2002) found that for students with or at-risk for mathematics difficulty, peer-assisted learning, explicit instruction, and providing data and feedback were all effective techniques (ES = 0.51–0.66), but contextualized teacher-facilitated instruction (e.g., focused on broad concepts and real-world applications) yielded negligible effect sizes (0.01). Later, Dennis et al. (2016), in a meta-analysis of 25 intervention studies for students with MD published between 2000 and 2014, found that peer-assisted learning and explicit instruction yielded the strongest ESs (0.82 and 0.76), and technology-focused interventions the weakest (ES = 0.39). For students in grades 4 through 12, Stevens et al. (2018) found that for studies evaluating fractions, moderate ESs were found, 0.41 to 0.74. Hughes et al. (2014), in a meta-analysis of algebraic interventions for students struggling in math, found an overall ES of 0.62, with somewhat better effects for systematic and explicit studies (0.68) relative to those emphasizing a concrete–representational–abstract framework (0.52). Even outside of an intervention context, Morgan, Farkas, and Maczuga (2015), using nationally representative data, found that for students with MD, teacher-directed instruction was associated with improvements, but student-centered instruction was not. Such findings are in line with the prior iteration of this chapter (Barnes, Fuchs, & Ewing-Cobbs, 2010) that constructivist or discovery learning is not as effective an approach for students with MD relative to systematic and explicit instruction. Overall, the results of these meta-analyses demonstrate that effective math interventions do exist but need to be tailored to specific outcomes (some of which have been much more extensively evaluated) and to consider important moderating factors.

Based on numerous intervention studies for students with MD, Fuchs et al. (2008a) describe general effective intervention practices. These include instructional explicitness; instructional design that is efficient, sequenced, and integrated, so that the burden on the learner is reduced; a strong conceptual foundation; drill and practice; cumulative review; motivation to support self-regulation of the learner; and ongoing progress monitoring. These principles can be applied over many outcomes, including number combinations, word problems, and fractions (for detailed examples, see Fuchs et al., 2010b; Fuchs, Malone, Schumacher, Namkung, & Wang, 2017). It should also be noted that many of these features are relevant for RD intervention as well.

Most intervention literature for MD focuses directly on a targeted mathematical skill, but there are fewer data that speak to the way *cognitive processes* are used for intervention, and many of those data are less than encouraging. For example, working memory is one of the strongest correlates of math, yet a meta-analysis of Schwaighofer, Fischer, and Bühner (2015) specifically focused on transfer found that across 15 ESs evaluating transfer of working memory training to math, 12 were nonsignificant, and though three were significant, one of these was negative; additionally, none of the eight ESs for delayed effects were significant. Therefore, intervention that directly/only focuses on a cognitive process is unlikely to improve mathematical outcomes.

Such findings may seem counter to expectations for many neuropsychologists, where the interpretation of neurocognitive data is paramount. However, similar to the literature for RD, and as reviewed in the first section of this chapter regarding classification and identification, there is not strong evidence to suggest that cognitive profiling plays a strong role in optimizing outcomes for students with MD. Two points are highly relevant. First, none of the above should be taken to mean that neurocognitive factors are irrelevant to mathematical performance—they clearly are, many robustly so (see earlier discussion in of this chapter). But if assessments of cognitive measures are used to inform intervention, the most effective measures are likely those that are not only very closely tied to the particular outcome of interest but whose effect is also demonstrated to be of added value over initial skill level. Similar conclusions were drawn from a meta-analysis of studies that used cognitive processes for achievement interventions (Burns et al., 2016).

Second, such results also do not preclude a cognitive focus for MD interventions. It is important though, that such attempts be clear in (1) considering the math hierarchy and lower-level skills that might function as strong predictors of outcome (including initial skill level), and in (2) recognizing that training for cognitive skills of any kind is only likely to be effective in the context of a math-focused intervention. Probably the most common way to incorporate cognitive factors is to explicitly design interventions to minimize working memory, language, or other cognitive demands. However, effects are not often disaggregated by manipulating intervention variables, or by evaluating potential mediators (but see Fuchs et al., 2013, 2014b). Cognitive strategies are also often used in math interventions to scaffold performance. For example, in mathematics schema-based instruction, a template is provided as a basis for understanding a variety of mathematical functions, while schema broadening additionally designs intervention specifically to allow for transfer to different math problem types (Fuchs et al., 2010c; Jitendra & Hoff, 1996).

But how might a cognitive focus be enacted more directly? For one, cognitive training might occur in parallel (e.g., over the same 6-month period, working memory or attention is trained, and at the same time, a separate math intervention is employed), or training might be embedded. In fact, some examples can be found in recent literature. Barnes et al. (2016) provide an example of separate training of attention and/or math in preschoolers, whereas Wang et al. (2019) provide an example of a contrast between an effective base fractions intervention versus an intervention that also embeds an explicit self-regulatory focus. An excellent example of a recent study that embeds specific language comprehension instruction for word problems intervention is given by Fuchs et al. (2021).

CONCLUSIONS AND FUTURE DIRECTIONS

Critique

The literature on MD has a long history, though with rapid developments in terms of both depth and breadth over the past 25 years. A central issue for MD and learning disabilities more generally is that of definition, with a key debate surrounding the level of performance and degree of persistence needed to be considered to have MD. There is increasing solidification around the key neural networks involved in processing mathematical information, both structurally and functionally, particularly with regard to basic arithmetic operations, with active investigation around genetic contributions, and some interesting developments with regard to the use of imaging as external validity for classification or intervention. Similarly, the neurocognitive concomitants of mathematical processing are diverse; although working memory is a common focus of study, in fact, a number of domain-specific and domain-general processes have been implicated, and their relative importance for different mathematical domains is still evolving. Developmental aspects of MD dominate the literature, as educational content is hierarchical and varies with age and grade, but specific curricular foci also differ across districts, states, and countries. This means that history and context for a student with suspected MD is highly important for determining recommended courses of action. Finally, particularly over the past 10–15 years, there has been a systematic increase in the number of strong intervention studies focused on basic facts and word problems, but also expanding to earlier (e.g., numerosity) and later (e.g., fractions) topics. There is no doubt that the near future will continue to elaborate on these exciting developments.

Future Directions

There remain a number of areas in which the field of MD will benefit from increased study. First, from the perspective of neurocognitive concomitants, neural concomitants, and intervention, it will be important to continue to expand this knowledge to different developmental stages, and in corollary, to different mathematical outcomes. This is especially true for students in secondary school and young adults in postsecondary contexts. Second, there remains substantial debate about whether cognitive data can help inform diagnosis and treatment; though some recent studies provide examples of how this might occur, much more data are needed. More data are also needed regarding how imaging can provide external validity data for treatment. Third, arguments for some points made throughout earlier sections (e.g., definitions; role of cognitive measures/treatment) relied in part on analogies to the RD literature, though, of course, it will be important for the MD literature to evaluate these issues independently to establish both similarities and differences. Finally, there are increasing, but not yet enough, data regarding how MD manifests in neurodevelopmental disorders with which it is commonly comorbid, including not only RD and ADHD but also more specific disorders that have distinct mathematical profiles (e.g., spina bifida). Understanding the ways that the math issues are similar versus different across populations has implications for treatment recommendations.

ACKNOWLEDGMENTS

This work was supported in part by National Science Foundation (Grant No. 1760760) awarded to the University of Houston. The views expressed herein are those of the author alone.

REFERENCES

American Psychiatric Association. (2013). *Diagnostic and statistical manual of mental disorders* (5th ed.). Arlington, VA: Author.

Andersson, U., & Lyxell, B. (2007). Working memory deficit in children with mathematical difficulties: A general or specific deficit? *Journal of Experimental Child Psychology, 96*(3), 197–228.

Ansari, D., & Dhital, B. (2006). Age-related changes in the activation of the intraparietal sulcus during nonsymbolic magnitude processing: An event-related functional magnetic resonance imaging study. *Journal of Cognitive Neuroscience, 18*(11), 1820–1828.

Ashkenazi, S., Black, J. M., Abrams, D. A., Hoeft, F., & Menon, V. (2013). Neurobiological underpinnings of math and reading learning disabilities. *Journal of Learning Disabilities, 46*(6), 549–569.

Ashkenazi, S., Rosenberg-Lee, M., Tenison, C., & Menon, V. (2012). Weak task-related modulation and stimulus representations during arithmetic problem solving in children with developmental dyscalculia. *Developmental Cognitive Neuroscience,* 2(Suppl.), S152–S166.

Badian, N. A. (1999). Persistent arithmetic, reading, or arithmetic and reading disability. *Annals of Dyslexia, 49*(1), 43–70.

Bailey, T., Jeong, D. W., & Cho, S. W. (2010). Referral, enrollment, and completion in developmental education sequences in community colleges. *Economics of Education Review, 29*(2), 255–270.

Baker, S., Gersten, R., & Lee, D. S. (2002). A synthesis of empirical research on teaching mathematics to low-achieving students. *Elementary School Journal, 103*(1), 51–73.

Barbaresi, W. J., Katusic, S. K., Colligan, R. C., Weaver, A. L., & Jacobsen, S. J. (2005). Math learning disorder: Incidence in a population-based birth cohort, 1976–1982, Rochester, Minn. *Ambulatory Pediatrics, 5*(5), 281–289.

Barnes, M. A., Fuchs, L. S., & Ewing-Cobbs, L. (2010). Math disabilities. In K. O. Yeates, M. D. Ris, H. G. Taylor, & B. F. Pennington (Eds.), *Pediatric neuropsychology: Research, theory, and practice* (pp. 297–323). New York: Guilford Press.

Barnes, M. A., Klein, A., Swank, P., Starkey, P., McCandliss, B., Flynn, K., . . . Roberts, G. (2016). Effects of tutorial interventions in mathematics and attention for low-performing preschool children. *Journal of Research on Educational Effectiveness, 9*(4), 577–606.

Barnes, M. A., Stubbs, A., Raghubar, K. P., Agostino, A., Taylor, H., Landry, S., . . . Smith-Chant, B. (2011). Mathematical skills in 3-and 5-year-olds with spina bifida and their typically developing peers: A longitudinal approach. *Journal of the International Neuropsychological Society, 17*(3), 431–444.

Blankenship, T. L., Keith, K., Calkins, S. D., & Bell, M. A. (2018). Behavioral performance and neural areas associated with memory processes contribute to math and reading achievement in 6-year-old children. *Cognitive Development, 45*, 141–151.

Branum-Martin, L., Fletcher, J. M., & Stuebing, K. K. (2013). Classification and identification of reading and math disabilities: The special case of comorbidity. *Journal of Learning Disabilities, 46*(6), 490–499.

Bugden, S., & Ansari, D. (2015). How can cognitive developmental neuroscience constrain our understanding of developmental dyscalculia? In S. Chinn (Ed.), *The Routledge international handbook of dyscalculia and mathematical learning difficulties* (pp. 18–43). New York: Routledge.

Burns, M. K., Petersen-Brown, S., Haegele, K., Rodriguez, M., Schmitt, B., Cooper, M., . . . VanDerHeyden, A. M. (2016). Meta-analysis of academic interventions derived from neuropsychological data. *School Psychology Quarterly, 31*(1), 28–42.

Butterworth, B. (1999). *The mathematical brain*. London: Macmillan.

Carey, E., Hill, F., Devine, A., & Szücs, D. (2016). The chicken or the egg?: The direction of the relationship between mathematics anxiety and mathematics performance. *Frontiers in Psychology, 6*, Article 1987.

Carlson, A. G., Rowe, E., & Curby, T. W. (2013). Disentangling fine motor skills' relations to academic achievement: The relative contributions of visual–spatial integration and visual-motor coordination. *Journal of Genetic Psychology, 174*(5), 514–533.

Casey, M. B., Pezaris, E., & Nuttall, R. L. (1992). Spatial ability as a predictor of math achievement: The importance of sex and handedness patterns. *Neuropsychologia, 30*(1), 35–45.

Chiaravalloti, N. D., Christodoulou, C., Demaree, H. A., & DeLuca, J. (2003). Differentiating simple versus complex processing speed: Influence on new learning and memory performance. *Journal of Clinical and Experimental Neuropsychology, 25*(4), 489–501.

Cho, S., Metcalfe, A. W., Young, C. B., Ryali, S., Geary, D. C., & Menon, V. (2012). Hippocampal–prefrontal engagement and dynamic causal interactions in the maturation of children's fact retrieval. *Journal of Cognitive Neuroscience, 24*(9), 1849–1866.

Cirino, P. T. (2011). The interrelationships of mathematical precursors in kindergarten. *Journal of Experimental Child Psychology, 108*(4), 713–733.

Cirino, P. T., Child, A. E., & Macdonald, K. T. (2018). Longitudinal predictors of the overlap between reading and math skills. *Contemporary Educational Psychology, 54*, 99–111.

Cirino, P. T., Fuchs, L. S., Elias, J. T., Powell, S. R., & Schumacher, R. F. (2015). Cognitive and mathematical profiles for different forms of learning difficulties. *Journal of Learning Disabilities, 48*(2), 156–175.

Cirino, P. T., Morris, M. K., & Morris, R. D. (2002). Neuropsychological concomitants of calculation skills in college students referred for learning difficulties. *Developmental Neuropsychology, 21*(2), 201–218.

Cirino, P. T., Morris, M. K., & Morris, R. D. (2007). Semantic, executive, and visuospatial abilities in mathematical reasoning of referred college students. *Assessment, 14*(1), 94–104.

Cirino, P. T., Tolar, T., & Fuchs, L. S. (2022). Domain general and specific contributions to algebra: A sequenced longitudinal path model. *Contemporary Educational Psychology, 68*, 102026.

Claessens, A., & Dowsett, C. (2014). Growth and change in attention problems, disruptive behavior, and achievement from kindergarten to fifth grade. *Psychological Science, 25*(12), 2241–2251.

Dehaene, S., & Cohen, L. (1995). Towards an anatomical and functional model of number processing. *Mathematical Cognition, 1*(1), 83–120.

Dehaene, S., Piazza, M., Pinel, P., & Cohen, L. (2003). Three parietal circuits for number processing. *Cognitive Neuropsychology, 20*(3–6), 487–506.

Dennis, M. S., Sharp, E., Chovanes, J., Thomas, A., Burns, R. M., Custer, B., & Park, J. (2016). A meta-analysis of empirical research on teaching students with mathematics learning difficulties. *Learning Disabilities Research and Practice, 31*(3), 156–168.

Devine, A., Hill, F., Carey, E., & Szücs, D. (2018). Cognitive and emotional math problems largely dissociate: Prevelance of developmental dyscalculia and mathematics anxiety. *Journal of Educational Psychology, 110*(3), 431–444.

Docherty, S. J., Davis, O. S. P., Kovas, Y., Meaburn, E. L., Dale, P. S., Petrill, S. A., . . . Plomin, R. (2010). A genome-wide association study identifies multiple loci associated with mathematics ability and disability. *Genes, Brain and Behavior, 9*(2), 234–247.

Docherty, S. J., Kovas, Y., & Plomin, R. (2011). Gene–environment interaction in the etiology of mathematical ability using SNP sets. *Behavior Genetics, 41*(1), 141–154.

Dowker, A., Sarkar, A., & Looi, C. Y. (2016). Mathematics anxiety: What have we learned in 60 years?. *Frontiers in Psychology, 7*, Article 508.

Duckworth, A. L., & Yeager, D. S. (2015). Measurement matters: Assessing personal qualities other than cognitive ability for educational purposes. *Educational Researcher, 44*(4), 237–251.

Duncan, G. J., Dowsett, C. J., Claessens, A., Magnuson, K., Huston, A. C., Klebanov, P., &Brooks-Gunn, J. (2007). School readiness and later achievement. *Developmental Psychology, 43*(6), 1428–1446.

Emerson, R. W., & Cantlon, J. F. (2015). Continuity and change in children's longitudinal neural responses to numbers. *Developmental Science, 18*(2), 314–326.

Every Student Succeeds Act (ESSA), PL 114-95 (2015).

Fias, W., Menon, V., & Szücs, D. (2013). Multiple components of developmental dyscalculia. *Trends in Neuroscience and Education, 2*(2), 43–47.

Flanagan, D. P., Ortiz, S. O., & Alfonso, V. C. (Eds.). (2013). *Essentials of cross-battery assessment* (3rd ed.). New York: Wiley.

Fletcher, J. M., & Miciak, J. (2017). Comprehensive cognitive assessments are not necessary for the identification and treatment of learning disabilities. *Archives of Clinical Neuropsychology, 32*(1), 2–7.

Fletcher, J. M., Shaywitz, S. E., Shankweiler, D. P., Katz, L., Liberman, I. Y., Stuebing, K. K., . . . Shaywitz, B. A. (1994). Cognitive profiles of reading disability: Comparisons of discrepancy and low achievement definitions. *Journal of Educational Psychology, 86*(1), 6–23.

Francis, D. J., Shaywitz, S. E., Stuebing, K. K., Shaywitz, B. A., & Fletcher, J. M. (1996). Developmental lag versus deficit models of reading disability: A longitudinal, individual growth curves analysis. *Journal of Educational Psychology, 88*(1), 3–17.

Friso-van den Bos, I., van der Ven, S. H., Kroesbergen, E. H., & van Luit, J. E. (2013). Working memory and mathematics in primary school children: A meta-analysis. *Educational Research Review, 10*, 29–44.

Fuchs, L. S., Compton, D. L., Fuchs, D., Powell, S. R., Schumacher, R. F., Hamlett, C. L., & Vukovic, R. K. (2012). Contributions of domain-general cognitive resources and different forms of arithmetic development to pre-algebraic knowledge. *Developmental Psychology, 48*(5), 1315–1326.

Fuchs, L. S., Fuchs, D., Compton, D. L., Hamlett, C. L., & Wang, A. Y. (2015). Is word-problem solving a form of text comprehension? *Scientific Studies of Reading, 19*(3), 204–223.

Fuchs, L. S., Fuchs, D., Powell, S. R., Seethaler, P. M., Cirino, P. T., & Fletcher, J. M. (2008a). Intensive intervention for students with mathematics disabilities: Seven principles of effective practice. *Learning Disability Quarterly, 31*(2), 79–92.

Fuchs, L. S., Fuchs, D., Stuebing, K., Fletcher, J. M., Hamlett, C. L., & Lambert, W. (2008b). Problem solving and computational skill: Are they shared or distinct aspects of mathematical cognition? *Journal of Educational Psychology, 100*(1), 30–47.

Fuchs, L. S., Geary, D. C., Compton, D. L., Fuchs, D., Hamlett, C. L., & Bryant, J. D. (2010a). The contributions of numerosity and domain-general abilities to school readiness. *Child Development, 81*(5), 1520–1533.

Fuchs, L. S., Gilbert, J. K., Powell, S. R., Cirino, P. T., Fuchs, D., Hamlett, C. L., . . . Tolar, T. D. (2016). The role of cognitive processes, foundational math skill, and calculation accuracy and fluency in word-problem solving versus prealgebraic knowledge. *Developmental Psychology, 52*(12), 2085–2098.

Fuchs, L. S., Malone, A. S., Schumacher, R. F., Namkung, J., & Wang, A. (2017). Fraction intervention for students with mathematics difficulties: Lessons learned from five randomized controlled trials. *Journal of Learning Disabilities, 50*(6), 631–639.

Fuchs, L. S., Powell, S. R., Cirino, P. T., Schumacher, R. F., Marrin, S., Hamlett, C. L., . . . Changas, P. C. (2014a). Does calculation or word-problem instruction provide a stronger route to prealgebraic knowledge?. *Journal of Educational Psychology, 106*(4), 990–1006.

Fuchs, L. S., Powell, S. R., Seethaler, P. M., Fuchs, D., Hamlett, C. L., Cirino, P. T., & Fletcher, J. M. (2010b). A framework for remediating number combination deficits. *Exceptional Children, 76*(2), 135–156.

Fuchs, L. S., Schumacher, R. F., Long, J., Namkung, J., Hamlett, C. L., Cirino, P. T., . . . Changas, P. (2013). Improving at-risk learners' understanding of fractions. *Journal of Educational Psychology, 105*(3), 683–700.

Fuchs, L. S., Schumacher, R. F., Sterba, S. K., Long, J., Namkung, J., Malone, A., . . . Changas, P. (2014b). Does working memory moderate the effects of fraction intervention?: An aptitude-treatment interaction. *Journal of Educational Psychology, 106*(2), 499–514.

Fuchs, L. S., Seethaler, P. M., Sterba, S. K., Craddock, C., Fuchs, D., Compton, D. L., Geary, D. C., & Changas, P. (2021). Closing the word problem achievement gap in first grade: Schema-based word-problem intervention with embedded language comprehension instruction. *Journal of Educational Psychology, 113*(1), 86–103.

Fuchs, L. S., Zumeta, R. O., Schumacher, R. F., Powell, S. R., Seethaler, P. M., Hamlett, C. L., & Fuchs, D. (2010c). The effects of schema-broadening instruction on second graders' word-problem performance and their ability to represent word problems with algebraic equations: A randomized control study. *Elementary School Journal, 110*(4), 440–463.

Fuhs, M. W., Farran, D. C., & Nesbitt, K. T. (2015). Prekindergarten children's executive functioning skills and achievement gains: The utility of direct assessments and teacher ratings. *Journal of Educational Psychology, 107*(1), 207–222.

Geary, D. C. (1993). Mathematical disabilities: Cognitive, neuropsychological, and genetic components. *Psychological Bulletin, 114*(2), 345–362.

Geary, D. C., & Hoard, M. K. (2002). Learning disabilities in basic mathematics: Deficits in memory and cognition. In J. M. Royer (Ed.), *Mathematical cognition* (pp. 93–115). Greenwich, CT: Information Age.

Geary, D. C., Hoard, M. K., & Hamson, C. O. (1999). Numerical and arithmetical cognition: Patterns of functions and deficits in children at risk for a mathematical disability. *Journal of Experimental Child Psychology, 74*, 213–239.

Gerst, E. H., Cirino, P. T., Fletcher, J. M., & Yoshida, H. (2017). Cognitive and behavioral rating measures of executive function as predictors of academic outcomes in children. *Child Neuropsychology, 23*(4), 381–407.

Gerst, E. H., Cirino, P. T., Macdonald, K. T., Miciak, J., Yoshida, H., Woods, S. P., & Gibbs, M. C. (2021). The structure of processing speed in children and its impact on reading. *Journal of Cognition and Development, 22*(1), 84–107.

Gerstmann, J. (1940). Syndrome of finger agnosia, disorientation for right and left, agraphia and acalculia: Local diagnostic value. *Archives of Neurology and Psychiatry, 44*(2), 398–408.

Gold, A. B., Ewing-Cobbs, L., Cirino, P., Fuchs, L. S., Stuebing, K. K., & Fletcher, J. M. (2013). Cognitive and behavioral attention in children with math difficulties. *Child Neuropsychology, 19*(4), 420–437.

Hansen, N., Jordan, N. C., & Rodrigues, J. (2017). Identifying learning difficulties with fractions: A longitudinal study of student growth from third through sixth grade. *Contemporary Educational Psychology, 50*, 45–59.

Hartje, W. (1987). The effect of spatial disorders on arithmetical skills. In G. Deloche & X. Seron (Eds.), *Mathematical disabilities: A cognitive neuropsychological perspective* (pp. 121–135). Hillsdale, NJ: Erlbaum.

Hécaen, H. Angelerges, T., & Houiller, S. (1961). Les varietes cliniques des acalculies au cours des lesions retrorolandiques. *Revue Neurologique, 105*, 85–103.

Hughes, E. M., Witzel, B. S., Riccomini, P. J., Fries, K. M., & Kanyongo, G. Y. (2014). A meta-analysis of algebra interventions for learners with disabilities and struggling learners. *Journal of the International Association of Special Education, 15*(1), 36–47.

Individuals with Disabilities Education Act (IDEA) Regulations, 34 C.F.R. §§ 300 (2004).

Jitendra, A. K., & Hoff, K. (1996). The effects of schema-based instruction on the mathematical word-problem-solving performance of students with learning disabilities. *Journal of Learning Disabilities, 29*(4), 422–431.

Kaufmann, L., Wood, G., Rubinsten, O., & Henik, A. (2011). Meta-analyses of developmental fMRI studies investigating typical and atypical trajectories of number processing and calculation. *Developmental Neuropsychology, 36*(6), 763–787.

Koponen, T., Georgiou, G., Salmi, P., Leskinen, M., & Aro, M. (2017). A meta-analysis of the relation between RAN and mathematics. *Journal of Educational Psychology, 109*(7), 977–992.

Kovas, Y., Haworth, C. M., Harlaar, N., Petrill, S. A., Dale, P. S., & Plomin, R. (2007). Overlap and specificity of genetic and environmental influences on mathematics and reading disability in 10-year-old twins. *Journal of Child Psychology and Psychiatry, 48*(9), 914–922.

Kovas, Y., Voronin, I., Kaydalov, A., Malykh, S. B., Dale, P. S., & Plomin, R. (2013). Literacy and numeracy are more heritable than intelligence in primary school. *Psychological Science, 24*(10), 2048–2056.

Kroesbergen, E. H., & Van Luit, J. E. (2003). Mathematics interventions for children with special educational needs: A meta-analysis. *Remedial and Special Education, 24*(2), 97–114.

Kucian, K., von Aster, M., Loenneker, T., Dietrich, T., & Martin, E. (2008). Development of neural networks for exact and approximate calculation: A FMRI study. *Developmental Neuropsychology, 33*(4), 447–473.

Lusardi, A. (2015). Financial literacy skills for the 21st century: Evidence from PISA. *Journal of Consumer Affairs, 49*(3), 639–659.

Ma, J., & Baum, S. (2016). Trends in community colleges: Enrollment, prices, student debt, and completion. *College Board Research Brief, 4*, 1–23.

Ma, X. (1999). A meta-analysis of the relationship between anxiety toward mathematics and achievement in mathematics. *Journal for Research in Mathematics Education, 30*(5), 520–540.

Martin, R. B., Cirino, P. T., Barnes, M. A., Ewing-Cobbs, L., Fuchs, L. S., Stuebing, K. K., & Fletcher, J. M. (2013). Prediction and stability of mathematics skill and difficulty. *Journal of Learning Disabilities, 46*(5), 428–443.

Martin, R. B., Cirino, P. T., Sharp, C., & Barnes, M. (2014). Number and counting skills in kindergarten as predictors of grade 1 mathematical skills. *Learning and Individual Differences, 34*, 12–23.

Mazzocco, M. M., & Myers, G. F. (2003). Complexities in identifying and defining mathematics learning disability in the primary school-age years. *Annals of Dyslexia, 53*(1), 218–253.

McGrath, L. M., Pennington, B. F., Shanahan, M. A., Santerre-Lemmon, L. E., Barnard, H. D., Willcutt, E. G., . . . Olson, R. K. (2011). A multiple deficit model of reading disability and attention-deficit/hyperactivity disorder: Searching for shared cognitive deficits. *Journal of Child Psychology and Psychiatry, 52*(5), 547–557.

Menon, V. (2016). A neurodevelopmental perspective on the role of memory systems in children's math learning. In D. B. Berch, D. C. Geary, & K. Mann Koepke (Eds.), *Development of mathematical cognition* (pp. 79–107). San Diego, CA: Academic Press.

Mix, K. S., & Cheng, Y. L. (2012). The relation between space and math: Developmental and educational implications. In J. B. Benson (Ed.), *Advances in child development and behavior* (Vol. 42, pp. 197–243). London: Academic Press.

Miyake, A., Friedman, N. P., Rettinger, D. A., Shah, P., & Hegarty, M. (2001). How are visuospatial working memory, executive functioning, and spatial abilities related?: A latent-variable analysis. *Journal of Experimental Psychology: General, 130*(4), 621–640.

Moll, K., Göbel, S. M., Gooch, D., Landerl, K., & Snowling, M. J. (2016). Cognitive risk factors for specific learning disorder: Processing speed, temporal processing, and working memory. *Journal of Learning Disabilities, 49*(3), 272–281.

Morgan, P. L., Farkas, G., Hillemeier, M. M., & Maczuga, S. (2016). Who is at risk for persistent mathematics difficulties in the United States? *Journal of Learning Disabilities, 49*(3), 305–319.

Morgan, P. L., Farkas, G., & Maczuga, S. (2015). Which instructional practices most help first-grade students with and without mathematics difficulties? *Educational Evaluation and Policy Analysis, 37*(2), 184–205.

Morgan, P. L., Farkas, G., & Wu, Q. (2009). Five-year growth trajectories of kindergarten children with learning difficulties in mathematics. *Journal of Learning Disabilities, 42*(4), 306–321.

Morsanyi, K., van Bers, B. M., McCormack, T., & McGourty, J. (2018). The prevalence of specific learning disorder in mathematics and comorbidity with other developmental disorders in primary school-age children. *British Journal of Psychology, 109*(4), 917–940.

Murphy, M. M., Mazzocco, M. M., Hanich, L. B., & Early, M. C. (2007). Cognitive characteristics of children with mathematics learning disability (MLD) vary as a function of the cutoff criterion used to define MLD. *Journal of Learning Disabilities, 40*(5), 458–478.

Organisation for Economic Cooperation and Development. (2009). *PIAAC numeracy: A conceptual framework* (Working Paper No. 35). Paris: OECD Publishing.

Organisation for Economic Cooperation and Development. (2013). *Time for the US to Reskill? What the Survey of Adult Skills says*. Paris: OECD Publishing.

Peng, P., Namkung, J., Barnes, M., & Sun, C. (2016). A meta-analysis of mathematics and working memory: Moderating effects of working memory domain, type of mathematics skill, and sample characteristics. *Journal of Educational Psychology, 108*(4), 455–473.

Peng, P., Wang, C., & Namkung, J. (2018). Understanding the cognition related to mathematics difficulties: A meta-analysis on the cognitive deficit profiles and the bottleneck theory. *Review of Educational Research, 88*(3), 434–476.

Penner-Wilger, M., & Anderson, M. L. (2013). The relation between finger gnosis and mathematical ability: Why redeployment of neural circuits best explains the finding. *Frontiers in Psychology, 4*, Article 877.

Peters, L., & De Smedt, B. (2018). Arithmetic in the developing brain: A review of brain imaging studies. *Developmental Cognitive Neuroscience, 30,* 265–279.

Peterson, R. L., Boada, R., McGrath, L. M., Willcutt, E. G., Olson, R. K., & Pennington, B. F. (2017). Cognitive prediction of reading, math, and attention: Shared and unique influences. *Journal of Learning Disabilities, 50*(4), 408–421.

Petrill, S., Logan, J., Hart, S., Vincent, P., Thompson, L., Kovas, Y., & Plomin, R. (2012). Math fluency is etiologically distinct from untimed math performance, decoding fluency, and untimed reading performance: Evidence from a twin study. *Journal of Learning Disabilities, 45*(4), 371–381.

Petrill, S. A., & Kovas, Y. (2016). Individual differences in mathematics ability: A behavioral genetic approach. In D. B. Berch, D. C. Geary, & K. Mann Koepke (Eds.), *Development of mathematical cognition* (pp. 299–323). San Diego, CA: Academic Press.

Pitchford, N. J., Papini, C., Outhwaite, L. A., & Gulliford, A. (2016). Fine motor skills predict maths ability better than they predict reading ability in the early primary school years. *Frontiers in Psychology, 7,* Article 783.

Plomin, R., & Kovas, Y. (2005). Generalist genes and learning disabilities. *Psychological Bulletin, 131*(4), 592–617.

Qin, S., Cho, S., Chen, T., Rosenberg-Lee, M., Geary, D. C., & Menon, V. (2014). Hippocampal-neocortical functional reorganization underlies children's cognitive development. *Nature Neuroscience, 17*(9), 1263–1272.

Raghubar, K. P., Barnes, M. A., Dennis, M., Cirino, P. T., Taylor, H., & Landry, S. (2015). Neurocognitive predictors of mathematical processing in school-aged children with spina bifida and their typically developing peers: Attention, working memory, and fine motor skills. *Neuropsychology, 29*(6), 861–873.

Raghubar, K. P., Barnes, M. A., & Hecht, S. A. (2010). Working memory and mathematics: A review of developmental, individual difference, and cognitive approaches. *Learning and Individual Differences, 20*(2), 110–122.

Ranpura, A., Isaacs, E., Edmonds, C., Rogers, M., Lanigan, J., Singhal, A., . . . Butterworth, B. (2013). Developmental trajectories of grey and white matter in dyscalculia. *Trends in Neuroscience and Education, 2*(2), 56–64.

Richard, A. E., Hodges, E. K., & Heinrich, K. P. (2018). Visual attention and math performance in survivors of childhood acute lymphoblastic leukemia. *Archives of Clinical Neuropsychology, 33*(8), 1015–1023.

Richardson, M., Abraham, C., & Bond, R. (2012). Psychological correlates of university students' academic performance: A systematic review and meta-analysis. *Psychological Bulletin, 138*(2), 353–387.

Rivera, S. M., Reiss, A. L., Eckert, M. A., & Menon, V. (2005). Developmental changes in mental arithmetic: Evidence for increased functional specialization in the left inferior parietal cortex. *Cerebral Cortex, 15*(11), 1779–1790.

Robinson, C. S., Menchetti, B. M., & Torgesen, J. K. (2002). Toward a two-factor theory of one type of mathematics disabilities. *Learning Disabilities Research and Practice, 17*(2), 81–89.

Rykhlevskaia, E., Uddin, L. Q., Kondos, L., & Menon, V. (2009). Neuroanatomical correlates of developmental dyscalculia: Combined evidence from morphometry and tractography. *Frontiers in Human Neuroscience, 3,* Article 51.

Schneider, M., Beeres, K., Coban, L., Merz, S., Susan Schmidt, S., Stricker, J., & De Smedt, B. (2016). Associations of nonsymbolic and symbolic numerical magnitude processing with mathematical competence: A meta-analysis. *Developmental Science, 20*(3), e12372.

Schneider, W. J., & Kaufman, A. S. (2017). Let's not do away with comprehensive cognitive assessments just yet. *Archives of Clinical Neuropsychology, 32*(1), 8–20.

Schwaighofer, M., Fischer, F., & Bühner, M. (2015). Does working memory training transfer?: A meta-analysis including training conditions as moderators. *Educational Psychologist, 50*(2), 138–166.

Sella, F., Berteletti, I., Lucangeli, D., & Zorzi, M. (2017). Preschool children use space, rather than counting, to infer the numerical magnitude of digits: Evidence for a spatial mapping principle. *Cognition, 158,* 56–67.

Shalev, R. S., Manor, O., Auerbach, J., & Gross-Tsur, V. (1998). Persistence of developmental dyscalculia: What counts?: Results from a 3-year prospective follow-up study. *Journal of Pediatrics, 133*(3), 358–362.

Singer, H. D., & Low, A. A. (1933). Acalculia (Henschen): A clinical study. *Archives of Neurology and Psychiatry, 29*(3), 467–498.

St Clair-Thompson, H. L., & Gathercole, S. E. (2006). Executive functions and achievements in school: Shifting, updating, inhibition, and working memory. *Quarterly Journal of Experimental Psychology, 59*(4), 745–759.

Stankov, L. (2013). Noncognitive predictors of intelligence and academic achievement: An important role of confidence. *Personality and Individual Differences, 55*(7), 727–732.

Stankov, L., & Lee, J. (2014). Quest for the best non-cognitive predictor of academic achievement. *Educational Psychology, 34*(1), 1–8.

Stevens, E. A., Rodgers, M. A., & Powell, S. R. (2018). Mathematics interventions for upper elementary and secondary students: A meta-analysis of research. *Remedial and Special Education, 39*(6), 327–340.

Stuebing, K. K., Fletcher, J. M., LeDoux, J. M., Lyon, G. R., Shaywitz, S. E., & Shaywitz, B. A. (2002). Validity of IQ-discrepancy classifications of reading disabilities: A meta-analysis. *American Educational Research Journal, 39*(2), 469–518.

Supekar, K., Swigart, A. G., Tenison, C., Jolles, D. D., Rosenberg-Lee, M., Fuchs, L., & Menon, V. (2013). Neural predictors of individual differences in response to math tutoring in primary-grade school children. *Proceedings of the National Academy of Sciences USA, 110*(20), 8230–8235.

Tolar, T. D., Lederberg, A. R., & Fletcher, J. M. (2009). A structural model of algebra achievement: Computational fluency and spatial visualisation as mediators of the effect of working memory on algebra achievement. *Educational Psychology, 29*(2), 239–266.

U.S. Office of Education. (1968). *First annual report of the National Advisory Committee on Handicapped Children*. Washington, DC: U.S. Department of Health, Education and Welfare.

Vanbinst, K., Ansari, D., Ghesquière, P., & De Smedt, B. (2016). Symbolic numerical magnitude processing is as important to arithmetic as phonological awareness is to reading. *PLOS ONE, 11*(3), e0151045.

Van der Ven, S. H., Kroesbergen, E. H., Boom, J., & Leseman, P. P. (2012). The development of executive functions and early mathematics: A dynamic relationship. *British Journal of Educational Psychology, 82*(1), 100–119.

Van Hoof, J., Vamvakoussi, X., Van Dooren, W., & Verschaffel, L. (2017). The transition from natural to rational number knowledge. In D. Geary, D. Berch, R. Ochsendorf, & K. Mann Koepke (Eds.), *Acquisition of complex arithmetic skills and higher-order mathematics concepts* (pp. 101–123). San Diego, CA: Academic Press.

Vogel, S. E., Grabner, R. H., Schneider, M., Siegler, R. S., & Ansari, D. (2013). Overlapping and distinct brain regions involved in estimating the spatial position of numerical and non-numerical magnitudes: An fMRI study. *Neuropsychologia, 51*(5), 979–989.

Von Aster, M. G., & Shalev, R. S. (2007). Number development and developmental dyscalculia. *Developmental Medicine and Child Neurology, 49*(11), 868–873.

Vukovic, R. K., & Lesaux, N. K. (2013). The relationship between linguistic skills and arithmetic knowledge. *Learning and Individual Differences, 23*, 87–91.

Wang, A. Y., Fuchs, L. S., Fuchs, D., Gilbert, J. K., Krowka, S., & Abramson, R. (2019). Embedding self-regulation instruction with fractions intervention for third graders with mathematics difficulties. *Journal of Learning Disabilities, 52*(4), 337–348.

Yeniad, N., Malda, M., Mesman, J., van IJzendoorn, M. H., & Pieper, S. (2013). Shifting ability predicts math and reading performance in children: A meta-analytical study. *Learning and Individual Differences, 23*, 1–9.

CHAPTER 14

Autism Spectrum Disorder

Kirsty L. Coulter
Mary F. S. Dieckhaus
Rebecca P. Thomas
Deborah Fein

HISTORICAL OVERVIEW

Although the diagnostic criteria for autism have shifted over time, autism was first identified in the 1940s by two clinicians who described similar clinical phenomena. In 1943, Leo Kanner described young patients as "autistic" to connote their isolated, self-circumscribed demeanor. The presentation of these children included pronoun reversals and "literal, inflexible" word usage (Kanner, 1943). In 1944, Hans Asperger described "little professors" with high intelligence but social difficulties (Asperger, 1991).

Autism was first considered a subset of childhood schizophrenia, but in DSM-III (American Psychiatric Association, 1980), autism was reconceptualized not as related to schizophrenia but instead as a "pervasive developmental disorder" (PDD). DSM-IV and DSM-IV-TR (American Psychiatric Association, 1994, 2000) conceptualized PDDs as a spectrum of severity, defined by social interaction and communication impairments, as well as restricted, repetitive, and stereotyped patterns of behavior. For a diagnosis of autistic disorder, an individual needed at least six of 12 symptoms across the domains of social interaction, communication, and restricted, repetitive, and stereotyped patterns of behavior, before age 3. PDD-not otherwise specified (PDD-NOS) required fewer symptoms and included a more heterogeneous group of children, all of whom had social interaction impairments.

In an attempt to improve specificity, the three disorders in DSM-IV-TR (autistic disorder, Asperger's disorder, and PDD-NOS) were reclassified in DSM-5 (American Psychiatric Association, 2013) as a single category: Autism spectrum disorder (ASD), defined by impairments in social communication and interaction, paired with restricted, repetitive patterns of behavior or interests. Some symptoms must be present during early development, but others may appear when social demands outweigh a person's abilities.

To meet DSM-5 criteria for ASD, an individual must display persistent social communication and interaction impairments, including deficits in social–emotional reciprocity (e.g., back-and-forth conversations, approach in social situations, sharing of affect or interests), nonverbal communicative behaviors (e.g., gestures, integrating eye contact and vocalizations, facial expressions), and development and maintenance of interpersonal relationships (e.g., adjusting behavior to the situation, interest in peers, imaginative play). Additionally, an individual must have two or more restricted and repetitive behaviors (e.g., hand flapping, lining up toys, spinning wheels of car, echolalia, idiosyncratic/novel word use), rigid adherence to routine or insistence on sameness, intense fixation on specific interests, and hyper- or hyporeactivity to sensory stimuli. DSM-5 also requires specifying the level of severity based on the amount of support an individual requires.

The diagnosis of ASD requires stricter criteria than the earlier PDD-NOS and Asperger's disorder diagnoses. The current DSM-5 criteria have been criticized for excluding those with less severe impairments, very young children, those with an IQ in the average range, and females (Barton, Robins, Jashar, Brennan, & Fein, 2013; Wiggins et al., 2019). A systematic review found that the overall reduction in diagnostic identification is between 20 and 31% (Kulage et al., 2020).

EPIDEMIOLOGY

Kanner's and Asperger's early epidemiological observations of ASD included a preponderance of males with varied intellectual capacities and suggested a prevalence of 3 or 4 in 10,000 (Wing, Leekam, Libby, Gould, & Larcombe, 2002). The most recent estimate of ASD prevalence, with more modern methods, is 70 per 10,000 (Myers, Presmanes Hill, Zuckerman, & Fombonne, 2018). However, other studies report significantly higher rates (e.g., Baird et al., 2006). A worldwide systematic review identified a median global prevalence estimate of 62 per 10,000 and did not demonstrate significantly different rates based on geography (Elsabbagh et al., 2012). However, the lack of studies in developing countries limits prevalence comparisons across geographic regions. Some evidence suggests cultural differences in the manifestation of ASD symptoms, which may influence prevalence rates in different regions (Matson et al., 2011). Since 2000, prevalence rates have ranged from 1.4 to 264 per 10,000; prevalence was negatively associated with sample size and positively associated with publication year (Myers et al., 2018). A U.S. study that reviewed educational and service provider records of 8-year-old children identified a prevalence rate of 168 per 10,000, which is significantly higher than the estimates described earlier (Baio et al., 2018). However, this sample was not nationally representative, and significant methodological flaws have been identified (Durkin, Bilder, Pettygrove, & Zahorodny, 2015; Fombonne, 2018). It should be noted that surveys or screens done in early childhood (ages 12 to 36 months) and at school age (e.g., age 8) will identify children who differ widely in severity and type of symptoms, and in degrees of developmental delay and therefore in prevalence. Although each of these time points has its own validity, they should not be directly compared.

An apparent increase in the prevalence of ASD in the past few decades has prompted attempts to ascertain whether the increase is real or a result of changing definitions, increased awareness, and other social factors. As the definition of ASD evolves and identification strategies and services improve, prevalence rates may continue to change. The ASD and Developmental Disabilities Monitoring Network found considerable variation in ASD prevalence in 8-year-olds among 11 U.S. sites but identified an overall 150% rise in prevalence of ASD from 2000 to 2014 (Baio et al., 2018). However, changes in data collection at some sites make interpretation of this increase challenging. Increased prevalence in many regions is likely due to broadened diagnostic criteria, increased efficiency of case identification, and diagnostic substitution (Elsabbagh et al., 2012). Studies with more rigorous methodologies have failed to find significant increases. A study that maintained identical methods for case identification and ascertainment found comparable prevalence rates over time (Chakrabarti & Fombonne, 2001, 2005). Similarly, a study examining the prevalence of ASD in adults found stable rates over time (Brugha et al., 2011).

Epidemiological studies of ASD have methodological challenges that may contribute to variation in prevalence estimates. Pertinent factors include screening challenges, diagnostic classifications, diagnostic substitution, and public perception of diagnosis, all of which complicate precise measurement and contribute to variations in prevalence. Such challenges have yet to be solved; the ASD and Developmental Disabilities Monitoring Network continues to find significant differences across states, in large part due to geographically dependent data acquisition (Baio et al., 2018). Large educational or medical databases are often used for estimates of ASD prevalence but exclude those who manage without substantial support, or those who lack access to health care.

Changes in diagnostic criteria have significant effects on prevalence and may cloud longitudinal estimates. For example, as ASD became more well-known in the early 1990s, concern about an "Autism epidemic" grew. However, as ASD rates increased, rates of mental retardation and learning disabilities decreased, suggesting that some degree of diagnostic substitution was responsible for growing ASD prevalence (Shattuck, 2006).

ETIOLOGY, NEUROPATHOLOGY, AND NEURAL SUBSTRATES

Genetics, sex, and neurodevelopmental characteristics are biological factors that influence risk and resilience in ASD (Szatmari, 2018). Twin studies indicate that ASD is highly heritable, with estimates ranging from 64% to 91% (Tick, Bolton, Happé, Rutter, & Rijsdijk, 2016). Family members sometimes demonstrate subclinical ASD symptoms, or the broader Autism phenotype, providing support for phenotypic heritability. However, identifying specific genetic factors associated with ASD is difficult. More than 100 potential genes have been identified, and almost all known genetic risk factors exist in unaffected members of the population, as well as those with other disorders (Robinson et al., 2016). Approximately 80% of younger siblings of children with ASD do not meet diagnostic criteria, even though they may present with socialization and communication problems, suggesting the existence of protective factors (Szatmari, 2018). In general, proposed genetic factors do not map well onto the phenotype; monozygotic twins concordant for ASD can still show very different phenotypes (Le Couteur et al., 1996), and as many as 70% of affected sibling pairs do not share known ASD risk genes (Yuen et al., 2015). A study of genomewide links supports a continuum model of how different types of genetic risk affect traits associated with ASD (Robinson et al., 2016), with additive influences of polygenic factors. Evidence suggests a female protective effect in which a greater number of genetic abnormalities are required before an ASD phenotype emerges in females (Jacquemont et al., 2014).

Genetic causes are insufficient to explain all cases of ASD (Gaugler et al., 2014). Environmental factors have been implicated with varying empirical support (Szatmari, 2018). Symptoms of ASD are present early in life, suggesting the early or even prenatal involvement of environmental factors. Though vaccines have long been targeted as potential causes of ASD, the proposed mechanisms have not been shown to increase risk (Gerber & Offit, 2009). Evidence exists for an association between air pollutants and risk for ASD, though more research is required (Dickerson et al., 2016; Modabbernia, Velthorst, & Reichenberg, 2017). Pesticide exposure and ASD are also linked, though the effects of different pesticides have yet to be clearly identified (Roberts, Dawley, & Reigart, 2019).

Older parental age (Modabbernia et al., 2017), as well as low birth weight (Lampi et al., 2012) and the occurrence of pre- or peri-natal adverse events (Gardener, Spiegelman, & Buka, 2011), are associated with increased rates of ASD. Additional proposed environmental influences include those affecting the gastrointestinal (Neuhaus, Bernier, Tham, & Webb, 2018) and immune systems (Bölte, Girdler, & Marschik, 2019). Maternal diet and lifestyle, including hypothyroidism (Getahun et al., 2018), have been linked to ASD; vitamins including folic acid are associated with reduced ASD occurrence (Surén et al., 2013). Maternal prenatal medication use has been studied, implicating some antidepressants (Andalib et al., 2017), antiasthmatics (Croen et al., 2011), and antiepileptics (Bromley et al., 2013) in ASD risk. Maternal fever and infection have also been linked to ASD (Lee et al., 2015; Zerbo et al., 2013), with differential effects found in response to exposure at different points of gestation. Involvement of immune factors is further supported by higher rates of autoimmune diseases in families of individuals with ASD (Atladottir et al., 2009). Another little understood biological factor associated with ASD is early, severe blindness (Hobson & Lee, 2010; Jure, Pogonza, & Rapin, 2016). A high prevalence of ASD, with generally positive prognosis, is found in blind children and seems to depend on the severity and timing of blindness rather than a biological cause, suggesting that early impaired input from the environment can lead to ASD or ASD features.

Neuropathology and Neural Substrates

Individuals with ASD tend to have larger head sizes, with 16% meeting criteria for macrocephaly (Sacco, Gabriele, & Persico, 2015). Accelerated brain volume growth has been observed in young children (Amaral, Schumann, & Nordahl, 2008). White matter development shows differences emerging in infants prior to behavioral symptoms (Wolff et al., 2012), though it is unclear whether these neural differences persist past childhood (Hazlett, Poe, Gerig, Smith, & Piven, 2006).

Some work has identified neural differences very early in life that successfully predict both behaviors associated with ASD (Wolff et al., 2017) and the diagnosis itself (Emerson et al., 2017). Infants with high family risk of ASD who were later diagnosed with ASD showed cortical surface area hyperexpansion as early as ages 6–12 months followed by brain volume overgrowth between the first and second years of life (Hazlett et al., 2017). Additionally, regional hyperconnectivity and hypoconnectivity of subcortical and cortical connections have been shown (Di Martino et al., 2014).

The diversity and relative independence of these neuropathologies suggest that, from a causal perspective, there may in fact be "many ASDs." The lack of correspondence between the proposed causes and the phenotype (with the exception of some specific genetic disorders) has impeded clarification (Rapin, 2014; Waterhouse, 2013; Waterhouse, London, & Gillberg, 2016). Clarity about neuropathology may emerge with a refined characterization of ASD (Amaral et al., 2008).

NEUROPSYCHOLOGICAL CONSEQUENCES

While we describe general findings here, we caution against broad interpretation given the immense heterogeneity of the neuropsychological profile of ASD.

General Intellectual Functioning

In the late 20th century, the majority (70%) of individuals with ASD were thought to exhibit comorbid intellectual disability (ID; IQ < 70), (Fombonne, 2002) but more recent estimates suggest one-third to one-half (Baio et al., 2018). Efforts to describe the developmental trajectory of IQ in ASD populations have identified distinct patterns of development and stability (Solomon et al., 2018). Longitudinal data suggest that IQ stabilizes in adolescence (Joseph, 2011; Sigman & McGovern, 2005). Significant discrepancies exist between Verbal and Nonverbal IQ in children with ASD in either direction (Joseph, 2011; Ryland, Hysing, Posserud, Gillberg, & Lundervold, 2014). Early IQ is predictive of later intellectual ability (Anderson, Liang, & Lord, 2014).

Perceptual and Sensorimotor Skills

Although atypical sensory experiences were not considered core symptoms of ASD until DSM-5, they are common in affected individuals. Neurophysiological data indicate abnormalities in basic sensory processing, as well as multisensory integration (Marco, Hinkley, Hill, & Nagarajan, 2011). Individuals with ASD display worse audiovisual integration relative to typically developing (TD) peers; better audiovisual integration is related to better language and communication, and reduced symptom severity (Feldman et al., 2018).

Hyporesponsiveness, hyperresponsiveness, sensory interests, sensory-seeking behaviors, and enhanced perception are commonly observed in ASD (Ausderau et al., 2014). Sensory processing differences in children with ASD are relatively stable 2 years later, with some decline in severity that may be due to neural maturation, improved coping, therapy, or exposure to positive social experiences (Baranek et al., 2019). Studies suggest that individuals with ASD consistently perform better on visual search and pitch discrimination tasks (Eigsti & Fein, 2013; Kaldy, Giserman, Carter, & Blaser, 2016). Enhanced early pitch discrimination may impair language development, as affected children may focus on auditory differences rather than similarities in phonemes produced by different speakers (Eigsti & Fein, 2013).

Language

ASD is associated with atypical communication characteristics (ACCs), including being nonverbal, having receptive or expressive language delays, pronoun reversal, neologisms, and atypical prosody and facial expressions (Kang, Gadow, & Lerner, 2020). In one study, 91% of youth with ASD displayed at least one ACC, compared to 39% in a non-ASD group. Some children show only moderate pragmatic difficulty, while a smaller subset faces pervasive challenges, including severe speech delay, repetitive or scripted language, and unusual prosody (Kang et al., 2020). Impairments in pragmatics and discourse are most common in ASD (Eigsti, De Marchena, Schuh, & Kelley, 2011).

Attention

Individuals with ASD often struggle with shifting their attention and refocusing on a novel stimulus. In particular, children with ASD take longer to disengage their attention than do TD peers (Sacrey, Bryson, & Zwaigenbaum, 2013). This may influence later deficits in social orienting, as children with ASD preferentially attend to nonsocial images rather than social images, such as faces (Pierce, Conant, Hazin, Stoner, & Desmond, 2011). Reduced social orienting can lead to drastically fewer learning opportunities in early life. Furthermore, visual orienting influences not only social-communicative skills but also emotion regulation, as children learn to disengage or distract themselves from upsetting stimuli. Some findings suggest deficits in controlled attention (Craig et al., 2016); however, significant differences between ASD and TD groups have not been consistently observed on objective measures.

Memory

Challenges with memory in ASD populations primarily derive from problems with encoding and organizing information rather than long-term storage (Ozonoff, 2009). Individuals with ASD often do not demonstrate the typical improvements in working memory between adolescence and adulthood (Luna, Doll, Hegedus, Minshew, & Sweeney, 2007).

Researchers hypothesize that memory ability varies with language and IQ. Individuals with low IQ and impaired language may have pervasive problems with declarative memory, affecting both recognition and recall (Boucher, Mayes, & Bigham, 2008). Individuals with ASD also tend to rely on semantic and procedural memory rather than episodic memory and perceptual learning (Boucher & Anns, 2018). They may show deficits on memory tasks with higher cognitive and attentional demands (Sheppard, Bruineberg, Kretschmer-Trendowicz, & Altgassen, 2018).

Executive Functions

Individuals with ASD exhibit deficits on both objective and self-report measures of executive function (EF). A meta-analysis found a moderate effect for global EF impairments in individuals with ASD, with no significant difference between subdomains (Demetriou et al., 2018). ASD is often associated with cognitive inflexibility (Craig et al., 2016). Laboratory-based data also reveal impaired response inhibition, flexibility and switching, working memory, planning, and vigilance compared to TD individuals (Corbett, Constantine, Hendren, Rocke, & Ozonoff, 2009). Fewer difficulties with EF predict better adaptive behavior outcomes, beyond age and Nonverbal IQ (Bertollo & Yerys, 2019).

Social Cognition

Individuals with ASD demonstrate difficulty with aspects of social cognition, including theory of mind, which involves attributing internal mental states to other people and understanding the intentions of others (Baron-Cohen, Leslie, & Frith, 1985). Young children with ASD struggle with the fundamental skills linked to theory of mind, including joint attention and initiation of sharing of interests by pointing or gaze shifting. Deficits in responses to joint attention typically fade around age 3 (Mundy, Sigman, & Kasari, 1994), while deficits in initiation of joint attention persist (Franchini, Armstrong, Schaer, & Smith, 2019).

Some researchers hypothesize that social impairments derive from reduced sensitivity to social rewards (Dawson, Webb, & McPartland, 2005). Impairments in social cognition, particularly in face processing, may derive from perceptual and cognitive deficits that hinder interpretation of social stimuli (Dawson et al., 2005). Behavioral and neurological data collected using techniques with increasing precision, such as eye tracking, are being integrated to continue to test these theories.

Adaptive and Social Functioning

Evidence suggests that adaptive behavior (i.e., independence; social/communication skills) develops atypically in ASD, increasing during childhood and then plateauing, regardless of IQ (Meyer, Powell, Butera, Klinger, & Klinger, 2018). About 20% of children display improvements in adaptive functioning over time, while others show stable or worsening trajectories (Szatmari et al., 2015).

Age, IQ, ASD symptom severity, and adaptive behavior have been examined in numerous studies, drawing mixed conclusions about the relationship between these factors. The link between adaptive skills and ASD symptom severity is relatively weak and may be moderated by IQ and age (Hill, Gray, Kamps, & Enrique Varela, 2015).

Emotional and Behavioral Adjustment

Emotional and behavioral problems are often present in ASD, including self-injury, aggression, low frustration tolerance, and lack of compliance (Matson & Nebel-Schwalm, 2007). Increased emotion reactivity, coupled with less frequent use of cognitive reappraisal strategies, is found in ASD and is associated with maladaptive behaviors (Mazefsky, 2015). Individuals with ASD commonly present with comorbid disorders, including social anxiety, attention-deficit/hyperactivity disorder (ADHD), and oppositional defiant disorder (Simonoff et al., 2008). Anxiety problems are especially common in children and adolescents with ASD (White, Oswald, Ollendick, & Scahill, 2009).

DEVELOPMENTAL CONSIDERATIONS

While ASD can be reliably diagnosed by age 2, the average age of diagnosis is closer to 5 years (Baio et al., 2018; Stone et al., 1999). Reliable diagnostic tools exist for toddlers with a mental age as young as 12 months (second edition of the Autism Diagnostic

Observation Schedule [ADOS-2] Toddler Module; Luyster et al., 2009). Prospective studies suggest diagnostic stability of an early ASD diagnosis by around 14 months (Pierce et al., 2019). The discrepancy between the average age of diagnosis and the age at which a stable diagnosis can be made highlights the need for health professionals to consistently screen all children for early symptoms of ASD, and refer them for a developmental evaluation when indicated by the screening tool.

Early signs of ASD can appear as early as the first year of life (Ozonoff et al., 2008). Infants who eventually receive an ASD diagnosis show declining, but not absent, attention to the eyes of human faces between ages 2 and 6 months (W. Jones & Klin, 2013). By 6 months of age, children later diagnosed with ASD show delayed responses to faces and atypical patterns of visual disengagement (E. Jones et al., 2016). Additional early warning signs of ASD in children under 1 year of age include atypical eye contact, diminished social smiling, and a tendency to fixate on specific objects (Zwaigenbaum et al., 2005). Children with ASD often show atypical language skills by 12–18 months, including difficulties understanding single words and lack of saying words (Lazenby et al., 2016). Behaviors that differentiate children with ASD from other infants include decreased orientation to visual stimuli, delayed or absent response to name, and diminished communicative gestures (Baranek, 1999; Miller et al., 2017). These impairments indicate a fundamental, early difference in response and engagement with social stimuli (E. Jones et al., 2016; Merin, Young, Ozonoff, & Rogers, 2007).

At around 2 years of age, children with ASD show fewer directed facial expressions and vocalizations during social games than do TD children or children with language delays. By 24 months of age, children with ASD show delays across cognitive domains, except for receptive language (Landa & Garrett-Mayer, 2006), and attend to different auditory and visual information than peers. Rather than relying on the eyes or upright, biological motion to infer important information from their environment, children with ASD tend to prefer nonsocial patterns (Klin, Lin, Gorrindo, Ramsay, & Jones, 2009).

Developmental regression, or the loss of a previously acquired skill, occurs in about one-third of children with ASD, typically before age 2, and at similar rates across sexes. Typically, children lose both language and social skills. After 36 months, the most common type of regression is loss of social skills (Parr et al., 2011). Regression is associated with poorer development across language and cognitive domains (Parr et al., 2011).

By age 4, most children with ASD demonstrate some gains in expressive language, which may co-occur with unusual features of speech, such as echolalia, atypical prosody, or restricted content of conversations. The average age of first words spoken in children with ASD is around 38 months, although about 30% of children with ASD do not develop spoken language (Wodka, Mathy, & Kalb, 2013). The best predictors of later language acquisition in children who lack phrase speech at age 4 are average nonverbal intelligence and social engagement. This highlights the need for early, intensive, evidence-based interventions that target early communication deficits in ASD. By age 5, verbal children with ASD use less complex speech and shorter utterances but understand and produce the same number of different word types as TD peers (Eigsti, Bennetto, & Dadlani, 2007). Children with ASD continue to show restricted and repetitive behaviors around ages 4–5, and often show the highest rates of stereotyped motor movements, insistence on sameness, adherence to rituals, and restricted interests during this time (Esbensen, Seltzer, Lam, & Bodfish, 2009). A subgroup of children with clear ASD symptoms in early childhood appear to lose their symptoms and catch up developmentally (Anderson et al., 2014; Fein et al., 2013; Fountain, Winter, & Bearman, 2012); they have been variably termed *optimal outcome, very positive outcome,* and *bloomers*. This outcome is estimated at 10–20% in these three cohorts, usually in response to intensive intervention and tends to be manifested by around age 7 or 8 years (Fein, Dixon, Paul, & Levin, 2005).

Adolescents with ASD tend to have difficulty completing postsecondary education, obtaining stable full-time jobs, and living independently (Sosnowy, Silverman, & Shattuck, 2018). Recent analyses suggest that adolescents with ASD who have fewer symptoms are more independent as adults (Eaves & Ho, 2008). About 50% of youth with ASD without a comorbid intellectual disability pursue postsecondary education, far below the national average for TD young adults. Evidence on vocational training programs suggest an unmet need to understand individual factors that contribute to the transition to adulthood (Taylor et al., 2012).

PREDICTORS AND MODERATORS

Biological Factors

Data suggest that the development of neural structure and function may contribute to phenotypic diversity and variable outcomes in ASD (Inui, Kumagaya, & Myowa-Yamakoshi, 2017). For example, megalencephaly, found in 15% of male children, is associated with increased severity of symptoms and poorer outcome (Amaral et al., 2017).

Sex differences may also influence symptoms and outcome. Compared to their male counterparts, females display more internalizing problems (Hull, Mandy, & Petrides, 2017), fewer stereotyped and repetitive behaviors (Kreiser & White, 2014), better executive functioning (Lehnhardt et al., 2015), and better interpersonal skills (Dean, Harwood, & Kasari, 2017), which may lead to under-diagnosis (Szatmari, 2018). Recently, there has been rising interest in "social camouflaging," especially among females with ASD, where they expend cognitive effort to express social behaviors that hide their residual social communication difficulties; this "camouflaging" may enable them to blend in with TD peers, but may come at a cost in increased stress and anxiety (Lai et al., 2017).

Psychological Factors

Psychological characteristics may affect the presentation of core ASD symptoms. Only 4–12% of adults with ASD achieve an independent lifestyle, and unemployment or underemployment is common (Ratto & Mesibov, 2015). Higher IQ and better language ability are predictors of favorable outcome (Seltzer, Shattuck, Abbeduto, & Greenberg, 2004). Some communicative language by age 5 has been frequently cited as a powerful predictor of later outcome (Rutter, 1970). Mayo, Chlebowski, Fein, and Eigsti (2013) found that some communicative language at any age examined was associated with better outcome, but that some words by age 24 months was the most predictive. Comorbid conditions, such as anxiety, depression, and ADHD, are found in up to 64% of adolescents and adults with ASD, and may also affect outcome (Seltzer et al., 2004).

EF skills may influence the development of comorbid psychopathology (Lawson et al., 2015), adaptive skills (Pugliese et al., 2015), play (Faja et al., 2016), and quality of life (de Vries & Geurts, 2015), making EF a critical target for intervention. EF challenges account for variance in adaptive skills (Pugliese et al., 2015).

Social Factors

More advanced maternal age and education may predict greater response to treatment (Ben-Itzchak & Zachor, 2011). Early intervention has positive effects, and social factors play an important role in accessing these services. In the United States, low socioeconomic status (SES) is associated with lower rates of ASD diagnosis (Baio et al., 2018), likely driven by inequities in health care access. In countries where access to health care is independent of wealth, no differences in SES groups (Larsson et al., 2005) are found, or rates of ASD are higher in lower SES groups (Rai et al., 2012), in contrast to findings in the United States.

Cross-Cultural or International Factors

While the presentation of ASD does not differ across races and ethnicities (Mandell, Ittenbach, Levy, & Pinto-Martin, 2007), evidence suggests that differences in caregiver reports of symptoms across races and ethnicities, as well as provider perceptions, may contribute to delayed diagnosis in minority children (Mandell et al., 2007, 2009). Early universal screening may reduce disparities in age of diagnosis (Herlihy et al., 2014).

Response to Treatment

In addition to the tremendous heterogeneity of symptoms in ASD, substantial individual differences are also observed in response to interventions (Howlin, Magiati, & Charman, 2009). Children who no longer met diagnostic criteria for ASD, as described earlier, received much more applied behavior analysis intervention than those with persisting ASD, with the biggest difference at age 2–3 years (Orinstein et al., 2014). In another group of "very positive outcome" children, the strongest predictor of group membership was reduction in repetitive behaviors between ages 2 and 3 (Anderson et al., 2014). Understanding the interventions that work best for specific child characteristics is understudied. Few studies report substantial information on moderators or evaluate moderators of only one treatment, and many use "broad-based" measures such as IQ that may fail to pick up on fine-grained predictors of response (Vivanti, Prior, Williams, & Dissanayake, 2014). Furthermore, the field lacks a clear measure of change in ASD symptoms (Smith & Iadarola, 2015), though novel measures attempt to address this gap (Cohen & Sudhalter, 2005; Grzadzinski et al., 2016). Future work that describes moderators and phenotypic factors that influence response to intervention will be important.

Predictors of improvement in ASD symptoms and development of cognitive and adaptive skills have been identified. These include younger age at the start of intervention (MacDonald, Parry-Cruwys, Dupere, & Ahearn, 2014; Rogers et al., 2014), better language and communication skills (Magiati, Charman, & Howlin, 2007; Sallows & Graupner, 2005), better social motivation and joint attention (Kasari, Paparella, Freeman, & Jahromi, 2008), imitation (Sallows & Graupner, 2005; Vivanti, Dissanayake, Zierhut, & Rogers, 2013), higher cognitive or adaptive skills (Magiati et al., 2007), and play skills

(Kasari et al., 2008; Vivanti et al., 2013). Later language abilities are predicted by early joint attention (Mundy, Sigman, & Kasari, 1990).

TREATMENT AND INTERVENTION

Lovaas's demonstration of "recovery" in 50% of children in 1987 changed the prognostic possibilities and redefined ASD as a condition far more malleable than previously believed. Lovaas used behavioral principles based in operant conditioning to reduce challenging behaviors and increase communication, an approach now known as applied behavior analysis (ABA). He posited that people with ASD have difficulty learning from their natural environment, and structured his intervention to provide salient reinforcers and frequent learning opportunities.

Interventions for Infants and Toddlers

Several research groups have confirmed what neurodevelopment and neural plasticity suggest—that early intervention is best. Research on cross-domain outcomes of an early intensive behavioral intervention approach showed that children beginning intervention prior to age 24 months had the greatest gains in skills including joint attention, play, and imitation (MacDonald et al., 2014). Using home-delivered, ABA-based treatment, MacDonald et al. showed that children beginning intervention prior to age 2 had better outcomes than children beginning before age 3, who in turn had better outcomes than those beginning before age 4. The Early Start Denver Model (ESDM) has also demonstrated that intervention applied prior to the first birthday results in more positive outcomes at ages 2 and 3 years when compared to intervention started later (Rogers et al., 2014).

Recommendations for research and practice suggest that (1) intervention begin as early as possible, employing both behavioral and developmental approaches, (2) caregivers be actively involved in treatment, and (3) intervention address both core and associated ASD symptoms (Zwaigenbaum et al., 2015). While Lovaas's model of ABA, also known as Early Intensive Behavioral Intervention (EIBI), is generally regarded as the most evidence-based method (Rogers & Vismara, 2008), a range of other approaches has emerged. Many of these approaches fall under the category of "Naturalistic Developmental Behavioral Interventions" (NDBIs), which integrate behavioral interventions with child-led methods developed for other intervention models (Schreibman et al., 2015). In recent years, behavioral approaches have been adjusted to more uniformly stress using positive affect and enthusiasm, selecting reinforcers to match the child's preference, tailoring session length to the child's tolerance, building compliance by giving instructions likely to be followed ("Eat your cookie, Johnny"), ensuring success by starting at the child's current level, focusing on functional skills (e.g., requesting, social attention), teaching in the child's natural environment, and eliminating punishment except for dangerous behavior. At the same time, developmental approaches (e.g., the ESDM) have incorporated behavioral approaches including defining goals, prompting, fading, and shaping. In fact, ABA and NDBI interventions now share more similarities than differences (see Schreibman et al., 2015, for a review).

Both ABA and ESDM are appropriate for children as young as 12 months (Rogers & Dawson, 2010). ESDM aims to make social engagement rewarding by offering the child increased learning opportunities in the natural environment; ABA accomplishes the same goal by pairing the adult's positive response with primary reinforcement, making activities short and fun, and providing primarily positive reinforcement. Children who received 20 hours per week of ESDM for 2 years demonstrated greater improvement in adaptive skills, cognitive abilities, severity of ASD symptoms, and language when compared with children randomized to community services as usual (Dawson et al., 2010). These children also showed better adaptive skills and fewer ASD symptoms at age six (Estes et al., 2015).

ESDM and ABA comprehensively address the child's functioning, consider skills across domains, and often address behavioral deficits related to the core symptoms of ASD. Comprehensive approaches usually have a curriculum that covers a range of skills across domains. ESDM has a curriculum checklist used to evaluate a child's skills and identify foci of intervention, and many ABA therapists use the Assessment of Basic Language and Learning Skills—Revised (ABLLS-R; Partington, 2006) for a similar purpose. Comprehensive approaches are often ideal, because they are based in theory and are appropriate for a range of abilities. However, their effects are more difficult to evaluate than focused interventions, which are designed to address a single, specific skill or goal (Odom, Boyd, Hall, & Hume, 2010). Focused interventions are more easily tested in experimental settings, are more easily learned by therapists and parents, and have proximal effects. Wong and colleagues (2015) identified 27 evidence-based, focused interventions that are often components of comprehensive interventions. These include fundamental ABA techniques (e.g., differential reinforcement, discrete trial teaching, extinction, prompting, task analysis), as well as functional communication training, peer mediated instruction, cognitive behavioral interventions, and structured play groups.

While these interventions have been demonstrated to be effective, the challenge of testing and comparing the efficacy of comprehensive interventions remains. Studies with random assignment to different treatments are difficult to run and require significant resources. Consistent methodology and large groups of well-characterized children are necessary to compare intervention efficacy and identify child factors that best suit a specific intervention.

Other interventions lack strong empirical support. One of the most well-known is DIRFloortime, which proposes that a child's ability to connect with others is a key skill that leads to overall improvement. This approach incorporates research on child development to encourage refined relationship and communication skills but does not use the teaching principles of ABA or other evidence-based approaches to learning (Greenspan & Wieder, 2006).

Interventions for School-Age Children

ASD is present across the lifespan, and interventions for school-age children have notably different goals than interventions for toddlers. As described earlier, interventions for very young children are directed toward improving communication and language, play, social engagement, and adaptive skills. In school-age children, many interventions address challenging behaviors, adaptive skills, social skills, functional language and communication, as well as a child's ability to engage in age-appropriate schooling, routines, and activities.

Behavioral teaching strategies, as described earlier, are frequently used in school-based settings with older children to address many of these teaching goals.

While many school-based social skills interventions have been demonstrated to be minimally effective (Rao, Beidel, & Murray, 2008), one intervention (Program for the Education and Enrichment of Relational Skills [PEERS]) has been shown to increase social skills and decrease social anxiety and problem behaviors in adolescents without ID (Laugeson, Frankel, Mogil, & Dillon, 2009). Other commonly applied interventions for school-age children are those addressing sensory symptoms of ASD. Sensory integration therapy (SIT), which seeks to provide sensory stimulation at levels that help the child better tolerate these stimuli, also lacks empirical support (Lang et al., 2012).

For children with ASD and comorbid anxiety or depression, cognitive-behavioral therapy (CBT) has resulted in reductions in symptoms (Ung, Selles, Small, & Storch, 2015). Some CBT programs, modified to reduce the reliance on recognition of one's own thoughts and emotions, have demonstrated positive treatment effects (Lang, Regester, Lauderdale, Ashbaugh, & Haring, 2010).

Medical Interventions

While no medical interventions have been shown to affect the core symptoms of ASD, nearly 50% of individuals with ASD are prescribed a psychopharmaceutical to address other symptoms (Jobski, Höfer, Hoffmann, & Bachmann, 2017). Aripiprazole and risperidone have the most empirical support in reducing challenging and repetitive behaviors, though both drugs also have significant adverse effects (McPheeters et al., 2011). Interested readers are encouraged to read Chapters 3–7 in the *Clinical Manual for the Treatment of Autism* (Hollander & Anagnostou, 2007).

CONCLUSIONS AND FUTURE DIRECTIONS

In this last section, we attempt to highlight the most successful threads of research over the past 35 to 40 years, the obstacles that have been faced and still remain, and some proposals for possible directions that will yield scientific and clinical advances. We wish to acknowledge the contributions of Molly Helt in an article in which we addressed these topics in more detail (Fein & Helt, 2017).

Rimland's 1964 book was arguably the beginning of scientific research into autism, despite much earlier clinical descriptions by Kanner (1943) and Asperger (1944) (for a description of the latter's questionable activities with the Third Reich, and the possible knowledge of each other's work, see Silberman's *Neurotribes*, 2015). Since that time, biological and behavioral research into the autism spectrum has expanded, as have journals and international meetings devoted to autism and related neurodevelopmental conditions. The areas of major growth in research are seen in the huge number of articles documenting heterogeneity in rates of development, acquisition of language and other skills, memory, motor development and performance, social interaction and cognition, and other aspects of the phenotype.

Another intensive focus of research has been the genetic/chromosomal/metabolic underpinnings of autism. Identification of specific and defined genetic disorders associated with an autism phenotype gave rise to the hope that a limited and manageable set of genetic etiologies would be identified, and would lead to biological treatments in early childhood or in the neonatal or even prenatal period. A set of such syndromes is described by Artigas Pallarés, Gabau-Vila, and Guitart-Feliubadaló (2005) and includes relatively common disorders such as Down, Prader–Willi, Angelman, and fragile X syndromes, as well as deletions of specific areas of specific chromosomes. However, the promise that this approach would map out causes for autism has not been realized. Although documented and suspected specific genetic syndromes may account for as many as 20% of cases, these tend to be cases associated with ID and often with dysmorphology. As of this writing, the Simons Foundation Autism Research Initiative (SFARI; n.d.) website lists 1,089 genes with associations with autism, 91 with strong associations, 2,291 Copy Number Variation loci, and over 2,000 genetic animal models of autism. In addition to genetic research, other studies have documented possible environmental exposures or deprivation in prenatal or early postnatal life.

Another area of research that has burgeoned in the last 20 years is brain imaging, with structural and functional magnetic resonance imaging (MRI), positron emission tomography (PET), and structural and functional connectivity studies. In addition to anatomical studies that measure the volume of specific area and gray matter tracts, a recent focus has been on identifying functional networks (e.g., Uddin et al., 2013). Here again, although very impressive results have been achieved, the linking of specific structural and functional findings with specific etiologies or phenotypes remains in its infancy.

Perhaps the most clinically relevant work in the past three decades has concerned treatment. Medical treatment has not yet connected with biological findings, and the only recognized effective medical treatments are medications for ancillary symptoms (e.g., mood, sleep, hyperactivity) or those that may reduce very challenging behaviors (extreme irritability and repetitive behaviors). Antipsychotic medications are used primarily for irritability, aggression, and self-injury, and secondarily for repetitive behaviors. Their sedating and weight gain effects limit their use to individuals with very challenging behavior (McPheeters et al., 2011). Behavioral treatments have met with significant success in ameliorating core symptoms. As described earlier in this chapter, a plethora of such treatments is available, often sharing critical components. In our clinical experience, all of the well-supported techniques allow virtually all children to make some progress in skills and behavior. However, only a minority of children make so much progress that they lose the limiting symptoms, and the biology of many children clearly limits the progress they can make, although the specifics of these biological factors are not yet known. Earlier implementation of treatment is well documented to result in better outcomes, leading to the premise that universal screening can lead to improved early detection and intervention (Robins et al., 2014).

Several obstacles to developing a more coherent picture of the many syndromes included in ASD, which would lead to deeper understanding of etiology and treatment, have led to a proliferation of findings that have not yet been integrated in a useful way. First is a lack of certainty about the way social deficits and repetitive behaviors co-occur to form the syndrome defined as ASD. Despite decades of research including only individuals who show both social and communicative deficits and some form of repetitive behavior or resistance to change, some recent theorists suggest that these areas are separable and need to be investigated and treated independently (Robins et al., 2014). The second obstacle is that biological findings have not mapped clearly onto phenotypic features (Frazier, Georgiades, Bishop, & Hardan, 2014; Ronald, Happe, & Plomin, 2005). Even monozygotic twins concordant for autism can show tremendous variation between the two phenotypes, and siblings with autism can show different genetic risk factors (Le Couteur et al., 1996).

Fein and Helt (2017) suggest several lines of research that may help in resolving some of these very difficult research issues. First, the question of the coherence of the autism syndrome itself might be illuminated by studying widely inclusive samples of young children with autistic-type social deficits, and determining what percent of them show repetitive behaviors (as defined in DSM-IV-TR or DSM-5) over the course of early and middle childhood. Second, as suggested by Waterhouse and Gillberg (2014), studies should include very narrowly defined phenotypic subgroups, which have a better chance of linking to a biological cause or correlate than the very heterogeneous samples of individuals who meet formal criteria. Third, features that appear very early in childhood (before intervention) and may be relatively resistant to the social environment may produce more biologically heterogeneous groups (e.g., presence or absence of high threshold for pain, disorganized sleep cycles, delayed motor development, head and brain growth, improvements in behavior in response to a high fever). Not only are these traits often not targeted for intervention, they are difficult to influence directly; therefore, their presence and severity may reflect innate features of the child rather than reflecting environmental differences in parenting and therapy. Finally, given the possibility of hundreds of syndromes with varied etiology and pathology that meet criteria for ASD, large databases from multiple research cites sharing genetic, brain imaging, and phenotypic data may be needed to allow small subgroups to be identified; such aggregates are underway (Di Martino et al., 2014) and hold significant promise for the future.

REFERENCES

Amaral, D. G., Li, D., Libero, L., Solomon, M., Van de Water, J., Mastergeorge, A., . . . Nordahl, C. W. (2017). In pursuit of neurophenotypes: The consequences of having autism and a big brain. *Autism Research, 10*(5), 711–722.

Amaral, D. G., Schumann, C. M., & Nordahl, C. W. (2008). Neuroanatomy of autism. *Trends in Neurosciences, 31*(3), 137–145.

American Psychiatric Association. (1980). *Diagnostic and statistical manual of mental disorders* (3rd ed.). Washington, DC: Author.

American Psychiatric Association. (1994). *Diagnostic and statistical manual of mental disorders* (4th ed.). Washington, DC: Author.

American Psychiatric Association. (2000). *Diagnostic and statistical manual diagnostic and statistical manual of mental disorders* (4th ed., text rev.). Washington, DC: Author.

American Psychiatric Association. (2013). *Diagnostic and statistical manual of mental disorders* (5th ed.). Arlington, VA: Author.

Andalib, S., Emamhadi, M. R., Yousefzadeh-Chabok, S., Shakouri, S. K., Høilund-Carlsen, P. F., Vafaee, M. S., & Michel, T. M. (2017). Maternal SSRI exposure increases the risk of autistic offspring: A meta-analysis and systematic review. *European Psychiatry, 45,* 161–166.

Anderson, D. K., Liang, J. W., & Lord, C. (2014). Predicting young adult outcome among more and less cognitively able individuals with autism spectrum disorders. *Journal of Child Psychology and Psychiatry, 55*(5), 485–494.

Artigas-Pallarés J., Gabau-Vila, E., & Guitart-Feliubadaló, M. (2005). [Syndromic autism: II. Genetic syndromes associated with autism]. *Revista de Neurologia, 40*(1), S151–S162.

Asperger, H. (1944). Die "Autistisehen Psychopathen" im Kindesalter [The "autistic psychopaths" in childhood]. *Archiv für Psychiatrie und Nervenkrankheiten, 117,* 76–136.

Asperger, H. (1991). "Autistic psychopathy" in childhood. In U. Frith (Ed.), *Autism and Asperger syndrome* (pp. 37–92). Cambridge, UK: Cambridge University Press.

Atladottir, H. O., Pedersen, M. G., Thorsen, P., Mortensen, P. B., Deleuran, B., Eaton, W. W., & Parner, E. T. (2009). Association of family history of autoimmune diseases and autism spectrum disorders. *Pediatrics, 124*(2), 687–694.

Ausderau, K. K., Furlong, M., Sideris, J., Bulluck, J., Little, L. M., Watson, L. R., . . . Baranek, G. T. (2014). Sensory subtypes in children with autism spectrum disorder: Latent profile transition analysis using a national survey of sensory features. *Journal of Child Psychology and Psychiatry, 55*(8), 935–944.

Baio, J., Wiggins, L., Christensen, D. L., Maenner, M. J., Daniels, J., Warren, Z., . . . Dowling, N. F. (2018). Prevalence of autism spectrum disorder among children aged 8 years—Autism and Developmental Disabilities Monitoring Network, 11 Sites, United States, 2014. *MMWR Surveillance Summaries, 67*(6), 1–23.

Baird, G., Simonoff, E., Pickles, A., Chandler, S., Loucas, T., Meldrum, D., & Charman, T. (2006). Prevalence of disorders of the autism spectrum in a population cohort of children in South Thames: The Special Needs and Autism Project (SNAP). *Lancet, 368*(9531), 210–215.

Baranek, G. T. (1999). Autism during infancy: A retrospective video analysis of sensory–motor and social behaviors at 9–12 months of age. *Journal of Autism and Developmental Disorders, 29*(3), 213–224.

Baranek, G. T., Carlson, M., Sideris, J., Kirby, A. V., Watson, L. R., Williams, K. L., & Bulluck, J. (2019). Longitudinal assessment of stability of sensory features in children with autism spectrum disorder or other developmental disabilities. *Autism Research, 12*(1), 100–111.

Baron-Cohen, S., Leslie, A. M., & Frith, U. (1985). Does the autistic child have a "theory of mind"? *Cognition, 21*(1), 37–46.

Barton, M. L., Robins, D. L., Jashar, D., Brennan, L., & Fein, D. A. (2013). Sensitivity and specificity of proposed DSM-5 criteria for autism spectrum disorder in toddlers. *Journal of Autism and Developmental Disorders, 43*(5), 1184–1195.

Ben-Itzchak, E., & Zachor, D. A. (2011). Who benefits from early intervention in autism spectrum disorders? *Research in Autism Spectrum Disorders, 5*(1), 345–350.

Bertollo, J. R., & Yerys, B. E. (2019). More than IQ: Executive function explains adaptive behavior above and beyond Nonverbal IQ in youth with autism and lower IQ. *American Journal on Intellectual and Developmental Disabilities, 124*(3), 191–205.

Bölte, S., Girdler, S., & Marschik, P. B. (2019). The contribution of environmental exposure to the etiology of autism spectrum disorder. *Cellular and Molecular Life Sciences, 76*(7), 1275–1297.

Boucher, J., & Anns, S. (2018, February 13). Memory, learning and language in autism spectrum disorder. *Autism and Developmental Language Impairments, 3.*

Boucher, J., Mayes, A., & Bigham, S. (2008). Memory, language and intellectual ability in low-functioning autism. In J. Boucher & D. Bowler (Eds.), *Memory in autism: Theory and evidence* (pp. 268–290). Cambridge, UK: Cambridge University Press.

Bromley, R. L., Mawer, G. E., Briggs, M., Cheyne, C., Clayton-Smith, J., Garcia-Finana, M., . . . Shallcross, R. (2013). The prevalence of neurodevelopmental disorders in children prenatally exposed to antiepileptic drugs. *Journal of Neurology, Neurosurgery and Psychiatry, 84*(6), 637–643.

Brugha, T. S., McManus, S., Bankart, J., Scott, F., Purdon, S., Smith, J., . . . Meltzer, H. (2011). Epidemiology of autism spectrum disorders in adults in the community in England. *Archives of General Psychiatry, 68*(5), 459–465.

Chakrabarti, S., & Fombonne, E. (2001). Pervasive developmental disorders in preschool children. *Journal of the American Medical Association, 285*(24), 3093–3099.

Chakrabarti, S., & Fombonne, E. (2005). Pervasive developmental disorders in preschool children: Confirmation of high prevalence. *American Journal of Psychiatry, 162,* 1133–1141.

Cohen, I. L., & Sudhalter, V. (2005). *PDD Behavior Inventory (PDDBI).* Lutz, FL: Psychological Assessment Resources.

Corbett, B. A., Constantine, L. J., Hendren, R., Rocke, D., & Ozonoff, S. (2009). Examining executive functioning in children with autism spectrum disorder, attention deficit hyperactivity disorder and typical development. *Psychiatry Research, 166*(2–3), 210–222.

Craig, F., Margari, F., Legrottaglie, A. R., Palumbi, R., De Giambattista, C., & Margari, L. (2016). A review of executive function deficits in autism spectrum disorder and attention-deficit/hyperactivity disorder. *Neuropsychiatric Disease and Treatment, 6*(617), 1191–1202.

Croen, L. A., Connors, S. L., Matevia, M., Qian, Y., Newschaffer, C., & Zimmerman, A. W. (2011). Prenatal exposure to β2-adrenergic receptor agonists and risk of autism spectrum disorders. *Journal of Neurodevelopmental Disorders, 3*(4), 307–315.

Dawson, G., Rogers, S., Munson, J., Smith, M., Winter, J., Greenson, J., . . . Varley, J. (2010). Randomized, controlled trial of an intervention for toddlers with autism: The Early Start Denver Model. *Pediatrics, 125*(1), e17–e23.

Dawson, G., Webb, S. J., & McPartland, J. (2005). Understanding the nature of face processing impairment in autism: Insights from behavioral and electrophysiological studies. *Developmental Neuropsychology, 27*(3), 403–424.

Dean, M., Harwood, R., & Kasari, C. (2017). The art of camouflage: Gender differences in the social behaviors of girls and boys with autism spectrum disorder. *Autism, 21*(6), 678–689.

Demetriou, E. A., Lampit, A., Quintana, D. S., Naismith, S. L., Song, Y. J. C., Pye, J. E., . . . Guastella, A. J. (2018). Autism spectrum disorders: A meta-analysis of executive function. *Molecular Psychiatry, 23*(5), 1198–1204.

de Vries, M., & Geurts, H. (2015). Influence of autism traits and executive functioning on quality of life in children with an autism spectrum disorder. *Journal of Autism and Developmental Disorders, 45*(9), 2734–2743.

Di Martino, A., Yan, C.-G., Li, Q., Denio, E., Castellanos, F. X., Alaerts, K., . . . Milham, M. P. (2014). The autism brain imaging data exchange: Towards a large-scale evaluation of the intrinsic brain architecture in autism. *Molecular Psychiatry, 19*(6), 659–667.

Dickerson, A. S., Rahbar, M. H., Bakian, A. V., Bilder, D. A., Harrington, R. A., Pettygrove, S., . . . Zahorodny, W. M. (2016). Autism spectrum disorder prevalence and associations with air concentrations of lead, mercury, and arsenic. *Environmental Monitoring and Assessment, 188*, Article 407.

Durkin, M. S., Bilder, D. A., Pettygrove, S., & Zahorodny, W. (2015). The validity and usefulness of public health surveillance of autism spectrum disorder. *Autism, 19*(1), 118–119.

Eaves, L. C., & Ho, H. H. (2008). Young adult outcome of autism spectrum disorders. *Journal of Autism and Developmental Disorders, 38*(4), 739–747.

Eigsti, I.-M., Bennetto, L., & Dadlani, M. B. (2007). Beyond pragmatics: Morphosyntactic development in autism. *Journal of Autism and Developmental Disorders, 37*(6), 1007–1023.

Eigsti, I.-M., De Marchena, A. B., Schuh, J. M., & Kelley, E. (2011). Language acquisition in autism spectrum disorders: A developmental review. *Research in Autism Spectrum Disorders, 5*, 681–691.

Eigsti, I.-M., & Fein, D. A. (2013). More is less: Pitch discrimination and language delays in children with optimal outcomes from autism. *Autism Research, 6*(6), 605–613.

Elsabbagh, M., Divan, G., Koh, Y.-J., Kim, Y. S., Kauchali, S., Marcín, C., . . . Fombonne, E. (2012). Global prevalence of autism and other pervasive developmental disorders. *Autism Research, 5*(3), 160–179.

Emerson, R. W., Adams, C., Nishino, T., Hazlett, H. C., Wolff, J. J., Zwaigenbaum, L., . . . Piven, J. (2017). Functional neuroimaging of high-risk 6-month-old infants predicts a diagnosis of autism at 24 months of age. *Science Translational Medicine, 9*(393), Article eaag2882.

Esbensen, A. J., Seltzer, M. M., Lam, K. S. L., & Bodfish, J. W. (2009). Age-related differences in restricted repetitive behaviors in autism spectrum disorders. *Journal of Autism and Developmental Disorders, 39*(1), 57–66.

Estes, A., Munson, J., Rogers, S. J., Greenson, J., Winter, J., & Dawson, G. (2015). Long-term outcomes of early intervention in 6-year-old children with autism spectrum disorder. *Journal of the American Academy of Child and Adolescent Psychiatry, 54*(7), 580–587.

Faja, S., Dawson, G., Sullivan, K., Meltzoff, A. N., Estes, A., & Bernier, R. (2016). Executive function predicts the development of play skills for verbal preschoolers with autism spectrum disorders. *Autism Research, 9*(12), 1274–1284.

Fein, D. A., Barton, M., Eigsti, I.-M., Kelley, E., Naigles, L., Schultz, R. T., . . . Tyson, K. (2013). Optimal outcome in individuals with a history of autism. *Journal of Child Psychology and Psychiatry, 54*(2), 195–205.

Fein, D. A., Dixon, P., Paul, J., & Levin, H. (2005). Brief report: Pervasive developmental disorder can evolve into ADHD: Case illustrations. *Journal of Autism and Developmental Disorders, 35*(4), 525–534.

Fein, D. A., & Helt, M. (2017). Facilitating autism research. *Journal of the International Neuropsychological Society, 23*(9–10), 903–915.

Feldman, J. I., Dunham, K., Cassidy, M., Wallace, M. T., Liu, Y., & Woynaroski, T. G. (2018). Audiovisual multisensory integration in individuals with autism spectrum disorder: A systematic review and meta-analysis. *Neuroscience and Biobehavioral Reviews, 95*, 220–234.

Fombonne, E. (2002). Epidemiological trends in

rates of autism. *Molecular Psychiatry, 7*(Suppl. 2), S4–S6.

Fombonne, E. (2018). Editorial: The rising prevalence of autism. *Journal of Child Psychology and Psychiatry, 59*(7), 717–720.

Fountain, C., Winter, A. S., & Bearman, P. S. (2012). Six developmental trajectories characterize children with autism. *Pediatrics, 129*(5), e1112–e1120.

Franchini, M., Armstrong, V. L., Schaer, M., & Smith, I. M. (2019). Initiation of joint attention and related visual attention processes in infants with autism spectrum disorder: Literature review. *Child Neuropsychology, 25*(3), 287–317.

Frazier, T. W., Georgiades, S., Bishop, S. L., & Hardan, A. Y. (2014). Behavioral and cognitive characteristics of females and males with autism in the Simons Simplex Collection. *Journal of the American Academy of Child and Adolescent Psychiatry, 53*(3), 329–340.

Gardener, H., Spiegelman, D., & Buka, S. L. (2011). Perinatal and neonatal risk factors for autism: a comprehensive meta-analysis. *Pediatrics, 128*(2), 344–355.

Gaugler, T., Klei, L., Sanders, S. J., Bodea, C. A., Goldberg, A. P., Lee, A. B., . . . Buxbaum, J. D. (2014). Most genetic risk for autism resides with common variation. *Nature Genetics, 46*(8), 881–885.

Gerber, J. S., & Offit, P. A. (2009). Vaccines and autism: A tale of shifting hypotheses. *Clinical Infectious Diseases, 48*(4), 456–461.

Getahun, D., Jacobsen, S. J., Fassett, M. J., Wing, D. A., Xiang, A. H., Chiu, V. Y., & Peltier, M. R. (2018). Association between maternal hypothyroidism and autism spectrum disorders in children. *Pediatric Research, 83*(3), 580–588.

Greenspan, S. I., & Wieder, S. (2006). *Engaging autism: Using the floortime approach to help children relate, communicate, and think.* Boston: Da Capo Press.

Grzadzinski, R., Carr, T., Colombi, C., McGuire, K., Dufek, S., Pickles, A., & Lord, C. (2016). Measuring changes in social communication behaviors: Preliminary development of the Brief Observation of Social Communication Change (BOSCC). *Journal of Autism and Developmental Disorders, 46*(7), 2464–2479.

Hazlett, H. C., Gu, H., Munsell, B. C., Kim, S. H., Styner, M., Wolff, J. J., . . . Piven, J. (2017). Early brain development in infants at high risk for autism spectrum disorder. *Nature, 542*(7641), 348–351.

Hazlett, H. C., Poe, M. D., Gerig, G., Smith, R. G., & Piven, J. (2006). Cortical gray and white brain tissue volume in adolescents and adults with autism. *Biological Psychiatry, 59*(1), 1–6.

Herlihy, L. E., Brooks, B., Dumont-Mathieu, T., Barton, M. L., Fein, D. A., Chen, C.-M., & Robins, D. L. (2014). Standardized screening facilitates timely diagnosis of autism spectrum disorders in a diverse sample of low-risk toddlers. *Journal of Developmental and Behavioral Pediatrics, 35*(2), 85–92.

Hill, T. L., Gray, S. A. O., Kamps, J. L., & Enrique Varela, R. (2015). Age and adaptive functioning in children and adolescents with ASD: The effects of intellectual functioning and ASD symptom severity. *Journal of Autism and Developmental Disorders, 45*(12), 4074–4083.

Hobson, R. P., & Lee, A. (2010). Reversible autism among congenitally blind children?: A controlled follow-up study. *Journal of Child Psychology and Psychiatry, 51*(11), 1235–1241.

Hollander, E., & Anagnostou, E. (Eds.). (2007). *Clinical manual for the treatment of autism.* Washington, DC: American Psychiatric Association Publishing.

Howlin, P., Magiati, I., & Charman, T. (2009). Systematic review of early intensive behavioral interventions for children with autism. *American Journal on Intellectual and Developmental Disabilities, 114*(1), 23–41.

Hull, L., Mandy, W., & Petrides, K. (2017). Behavioural and cognitive sex/gender differences in autism spectrum condition and typically developing males and females. *Autism, 21*(6), 706–727.

Inui, T., Kumagaya, S., & Myowa-Yamakoshi, M. (2017). Neurodevelopmental hypothesis about the etiology of autism spectrum disorders. *Frontiers in Human Neuroscience, 11,* 1–19.

Jacquemont, S., Coe, B. P., Hersch, M., Duyzend, M. H., Krumm, N., Bergmann, S., . . . Eichler, E. E. (2014). A higher mutational burden in females supports a "female protective model" in neurodevelopmental disorders. *American Journal of Human Genetics, 94*(3), 415–425.

Jobski, K., Höfer, J., Hoffmann, F., & Bachmann, C. (2017). Use of psychotropic drugs in patients with autism spectrum disorders: A systematic review. *Acta Psychiatrica Scandinavica, 135*(1), 8–28.

Jones, E. J. H., Venema, K., Earl, R., Lowy, R., Barnes, K., Estes, A., . . . Webb, S. J. (2016). Reduced engagement with social stimuli in 6-month-old infants with later autism spectrum disorder: A longitudinal prospective study of infants at high familial risk. *Journal of Neurodevelopmental Disorders, 8*, Article 7.

Jones, W., & Klin, A. (2013). Attention to eyes is present but in decline in 2–6-month-old infants later diagnosed with autism. *Nature, 504*(7480), 427–431.

Joseph, R. M. (2011). The significance of IQ and differential cogntive abilities. In D. Fein (Ed.), *The neuropsychology of autism* (pp. 281–294). New York: Oxford University Press.

Jure, R., Pogonza, R., & Rapin, I. (2016). Autism spectrum disorders (ASD) in blind children: Very high prevalence, potentially better outlook. *Journal of Autism and Developmental Disorders, 46*(3), 749–759.

Kaldy, Z., Giserman, I., Carter, A. S., & Blaser, E. (2016). The mechanisms underlying the ASD advantage in visual search. *Journal of Autism and Developmental Disorders, 46*(5), 1513–1527.

Kang, E., Gadow, K. D., & Lerner, M. D. (2020). Atypical communication characteristics, differential diagnosis, and the autism spectrum disorder phenotype in youth. *Journal of Clinical Child and Adolescent Psychology, 49*, 251–263.

Kanner, L. (1943). Autistic disturbances of affective contact. *Nervous Child, 2*, 217–250.

Kasari, C., Paparella, T., Freeman, S., & Jahromi, L. B. (2008). Language outcome in autism: Randomized comparison of joint attention and play interventions. *Journal of Consulting and Clinical Psychology, 76*(1), 125–137.

Klin, A., Lin, D. J., Gorrindo, P., Ramsay, G., & Jones, W. (2009). Two-year-olds with autism orient to non-social contingencies rather than biological motion. *Nature, 459*(7244), 257–261.

Kreiser, N. L., & White, S. W. (2014). ASD in females: Are we overstating the gender difference in diagnosis? *Clinical Child and Family Psychology Review, 17*(1), 67–84.

Kulage, K. M., Goldberg, J., Usseglio, J., Romero, D., Bain, J. M., & Smaldone, A. M. (2020). How has DSM-5 affected autism diagnosis?: A 5-year follow-up systematic literature review and meta-analysis. *Journal of Autism and Developmental Disorders, 50*, 2102 -2127.

Lai, M.-C., Lerch, J. P., Floris, D. L., Ruigrok, A. N. V., Pohl, A., Lombardo, M. V., & Baron-Cohen, S. (2017). Imaging sex/gender and autism in the brain: Etiological implications. *Journal of Neuroscience Research, 95*(1–2), 380–397.

Lampi, K. M., Lehtonen, L., Tran, P. L., Suominen, A., Lehti, V., Banerjee, P. N., . . . Sourander, A. (2012). Risk of autism spectrum disorders in low birth weight and small for gestational age infants. *Journal of Pediatrics, 161*(5), 830–836.

Landa, R., & Garrett-Mayer, E. (2006). Development in infants with autism spectrum disorders: A prospective study. *Journal of Child Psychology and Psychiatry, 47*(6), 629–638.

Lang, R., O'Reilly, M., Healy, O., Rispoli, M., Lydon, H., Streusand, W., . . . Giesbers, S. (2012). Sensory integration therapy for autism spectrum disorders: A systematic review. *Research in Autism Spectrum Disorders, 6*(3), 1004–1018.

Lang, R., Regester, A., Lauderdale, S., Ashbaugh, K., & Haring, A. (2010). Treatment of anxiety in autism spectrum disorders using cognitive behaviour therapy: A systematic review. *Developmental Neurorehabilitation, 13*(1), 53–63.

Larsson, H. J., Eaton, W. W., Madsen, K. M., Vestergaard, M., Olesen, A. V., Agerbo, E., . . . Mortensen, P. B. (2005). Risk factors for autism: Perinatal factors, parental psychiatric history, and socioeconomic status. *American Journal of Epidemiology, 161*(10), 916–925.

Laugeson, E. A., Frankel, F., Mogil, C., & Dillon, A. R. (2009). Parent-assisted social skills training to improve friendships in teens with autism spectrum disorders. *Journal of Autism and Developmental Disorders, 39*(4), 596–606.

Lawson, R. A., Papadakis, A. A., Higginson, C. I., Barnett, J. E., Wills, M. C., Strang, J. F., . . . Kenworthy, L. (2015). Everyday executive function impairments predict comorbid psychopathology in autism spectrum and attention deficit hyperactivity disorders. *Neuropsychology, 29*(3), 445–453.

Lazenby, D. W. C., Sideridis, G. D., Huntington, N., Prante, M., Dale, P. S., Curtin, S., . . . Tager-Flusberg, H. (2016). Language differences at 12 months in infants who develop autism spectrum disorder. *Journal of Autism and Developmental Disorders, 46*(3), 899–909.

Le Couteur, A., Bailey, A., Goode, S., Pickles, A., Robertson, S., Gottesman, I., & Rutter, M. (1996). A broader phenotype of autism: The clinical spectrum in twins. *Journal of Child Psychology and Psychiatry, 37*(7), 785–801.

Lee, B. K., Magnusson, C., Gardner, R. M., Blomström, Å., Newschaffer, C. J., Burstyn, I., . . . Dalman, C. (2015). Maternal hospitalization with infection during pregnancy and risk of autism spectrum disorders. *Brain, Behavior, and Immunity, 44*(6), 100–105.

Lehnhardt, F.-G., Tepest, R., Franklin, J., Falter, C. M., Vogeley, K., Gawronski, A., & Pfeiffer, K. (2015). Sex-related cognitive profile in autism spectrum disorders diagnosed late in life: Implications for the female autistic phenotype. *Journal of Autism and Developmental Disorders, 46*(1), 139–154.

Lovaas, O. I. (1987). Behavioral treatment and normal educational and intellectual functioning in young autistic children. *Journal of Consulting and Clinical Psychology, 55*(1), 3–9.

Luna, B., Doll, S. K., Hegedus, S. J., Minshew, N. J., & Sweeney, J. A. (2007). Maturation of executive function in autism. *Biological Psychiatry, 61*(4), 474–481.

Luyster, R., Gotham, K., Guthrie, W., Coffing, M., Petrak, R., Pierce, K., . . . Lord, C. (2009). The Autism Diagnostic Observation Schedule—Toddler Module: A new module of a standardized diagnostic measure for autism spectrum disorders. *Journal of Autism and Developmental Disorders, 39*(9), 1305–1320.

MacDonald, R., Parry-Cruwys, D., Dupere, S., & Ahearn, W. (2014). Assessing progress and outcome of early intensive behavioral intervention for toddlers with autism. *Research in Developmental Disabilities, 35*(12), 3632–3644.

Magiati, I., Charman, T., & Howlin, P. (2007). A two-year prospective follow-up study of community-based early intensive behavioural intervention and specialist nursery provision for children with autism spectrum disorders. *Journal of Child Psychology and Psychiatry and Allied Disciplines, 48*(8), 803–813.

Mandell, D. S., Ittenbach, R. F., Levy, S. E., & Pinto-Martin, J. A. (2007). Disparities in diagnoses received prior to a diagnosis of autism spectrum disorder. *Journal of Autism and Developmental Disorders, 37*(9), 1795–1802.

Mandell, D. S., Wiggins, L. D., Carpenter, L. A., Daniels, J., DiGuiseppi, C., Durkin, M. S., . . . Kirby, R. S. (2009). Racial/ethnic disparities in the identification of children with autism spectrum disorders. *American Journal of Public Health, 99*(3), 493–498.

Marco, E. J., Hinkley, L. B., Hill, S. S., & Nagarajan, S. S. (2011). Sensory processing in autism: A review of neuropsychologic findings. *Pediatric Research, 69*(5), 48–54.

Matson, J. L., & Nebel-Schwalm, M. S. (2007). Comorbid psychopathology with autism spectrum disorder in children: An overview. *Research in Developmental Disabilities, 28*(4), 341–352.

Matson, J. L., Worley, J. A., Fodstad, J. C., Chung, K. M., Suh, D., Jhin, H. K., . . . Furniss, F. (2011). A multinational study examining the cross cultural differences in reported symptoms of autism spectrum disorders: Israel, South Korea, the United Kingdom, and the United States of America. *Research in Autism Spectrum Disorders, 5*(4), 1598–1604.

Mayo, J., Chlebowski, C., Fein, D. A., & Eigsti, I.-M. (2013). Age of first words predicts cognitive ability and adaptive skills in children with ASD. *Journal of Autism and Developmental Disorders, 43*(2), 253–264.

Mazefsky, C. A. (2015). Emotion regulation and emotional distress in autism spectrum disorder: Foundations and considerations for future research. *Journal of Autism and Developmental Disorders, 45*(11), 3405–3408.

McPheeters, M. L., Warren, Z., Sathe, N., Bruzek, J. L., Krishnaswami, S., Jerome, R. N., & Veenstra-VanderWeele, J. (2011). A systematic review of medical treatments for children with autism spectrum disorders. *Pediatrics, 127*(5), e1312–e1321.

Merin, N., Young, G. S., Ozonoff, S., & Rogers, S. J. (2007). Visual fixation patterns during reciprocal social interaction distinguish a subgroup of 6-month-old infants at-risk for autism from comparison infants. *Journal of Autism and Developmental Disorders, 37*(1), 108–121.

Meyer, A. T., Powell, P. S., Butera, N., Klinger, M. R., & Klinger, L. G. (2018). Brief Report: Developmental trajectories of adaptive behavior in children and adolescents with ASD. *Journal of Autism and Developmental Disorders, 48*(8), 2870–2878.

Miller, M., Iosif, A.-M., Hill, M., Young, G. S., Schwichtenberg, A. J., & Ozonoff, S. (2017). Response to name in infants developing autism spectrum disorder: A prospective study. *Journal of Pediatrics, 183*, 141–146.

Modabbernia, A., Velthorst, E., & Reichenberg, A. (2017). Environmental risk factors for autism: an evidence-based review of systematic reviews and meta-analyses. *Molecular Autism, 8*(1), Article 13.

Mundy, P., Sigman, M., & Kasari, C. (1990). A longitudinal study of joint attention and language development in autistic children. *Journal of Autism and Developmental Disorders, 20*(1), 115–128.

Mundy, P., Sigman, M., & Kasari, C. (1994). Joint attention, developmental level, and symptom presentation in autism. *Development and Psychopathology, 6*(3), 389–401.

Myers, J., Presmanes Hill, A., Zuckerman, K., & Fombonne, E. (2018). Epidemiology. In E. Hollander, R. Hagerman, & D. A. Fein (Eds.), *Autism spectrum disorders* (1st ed., pp. 1–48). Washington,

DC.: American Psychiatric Association Publishing.

Neuhaus, E., Bernier, R. A., Tham, S. W., & Webb, S. J. (2018). Gastrointestinal and psychiatric symptoms among children and adolescents with autism spectrum disorder. *Frontiers in Psychiatry, 9*, 1–9.

Odom, S. L., Boyd, B. A., Hall, L. J., & Hume, K. (2010). Evaluation of comprehensive treatment models for individuals with autism spectrum disorders. *Journal of Autism and Developmental Disorders, 40*(4), 425–436.

Orinstein, A. J., Helt, M., Troyb, E., Tyson, K. E., Barton, M. L., Eigsti, I.-M., . . . Fein, D. A. (2014). Intervention for optimal outcome in children and adolescents with a history of autism. *Journal of Developmental and Behavioral Pediatrics, 35*(4), 247–256.

Ozonoff, S. (2009). Autism spectrum disorders. In K. O. Yeates, M. D. Ris, H. G. Taylor, & B. F. Pennington (Eds.), *Pediatric neuropsychology* (2nd ed., pp. 418–446). New York: Guilford Press.

Ozonoff, S., Macari, S., Young, G. S., Goldring, S., Thompson, M., Rogers, S. J. (2008). Atypical object exploration at 12 months of age is associated with autism in a prospective sample. *Autism, 12*(5), 457–472.

Parr, J. R., Le Couteur, A., Baird, G., Rutter, M., Pickles, A., Fombonne, E., & Bailey, A. J. (2011). Early developmental regression in autism spectrum disorder: Evidence from an international multiplex sample. *Journal of Autism and Developmental Disorders, 41*(3), 332–340.

Partington, J. W. (2006). *The Assessment of Basic Language and Learning Skills–Revised (the ABLLS-R)*. Pleasant Hill, CA: Behavior Analysts.

Pierce, K., Conant, D., Hazin, R., Stoner, R., & Desmond, J. (2011). Preference for geometric patterns early in life as a risk factor for autism. *Archives of General Psychiatry, 68*(1), 101–109.

Pierce, K., Gazestani, V. H., Bacon, E., Barnes, C. C., Cha, D., Nalabolu, S., . . . Courchesne, E. (2019). Evaluation of the diagnostic stability of the early autism spectrum disorder phenotype in the general population starting at 12 months. *JAMA Pediatrics, 173*(6), 578–587.

Pugliese, C. E., Anthony, L., Strang, J. F., Dudley, K., Wallace, G. L., & Kenworthy, L. (2015). Increasing adaptive behavior skill deficits from childhood to adolescence in autism spectrum disorder: Role of executive function. *Journal of Autism and Developmental Disorders, 45*(6), 1579–1587.

Rai, D., Lewis, G., Lundberg, M., Araya, R., Svensson, A., Dalman, C., . . . Magnusson, C. (2012). Parental socioeconomic status and risk of offspring autism spectrum disorders in a Swedish population-based study. *Journal of the American Academy of Child and Adolescent Psychiatry, 51*(5), 467–476.

Rao, P. A., Beidel, D. C., & Murray, M. J. (2008). Social skills interventions for children with Asperger's syndrome or high-functioning autism: A review and recommendations. *Journal of Autism and Developmental Disorders, 38*(2), 353–361.

Rapin, I. (2014). Classification of behaviorally defined disorders: Biology versus the DSM. *Journal of Autism and Developmental Disorders, 44*(10), 2661–2666.

Ratto, A. B., & Mesibov, G. B. (2015). Autism spectrum disorders in adolescence and adulthood: Long-term outcomes and relevant issues for treatment and research. *Science China Life Sciences, 58*(10), 1010–1015.

Rimland, B. (1964). *Infantile autism: The syndrome and its implications for a neural theory of behavior.* New York: Appleton-Century-Crofts.

Roberts, J. R., Dawley, E. H., & Reigart, J. R. (2019). Children's low-level pesticide exposure and associations with autism and ADHD: A review. *Pediatric Research, 85*(2), 234–241.

Robins, D. L., Casagrande, K., Barton, M., Chen, C.-M. A., Dumont-Mathieu, T., & Fein, D. (2014). Validation of the Modified Checklist for Autism in Toddlers, Revised with follow-up (M-CHAT-R/F). *Pediatrics, 133*(1), 37–45.

Robinson, E. B., Anttila, V., Kosmicki, J. A., Bulik-sullivan, B., Grove, J., Maller, J., . . . Daly, M. J. (2016). Genetic risk for autism spectrum disorders and neuropsychiatric variation in the general population. *Nature Genetics, 48*(5), 552–555.

Rogers, S. J., & Dawson, G. (2010). *Early Start Denver Model for Young Children with Autism: Promoting language, learning, and engagement*. New York: Guilford Press.

Rogers, S. J., & Vismara, L. A. (2008). Evidence-based comprehensive treatments for early autism. *Journal of Clinical Child and Adolescent Psychology, 37*(1), 8–38.

Rogers, S. J., Vismara, L., Wagner, A. L., McCormick, C., Young, G., & Ozonoff, S. (2014). Autism treatment in the first year of life: A pilot study of Infant Start, a parent-implemented intervention for symptomatic infants. *Journal of Autism and Developmental Disorders, 44*(12), 2981-2995.

Ronald, A., Happe, F., & Plomin, R. (2005). The

genetic relationship between individual differences in social and nonsocial behaviours characteristic of autism. *Developmental Science, 8*(5), 444–458.

Rutter, M. (1970). Autistic children: Infancy to adulthood. *Seminars in Psychiatry, 2*(4), 435–450.

Ryland, H. K., Hysing, M., Posserud, M.-B., Gillberg, C., & Lundervold, A. J. (2014). Autistic features in school age children: IQ and gender effects in a population-based cohort. *Research in Autism Spectrum Disorders, 8*(3), 266–274.

Sacco, R., Gabriele, S., & Persico, A. M. (2015). Head circumference and brain size in autism spectrum disorder: A systematic review and meta-analysis. *Psychiatry Research: Neuroimaging, 234*(2), 239–251.

Sacrey, L.-A. R., Bryson, S. E., & Zwaigenbaum, L. (2013). Prospective examination of visual attention during play in infants at high-risk for autism spectrum disorder: A longitudinal study from 6 to 36 months of age. *Behavioural Brain Research, 256*, 441–450.

Sallows, G. O., & Graupner, T. D. (2005). Intensive behavioral treatment for children with autism: Four-year outcome and predictors. *American Journal of Mental Retardation, 110*(6), 417–438.

Schreibman, L., Dawson, G., Stahmer, A. C., Landa, R., Rogers, S. J., McGee, G. G., . . . Halladay, A. (2015). Naturalistic developmental behavioral interventions: Empirically validated treatments for autism spectrum disorder. *Journal of Autism and Developmental Disorders, 45*(8), 2411–2428.

Seltzer, M. M., Shattuck, P., Abbeduto, L., & Greenberg, J. S. (2004). Trajectory of development in adolescents and adults with autism. *Mental Retardation and Developmental Disabilities Research Reviews, 10*(4), 234–247.

Shattuck, P. T. (2006). The contribution of diagnostic substitution to the growing administrative prevalence of autism in US special education. *Pediatrics, 117*(4), 1028–1037.

Sheppard, D. P., Bruineberg, J. P., Kretschmer-Trendowicz, A., & Altgassen, M. (2018). Prospective memory in autism: Theory and literature review. *Clinical Neuropsychologist, 32*(5), 748–782.

Sigman, M., & McGovern, C. W. (2005). Improvement in cognitive and language skills from preschool to adolescence in autism. *Journal of Autism and Developmental Disorders, 35*(1), 15–23.

Silberman, S. (2015). *Neurotribes: The legacy of autism and the future of neurodiversity*. New York: Penguin.

Simonoff, E., Pickles, A., Charman, T., Chandler, S., Loucas, T., & Baird, G. (2008). Psychiatric disorders in children with autism spectrum disorders: Prevalence, comorbidity, and associated factors in a population-derived sample. *Journal of the American Academy of Child and Adolescent Psychiatry, 47*(8), 921–929.

Simons Foundation Autism Research Initiative. (n.d.). SFARI gene. Retrieved from *www.sfari.org/resource/sfari-gene*.

Smith, T., & Iadarola, S. (2015). Evidence base update for autism spectrum disorder. *Journal of Clinical Child and Adolescent Psychology, 44*(6), 897–922.

Solomon, M., Iosif, A.-M., Reinhardt, V. P., Libero, L. E., Nordahl, C. W., Ozonoff, S., . . . Amaral, D. G. (2018). What will my child's future hold?: Phenotypes of intellectual development in 2–8-year-olds with autism spectrum disorder. *Autism Research, 11*(1), 121–132.

Sosnowy, C., Silverman, C., & Shattuck, P. (2018). Parents' and young adults' perspectives on transition outcomes for young adults with autism. *Autism, 22*(1), 29–39.

Stone, W. L., Lee, E. B., Ashford, L., Brissie, J., Hepburn, S. L., Coonrod, E. E., & Weiss, B. H. (1999). Can autism be diagnosed accurately in children under 3 years? *Journal of Child Psychology and Psychiatry, 40*(2), 219–226.

Surén, P., Roth, C., Bresnahan, M., Haugen, M., Hornig, M., Hirtz, D., . . . Stoltenberg, C. (2013). Association between maternal use of folic acid supplements and risk of autism spectrum disorders in children. *Journal of the American Medical Association, 309*(6), 570–577.

Szatmari, P. (2018). Risk and resilience in autism spectrum disorder: A missed translational opportunity? *Developmental Medicine and Child Neurology, 60*(3), 225–229.

Szatmari, P., Georgiades, S., Duku, E., Bennett, T. A., Bryson, S., Fombonne, E., . . . Thompson, A. (2015). Developmental trajectories of symptom severity and adaptive functioning in an inception cohort of preschool children with autism spectrum disorder. *JAMA Psychiatry, 72*(3), 276–283.

Taylor, J. L., McPheeters, M. L., Sathe, N. A., Dove, D., Veenstra-VanderWeele, J., & Warren, Z. (2012). A systematic review of vocational interventions for young adults with autism spectrum disorders. *Pediatrics, 130*(3), 531–538.

Tick, B., Bolton, P., Happé, F., Rutter, M., & Rijsdijk, F. (2016). Heritability of autism spectrum disorders: A meta-analysis of twin studies. *Journal of Child Psychology and Psychiatry, 57*(5), 585–595.

Uddin, L. Q., Supekar, K., Lynch, C. J., Khouzam, A., Phillips, J., Feinstein, C., . . . Menon, V. (2013). Salience network-based classification and prediction of symptom severity in children with autism. *JAMA Psychiatry, 70*(8), 869–879.

Ung, D., Selles, R., Small, B. J., & Storch, E. A. (2015). A systematic review and meta-analysis of cognitive-behavioral therapy for anxiety in youth with high-functioning autism spectrum disorders. *Child Psychiatry and Human Development, 46*(4), 533–547.

Vivanti, G., Dissanayake, C., Zierhut, C., & Rogers, S. J. (2013). Brief Report: Predictors of outcomes in the early start denver model delivered in a group setting. *Journal of Autism and Developmental Disorders, 43*(7), 1717–1724.

Vivanti, G., Prior, M., Williams, K., & Dissanayake, C. (2014). Predictors of outcomes in autism early intervention: Why don't we know more? *Frontiers in Pediatrics, 2,* 1–10.

Waterhouse, L. (2013). *Rethinking autism: Variation and complexity*. San Diego, CA: Academic Press.

Waterhouse, L., & Gillberg, C. (2014). Why autism must be taken apart. *Journal of Autism and Developmental Disorders, 44*(7), 1788–1792.

Waterhouse, L., London, E., & Gillberg, C. (2016). ASD Validity. *Review Journal of Autism and Developmental Disorders, 3*(4), 302–329.

White, S. W., Oswald, D., Ollendick, T., & Scahill, L. (2009). Anxiety in children and adolescents with autism spectrum disorders. *Clinical Psychology Review, 29*(3), 216–229.

Wiggins, L. D., Rice, C. E., Barger, B., Soke, G. N., Lee, L.-C., Moody, E., . . . Levy, S. E. (2019). DSM-5 criteria for autism spectrum disorder maximizes diagnostic sensitivity and specificity in preschool children. *Social Psychiatry and Psychiatric Epidemiology, 54*(6), 693–701.

Wing, L., Leekam, S. R., Libby, S. J., Gould, J., & Larcombe, M. (2002). The Diagnostic Interview for Social and Communication Disorders: Background, inter-rater reliability and clinical use. *Journal of Child Psychology and Psychiatry, 43*(3), 307–325.

Wodka, E. L., Mathy, P., & Kalb, L. (2013). Predictors of Phrase and Fluent Speech in Children With Autism and Severe Language Delay. *Pediatrics, 131*(4), e1128–e1134.

Wolff, J. J., Gu, H., Gerig, G., Elison, J. T., Styner, M., Gouttard, S., . . . Piven, J. (2012). Differences in white matter fiber tract development present from 6 to 24 months in infants with autism. *American Journal of Psychiatry, 169*(6), 589–600.

Wolff, J. J., Swanson, M. R., Elison, J. T., Gerig, G., Pruett, J. R., Styner, M. A., . . . Piven, J. (2017). Neural circuitry at age 6 months associated with later repetitive behavior and sensory responsiveness in autism. *Molecular Autism, 8*(1), Article 8.

Wong, C., Odom, S. L., Hume, K. A., Cox, A. W., Fettig, A., Kucharczyk, S., . . . Schultz, T. R. (2015). Evidence-based practices for children, youth, and young adults with autism spectrum disorder: A comprehensive review. *Journal of Autism and Developmental Disorders, 45*(7), 1951–1966.

Yuen, R. K. C., Thiruvahindrapuram, B., Merico, D., Walker, S., Tammimies, K., Hoang, N., . . . Scherer, S. W. (2015). Whole-genome sequencing of quartet families with autism spectrum disorder. *Nature Medicine, 21*(2), 185–191.

Zerbo, O., Iosif, A.-M., Walker, C., Ozonoff, S., Hansen, R. L., & Hertz-Picciotto, I. (2013). Is maternal influenza or fever during pregnancy associated with autism or developmental delays?: Results from the CHARGE (CHildhood Autism Risks from Genetics and Environment) study. *Journal of Autism and Developmental Disorders, 43*(1), 25–33.

Zwaigenbaum, L., Bauman, M. L., Choueiri, R., Kasari, C., Carter, A., Granpeesheh, D., . . . Natowicz, M. R. (2015). Early intervention for children with autism spectrum disorder under 3 years of age: Recommendations for practice and research. *Pediatrics, 136*(Suppl.), S60–S81.

Zwaigenbaum, L., Bryson, S., Rogers, T., Roberts, W., Brian, J., & Szatmari, P. (2005). Behavioral manifestations of autism in the first year of life. *International Journal of Developmental Neuroscience, 23*(2–3), 143–152.

CHAPTER 15

Movement Disorders

E. Mark Mahone

OVERVIEW

In the practice of pediatric neuropsychology, assessment of movement and motor function is essential to identifying and understanding brain–behavior relationships in children. Neuropsychologists assess movement and motor skills in children because these functions provide insight into brain mechanisms in a more direct way than does assessment of other, "higher" cognitive functions; that is, the neurological basis for tests of motor function is relatively well characterized compared with other types of neuropsychological tests (Denckla, 2004). Moreover, in children, motor skills serve as markers for deficits in parallel brain systems important for social and communication skill. While motor skill deficits were once considered to be relatively preserved in many neurodevelopmental conditions (e.g., intellectual disability, autism, learning disorders), it is now clear that most children with neurodevelopmental disorders manifest motor skill difficulties that affect life function if one looks carefully (Denckla & Mahone, 2018).

Assessment of motor function is critical to neuropsychological assessment within the developmental framework. As the child matures, so does the motor system, marked by improved efficiency, coordination, and speed of movements critical for both the assessment itself, and for life function (Garvey et al., 2003; Roeder et al., 2008). Additionally, careful assessment of basic motor function in children can uncover subtle motor deficits (described below) that contribute importantly to the overall neuropsychological formulation. Such neurological *subtle signs* can include overflow (also called *associated* or *extraneous*) movements, involuntary movements (e.g., tremor, dystonia, or choreiform), or dysrhythmia. These subtle signs, when interpreted in the context of the overall neuropsychological examination, can serve as markers for inefficiency in neighboring parallel brain systems important for control of cognition and behavior (Mahone et al., 2006). While subtle signs are common in typically developing younger children, their presence in later childhood and adolescence suggests motor dysfunction and is associated with atypical neurological function (Cole et al., 2008; Denckla, 2005).

Motor skills and "higher" neuropsychological functions (e.g., executive functions) are observed to develop in a parallel manner. Both display a similar protracted developmental trajectory, with periods of rapid growth in elementary years and continued maturation into young adulthood (Diamond, 2000; Mahone et al., 2006). Functional development of each system is dependent on the maturation of associated brain regions, suggesting shared neural circuitry involving cortical–striatal–thalamo–cortical (CSTC) pathways (Mahone, Slomine, & Zabel, 2018b). Importantly, when *cognitive* deficits are observed in children with neurological or other neurodevelopmental disorders, they frequently co-exist with difficulties in *motor* functioning. For example, as many as half of children with attention-deficit/hyperactivity disorder, or ADHD (especially males) demonstrate problems with motor coordination (Pitcher, Piek, & Hay, 2003) and approximately half of children with developmental coordination disorder manifest problems with attention (Kadesjo & Gillberg, 1998). Given these observations, the motor examination should be considered central to the comprehensive pediatric neuropsychological assessment. Unfortunately, the motor examination component of pediatric neuropsychological assessments is often limited in scope (Denckla, 2019). This chapter is organized to cover the breadth of motor functions and disorders likely to be encountered by pediatric neuropsychologists and other pediatric specialists. Sections below address the core features and development of the motor system, types and descriptions of abnormal movements (including subtle signs), and praxis and disorders of coordination. The chapter concludes with descriptions of specific movement disorders, including common conditions such tic disorders and stereotypic movement disorders.

APPROACH TO THE NEUROMOTOR EXAMINATION IN CHILDREN

The approach to the neuromotor examination in children is guided by the observation that virtually all behavior has a motor component. The human motor system is able to direct muscles to perform an almost infinite number of movements (Heilman & Rothi, 2003). In the context of the broader neuropsychological assessment, motor function thus serves as the template for cognition. Traditionally, the adult neurological examination emphasizes the search for *hard neurological signs* (e.g., paralysis, abnormal reflexes, or loss of previously acquired skill, like aphasia or alexia), thought to imply an acquired lesion. In children, however, such signs are more often observed with a more "pastel" or subtle presentation (Bernstein & Waber, 1990; Denckla, 2004), in conjunction with anomalous developmental trajectories in other neurobehavioral domains. Also, unlike adults, who more often present with "pure" syndromes, children are more likely to present with mixed movement disorders (Pearson & Pons, 2019). As such, assessment for the presence of unexpected-for-age motor subtle signs plays a central role in the pediatric neuropsychological examination. Interpretation of these and other motor signs sets the stage for the generation of hypotheses related to anomalous developmental trajectories of parallel or *neighborhood* brain systems, informing recommendations related to inefficiency of function (Denckla, 2005a, 2019). For example, when the pediatric neuropsychologist observes contralateral orofacial motor overflow (i.e., unintentional movement of the mouth) during a unimanual motor task in a child for whom the behavior is unexpected for age, hypotheses can be developed regarding the integrity of "neighboring" motor cortex regions involving mouth and hand representations, and their functional maturity.

The developmental approach to pediatric neuropsychological assessment draws information from four primary sources—history, observations, formal psychometric testing, and relevant research literature—in generating neuropsychological formulations (Mahone et al., 2018b), taking into account each individual's unique characteristics and life circumstances. Within this framework, data from the (often separate) neurological examination become critical to the interpretation of motor skill function assessed in the pediatric neuropsychological examination. As such, it is critical for the pediatric neuropsychologist to be familiar with the ways motor skills and movements are assessed and reported in the pediatric neurological examination.

THE CORTICOSPINAL SYSTEM AND MOTOR FUNCTION

The corticospinal or pyramidal system, the main motor pathway in the central nervous system (CNS), extends from the motor area of the cortex through the brainstem and into the spinal cord. The pathways cross in the "pyramids," which are in the medulla, just at the junction between brainstem and spinal cord. The tract terminates and synapses in anterior horn cells of the spinal cord, which give rise to the peripheral nerves. The corticospinal tracts are divided functionally into upper and lower motor neurons. *Upper motor neurons* include the motor neurons above the level of the synapse in the anterior horn (i.e., motor strip), while the *lower motor neurons* involve motor neurons below the level of the anterior horn. As the CNS develops, muscle movements become more discrete, with myelination of corticospinal tract and anterior horn cells. The corticospinal (pyramidal) tracts are critical for generating voluntary movements, while the extrapyramidal tracts, involving basal ganglia projections and associated circuitry, are important for selecting, inhibiting, and sequencing complex movements (Lohia & McKenzie, 2019). As part of their examinations, neurologists commonly assess for increases or decreases in *tone* (i.e., the normal state of muscle tension). Abnormalities in increased tone are thought to implicate anomalous development of the corticospinal tract; conversely, rigidity is considered to be an extrapyramidal sign. For example, *spasticity* is a condition involving continuous contraction of muscles thought to reflect upper motor neuron dysfunction. In children, spasticity can be observed early in life in the form of persistent toe walking (Schlough et al., 2020), and spasticity in more severe forms serves as one element of the diagnosis of many forms of cerebral palsy.

In children, spasticity is the most common sign of upper motor neuron dysfunction. *Fasciculations* (involuntary twitches) and *fibrillations* (irregular contractions) are usually not present in upper motor neuron disorders, nor is there typically significant muscle atrophy (Johnson, Hoon, & Kaufmann, 2008). On neurological examination, hyperreflexia (i.e., increased deep tendon reflexes) and the Babinski reflex may be present. The *Babinski reflex* is a plantar reflex in which an upward toe deviation is observed upon stimulation of the bottom of the foot. This reflex is normal in children up to around 12 months of age, but afterward is associated with atypical development of the corticospinal tracts (Lohia & McKenzie, 2019). Lower motor neuron dysfunction is more likely to involve flaccid paralysis and muscle atrophy, and can be seen in children with acquired conditions such as postpolio syndrome (Lambert, Giannouli, & Schmidt, 2005) or congenital genetic diseases (e.g., spinocerebellar atrophy; Ross & Kwon, 2019). In lower motor neuron dysfunction, fasciculations and fibrillations are more commonly present, and examination of deep tendon reflexes reveals hyporeflexia, such that spasticity and the Babinski reflex are not typically observed. Decreased reflexes in lower motor neuron disorders are not localizing and can also reflect abnormalities in the peripheral nervous system, or perhaps the muscle itself (Johnson et al., 2008).

ABNORMAL MOVEMENTS

Overview

While the pediatric neuropsychologist should be familiar with the variety of abnormal movements observed in childhood, the classification of these movements, and the neurological diagnoses associated with them, should usually be completed in conjunction with a pediatric movement disorder specialist—typically a child neurologist. Abnormal movements occur commonly in children, and can be transient and part of normal development (Pearson & Pons, 2019). Alternatively, these movements can represent signs of anomalous (delayed) development, medical or neurological conditions (environmental, toxic, viral, genetic), or a reaction to foods or medication. For example, "feet-to-hand" overflow (i.e., involuntary upward deviation of the hands observed while walking on heels) is observed as part of normal development among 5-year olds; however, this sign is considered abnormal, reflecting delayed motor development, in a 9-year old (Denckla, 1985). Recognition of abnormal movements, when they occur, can be critical to the developmental neuropsychological formulation, since many of the movements reflect anomalous function of CTSC pathways—especially involving the basal ganglia and cerebellum (Riva, Taddei, & Bulgheroni, 2018). When characterizing movement, the approach to assessment of children is to characterize whether there is too much (*hyperkinetic*) or too little (*hypokinetic*) activity, and whether the observed behavior is abnormal for age (i.e., a developmental phenomenon), versus abnormal for any age (Wolf & Singer, 2008). Additionally, the observation of normal and abnormal movements allows for direct assessment of motor asymmetry, allowing for hypotheses about lateralization of the underlying neural substrate, which is critical as more global coordination problems tend to be nonlocalizing. An important clinical consideration when examining abnormal movements is that they can be exacerbated by exertion, fatigue, excitement, anxiety, and stimulant medications (including caffeine). At the same time, many of the movements can be temporarily suppressed by concentration, or when the child is engrossed in another activity, and are commonly (although not always) absent in sleep (Singer, 2010). The more commonly observed abnormal movements are described below and may be considered signs of underlying neurological dysfunction.

Dystonia

Dystonia is one of the more common types of abnormal movements in childhood, and involves abnormal posturing (contractions) due to simultaneous activation of agonist and antagonist muscles (Pearson & Pons, 2019). Dystonic postures can occur in brief intervals or can be sustained over longer periods of time. When sustained posturing occurs, it is often difficult to distinguish from chorea and athetosis. Overflow movements are sometimes characterized as a form of dystonic posturing. Dystonia, which can occur as a feature of many disorders, or as a side effect of some medications, has been associated with injury to the putamen and globus pallidus (Sanger et al., 2010). Dystonic cerebral palsy can be observed as a secondary complication to premature birth, and/or hypoxic-ischemic encephalopathy.

Chorea and Athetosis

Chorea is a form of involuntary hyperkinetic movement disorder that involves random, discrete, dance-like jerking movements that are largely distal (limbs) but can also be seen in trunk and pelvis movements. In children, acute chorea can be observed as part of a postinfectious or encephalitic syndrome (e.g., Sydenham's chorea, which can occur postrheumatic fever), for which symptoms develop rapidly and are often asymmetric or unilateral. In contrast, chorea associated with genetic syndromes tends to develop more slowly, with movements observed bilaterally (Pearson & Pons, 2019). The most notorious genetic cause of chorea is *Huntington's disease*, characterized by chorea and dementia, which is associated with degeneration of the caudate nucleus. While Huntington's disease most often develops in adulthood, approximately 5% of cases begin with juvenile onset (Cronin, Rosser, & Massey, 2019). Chorea occurs on a continuum and can present in a milder *choreiform* presentation, which is usually undirected and nonrepetitive, and associated with postural instability. Choreiform movements can be elicited during the pediatric motor examination or during graphomotor activities, and are associated with inefficiency of written expression (Denckla, 1997). Choreiform movements can also be observed on common neuropsychological tests, such as the Developmental Test of Visuomotor Integration (Beery, Buktenica, & Beery, 2010), or the NEPSY-2 Visuomotor Precision (Korkman, Kirk, & Kemp, 2007). Chorea is often accompanied by *athetosis*, another type of abnormal hyperkinetic movement, characterized by slow, continuous, involuntary writhing movements that are primarily distal and impede postural stability (Pearson & Pons, 2019). *Ballism*, characterized by flinging (ballistic) movements, is a type of chorea in which the individual produces rapid, abrupt, large-amplitude movements, usually on one side of the body (*hemiballismus*). Hemiballistic movements are seen in individuals who have had lesions to the contralateral subthalamic nucleus.

Myoclonus

Myoclonus is a type of hyperkinetic movement characterized by repeated, irregular, nonrhythmic, shock-like jerks in the context of involuntary muscle contractions. The movements are considered to originate from upper motor neuron abnormalities in the cortex, brainstem, or spinal cord and are characterized accordingly (Sanger et al., 2010). In children, myoclonic jerks can be focal, multifocal, or generalized, and are observed as a benign condition, or part of a wide range of neurological disorders including partial epilepsy, hypoxic injury, encephalitis, or autoimmune disorders (Eberhardt & Topka, 2017).

Tremor

Tremor involves rhythmic oscillations around a joint axis, usually the wrist, fingers, and hands. The back-and-forth motions are typically symmetric. Tremor is characterized by its appearance at rest (as in Parkinson's disease), or as an action/postural tremor (as in essential tremor). *Resting* tremor is relatively slow (4–6 Hz), and is most apparent when the individual is sitting comfortably. *Action* tremor in the context of essential tremor is slightly faster (6–9 Hz), and is observed when individuals are performing routine tasks (handwriting, drinking from a glass). *Intention* tremor is a specific type of abnormal movement that is considered to be a sign of cerebellar dysfunction (Sanger et al., 2010). With intention tremor, the oscillatory movements are commonly side to side, and increase in amplitude as the hand is moved closer to the target and more distally from the body. A more global term for inaccurate movements associated with cerebellar dysfunction is *dysmetria*, characterized by overshooting and overcorrecting attempts to come in contact with a target. Both dysmetria and intention tremor can be observed on structured motor examination (e.g., Physical and Neurological Examination for Subtle Signs—PANESS; Denckla, 1985), and are seen in children with known cerebellar injury, especially to the cerebellar hemispheres, as well as other neurodevelopmental disorders without overt pathology (e.g., autism spectrum disorder [ASD]; Gill & Sillitoe, 2019).

Ataxia

Ataxia involves difficulties with muscle control or coordination of voluntary movements that is not due to muscle weakness or other involuntary movements (Petley, Prasad, Ojha, & Whitehouse, 2020). The movements are typically jerky and unsteady, and the individual often attempts to compensate for the difficulties. Ataxia, which is derived from the Greek terms meaning "lack of" and "order," can be observed in speech, eye movements, head and trunk stability, or gait, depending on the etiology. Ataxia can be characterized as acute, episodic, or chronic (progressive or nonprogressive), and the abnormal movements are typically attributed to cerebellar dysfunction (Pavone et al., 2017). Acute onset of ataxia can occur in children in the context of toxic exposure (including drug and alcohol intoxication), infections, acquired brain injury, brain tumors, or autoimmune disease (e.g., acute disseminated encephalomyelitis—ADEM). Conversely, chronic ataxia in children most often occurs in the context of genetic or neurodegenerative disease (Pearson & Pons, 2019).

Subtle Signs

Careful and informed assessment of motor function is likely to uncover subtle motor deficits in the pediatric neuropsychological exam. Such *subtle signs* include overflow, involuntary movements, and dysrhythmia, and, when present, can complicate the interpretation of cognitive tasks, especially those for which there is a motor component. Subtle signs can serve as markers for inefficiency in neighboring parallel brain systems important for control of cognition and behavior, and provide insight into the maturation of the corticospinal tracts.

Gaits and Stations

The pediatric neuropsychologist is most likely to encounter ataxia, as well as other subtle signs, when observing a child's *gait* either informally or as part of a structured motor examination (i.e., PANESS). During observation of routine gait, the neuropsychologist can assess for ataxia, asymmetrically decreased arm swing, or dystonic posturing, the presence of which can lead to hypotheses about anomalous neurodevelopmental function. The examiner may also seek to elicit these movements during *stressed gaits* tasks, which require the child to walk 10 paces on the toes, heels, or sides of the feet, or *tandem gaits*, requiring 10 paces of heel-to-toe walking forward and backward (Denckla, 1985). During the stressed gaits, the examiner assesses whether the child can perform the task, whether the task elicits ataxic or overflow movements ("feet-to-hand" overflow, i.e., mirrored movements of the hands occurring simultaneously with foot movements), and whether these signs are unexpected for age (Larson et al., 2007). *Stations* tasks involve assessment of motor persistence, balance, and cerebellar function (Gill & Sillitoe, 2019; Sweeney et al., 2018). Motor persistence is examined during stationary tandem stance, standing on one leg, and hopping on one foot—all of which are considered to assess *axial* cerebellar function, with errors assessed for task completion, falls, and presence of (basal ganglia implicating) choreiform movements. The *finger-to-nose* cerebellar task, in which the child is asked to make alternating touches to his or her nose and the examiner's finger (in four separate visual quadrants) assesses for appendicular cerebellar dysfunction, including presence of dysmetria, limb tremor, intention tremor, and past pointing (Denckla, 1985).

Overflow

Overflow movements are subtle motor signs that involve comovement of body parts not specifically needed to complete a task, and can represent a failure of inhibition of prepotent movement (Hoy, Fitzgerald, Bradshaw, Armatas, & Georgiou-Karistianis, 2004). When unexpected for age, overflow movements are considered to be a sign of anomalous or immature development of CTSC brain systems critical for *inhibitory control*, a fundamental component of executive function (Cohen, Taft, Mahadeviah, & Birch, 1967; Cole, Mostofsky, Gidley Larson, Denckla, & Mahone, 2008; O'Brien, Dowell, Mostofsky, Denckla, & Mahone, 2010). Overflow is categorized by the proximity of the extraneous movement to the intended movement. *Proximal overflow* involves movement of a muscle group in close proximity to the intended movement, and also includes exaggerated movement of the intended body part (e.g., lifting at elbow rather than wrist during hand patting; movement of ring and pinkie finger when tapping index finger to thumb). *Orofacial overflow* is characterized by the movement of mouth, tongue, and facial muscles during hand and/or leg movements. *Mirror overflow* involves unintended contralateral movements of homologous muscles, often observed in distal limbs, which accompany voluntary movements (Cole et al., 2008). A related cerebellar sign, *dysrhythmia*, can be also observed during speeded motor tasks when a child fails to maintain a steady pace after starting.

Physical and Neurological Examination for Subtle Signs

To better describe and quantify the range of subtle signs and speed-related skills in children, neurologist Martha Denckla published the Revised Physical and Neurological Examination for Subtle Signs (PANESS; Denckla, 1985). Requiring no specialized equipment, this 20-minute assessment tool allows for detailed examination of subtle signs via gaits, stations, and timed basic motor function. The PANESS quantifies not only mirror but also the additional types of overflow (proximal, orofacial, feet-to-hand), and also delineates dysrhythmia, dysmetria, and choreiform movements. Included in the PANESS

TABLE 15.1. Scoring Criteria for the PANESS

Exam	Task	Scoring
Gaits	*Walking:* • On heels • On toes • On sides of feet • Tandem (forward and backward)	*Errors:* Score 0, 1, 2 *Overflow:* Score right, left, both
Stations	*Standing (20 seconds):* • Tandem—One foot in front of another • Feet together, eyes closed, arms outstretched • Feet comfortable, eyes closed, tongue protruding • Stand on one foot (separately for left and right feet) *Hopping:* • Hop on one foot 50 times (separately for left and right feet) *Finger-to-nose*	*Standing tasks:* Score 0 (20 seconds), 1 (10–19 seconds), 2 (< 10 seconds) *Hopping:* Score 0 (50 hops), 1 (25–49 hops), 2 (< 25 hops) *Finger-to-nose:* Score 0 (normal), 1 (clumsy, mild dysmetria, mild limb tremor), 2 (intention tremor, past pointing) *Errors* (e.g., choreiform movements, falls, arms outstretched): Score 0, 1, 2
Timed Motor Exam	• Foot tap • Hand pat • Finger tap • Heel–toe tap • Hand pronation–supination • Finger sequences • Tongue wiggles	*Time to do 20 touches:* Score in seconds *Overflow:* Score 0, 1 (present/not present) *Dysrhythmia:* Score 0, 1 (present/not present)

Note. PANESS, Revised Physical and Neurological Assessment of Subtle Signs. Adapted with permission from Denckla (1985).

are the following: (1) praxis examination; (2) untimed motor tasks (gaits on heels, toes, and sides of feet; tandem gait forward/backward; standing/hopping on one foot; standing heel-to-toe with eyes closed; standing both feet together, arms outstretched with eyes closed (and choreiform); and (3) timed motor tasks, including a sequence of 20 toe taps, hand pats, and finger taps; 10 "heel-toe," 10 hand pronate–supinate and tongue side-to-side; and 5 sequences of finger appositions (left and right sides). A summary of PANESS administration and scoring is included in Larson et al. (2007) and in Table 15.1.

PRAXIS AND COORDINATION

While assessment of motor speed, strength, and coordination are commonly included in pediatric neuropsychological examinations, the direct assessment of praxis is often a less central component of the assessment (Denckla, 2019). This omission is unfortunate given the importance of motor learning and motor skill acquisition to success in school. The term *praxis* originates from the word *doing* in ancient Greek (Baxter, 2012), leading to words like *practical* and *practice* (Denckla, 2019). From the perspective of the child neurologist, *praxis* refers to the ability to formulate and perform skilled (nonhabitual) motor behaviors given that (1) the task has been previously learned and (2) the individual has the basic motor skill to perform the required behavior; that is, observed problems are *not* attributable to basic deficits in tone, posture, or other movement disorders (Dewey, 1995; Dowell, Mahone, & Mostofsky, 2009).

In order to perform nonhabitual behaviors involving motor function, a child needs to have acquired not only the basic motor skill but also the *knowledge* of the representations of movement, and the ability to transcode these representations into a purposeful *movement plan* (Chang & Yu, 2018; Dowell et al., 2009). Since virtually all behavior is motor, praxis is central to nearly all aspects of childhood functioning. Development of this set of skills is orderly over the childhood period, in parallel with skills development in other functional neurobehavioral domains. Developmentally, cortical maturation progresses from primary sensorimotor areas and spreads rostrally over the frontal cortex, and caudally and laterally over the parietal, occipital, and finally to the temporal cortex (Gogtay et al., 2004). In children, progressive myelination and associated cortical thinning is associated with improved neurobehavioral function. Luria (1980) argued that in children, the primary motor cortex (required for simple one-step actions) is "fully developed" by age 4 years, while the premotor cortex (essential for more complex movements) is not developed until age 6–7 years (Dewey, 1995). These observations are consistent with the functional development described by Piaget (Piaget & Inhelder, 1967), and have contributed to, until recently, policies involving start of formal elementary school education.

In her doctoral dissertation, Edith Kaplan (1968) reported on the early development of praxis in typically developing children. She noted a progression of skills development marked by an increase in the ability to perform skilled tasks, along with a decrease in errors committed while performing the tasks. These skills were observed to progress up to age 12 years, when they were found to be similar to adults. A similar pattern of development was observed by Dewey (1993) in children with developmental motor deficits. In both studies, the "developmental" errors of praxis included body part substitution (i.e., body part as object/tool), temporal (timing), spatial (posturing), and perseverative errors. More recently, Chang and Yu (2018) provided initial validation of a praxis measurement for children ages 6–8 years, showing a similar developmental progression and the ability to separate imagery, verbal gesture production, imitation, and knowledge of object use.

In the developmental context, neuropsychologists are more likely to encounter (or use) the term *dyspraxia*, as opposed to *apraxia*, with the intention of distinguishing a developmental disorder from an acquired condition. As is the case in other childhood disorders, the *dys-* prefix refers to "abnormal" (or out or proportion to the motor problem), while the *a-* prefix refers to "lack of" (Steinman, Mostofsky, & Denckla, 2010). Within this framework, the term *developmental dyspraxia* is used to specify the abnormal development of the ability to perform complex motor actions that is not otherwise explained by lack of exposure, basic motor strength, or skill. This usage is at times confusing, because the terms *developmental dyspraxia* and *developmental coordination disorder* (DCD) are often used interchangeably (Baxter, 2011). Developmental dyspraxia has been operationalized by Dewey (1995) as a disorder of *gesture* and differentiated from other disorders of motor function and control (e.g., cerebral palsy, ataxia, choreiform). In the pediatric assessment, analysis of errors committed during skilled movements helps to determine whether error patterns are similar to those at a younger age (suggesting *delay*) versus unique patterns specific to those with developmental dyspraxia (suggesting *deviance*). In the latter model, developmental dyspraxia is considered a neurological sign, with clumsiness as one possible associated symptom rather than a disorder unto itself (Steinman et al., 2010).

Observations from acquired apraxia in the adult literature help to inform the functional impact and neighborhood signs related to left-hemisphere development in developmental dyspraxia. The disproportionate prevalence of right-handedness leads to belief that the contralateral left hemisphere is specialized for complex motor movements (i.e., praxis), and acquired apraxia is common after left-hemisphere damage in adults (Mesulam, 2000). In adults, limb apraxia is considered an example of left-hemisphere dominance for action (Haaland, 2006), and *cognitive* motor disorder (Heilman & Rothi, 2003). In right-handers, the right motor cortex shows activation when complex motor actions are performed with the left hand, while the left motor cortex shows activation when complex motor actions are done with either hand. The same pattern is not true for simple motor movements (Rao et al., 1993). Moreover, one-third of adult patients with aphasia also present with apraxia (Mesulam, 2000). These observations highlight the hemispheric specialization and functional dissociations for both complex motor movements and language, leading clinicians to consider acquired apraxia as the motor system parallel to nonfluent aphasia. In children, Dewey and Kaplan (1994) found that those with deficits in praxis rarely occurred without coexisting deficits in language, reading, arithmetic, and visual perceptual skills. These associations highlight the need for the pediatric neuropsychologist to use assessments of praxis and language concurrently, and to look for problems with developmental dyspraxia whenever developmental problems with language (including dyslexia) are observed.

Praxis examination should exclude primary motor and sensory impairments, as well as language, behavioral, or other intellectual disabilities that would preclude a child from carrying out non-habitual skilled movements. Once these conditions have been ruled out, the examination then requires consideration of two parallel systems: *conceptual* (i.e., the representation or "praxicon"), and *production* (i.e., the sensory-motor component). These systems underlie the three types of limb apraxia originally described by Liepmann (1900): *ideational* (impaired object use due to difficulty sequencing complex actions), *ideomotor* (production errors for single acts most obvious when pantomiming to verbal command), and *limb-kinetic* (trouble with fast and smooth independent finger movements; Njiokiktjien, Verschoor, Vranken, & Vroklage, 2000). Gestures can further be representational/symbolic, that is, related to meaningful acts (e.g., waving goodbye) or nonrepresentational/nonsymbolic, that is, for nonmeaningful acts (e.g., imitating postures, such as those required for the Imitating Hand Positions subtest of the NEPSY-2 [a developmental NEuroPSYchological assessment]; Korkman et al., 2007). Symbolic gestures can also be divided into those that are *transitive*, or related to a specific tool (e.g., using a toothbrush) or *intransitive* (e.g., a salute). Assessment of movement in praxis examination necessarily includes both gestures (to command and by imitation) and via tool/object use. This framework then sets the stage for parallel examination of praxis and language function in children (see Table 15.2).

When praxis is directly assessed, over and above motor coordination in general, group studies have found deficits in skilled gestures in response to verbal command, imitation, and actual object use among children with ASD (Mostofsky et al., 2006). These findings persist, even when accounting for basic motor skill performance, with praxis

TABLE 15.2. Praxis and Language: Examples of Parallel Assessments

Function	Skill	Stimuli	Response	Examples
Language	Naming	Visual input (picture, object)	Spoken	Boston Naming Test, Rapid Automatized Naming (RAN)
Praxis	Naming	Gesture (postural knowledge)	Spoken	"What is this?" (demonstrates a salute)
Language	Repetition	Spoken language	Spoken	Digit Span, Sentence Memory
Praxis	Repetition	Visual input–gesture to imitation	Gesture	Pantomime hammering a nail
Language	Comprehension	Spoken language	Spoken	Story Memory
Language	Comprehension	Written language	Spoken	Gray Oral Reading Test–5
Praxis	Comprehension	Pantomime—complex gestures	Spoken	"What am I doing?" (demonstrates making a sandwich)
Praxis	Comprehension	Gesture to command	Gesture	"Show me how you brush your teeth."
Language	Fluency	Spoken language	Spoken	Verbal Fluency (semantic, letter)
Language	Fluency	Visual input (picture)	Written	Test of Written Language
Praxis	Fluency	Spoken language; ideational apraxia	Sequencing of gestures	"Demonstrate how to make a peanut butter and jelly sandwich."
Praxis	Fluency	Tool use–visual and somatosensory	Gesture	Examiner gives examinee a hammer. "Show me how this is used."

performance predictive of ASD symptomatology (Dziuk et al., 2007), suggesting a relationship between praxis and core symptoms of the disorder (Steinman et al., 2010). Children with ASD also demonstrate deficits in postural knowledge (understanding gestural postures), in addition to deficits in performing the gestures themselves (Dowell, Mahone, & Mostofsky, 2009). Of note, these specific deficits in praxis have been demonstrated to be present in children with ASD when contrasted to those with ADHD, DCD, and ADHD+DCD (Dewey, Cantell, & Crawford, 2007), suggesting some specificity of this sign in children with autism. *Limb-kinetic praxis*, as originally described, most closely parallels the finger sequencing elements of the developmental neurological examination (e.g., Denckla, 1985), in which performance on sequenced (skilled) movements (heel–toe, hand pronation–supination, finger sequencing) is contrasted with performance on repetitive (simple) movements (toe tapping, hand patting, finger repetition). Using elements of the PANESS (Denckla, 1985), Martin, Tigera, Denckla, and Mahone (2010) showed an association between development of IQ and sequenced (but not repetitive) movements in both typically developing and clinical samples. Using the PANESS examination Berninger and colleagues (1992) demonstrated the associations between finger sequencing and handwriting skills on behavioral examinations, and dissociations in functional magnetic resonance imaging (fMRI) activation during finger sequencing between good writers and those with written expression disorders (Richards et al., 2009).

TICS AND TOURETTE SYNDROME

Overview

When a child begins to make strange or unusual movements, the behaviors can be very concerning to parents. To the untrained eye, it is often unclear whether the movements are indeed abnormal, or otherwise a part of typical development. *Tics* represent one of the most commonly observed types of unusual movements in children (Singer, 2011). Tics are rapid, sudden, recurrent, nonrhythmic motor movements or vocalizations that are explosive in nature. They tend to wax and wane over time, and are exacerbated by sensory stimuli, stress, anxiety, and fatigue, and are often preceded by a premonitory urge. Phenomenologically, tics have been classified as *habits* (Delorme, Gras, Fabre-Teste, & Roze, 2016; Singer, 2016), as they are performed without apparent gain and are unrelated to a clear outcome.

Tics may be mild and relatively unobtrusive, or complex, forceful, intrusive, and even self-injurious (Singer, 2019). For many children, initial presentation of tics is confused with allergies (e.g., eye blinking, coughing, throat clearing), skin irritations (e.g., skin picking, face touching), or simple habits (e.g., cracking knuckles, nail biting). Nevertheless, the presence of tics can lead to psychosocial issues, bullying, physical discomfort, disruptions in school, and a poor quality of life (Singer, 2011). When the pediatric neuropsychologist works with a child with a history of tics, examination for other coexisting conditions should be emphasized. The presence of tics, with no other comorbid neuropsychiatric conditions, is the exception rather than the rule (Dale, 2017). In addition to tics, as many as 90% of affected children have some degree of coexisting behavioral difficulties, including ADHD (~50%), obsessive–compulsive behaviors (50%), autistic features (10–20%), mood difficulties (20–50%), and a variety of other disruptive behaviors that can interfere with social and academic development (Hirschtritt et al., 2015). Clinically, the presence of these comorbidities can be more troubling for parents and families than the tics themselves. As such, the care of children with tic disorders nearly always includes intervention and accommodations for comorbid conditions (Mahone, 2011).

Description and Diagnosis

Tics are usually described along two dimensions—simple versus complex, and motor versus vocal (phonic). *Simple motor tics* typically involve small muscle groups and discrete or focal movements (e.g., eye blinks, head jerks, or nose twitching), and are abrupt and rapid (clonic). *Complex motor tics* involve coordinated and sequenced movements involving multiple muscle groups and can at times look like purposeful gestures (e.g., scratching, gesturing), and include imitation of others (echopraxia), imitation of one's own movements (palipraxia), and production of offensive or obscene gestures (copropraxia). *Simple vocal tics* involve short, meaningless noises (e.g., grunts, snorts, squeals), whereas *complex vocal tics* involve utterances involving multiple syllables and meaningful words or phrases (e.g., *OK*, *goodbye*), repetition of others' words (echolalia), repetition of one's own speech (palilalia), or obscene or offensive utterances (coprolalia; Robertson et al., 2017).

Transient tics are common in typical development among children under age 10 years, with prevalence estimates ranging from 4 to 24% (Robertson, 2015). Most often, tic onset involves simple motor tics around the head and neck area, occurring by age 5–7 years. Motor tics usually precede onset of vocal tics, and simple tics usually precede onset of complex tics (Peterson & Leckman, 1998; Robertson et al., 2017). That being said, tics can occur for months at a time, then disappear, only to reoccur later as similar tics or entirely different tic patterns. This waxing and waning pattern is ubiquitous to tic disorders, and makes the assessment of the "typical" developmental course and responses to interventions more challenging than in other neurodevelopmental conditions (Mahone, 2011). Additionally, tics must be differentiated from other behaviors, such as drug-induced movements (akathisia, dystonia, parkinsonism), stereotypies (described below), hyperactivity, or antisocial behaviors (Kompoliti & Goetz, 1998). Tics are also differentiated from *mannerisms* (i.e., repetitive, distinctive behavioral traits, that have no noticeable interference with life functioning), *habits* (noninterfering routines or behaviors—not necessarily motor—that are repeated regularly but can lack the distinctiveness of mannerisms), and *compulsions* (behaviors associated with an overwhelming urge to perform an act or ritual; Barry, Baird, Lascelles, Bunton, & Hedderly, 2011). The distinction between tics and compulsions is often difficult, since both are commonly preceded by urges that appear to be satisfied following the completion of the action. Compulsions, however, are typically preceded by *obsessions*—which are *cognitive* and ruminative in nature—leading to an anxiety state that is reduced temporarily by the completion of the compulsive act. Conversely, tics are commonly preceded by *premonitory urges*—typically more *sensory* than cognitive—and present as feelings of tension, tightness, or itching, and a progressive feeling of discomfort (i.e., like the sensation prior to a sneeze; Robertson et al., 2017). Like compulsions, the production of the tic often reduces the distress associated with the premonitory urge (Hartmann & Millet, 2018).

When tics persist over time, either continuously or recurring, then the diagnosis of a chronic tic disorder should be considered. The fifth edition of the *Diagnostic and Statistical Manual of Mental Disorders* (DSM-5; American Psychiatric Association, 2013) delineates five categories of tic disorders. In all categories, tic disorders are not diagnosed when tics occur only in the presence of a substance (drug) or another neurological disorder. Additionally, onset of tics by age 18 years is required for the first three conditions listed below. A *provisional tic disorder* is the term used for a person whose tics have been present for less than 1 year. *Chronic motor or vocal tic disorders* are diagnosed in those individuals who have had motor or vocal tics (but not both) for more than 1 year. *Tourette disorder* (sometimes used interchangeably with Tourette syndrome) is diagnosed in individuals who have multiple motor tics and at least one vocal tic, a waxing and waning course, and duration longer than 1 year. The definition for *Tourette syndrome* is similar, but has age of onset before 21 years, and less emphasis on functional impairment associated with the presence of tics (Tourette Syndrome Classification Group, 1993). DSM-5 includes two other conditions: *other specified tic disorder* and *unspecified tic disorder*, which can be used when the individual does not meet criteria for the other tic disorders but has some functional impact in the context of a known or unknown etiology.

Epidemiology

Tourette syndrome (TS), also known as also known as Gilles de la Tourette syndrome, is named after Georges Gilles de la Tourette (1885), the French physician who initially described the condition in a sample of nine patients. TS occurs worldwide with an estimated prevalence of about 1%, although population estimates vary by region and by diagnostic methods. Two meta-analyses in children reported the prevalence rates at 0.52% (Scharf et al., 2015) and 0.77% (Knight et al., 2012). Tic disorders are also more common in males than in females (ratio of 3:1 to 4:1). A recent Norwegian population study examining national data from 2008–2016 (Surén et al., 2019) found that by the age of 12 years, 0.43% of children had received a diagnosis of TS (0.71% for boys, 0.15% for girls), and that among those diagnosed with TS, 50% were also diagnosed with ADHD, and 11% diagnosed with ASD.

Etiology

Genetic predisposition is the most salient risk factor for TS (Robertson et al., 2017). In studies of twins and families, the heritability is calculated at around 77%; concordance between monozygotic twins is consistently greater than 80%, while concordance rate for dizygotic twins is around 20% (Hyde, Aaronson, Randolph, Rickler, & Weinberger, 1992). The neurobiological substrate of TS is not fully established, although MRI studies suggest that individuals with TS have functional disturbances in the neural pathways involving CSTC pathways (Albin & Mink, 2006; Robertson et al., 2017). Evidence supports the influence of the dopaminergic system in the pathophysiology of TS given the observation that dopaminergic medications can induce tics, while blockade of dopaminergic transmission is effective in tic suppression (Mahone, 2011). However, since multiple other neurotransmitters are active within the CTSC circuitry, including glutamate, gamma-aminobutyric acid (GABA), serotonin, acetylcholine, norepinephrine, endogenous cannabinoids, opioids, histamine, and adenosine (Robertson et al., 2017), these agents have also been the source of investigations into the pathophysiology and treatment of TS.

Treatments

There is no established cure for tics, and therapeutic plans should address not only the tics themselves but also the co-occurring conditions and the impairment associated with each (Singer, 2019). Specific treatments should also be proportional to tic frequency, severity, and the degree to which they (rather than other comorbid conditions) are causing functional or psychosocial difficulties. In children whose tics are relatively mild, reassurance, education, and monitoring may be sufficient. More active treatments, either behavioral or pharmacological, are considered when the tics interfere with psychosocial development, participation in academic activities, or when the tics are severe enough to induce physical or musculoskeletal problems (Singer, 2019). The goal of treatment is to reduce tics to levels where they no longer cause functional life problems; however, the urgency of treatment can also be driven by parent, teacher, or patient concern, as in situations when a child's tics (often vocal) cause significant disruption in a classroom setting (Mahone, 2011).

The two primary therapeutic methods for tics involve behavioral treatments and pharmacotherapy. Given the data suggesting the effectiveness of habit reversal therapy and other behavioral methods (Wile & Pringsheim, 2013), these nonpharmacological treatments are now recommended as first-tier or front-line therapies for tic disorders in children (Singer, 2019). Habit reversal therapy is a multicomponent behavioral treatment based on the premise that reduction in tics (or other habits) can occur when the individual becomes more aware and is able to perform a competing response. Comprehensive habit reversal treatments involve training in the following: awareness of habits, self-monitoring, relaxation, development of competing responses, and motivational techniques (Himle, Woods, Piacentini, & Walkup, 2006). Comprehensive behavior therapy for tics (CBIT), a specific form of habit reversal therapy, has demonstrated effectiveness, with few side effects, in large-scale treatment studies (Piacentini et al., 2010), and is specifically recommended for children old enough to participate. Unfortunately, there is a dearth of individuals trained to provide CBIT (Cuenca et al., 2015), and as such, these methods may not be available to many families seeking nonpharmacological treatments (Singer, McDermott, Ferenc, Specht, & Mahone, 2020). Pharmacological approaches to treatment of chronic tic disorders involve multiple-tier approach, such that milder (but less effective) medications such as alpha-2 adrenergic agonists (e.g., guanfacine, clonidine) are employed as Tier 1 treatments, with more effective tic suppressants (e.g., antipsychotics) prescribed as Tier 2, in part because of the significant side effect profiles. For some individuals with severe, treatment-resistant tics, deep brain stimulation is a promising option (Martinez-Ramirez et al., 2018); however, its use and efficacy have not been established in children.

Neuropsychological Function

Neuropsychological function in TS is observed to vary widely, not surprisingly, depending on the presence of comorbid neuropsychiatric dysfunction. Given the high rates of comorbidities, the presence of "pure" TS in the clinical setting is rare, and most children with TS referred to the pediatric neuropsychologist are likely to have some combination of comorbid ADHD, obsessive–compulsive disorder (OCD; or obsessive–compulsive behaviors), and/or features of ASD. This tetrad of symptoms involving tics with or without ADHD, OCD, and ASD symptoms represents a common and highly complex neuropsychiatric syndrome that may require the involvement of multiple specialty disciplines (neuropsychology, behavioral psychology, neurology, psychiatry, speech–language pathology) for optimal care (Mahone, 2011).

In clinical settings, measurement of tic severity in children is accomplished via caregiver ratings and clinical interviews with the parent and the child. The most widely used measure of tic severity is the Yale Global Tic Severity Scale (Leckman et al., 1989), a semistructured interview that assesses severity (number, frequency, intensity, complexity, interference) and impairment (self-esteem, family life, social acceptance) of motor and vocal tics. In children, tic severity does not always predict functional impairment, and the association appears to be moderated by presence of comorbidities (Groth, Mol Debes, Rask, Lange, & Skov, 2017). Additional rating scales for tic severity and function are widely available and include the Parent Tic Questionnaire (PTQ; Chang, Himle, Tucker, & Woods, 2009), the patient-reported Health-Related Quality of Life Scale (Cavanna, Schrag, Morley, Orth, & Robertson, 2008), and the patient-reported Premonitory Urge for Tics Scale (Woods, Piacentini, Himle, & Chang, 2005).

In group studies, observed neuropsychological dysfunction in children with TS is most often associated with the presence of comorbidities (Mahone et al., 2002), whereas children with "pure" TS are more likely to have relatively preserved neuropsychological skills (Mahone, 2011; Termine et al., 2016). In fact, among studies of pure TS in which comorbidities have been carefully screened, several have reported *unexpectedly above average* performance relative to typically developing groups in the areas of IQ (Casey, Cohen, Schuerholz, Singer, & Denckla, 2000; Mahone, Koth, Cutting, Singer, & Denckla, 2001; Schuerholz, Baumgardner, Singer, Reiss, & Denckla, 1996), language skills (Harris et al., 1995), and motor speed (Schuerholz, Cutting, Mazzocco, Singer, & Denckla, 1997). A recent review of neuropsychological functioning in children with TS concluded that, at maximum, only slight neuropsychological impairments were observed in TS groups when comorbidities were considered (IQ, attention, executive functions), and that in several neurobehavioral domains (memory, motor skills, language, social cognition, academic skills), no conclusions about TS-specific neuropsychological dysfunction could be drawn, or that the evidence pointed to no TS-related dysfunction (Morand-Beaulieu et al., 2017). As such, when reviewing results of published studies of neuropsychological function in children with TS, it is critical to look carefully at whether comorbidities (especially ADHD, OCD, and ASD) are screened or measured in the TS sample. For those studies in which comorbidities are not clearly delineated in the TS group, conclusions of TS-related neuropsychological dysfunction should be interpreted with caution.

STEREOTYPIC MOVEMENT DISORDERS

Overview

Imagine the following: A 3-year-old boy, playing at home, suddenly rocks his head back, opens his mouth, and rhythmically flaps both hands and arms for 30 seconds. He seems aware of the activity, but not concerned, and appears unable to stop. These movements begin to occur repetitively through the day, especially when he is excited or engrossed in an activity. The behaviors are understandably upsetting to the parent, who may not understand why the child is making the movements. Other children may begin to tease the child, and other parents may start to raise questions, including whether the behaviors are a sign of autism (Freeman, Soltanifar, & Baer, 2010). This scenario is being reported more commonly to developmental specialists. These previously described movements may represent motor stereotypies.

Motor stereotypies are repetitive, rhythmic movements that have a predictable pattern and location (Barry, Baird, Lascelles, Bunton, & Hedderly, 2011). The movements seem purposeful but actually serve no obvious function. They tend to be prolonged when uninterrupted but will stop with distraction. It has been estimated that 3–4% of otherwise typically developing preschoolers have motor stereotypies (Foster, 1998). Motor stereotypies can be categorized based on whether the movements occur in an otherwise typically developing child (primary) or in the context of a specific neurological or neurodevelopmental condition (secondary) (Gao & Singer, 2013; Muthugovindan & Singer, 2009).

Within primary stereotypies, three types of motor stereotypies have been described in children: common, head nodding, and complex (Wolf & Singer, 2008). *Common motor stereotypies* include activities such as thumb sucking, nail/lip biting, hair twirling, body rocking, and teeth clenching/grinding. These behaviors are often labeled "habits" and typically dissipate with age. *Head nodding stereotypies* occur when the child nods his or her head from side to side (like saying "no"), up and down (like saying "yes"), or shoulder to shoulder. The nodding is occasionally accompanied by up-gaze eye deviations or movements of the hands or feet, and is often confused with tics. *Complex motor stereotypies* are movements that include hand/arm flapping or waving, wiggling the fingers in front of the face, rotating or opening and closing the hands. Generally, a child will simultaneously perform the movement bilaterally (Wolf & Singer, 2008).

Previously thought to be associated only with ASD, intellectual disability (ID), or sensory deprivation, complex motor stereotypies are now recognized to occur in a more primary form (Edwards, Lang, & Bhatia, 2012; Mahone, Bridges, Prahme, & Singer, 2004). Motor stereotypies also continue to be included as one of the criteria for diagnosis of ASD in DSM-5 (American Psychiatric Association, 2013). Similar to complex motor stereotypies observed in ASD, primary complex motor stereotypies typically begin before age 3 years, persist throughout childhood, and respond poorly to pharmacotherapy. Stereotypic movements that are secondary to known neurodevelopmental conditions such as ASD or Rett syndrome (*secondary* complex motor stereotypies) are, by direct observation, not easily distinguishable from those occurring in the primary form (Singer, 2010).

Phenomenology of Primary Complex Motor Stereotypies

Primary complex motor stereotypies (CMS) often begin in infancy (Mahone et al., 2004), persist into adulthood (Oakley, Mahone, Morris-Berry, Kline, & Singer, 2015), and are associated with increased psychiatric dysfunction (Harris, Mahone, & Singer, 2008). They show limited response to medication, and when chronic, the movements can adversely impact social, academic, and cognitive functions (Mahone, Ryan, Ferenc, Morris-Berry, & Singer, 2014). Children with primary CMS often show a pattern of comorbidities similar to that observed in TS—albeit at lower rates—including ADHD (~30%), and obsessive-compulsive behaviors (~10%), and as many as 18–20% of children with stereotypies also have TS (Harris et al., 2008).

Clinically, primary CMS are distinguishable from tics based on age of onset, movement patterns, ease of suppression, triggers, and response to medication (Table 15.3); however, tics and stereotypies can (and often do) co-occur in the same child (Mahone et al., 2004).

Neuropsychological Function

The majority of studies examining neuropsychological function in children with stereotypic behavior have been in those displaying secondary stereotypies (especially ASD, Rett syndrome, or other neurodevelopmental disorders), with relatively few investigations of children with primary CMS. The largest neuropsychological study to date compared 57 children with primary CMS (screened for ASD and ID), ages 4–12 years, to age- and sex-matched typically developing controls, using a targeted assessment emphasizing IQ, language, attention, executive function, and motor skills, as well as caregiver ratings of motor, behavioral, and psychiatric symptoms (Mahone et al., 2014). Frequency and severity of stereotypies were assessed using the Stereotypy Severity Scale (SSS) and the Stereotypy Linear Analog Scale (SLAS; Miller, Singer, Bridges, & Waranch, 2006). In this sample, children with stereotypies had largely intact neuropsychological function, with

TABLE 15.3. Characteristics of Tics versus Stereotypies

Characteristic	Tics	Stereotypies
Age of onset	Around school entry age	< 2 years
Pattern	Variable, wax and wane	Fixed, patterned, predictable
Movements	Initially facial (blinks, grimace)	Initially arms/hands, flap/wave
Rhythm	Rapid, sudden, abrupt, random	Rhythmic, "looped"
Duration	Brief, abrupt, unpredictable	Continuous, prolonged
Premonitory urge	Yes	No
Trigger	Stress, excitement	When engrossed or excited
Suppression	Brief, but with feeling of buildup	With distraction
Family history	Often positive	May be positive
Present in sleep	Usually not	No
Treatment	Alpha-2 agonists, CBIT	Poorly response to medication

Note. Reprinted with permission from Mahone et al. (2004). Copyright 2004 by Elsevier.

deficits observed only in core motor function (overflow movements and total score from the PANESS). Moreover, nearly one-third of the children with stereotypies were rated by their parents on the Developmental Coordination Disorder Questionnaire (DCDQ, Wilson, Kaplan, Crawford, Campbell, & Dewey, 2000) as being at risk for DCD. These findings point to a potentially specific deficit in motor skill acquisition and control in children with primary complex motor stereotypies.

Pathophysiology

The neurobiology of primary CMS is not fully understood; although the substrate is hypothesized to involve CTSC circuitry, based on functional similarities and comorbidity patterns observed in TS (Gao & Singer, 2013). Within these networks, data from animal and human studies suggest the delineation of distinct cortical–striatal pathways that are involved in goal-directed behaviors (ventromedial prefrontal cortex–caudate nucleus) and habitual behaviors (premotor cortex–putamen), and the functional balance between these networks may underlie the onset and persistence of motor stereotypies (Augustine, Nebel, Mostofsky, Mahone, & Singer, 2021). MRI studies of primary CMS have been limited but support the salience of these frontostriatal networks. A volumetric MRI study of 20 children with CMS, ages 8–12 years, showed significantly reduced putamen but not caudate or frontal volume relative to age- and sex-matched controls (Mahone et al., 2016). In a magnetic resonance spectroscopy study of a younger sample of children with primary CMS ages 5–10 years, Harris et al. (2016) identified reduced levels of GABA in the anterior cingulate cortex (ACC) and striatum, but not prefrontal or premotor cortex, with ACC GABA significantly associated with stereotypy severity (as measured by the SSS). More recently, a functional connectivity study of 24 children with primary CMS showed significantly *reduced* functional connectivity between the executive striatum (caudate) and orbitofrontal and dorsolateral prefrontal cortex; and between the limbic striatum and the orbitofrontal, dorsolateral, and medial prefrontal cortex. In contrast, no differences were observed in functional connectivity between the sensorimotor striatum (putamen) and any frontal lobe region (Augustine et al., 2021). Together, these findings support the concept of a required *optimal balance* between goal-directed and habitual pathways. The persistence of stereotypies observed in children with primary CMS may reflect anomalous development within the prefrontal–striatal networks required for the development of mature goal-directed behavior, rather than enhanced connectivity within premotor/motor to striatal pathways associated with habitual, patterned behaviors.

Treatments

Unlike treatments for tics, there are no known effective pharmacological therapies targeting primary CMS (Harris et al., 2008; Singer, 2013), although children may receive pharmacological treatments to target comorbidities, including ADHD, OCD, or tics. Conversely, behavioral therapy has been shown to be a promising approach to reducing the frequency and severity of the stereotypic movements. Behavioral treatments for primary CMS have been adapted from the habit reversal therapeutic approaches used to treat tic disorders (Miller et al., 2006). The challenge for children with CMS, however, is that the onset of the movements is typically in infancy or toddlerhood—well before the child is able to effectively participate in habit reversal treatments. The other challenge, as in TS, is the relative paucity of therapists trained to apply these variations on CBIT. To address these issues, a home-based, parent-administered, DVD-guided treatment was developed and successfully implemented in a sample of children (ages 7–14 years), showing effectiveness comparable to in-person behavioral treatments in reducing stereotypy frequency and severity (Specht et al., 2017). More recently, this home-based treatment was adapted and extended to younger children (ages 5–7 years). The adaptation involved the inclusion of regular therapist phone calls with the parent(s), in addition to the home-based, DVD-guided treatments, and resulted in 30–50% reduction in parent-reported CMS severity and frequency (Singer, Rajendran, Waranch, & Mahone, 2018).

CONCLUSIONS AND FUTURE DIRECTIONS

Examination of motor development and function is critical to the neuropsychological formulation, likely more because of its indirect, rather than direct, biological significance (Denckla, 2005b). In the developmental context, motor signs can serve as biomarkers, allowing the clinician to generate hypotheses that are then pursued via other components of the assessment using the "n-of-1" experimental approach (Bernstein & Waber, 1990; Mahone et al., 2018b). Motor development may serve as the "canary in the coal mine" to inform how myelination occurs in parallel manner, setting the stage for other critical cognitive and emotional control functions to follow (Denckla, 2019). The developmental approach to neuropsychological assessment can be framed through the lens of motor biomarkers that have direct relevance to "neighboring" neurobehavioral systems. This framework can and should be applied to assessment of both neurodevelopmental and acquired neurological conditions of childhood.

It is my hope that this chapter encourages pediatric neuropsychologists to look *beyond* the most straightforward assessment of motor speed (e.g., Grooved Pegboard, Finger Oscillation) in their examinations in order to take full advantage of the role that movement and motor development plays in neuropsychological formulation. Motor development (including the development of praxis) has direct significance for most critical life skills, including academics, sports, art, social skills, and functional communication. In order to effectively incorporate assessment of movement and motor skill into the neuropsychological examination, the clinician needs to know what to look for, how to elicit it, and what it means when it is observed. In my 30 years as a practicing clinician, teacher, and researcher, it has been my observation that this element of training among pediatric neuropsychologists often lags behind that of other elements of their skill sets.

The field has clearly begun to recognize the importance of motor biomarkers in pediatric research. Nevertheless, the neuropsychological contribution to this work and its translation back to clinical practice has room to grow. For example, the "gold standard" methods for assessment of ASD, both in research and clinical contexts, is considered to include the Autism Diagnostic Observation Schedule (ADOS-2; Lord et al., 2012). Recognizing the importance of informed and standardized ASD assessment, practitioners using the ADOS-2 are now able to access formal training (and booster sessions) that "certify" clinicians to provide clinical- and research-reliable assessments. Those engaging in research using the ADOS-2 are expected to have attained "research-reliable" status, based on the aforementioned training. This standardization is important, since the subtleties of ASD assessment are difficult to quantify without specific training and experience. In contrast, outside of a few select training programs, there is no such formalized training available to the practicing neuropsychologist in assessment of the full range of movement disorders and the quantified motor assessment (e.g., PANESS). The result is that pediatric neuropsychologists often refrain from using these more thorough methods, rely on motor assessments from neurologists (which may or may not be quantified), or implement components of the PANESS without specific training and reliability. In future research and training methods, it is my hope that the field of pediatric neuropsychology will see the value in training its clinicians and researchers in quantified motor examinations in the same manner that is now available for training on instruments such as the ADOS-2.

REFERENCES

Albin, R. L., & Mink, J. W. (2006). Recent advances in Tourette syndrome research. *Trends in Neuroscience, 29,* 175–182.

American Psychiatric Association. (2013). *Diagnostic and statistical manual of mental disorders* (5th ed.). Arlington, VA: Author.

Augustine, F., Nebel, M. B., Mostofsky, S. H., Mahone, E. M., & Singer, H. S. (2021). Aberrant prefrontal cortical–striatal functional connectivity in children with primary complex motor stereotypies. *Cortex, 142,* 272–282.

Barry, S., Baird, G., Lascelles, K., Bunton, P., & Hedderly, T. (2011). Neurodevelopmental movement disorders—an update on childhood motor stereotypies. *Developmental Medicine and Child Neurology, 53,* 979–985.

Baxter, P. (2012). Developmental coordination disorder and motor dyspraxia. *Developmental Medicine and Child Neurology, 54,* 3.

Beery, K. E., Buktenica, N. A., & Beery, N. A. (2010). *Beery–Buktenica Developmental Test of Visual–Motor Integration, Sixth Edition.* New York: Pearson.

Berninger, V., Yates, C., Cartwright, A., Rutberg, J., Remy, E., & Abbot, R. (1992). Lower-level developmental skills in beginning writing. *Reading and Writing, 4,* 257–280.

Bernstein, J., & Waber, D. (1990). Developmental neuropsychological assessment: The systemic approach. In A. Boulton, G. Baker, & M. Hiscock (Eds.), *Neuromethods: neuropsychology* (pp. 311–371). Clifton, NJ: Humana Press.

Casey, M. B., Cohen, M., Schuerholz, L. J., Singer, H. S., & Denckla, M. B. (2000). Language-based cognitive functioning in parents of offspring with ADHD comorbid for Tourette syndrome or learning disabilities. *Developmental Neuropsychology, 17,* 85–110.

Cavanna, A. E., Schrag, A., Morley, D., Orth, M., & Robertson, M. M. (2008). The Gilles de la Tourette Syndrome—Quality of Life Scale (GTS-QOL): Development and validation. *Neurology, 71,* 1410–1416.

Chang, S., Himle, M. B., Tucker, B. T. P., & Woods, D. W. (2009). Initial psychometric properties of a brief parent-reported instrument for assessing tic severity in children with chronic tic disorders. *Child and Family Behavior Therapy, 31,* 181–191.

Chang, S.-H., & Yu, N.-Y. (2018). Development and validation of the comprehensive praxis assessment for children 6–8. *Human Movement Science, 57,* 332–341.

Cohen, H. J., Taft, L. T., Mahadeviah, M. S., & Birch, H. G. (1967). Developmental changes in overflow in normal and aberrantly functioning children. *Journal of Pediatrics, 71,* 39–47.

Cole W., Mostofsky, S. H., Gidley Larson, J. C., Denckla, M. B., & Mahone, E. M. (2008). Age related change in motor subtle signs among girls and boys with ADHD. *Neurology, 71,* 1514–1520.

Cronin, T., Rosser, A., & Massey, T. (2019). Clinical presentation and features of juvenile-onset Huntington's disease: A systematic review. *Journal of Huntington's Disease, 8,* 171–179.

Cuenca, J., Glazebrook, C., Kendall, T., Hedderly, T., Heyman, I., Jackson, G., . . . Hollis, C. (2015). Perceptions of treatment for tics among young people with Tourette syndrome and their parents: A mixed methods study. *BMC Psychiatry, 15,* Article 46.

Dale, R. C. (2017). Tics and Tourette: A clinical, pathophysiological and etiological review. *Current Opinion in Pediatrics, 29,* 665–673.

Delorme, C., Gras, D., Fabre-Teste, J., & Roze, E. (2016). Forceful backbending stereotypies revealing MEF2C haploinsufficiency. *Pediatric Neurology, 60,* 90–91.

Delorme, C., Salvador, A., Valabrègue, R., Roze, E., Palminteri, S., Vidailhet, M., . . . Worbe, Y. (2016). Enhanced habit formation in Gilles de la Tourette syndrome. *Brain, 139,* 605–615.

Denckla, M. B. (1985). Revised neurological examination for subtle signs. *Psychopharmacology Bulletin, 21,* 773–779.

Denckla, M. B. (1997). The neurobehavioral examination in children. In T. E. Feinberg & M. J. Farah (Eds.), *Behavioral neurology and neuropsychology* (pp. 721–728). New York: McGraw-Hill.

Denckla, M. B. (2004). Neurodevelopmental disorders from a cognitive neurosciences perspective. In D. Riva, U. Bellugi, & M. B. Denckla (Eds.), *Neurodevelopmental disorders: Cognitive/behavioural phenotypes* (pp. 1–8). Arcueil, France: John Libbey Eurotext.

Denckla, M. B. (2005a). Executive function. In D. Gozal & D. L. Molfese (Eds.), *Attention deficit hyperactivity disorder: From genes to patients* (pp. 165–183). Totawa, NJ: Humana Press.

Denckla, M. B. (2005b). Why assess motor functions "early and often?" *Mental Retardation and Developmental Disabilities Research Reviews, 11,* Article 3.

Denckla, M. B. (2019). Motor coordination factors contributing to school problems. In M. B. Denckla (Ed.), *Understanding learning and related disabilities: Inconvenient brains* (pp. 32–43). Abingdon, UK: Routledge.

Denckla, M. B., & Mahone, E. M. (2018). Binding together the definitions of attention-deficit/hyperactivity disorder and learning disabilities. In L. Meltzer (Ed.), *Executive function in education* (2nd ed., pp. 5–24). New York: Guilford Press.

Dewey, D. (1993). Error analysis of limb and orofacial praxis in children with developmental motor deficits. *Brain and Cognition, 23,* 203–221.

Dewey, D. (1995). What is developmental dyspraxia? *Brain and Cognition, 29,* 254–274.

Dewey, D., Cantell, M., & Crawford, S. G. (2007). Motor and gestural performance in children with autism spectrum disorders, developmental coordination disorder, and/or attention deficit hyperactivity disorder. *Journal of the International Neuropsychological Society, 13,* 246–256.

Dewey, D., & Kaplan, B. J. (1994). Subtyping of

developmental motor deficits. *Developmental Neuropsychology, 8,* 267–379.

Diamond, A. (2000). Close interrelation of motor development and cognitive development and of the cerebellum and prefrontal cortex. *Child Development, 71,* 44–56.

Dowell, L. R., Mahone, E. M., & Mostofsky, S. H. (2009). Associations of postural knowledge and basic motor skill with dyspraxia in autism: Implication for abnormalities in distributed connectivity and motor learning. *Neuropsychology, 23,* 563–570.

Dziuk, M. A., Gidley Larson, J. C., Apostu, A., Mahone, E. M., Denckla, M. B., & Mostofsky, S. H. (2007). Dyspraxia in autism: Association with motor, social, and communicative deficits. *Developmental Medicine and Child Neurology, 49,* 734–739.

Eberhardt, O., & Topka, H. (2017). Myoclonic disorders. *Brain Sciences, 7,* Article E103.

Edwards, M. J., Lang, A. E., & Bhatia, K. P. (2012). Stereotypies: A critical appraisal and suggestion of a clinically useful definition. *Movement Disorders, 27,* 179–185.

Foster, L. G. (1998). Nervous habits and stereotyped behaviors in preschool children. *Journal of the American Academy of Child and Adolescent Psychiatry, 37,* 711–717.

Freeman, R. D., Soltanifar, A., & Baer, S. (2010). Stereotypic movement disorder: Easily missed. *Developmental Medicine and Child Neurology, 52,* 733–738.

Gao, S., & Singer, H. (2013). Complex motor stereotypies: An evolving neurobiological concept. *Future Neurology, 8,* 273–285.

Garvey, M. A., Ziemann, U., Bartko, J. J., Denckla, M. B., Barker, C. A., & Wassermann, E. M. (2003). Clinical cortical correlates of neuromotor development in healthy children. *Clinical Neurophysiology, 114,* 1662–1670.

Gill, J. S., & Sillitoe, R. V. (2019). Functional outcomes of cerebellar malformations. *Frontiers in Cellular Neuroscience, 13,* Article 441.

Gilles de la Tourette, G. (1885). *Étude sur une affection nerveuse caractérisée par de l'incoordination motrice accompagnée d'écholalie et de coprolalia (jumping, latah, myriachit) [Study on a nervous affection characterized by motor incoordination accompanied by echolalia and coprolalia (jumping, latah, myriachit)].* Paris: Aux bureaux du Progrès médical, V.-A. Delahaye et Lecrosnier.

Gogtay, N., Giedd, J. N., Lusk, L., Hayashi, K. M., Greenstein, D., Vaituzis, A. C., . . . Thompson, P. M. (2004). Dynamic mapping of human cortical development during childhood through early adulthood. *Proceedings of the National Academy of Sciences USA, 101,* 8174–8179.

Groth, C., Mol Debes, N., Rask, C. U., Lange, T., & Skov, L. (2017). Course of Tourette syndrome and comorbidities in a large prospective clinical study. *Journal of the American Academy of Child and Adolescent Psychiatry, 56,* 304–312.

Haaland, K. Y. (2006). Left hemisphere dominance for movement. *Clinical Neuropsychologist, 20,* 609–622.

Harris, A. D., Singer, H. S., Horska, A., Kline, T., Ryan, M., Edden, R. A. E., & Mahone, E. M. (2016). GABA and glutamate in children with primary complex motor stereotypies: A ^{1}H MRS study at 7T. *American Journal of Neuroradiology, 37,* 552–557.

Harris, E. L., Singer, H. S., Reader, M. J., Brown, J. E., Cox, C., Mohr, J., . . . Denckla, M. B. (1995). Executive function in children with Tourette syndrome and/or attention deficit hyperactivity disorder. *Journal of the International Neuropsychological Society, 1,* 511–516.

Harris, K. M., Mahone, E. M., & Singer, H. S. (2008). Nonautistic motor stereotypies: Clinical features and longitudinal follow-up. *Pediatric Neurology, 38,* 267–272.

Hartmann, A., & Millet, B. (2018). Repetitive movements and behaviors in neurological and psychiatric practice: Distinctions and similarities between Tourette disorder and obsessive–compulsive disorder. *Revue Neurologique, 174,* 199–202.

Heilman, K. M., & Rothi, L. J. G. (2003). Apraxia. In E. Valenstein & K. M. Heilman (Eds.), *Clinical neuropsychology* (4th ed., pp. 215–235). New York: Oxford University Press.

Himle, M. B., Woods, D. W., Piacentini, J. C., & Walkup, J. T. (2006). Brief review of habit reversal training for Tourette syndrome. *Journal of Child Neurology, 21,* 719–725.

Hirschtritt, M. E., Lee, P. C., Pauls, D. L., Dion, Y., Grados, M. A., Illmann, C., . . . Mathews, C. A. (2015). Lifetime prevalence, age of risk, and genetic relationships of comorbid psychiatric disorders in Tourette syndrome. *JAMA Psychiatry, 72,* 325–333.

Hoy, K. E., Fitzgerald, P. B., Bradshaw, J. L., Armatas, C. A., & Georgiou-Karistianis, N. (2004). Investigating the cortical origins of motor overflow. *Brain Research Reviews, 46,* 315–327.

Hyde, T., Aaronson, B., Randolph, C., Rickler, K., & Weinberger, D. (1992). Relationship of birth weight to phenotypic expression of Gilles de la

Tourette's syndrome in monozygotic twins. *Neurology, 42*, 652–658.

Johnson, M. W., Hoon, A. H., & Kaufmann, W. E. (2008). Neurobiology, diagnosis, and management of cerebral palsy. In P. J. Accardo (Ed.), *Capute & Accardo's neurodevelopmental disabilities in infancy and childhood* (3rd ed., pp. 61–81). Baltimore: Brookes.

Kadesjo, B., & Gillberg, C. (1998). Attention deficits and clumsiness in Swedish 7-year-old children. *Developmental Medicine and Child Neurology, 40*, 796–804.

Kaplan, E. (1968). *Gestural representation of implement usage: An organismic–developmental study.* Unpublished doctoral dissertation, Clark University, Worchester, MA.

Knight, T., Steeves, T., Day, L., Lowerison, M., Jette, N., & Pringsheim, T. (2012). Prevalence of tic disorders: A systematic review and meta-analysis. *Pediatric Neurology, 47*, 77–90.

Kompliti, K., & Goetz, C. G. (1998). Hyperkinetic movement disorders misdiagnosed as tics in Gilles de la Tourette syndrome. *Movement Disorders, 13*, 477–480.

Korkman, M., Kirk, U., & Kemp, S. (2007). *NEPSY* (2nd ed.). San Antonio, TX: Pearson.

Lambert, D. A., Giannouli, E., & Schmidt, B. J. (2005). Postpolio syndrome and anesthesia. *Anesthesiology, 103*, 638–644.

Larson, J. C., Mostofsky, S. H., Goldberg, M., Cutting, L., Denckla, M. B., & Mahone, E. M. (2007). Effects of gender and age on motor exam in typically developing children. *Developmental Neuropsychology, 32*, 543–562.

Leckman, J. F., Riddle, M. A., Hardin, M. T., Ort, S. I., Swartz, K. L., Stevenson, J., & Cohen, D. J. (1989). The Yale Global Tic Severity Scale: Initial testing of a clinician-rated scale of tic severity. *Journal of the American Academy of Child and Adolescent Psychiatry, 28*, 566–573.

Liepmann, H. (1900). Das krankheitsbild der apraxie ("motorischen asymbolie") auf grund eines falles von einseitiger apraxie [The clinical picture of apraxia ("motoric asymboly") due to a case of unilateral apraxia]. *Monatsschrift für Psycholgie und Neurologie, 8*, 117–132.

Lohia, A., & McKenzie, J. (2019). *Neuroanatomy, pyramidal tract lesions.* Treasure Island, FL: StatPearls Publishing.

Lord, C., Rutter, M., DiLavore, P. C., Risi, S., Gotham, K., Bishop, S. L. (2012). *Autism Diagnostic Observation Schedule, Second edition (ADOS-2)*. Los Angeles, CA: Western Psychological Services.

Luria, A. R. (1980). *Higher cortical functions in man.* New York: Basic Books.

Mahone, E. M. (2011). Tourette syndrome. In J. Morgan, I. S. Baron, & J. Ricker (Eds.), *Casebook of clinical neuropsychology* (pp. 60–77). New York: Oxford University Press.

Mahone, E. M., Bridges, D., Prahme, C., & Singer, H. S. (2004). Repetitive arm and hand movements (complex motor stereotypies) in children. *Journal of Pediatrics, 145*, 391–395.

Mahone, E. M., Cirino, P. T., Cutting, L. E., Cerrone, P. M., Hagelthorn, K. M., Hiemenz, J. R., . . . Denckla, M. B. (2002). Validity of the behavior rating inventory of executive function in children with ADHD and/or Tourette syndrome. *Archives of Clinical Neuropsychology, 17*, 643–662.

Mahone, E. M., Crocetti, D., Tochen, L., Kline, T., Mostofsky, S. H., & Singer, H. S. (2016). Anomalous putamen volume in children with complex motor stereotypies. *Pediatric Neurology, 65*, 59–63.

Mahone, E. M., Koth, C. W., Cutting, L., Singer, H. S., & Denckla, M. B. (2001). Executive function in fluency and recall measures among children with Tourette syndrome or ADHD. *Journal of the International Neuropsychological Society, 7*, 102–111.

Mahone, E. M., Powell, S., Loftis, C. W., Goldberg, M., Denckla, M. B., & Mostofsky, S. H. (2006). Motor persistence and inhibition in autism and ADHD. *Journal of the International Neuropsychological Society, 12*, 622–631.

Mahone, E. M., Puts, N. A., Edden, R. A. E., Ryan, M., & Singer, H. S. (2018). GABA and glutamate in children with Tourette syndrome: A 1 H MR spectroscopy study at 7 T. *Psychiatry Research-Neuroimaging, 273*, 46–53.

Mahone, E. M., Ryan, M., Ferenc, L., Morris-Berry, C., & Singer, H. S. (2014). Neuropsychological function in children with primary complex motor stereotypies. *Developmental Medicine and Child Neurology, 56*, 1001–1008.

Mahone, E. M., Slomine, B. S., & Zabel, T. A. (2018). Genetic and neurodevelopmental disorders. In J. Morgan & J. Ricker (Eds.), *Textbook of clinical neuropsychology* (2nd ed., pp. 127–140). New York: Psychology Press.

Martin, R., Tigera, C., Denckla, M. B., & Mahone, E. M. (2010). Factor structure of paediatric timed motor examination and its relationship with IQ. *Developmental Medicine and Child Neurology, 52*, e188–e194.

Martinez-Ramirez, D., Jimenez-Shahed, J., Leckman, J. F., Porta, M., Servello, D., Meng, F., . . .

Okun, M. S. (2018). Efficacy and safety of deep brain stimulation in Tourette syndrome: The international Tourette syndrome deep brain stimulation public database and registry. *JAMA Neurology, 75,* 353–359.

Mesulam, M. M. (2000). Hemispheric specialization and asymmetry. In *Principles of behavioral and cognitive neurology* (2nd ed., pp. 80–86). New York: Oxford University Press.

Miller, J. M., Singer, H. S., Bridges, D. D., & Waranch, R. H. (2006). Behavioral therapy for treatment of stereotypic movements in nonautistic children. *Journal of Child Neurology, 21,* 119–125.

Morand-Beaulieu, S., Leclerc, J., Valois, P., Lavoie, M., O'Connor, K., & Gauthier, B. (2017). A review of the neuropsychological dimensions of Tourette syndrome. *Brain Sciences, 7*(12), Article 106.

Mostofsky, S. H., Dubey, P., Jerath, V. K., Jansiewicz, E. M., Goldberg, M. C., & Denckla, M. B. (2006). Developmental dyspraxia is not limited to imitation in children with autism spectrum disorders. *Journal of the International Neuropsychological Society, 12,* 314–326.

Muthugovindan, D., & Singer, H. (2009). Motor stereotypy disorders. *Current Opinion in Neurology, 22,* 131–136.

Njiokiktjien, C., Verschoor, C. A., Vranken, M., & Vroklage, L. M. (2000). Development of ideomotor praxis representation. *Developmental Medicine and Child Neurology, 42,* 253–257.

Oakley, C., Mahone, E. M., Morris-Berry, C., Kline, T., & Singer, H. (2015). Primary complex motor stereotypies in older children and adolescents: Clinical features and longitudinal follow-up. *Pediatric Neurology, 52,* 398–403.

O'Brien, J. W., Dowell, L. R., Mostofsky, S. H., Denckla, M. B., Mahone, E. M. (2010). Neuropsychological profile of executive function in girls with attention-deficit/hyperactivity disorder. *Archives of Clinical Neuropsychology, 25,* 656–670.

Pavone, P., Praticò, A. D., Pavone, V., Lubrano, R., Falsaperla, R., Rizzo, R., & Ruggieri, M. (2017). Ataxia in children: Early recognition and clinical evaluation. *Italian Journal of Pediatrics, 43*(1), Article 6.

Pearson, T. S., & Pons, R. (2019). Movement disorders in children. *Continuum (Minneapolis, Minnesota), 25,* 1099–1120.

Peterson, B. S., & Leckman, J. F. (1998). The temporal dynamics of tics in Gilles de la Tourette syndrome. *Biological Psychiatry, 44,* 1337–1348.

Petley, E., Prasad, M., Ojha, S., & Whitehouse, W. P. (2020). Investigating ataxia in childhood. *Archives of Disability in Childhood Education Practice, 105,* 214–221.

Piacentini, J., Woods, D. W., Scahill, L., Wilhelm, S., Peterson, A. L., Chang, S., . . . Walkup, J. T. (2010). Behavior therapy for children with Tourette disorder: A randomized controlled trial. *Journal of the American Medical Association, 303,* 1929–1937.

Piaget, J., & Inhelder, B. (1967). *The child's conception of space.* New York: Norton.

Pitcher, T. M., Piek, J. P., & Hay, D. A. (2003). Fine and gross motor ability in males with ADHD. *Developmental Medicine and Child Neurology, 45,* 525–535.

Rao, S. M., Binder, J. R., Bandettini, P. A., Hammeke, T. A., Yetkin, F. Z., Jesmanowicz, A., . . . Hyde, J. S. (1993). Functional magnetic resonance imaging of complex human movements. *Neurology, 43*(11), 2311.

Richards, T. L., Berninger, V. W., Stock, P., Altemeier, L., Trivedi, P., & Maravilla, K. (2009). Functional magnetic resonance imaging sequential-finger movement activation differentiating good and poor writers. *Journal of Clinical and Experimental Neuropsychology, 31,* 967–983.

Riva, D., Taddei, M., & Bulgheroni, S. (2018). The neuropsychology of basal ganglia. *European Journal of Paediatric Neurology, 22,* 321–326.

Robertson, M. M. (2015). A personal 35-year perspective on Gilles de la Tourette syndrome: Prevalence, phenomenology, comorbidities, and coexistent psychopathologies. *Lancet Psychiatry, 2,* 68–87.

Robertson, M. M., Eapen, V., Singer, H. S., Martino, D., Scharf, J. M., Paschou, P., . . . Leckman, J. F. (2017). Gilles de la Tourette syndrome. *Nature Reviews Disease Primers, 3,* Article 16097.

Roeder, M. B., Mahone, E. M., Gidley Larson, J., Mostofsky, S. H., Cutting, L. E., Goldberg, M. C., & Denckla, M. B. (2008). Left–right differences on timed motor examination in children. *Child Neuropsychology, 14,* 249–262.

Ross, L. R., & Kwon, J. M. (2019). Spinal muscular atrophy: Past, present, and future. *NeoReviews, 20*(8), Article e4337.

Sanger, T. D., Chen, D., Fehlings, D. L., Hallett, M., Lang, A. E., Mink, J. W., . . . Valero-Cuevas, F. (2010). Definition and classification of hyperkinetic movements in childhood. *Movement Disorders, 25,* 1538–1549.

Scharf, J. M., Miller, L. L., Gauvin, C. A., Alabiso, J., Mathews, C. A., & Ben-Shlomo, Y. (2015).

Population prevalence of Tourette syndrome: A systematic review and meta-analysis: meta-analysis of TS prevalence. *Movement Disorders, 30,* 221–228.

Schlough, K., Andre, K., Owen, M., Adelstein, L., Hartford, M. C., Javier, B., & Kern, R. (2020). Differentiating between idiopathic toe walking and cerebral palsy: A systematic review. *Pediatric Physical Therapy, 32,* 2–10.

Schuerholz, L. J., Baumgardner, T. L., Singer, H. S., Reiss, A. L., & Denckla, M. B. (1996). Neuropsycological status of children with Tourette's syndrome with and without attention deficit hyperactivity disorder. *Neurology, 46,* 958–965.

Schuerholz, L. J., Cutting, L., Mazzocco, M. M., Singer, H. S., & Denckla, M. B. (1997). Neuromotor functioning in children with Tourette syndrome with and without attention deficit hyperactivity disorder. *Journal of Child Neurology, 12,* 438–442.

Singer, H. (2011). Tourette syndrome and other tic disorders. *Handbook of Clinical Neurology, 100,* 641–657.

Singer, H. S. (2010). Treatment of tics and Tourette syndrome. *Current Treatment Options in Neurology, 12,* 539–561.

Singer, H. S. (2013). Motor control, habits, complex motor stereotypies, and Tourette syndrome. *Annals of the New York Academy of Sciences, 1304,* 22–31.

Singer, H. S. (2016). Habitual and goal-directed behaviours and Tourette syndrome. *Brain, 139,* 312–316.

Singer, H. S. (2019). Tics and Tourette syndrome. *Continuum: Lifelong Learning in Neurology, 25*(4), 936–958.

Singer, H. S., McDermott, S., Ferenc, L., Specht, M., & Mahone, E. M. (2020). Efficacy of parent-delivered, home-based therapy for tics. *Pediatric Neurology, 106,* 17–23.

Singer, H. S., Rajendran, S., Waranch, H. R., & Mahone, E. M. (2018). Home-based, therapist-assisted, therapy for young children with primary complex motor stereotypies. *Pediatric Neurology, 85,* 51–57.

Specht, M. W., Mahone, E. M., Kline, T., Waranch, R., Brabson, L., Thompson, C. B., & Singer, H. S. (2017). Efficacy of parent-delivered behavioral therapy for primary complex motor stereotypies. *Developmental Medicine and Child Neurology, 59,* 168–173.

Steinman, K. J., Mostofsky, S. H., & Denckla, M. B. (2010). Toward a narrower, more pragmatic, view of developmental dyspraxia. *Journal of Child Neurology, 25,* 71–81.

Surén, P., Bakken, I. J., Skurtveit, S., Handal, M., Reichborn-Kjennerud, T., Stoltenberg, C. N., . . . Weidle, B. (2019, November 12). Tourette syndrome in children in Norway. *Tidsskrift for Den Norske Legeforening, 139*(17).

Sweeney, K., Ryan, M., Schneider, H., Ferenc, L., Denckla, M. B., & Mahone, E. M. (2018). Developmental trajectory of motor deficits in preschool children with ADHD. *Developmental Neuropsychology, 43,* 419–429.

Termine, C., Luoni, C., Fontolan, S., Selvini, C., Perego, L., Pavone, F., . . . Cavanna, A. E. (2016). Impact of co-morbid attention-deficit and hyperactivity disorder on cognitive function in male children with Tourette syndrome: A controlled study. *Psychiatry Research, 243,* 263–267.

Tourette Syndrome Classification Study Group. (1993). Definitions and classification of tic disorders. *Archives of Neurology, 50,* 1013–1016.

Wile, D. J., & Pringsheim, T. M. (2013). Behavior therapy for Tourette syndrome: A systematic review and meta-analysis. *Current Treatment Options in Neurology, 15,* 385–395.

Wilson, B. N., Kaplan, B. J., Crawford, S. G., Campbell, A., & Dewey, D. (2000). Reliability and validity of a parent questionnaire on childhood motor skills. *American Journal of Occupational Therapy, 54,* 484–493.

Wolf, D. S., & Singer, H. S. (2008). Pediatric movement disorders: An update. *Current Opinion in Neurology, 21,* 491–496.

Woods, D. W., Piacentini, J., Himle, M. B., & Chang, S. (2005). Premonitory Urge for Tics Scale (PUTS): Initial psychometric results and examination of the premonitory urge phenomenon in youths with tic disorders. *Journal of Developmental and Behavioral Pediatrics, 26,* 397–403.

PART IV

GENETIC DISORDERS

CHAPTER 16

Fragile X Syndrome

Andrea Schneider
Haleigh Scott
Rebecca Shields
David Hessl

Fragile X syndrome (FXS) is the most common identifiable, inherited cause of intellectual disability and the most common known single-gene mutation leading to autism. FXS is an inherited, X-linked disorder. Mutations in the fragile X mental retardation 1 gene (*FMR1*) are relatively common in the general population and create a spectrum of disorders, ranging from neurodevelopmental problems in childhood to neurodegenerative problems in aging. FXS is caused by expansions of a CGG repeat in the 5′ untranslated region (5′ UTR) of *FMR1* (Verkerk et al., 1991), which is located in the terminal portion (Xq27.3) of the long arm of the X chromosome. The normal range of the CGG repeat element is 5–44 CGG repeats. Expansions of 45–54 CGG repeats are classified as *intermediate* or *gray zone*, 55–200 CGG repeats define the *premutation*, and > 200 CGG repeats define the *full mutation* (Maddalena et al., 2001). FXS is caused by full mutation alleles as a result of methylation-coupled gene silencing, leading to a lack of the *FMR1* protein, FMRP (Loesch, Huggins, & Hagerman, 2004). Patients with FXS show distinct phenotypic features (Hagerman, 2002; Reiss & Dant, 2003; Sabaratnam, 2006): cognitive and language delay and intellectual disability, physiological and emotional hyperarousal, hyperactivity and impulsivity, attention deficits, autism or autistic features (avoiding eye contact, hand flapping and hand biting, sensory defensiveness, repetitive behaviors and speech, poor adaption to changes in routine), shyness, selective mutism, social anxiety, phobias and generalized anxiety, stereotypies and tics, aggressive outbursts, enuresis, and encopresis.

HISTORICAL OVERVIEW

In 1943, Martin and Bell published the first report of a family with intellectual disability and associated characteristic physical features that were transmitted transgenerationally in an X-linked fashion. The first report of the "marker X chromosome" in 1969 described two brothers with intellectual disability (Lubs, 1969). Later on, the Martin Bell pedigree with 11 males with cognitive disability (Martin & Bell, 1943) revealed the characteristic "fragile" appearing section on the distal end of the chromosome, giving the disorder its current name. Throughout the 1980s, individuals were diagnosed with FXS by cytogenetic testing until the *FMR1* gene was discovered in 1991 (Oberle et al., 1991; Verkerk et al., 1991) leading to a more widespread utilization of *FMR1* DNA testing. The FXS physical phenotype was then better characterized as involving a connective tissue dysplasia leading to soft velvety skin, hyperextensible joints, and prominent ears (Hagerman & McBogg, 1983), as well as a range of other physical features, including a long face, large head, prominent chin, high arched palate, single palmar crease, testicular enlargement during and after puberty, and epilepsy (Turk & Patton, 2000). In 1982, Brown et al. first reported the presence of autism in some individuals with FXS. The presence of *genetic anticipation*—increasing penetrance and/or severity of the phenotype in successive generations—was first described by Stephanie Sherman and has been referred to as "Sherman's paradox" (Sherman et al., 1985).

The characterization of molecular–clinical correlations accelerated during the 1990s, with a consensus that approximately 15% of males with FXS are high functioning (IQ ≥ 70), an observation that is now regarded as being due to the presence of CGG repeat- and/or methylation-mosaicism (Hagerman et al., 1994). *Mosaicism* refers to the presence of both premutation and full mutation alleles in the cells of an individual, or incomplete methylation patterns, resulting in a proportion of cells that produce the fragile X mental retardation protein (FMRP; Tassone et al., 1999).

FMR1 premutation involvement leading to premature ovarian insufficiency (POI) in female *FMR1* carriers was first described by Cronister et al. (1991). Fragile X-associated POI (FXPOI), characterized by ovaries that do not function to full capacity, a higher frequency of fertility problems, and premature menopause occurs in about 20% of adult female *FMR1* carriers, compared to about 1% of women in the general population.

The discovery of abnormal elevation of *FMR1* mRNA in premutation carriers was made several years later (Tassone et al., 2000a). For alleles in the premutation range, there is a strong positive correlation of mRNA levels with CGG repeat size. The finding of a molecular phenotype in the premutation range helped to validate the clinical phenotype of fragile X-associated tremor ataxia syndrome (FXTAS), a progressive neurodegenerative disorder characterized predominantly by intention tremor and/or ataxia (Hagerman et al., 2001) with associated age-related cognitive changes (Cornish et al., 2009). FXTAS was discovered because the mothers of children with FXS repeatedly expressed concern about the neurological problems of their own fathers, who were also premutation carriers. These fathers had never had developmental problems such as those in FXS, but they experienced a progressive tremor and ataxia in addition to cognitive decline in their later years. In a survey of families affected by FXS in California, the prevalence of FXTAS was found to be 17% in the male carriers in their 50s, 38% of those in their 60s, 47% in their 70s, and 75% in their 80s (Jacquemont et al., 2004). Although FXTAS also affects older female carriers (Hagerman et al., 2004), its prevalence (~8%) is less than that in males (Berry-Kravis et al., 2007; Coffey et al., 2008).

While premutation alleles produce normal or only slightly reduced FMRP, full mutation *FMR1* alleles are generally hypermethylated, or "silenced." This causes a lack of transcription and translation in the cell, resulting in the absence or near absence of FMRP. The lack of FMRP leads to FXS, characterized by the physical, cognitive, and behavioral features noted earlier. Females with full mutation alleles are generally less affected than males due to the presence of a second, normal X chromosome. In females, the amount of FMRP overall depends on the percentage of cells with the normal X as the active X chromosome (activation ratio; the processes that determine this ratio within individuals are not fully understood). As such, females with a favorable X activation pattern generally have higher FMRP expression and higher levels of intellectual and general functioning (Loesch et al., 2004; Tassone et al., 2000b).

EPIDEMIOLOGY

Prevalence rates of the FXS full mutation have generally been estimated at about 1 in 4,000 males and 1 in 8,000 females (Crawford, Acuna, & Sherman, 2001). In a 2014 systematic review and meta-analysis, Hunter et al. (2014) found more conservative rates of about 1 in 7,000 males and 1 in 11,000 females, which are the most current and representative estimates, though larger screening studies of general populations are needed. According to the Centers for Disease Control and Prevention (CDC), between 1 in 291 and 1 in 148 females and between 1 in 290 and 1 in 855 males in the United States have a fragile X premutation, although prevalence rates vary considerably by geographic region and race or ethnic background (Owens et al., 2018). Many carriers do not know of their status until they or a family member has a child diagnosed with FXS (Hunter et al., 2014).

Individuals with a family history of the premutation or full mutation are at risk of having FXS. CGG repeats in the premutation can become unstable as they are passed down through successive generations, with expansions occurring in transmission from mother to child. In maternal transmission, larger maternal CGG lengths are associated with increasing risk of expansion to the full mutation in the child (Nolin et al., 2011). AGG interruptions within the CGG expansion are also known to influence risk of transmission (Yrigollen et al., 2012) and as such, genetic counseling is important for families to obtain accurate information about transmission risk. Rarely, there are instances of an *FMR1* deletion causing FXS (fewer than 1% of FXS cases) (Hammond, Macias, Tarleton, & Shashidar Pai, 1997).

A mother with the altered gene (premutation or full mutation) has a 50% chance of passing the altered gene to each of her children. A father with the premutation or full mutation passes the altered gene on only to his daughters, and this can only result in the premutation (not full mutation) in the daughter except in extremely rare cases (Maddalena et al., 2001). As such, daughters of fathers with the premutation are referred to as "obligate carriers."

While FXS is reported worldwide, there appear to be some cultural and geographic differences in prevalence. One of the best examples of this is Ricaurte, Colombia, a small town of approximately 1,500 people. Ricaurte is known to have a cluster of FXS, with 1:19 men and 1:46 women carrying the full mutation; men and women in this town are hundreds of times more likely to have FXS than people in the general population (Saldarriaga et al., 2018). This clustering in a geographic region is likely due to a "founder effect," as it is hypothesized that some of the founding families of the small town were premutation carriers, and over time the limited influx of people and remoteness and relative isolation of the town have contributed to these increased rates. On the other hand, there have been some reports of populations that have decreased prevalence of FXS, most notably in

Canada, Estonia, Japan, and Taiwan as compared to other Western countries that have reported prevalence estimates (Peprah, 2012). Some studies on FXS prevalence in China suggested lower prevalence rates than in Western countries (Pang et al., 1999; Chen et al., 2015); however, this could be due at least in part to less common screening and clinical awareness (Niu et al., 2017).

ETIOLOGY, NEUROPATHOLOGY, AND NEURAL SUBSTRATES

FMRP is most commonly expressed in neurons, particularly at the dendritic spines, cytoplasm, and ribosomes bound to the endoplasmic reticulum (Bassell & Warren, 2008; Eberhart, Malter, Feng, & Warren, 1996; Weiler et al., 1997; Willemsen et al., 1996). However, this protein is diminished, or is essentially absent in individuals with FXS (Sutcliffe et al., 1992). Notably, many of the neuropsychological phenotypes described in this chapter correlate with area specific abnormalities in the FXS brain (Reiss, Abrams, Greenlaw, Freund, & Denckla, 1995a; Reiss, Lee, & Freund, 1994; Reiss, Patel, Kumar, & Freund, 1988).

The neuropathological consequences of a decreased FMRP level have been established in a mouse model of FXS that shows immature dendritic spines and a higher spine density compared to control mice (Bakker et al., 1994). These findings were confirmed in human postmortem brain studies (Irwin et al., 2001). After the formation of numerous dendritic spines during fetal cortical neurogenesis, the dendritic spines need to mature, or be pruned. Immature spines show malformations (e.g., too long "necks" or lack of "heads") and a significant impairment in signal transduction. Several studies show abnormalities in spine formation in FXS, which can be directly correlated to cognitive impairment. One mechanism for dendritic spine pruning is linked to the presence of FMRP in the cortical cells. FMRP is considered to be a repressor of specific messenger RNA (mRNA) translation and numerous proteins are up-regulated, particularly in the hippocampus, when FMRP is absent (Qin, Kang, Burlin, Jiang, & Smith, 2005). *FMR1* regulates the expression of many other genes implicated in synaptic formation and plasticity. Therefore, if FMRP is decreased or absent, there is significant dysregulation of various pathways that disrupts brain development, causing developmental delay and other phenotypic effects.

Regarding brain imaging findings, the research team of Allan Reiss has reported structural imaging abnormalities in patients with FXS since 1988, when he and his colleagues described hypoplasia of the cerebellar vermis (Reiss et al., 1988), a finding that was later replicated in several other studies. Nearly all patients with FXS have significant executive dysfunction, including deficits in attention, inhibitory control, planning/goal-directed behavior, and organization. It is perhaps not surprising, then, that structural abnormalities have been reported in brain regions important for mediating these functions, such as the many connections and circuits associated with the frontal lobes. Reiss and colleagues initially reported and then replicated the finding of larger caudate nuclei in young boys and girls with FXS (Eliez, Blasey, Freund, Hastie, & Reiss, 2001; Reiss, Mazzocco, Greenlaw, Freund, & Ross, 1995b). Results of a voxel-based morphometry study showed that the FXS group had significantly larger gray matter volume (GMV) in the bilateral caudate, but it had smaller GMV in several regions, including bilateral medial frontal, pregenual cingulate, gyrus rectus, insula, and superior temporal gyrus compared to healthy controls. Lower Full Scale IQ within the FXS group was associated with larger right caudate nucleus GMV (Sandoval et al., 2018). The authors concluded that the differences in brain anatomy likely result from reduced FMRP during early neurodevelopment, which in turn mediate deleterious effects on cognitive function.

The amygdala and related limbic structures are especially relevant to the study of the neurobiology of FXS because of the high rate of anxiety and socially avoidant behaviors demonstrated by many patients. Four fMRI studies in FXS have used human face stimuli to investigate the social–emotional deficits which are prominent features of the phenotype, such as eye gaze avoidance, anxiety, and hyperarousal. Two examined the effect of direct versus averted gaze (Garrett, Menon, MacKenzie, & Reiss, 2004; Watson, Hoeft, Garrett, Hall, & Reiss, 2008), one focused on emotion attribution (Hagan, Hoeft, Mackey, Mobbs, & Reiss, 2008), and one focused on face encoding (Holsen, Dalton, Johnstone, & Davidson, 2008). Females with FXS have difficulty determining the direction of social gaze, which appears to be mediated by deficits in activation of the fusiform gyrus, a brain region known to be critical for recognition of faces and other highly salient visual stimuli (Garrett et al., 2004). A similar task administered to males with FXS revealed elevated insula activation during direct gaze, as well as greater sensitization of the amygdala over successive exposures to direct gaze (Watson et al., 2008). The insula finding may have special relevance to the phenotype, as it was also strongly activated in the Garrett et al. (2004) study of females, and plays a critical limbic system role in conveying representations of fear and other strong emotions to the sympathetic nervous system and hypothalamic–pituitary–adrenal (HPA) axis, which are known to be hyperaroused in FXS and associated with social behavior and gaze abnormalities (Farzin, Rivera, & Hessl, 2009; Hessl et al., 2002; Hessl, Glaser, Dyer-Friedman, & Reiss, 2006; Miller et al., 1999; Roberts, Boccia, Bailey, Hatton, & Skinner, 2001a). In a study of 10 females with FXS and 10 female controls, Hagan et al. (2008) used emotional faces in an event-related fMRI study to demonstrate that emotion recognition and processing of human faces appear to be associated with aberrant activation of the anterior cingulate cortex, caudate nucleus, and insula, an emotional circuit recruited for processing emotional responses to social stimuli. Surprisingly, a study on emotion potentiated startle (a biobehavioral probe of amygdala responsiveness; Ballinger, Cordeiro, Chavez, Hagerman, & Hessl, 2014) showed significantly reduced potentiation to fearful faces in FXS compared to a neurotypical control group, with the interesting finding of a higher correlation of social avoidance to fearful-face potentiation in the female subgroup with FXS.

NEUROPSYCHOLOGICAL CONSEQUENCES

General Intellectual Functioning

Individuals with full mutation alleles usually function in the mild to moderate intellectual disability range, with a verbal–performance discrepancy favoring language skills over mathematical and visuospatial abilities (Kogan et al., 2004b; Roberts et al., 2005b). Over 90% of males and 50% of females have intellectual disability by the school-age years (Hessl et al., 2008). A gradual decline in IQ occurs as the gap between the child's lower rate of cognitive growth widens relative to the development of typical peers, particularly in males (Hall, Burns, Lightbody, & Reiss, 2008a; Bennetto & Pennington, 2002; Skinner et al., 2005). School-age children with FXS show difficulties across multiple domains, including visual–motor coordination, sequential processing, short-term memory, and arithmetic (Freund & Reiss, 1991; Rivera, Menon, White, Glaser, & Reiss, 2002; Tamm, Menon, Johnston, Hessl, & Reiss, 2002); attention, inhibitory control, and cognitive flexibility (Cornish, Sudhalter, & Turk, 2004a; Hagerman, Kemper, & Hudson, 1985); and fine and gross motor control/coordination (Bailey, Hatton, & Skinner, 1998; Zingerevich et al., 2009).

In addition to global deficits in cognitive functioning, a variety of studies have demonstrated a cognitive profile with relative strengths and weakness specific to FXS. Children with FXS tend to have relative strengths in vocabulary, visual–perceptual processes, and recall of relevant and simultaneous information. Areas of relative weakness are verbal and visual–spatial short-term memory, processing of linguistic or abstract information, and sequential information ordering and processing. This pattern of strengths and weakness is robust and persists even in differing levels of function (Van der Molen et al., 2010). Comparisons of children with FXS to controls matched for mental age have also indicated that children with FXS display deficits in executive functioning beyond what is expected for their intellectual functioning (e.g., Hessl et al., 2016). Executive functioning deficits include inhibition, working memory, cognitive flexibility, and planning (Hooper et al., 2008).

Perceptual and Sensorimotor Skills

Perceptual and sensorimotor impairments are closely related to social impairments in FXS. The high degree of social anxiety and gaze aversion is associated with a range of other visual, auditory, tactile, olfactory and gustatory sensitivities; self-injury (Hall, Lightbody, & Reiss, 2008b; Symons, Clark, Hatton, Skinner, & Bailey, 2003), usually in the form of hand biting in response to anxiety or excitement; and marked stereotypic repetitive behaviors including hand flapping, rocking, jumping, and running round in circles (Turk & Graham, 1997).

Language

The development of language, especially in males, is closely linked to IQ level and includes distinct speech abnormalities: delayed and distorted speech, perseveration, delayed echolalia, and cluttering of speech. In a longitudinal study by Fisch and colleagues, language and communication were the most affected adaptive behavior domains, compared to socialization or daily living skills (Fisch et al., 1996; Fisch, Simensen, & Schroer, 2002). Speech and language are usually highly characteristic with "jocular litanic phraseology" (a specific speech pattern with repeated, habitually jolly phrases), as well as perseverations, repetitions, echolalia, palilalia (involuntary repetitions), rapid utterances, and dysrhythmias (Abbeduto et al., 2003; Belser & Sudhalter, 2001; Cornish et al., 2004a; Roberts et al., 2005a). Young boys with FXS acquire expressive language skills at one-third the rate of normally developing children and receptive language skills at half the rate of normal

(Roberts, Mirrett, & Burchinal, 2001b). Compared to nonverbal cognitive ability in FXS, vocabulary skills and receptive grammar were areas of relative strength, whereas expressive grammar skills were weaker than nonverbal cognitive expectations (Thurman, McDuffie, Kover, Hagerman, & Abbeduto, 2015a). However, Oakes, Kover, and Aabbeduto (2013) reported that adolescents with FXS continued to show a weakness in grammatical comprehension relative to typically developing children matched on nonverbal cognitive ability. Oakes et al. proposed that individuals with FXS might have particular difficulty in processing sentences that are highly taxing of auditory sequential memory, as well as those that lack lexical supports for grammatical processing. Within the FXS population, better language skills are associated with fewer repetitive behaviors (Thurman et al., 2015a, 2015b; Thurman, McDuffie, Hagerman, Josol, & Abbeduto, 2017).

Attention

Challenges in attention are well established as part of the FXS profile and have been demonstrated both via objective neurocognitive tests and behavioral rating scales. Kogan and colleagues (2004a, 2004b) showed a specific impairment in the precortical magnocellular visual pathway in older children and adolescents with FXS and Farzin, Whitney, Hagerman, and Rivera (2008) reported deficits in the dorsal or magnocellular visual pathway already in infants and toddlers with FXS. These findings may help to explain the very common visual inhibitory control and attention problems clinically seen in individuals with FXS. Several studies have pointed out that the basic visuospatial and visual attention deficits are observable early in development (Farzin et al., 2008; Farzin & Rivera, 2010), especially the frontoparietally mediated attention processing (Chernenok, Burris, Owen, & Rivera, 2019).

Individuals with FXS commonly have severe symptoms of inattention, hyperactivity, and impulsivity, all of which can be aggravated by high levels of anxiety (Turk, 1998). In general, about 30–66% of individuals with FXS are reported to have a comorbid diagnosis of attention-deficit/hyperactivity disorder (ADHD; Cordeiro, Ballinger, Hagerman, & Hessl, 2011; Ciaccio et al., 2017; Sullivan et al., 2006).

Executive Functions

Neuropsychological impairments mediating the challenging developmental and behavioral features in FXS include deficits in working memory, inhibitory control, cognitive switching, sequential information processing, and arousal modulation (Cornish et al., 2004b). These phenomena have been identified in individuals with both premutation and full mutation alleles (Cornish et al., 2005; Grigsby et al., 2007), as well as across development in individuals with FXS.

Toddlers with FXS show particular problems inhibiting prior successful responses (Scerif, Cornish, Wilding, Driver, & Karmiloff-Smith, 2004), a reaction pattern that has also been shown in older children with FXS (Wilding, Cornish, & Munir, 2002). The poor ability to switch cognitive "set" was demonstrated with the National Institutes of Health Toolbox Dimensional Change Card Sort test (Hessl et al., 2016; Shields et al., 2020). Deficits in inhibiting inappropriate eye movements in an analogue of the antisaccade task were also demonstrated in infants with FXS as young as 12 months old (Scerif et al., 2005). In school-age children with FXS, deficits in goal-directed behavior, working memory, planning, and inhibitory control remain prevalent, and, in fact, executive functioning impairments persist over the lifespan (Cornish et al., 2009; Cornish, Munir, & Cross, 2001; Garner, Callias, & Turk, 1999; Munir, Cornish, & Wilding, 2000; Sobesky, Pennington, Porter, Hull, & Hagerman, 1994; Wilding et al., 2002).

Social Cognition

The association between the *etiological–genetic* diagnosis of FXS and the *clinical–phenomenological* diagnosis of autism is well evidenced yet complex (Cornish, Turk, & Levitas, 2007; Hatton et al., 2006; Kaufmann et al., 2004). Approximately 2–6% of people with autism have FXS (Hagerman, Rivera, & Hagerman, 2008; Reddy, 2005), and approximately one-third of boys with FXS have autism (Harris et al., 2008; Rogers, Wehner, & Hagerman, 2001). This proportion rises to almost two-thirds in young men (Das & Turk, 2002). However, a far higher proportion of individuals with FXS manifest the paradoxical juxtaposition of a friendly and sociable (albeit often shy and socially anxious) personality in the presence of multiple autistic-like communicatory and ritualistic qualitative impairments. In addition, there is usually a good understanding of facial expression (Turk & Cornish, 1998) and theory of mind abilities are typically as expected for an individual's general cognitive ability level (Garner et al., 1999). Kaufmann et al. (2004) have pointed out that the finding of autism in FXS depends on the severity of the social and communication deficits, not the severity of poor eye contact or unusual hand mannerisms. However, in a comparison study with an intellectually disabled control group without FXS, Grant, Apperly, and Oliver (2007) argued that theory of mind difficulties are an important aspect of the FXS clinical profile, but are most likely based on a more basic difficulty with working memory. For individuals with FXS and co-occurring autism spectrum disorder (ASD), longitudinal research indicates the ASD diagnosis is stable over time and in childhood is associated with clearly differentiated symptoms and behaviors as compared to people with FXS without ASD (Hernandez et al., 2009).

Social, Emotional, and Behavioral Adjustment

Several studies have indicated that the majority (70–82%) of children and adolescents with FXS meet criteria for at least one anxiety disorder, with social phobia and specific phobia being the most common (Cordeiro et al., 2011; Bailey, Raspa, Olmsted, & Holiday, 2008). Both males and females with FXS show anxiety reactions and overarousal that impair their social interactions. A major indicator of social anxiety is gaze avoidance, especially in males with FXS (Cohen et al., 1988; Dalton, Holsen, Abbeduto, & Davidson, 2008; Farzin et al., 2009; Garrett et al., 2004; Hessl et al., 2006; Holsen et al., 2008; Simon & Finucane, 1996; Watson et al., 2008). Females with FXS and social anxiety are at risk for developing symptoms of major depression (Angkustsiri, Wirojanan, Deprey, Gane, & Hagerman, 2008; Hagan et al., 2008; Reiss, Freund, Vinogradov, Hagerman, & Cronister, 1989; Tranebjaerg & Orum, 1991), which could be a secondary effect of the social neglect by peers or of growing self-awareness of having a disability.

As mentioned previously, over 50% of children with FXS meet behavioral criteria for ADHD (Sullivan et al., 2006). In addition, people with FXS often display challenging behaviors such as self-injury and aggression. Hessl and colleagues (2008) reported that 75% of males with FXS between ages 8 and 24 years demonstrated some aggression toward others during the 2-month reporting period. The most common aggressive behaviors were hitting others (49% of the sample) and kicking others (30%). Clinical experience suggests that aggression and irritability increase and reach a peak during late adolescence and early adulthood, perhaps as a result of central nervous system (CNS) changes related to puberty and stresses associated with leaving the stability and structure of the school system. Aggressive acts are often preceded by periods of overstimulation, anxiety, or stress. A national study on self-injurious behavior found that for males with the full mutation and self-injurious behavior, the behavior developed prior to the first birthday for 11% of the sample and between ages 1 and 3 for 52% of the sample (Symons, Byiers, Raspa, Bishop, & Bailey, 2010). Symons et al. also reported that 41% of males and 16.7% of females had self-injured at some point in their lifetime, while 32% percent of males and 11.4% of females had displayed self-injurious in the past 30 days. Aggression is also common, with one study revealing that over 90% of parents reported that their child with FXS had engaged in at least one aggressive act in the past year, with males being more likely to display severe aggressive behavior that results in injury to others (Wheeler, Raspa, Bishop, & Bailey, 2016).

DEVELOPMENTAL CONSIDERATIONS AND GENDER DIFFERENCES

Infants with FXS are rarely diagnosed prenatally. Instead, testing is recommended when they begin to exhibit developmental delays, such as impaired language development in toddlerhood. Genetic testing is recommended when there is a family history of FXS or when a child presents with developmental delay, autism, or other clinically significant features that may be related to the disorder. However, it is likely that some individuals with FXS never receive this diagnosis, as it requires genetic testing and they instead receive services and supports under another diagnostic category such as intellectual disability or autism spectrum disorder. Girls with FXS, especially those with only mild cognitive impairment, executive dysfunction, or anxiety, are often overlooked for DNA testing (Bartholomay, Lee, Bruno, Lightbody, & Reiss, 2019). While there is increased awareness of FXS and a push to recommend testing to all young children with developmental delay, the average age of FXS diagnosis is still 30–35 months for males and slightly higher for females (Bailey, Raspa, Bishop, & Holiday, 2009a).

Early Development

While both sexes can have the full mutation, resulting in complete inactivation of the *FMR1* protein, the X-linked nature of FXS results in differing developmental trajectories for males and females. Males with FXS exhibit developmental delays in infancy, usually failing to reach typical milestones in language and gross motor development (Bailey, Hatton, Mesibov, Ament, & Skinner, 2000). While females with FXS may also exhibit developmental delays, these tend to be milder and thus less noticeable at a young age (Garber, Visootsak, & Warren, 2008). Males with FXS often present with syndrome-specific facial features (long face with prominent ears) that are evident from a young age. Children with FXS are also more likely to have a variety of medical conditions such as cleft palates, orthopedic abnormalities, and seizure disorders. It is estimated that between 10 and 20% of males with FXS have epilepsy, with slightly lower numbers for females with FXS (Leung & Ring, 2013). For those affected, seizures generally begin in early childhood (Berry-Kravis et al., 2010).

People with FXS exhibit a wide variety of co-occurring mental and behavioral symptoms starting in infancy. Symptoms commonly associated with ASD (hand flapping, hand biting, and poor eye contact), self-injury, aggression, attentional concerns, and anxious behavior are all likely to be seen in early childhood (Hall et al., 2008b). Attentional bias toward threat, which has been linked with anxiety, was demonstrated in preschool-age children with FXS when compared to age- and mental-age-matched groups of children without FXS (Burris et al., 2017).

School Age

Male school-age children with FXS are extremely likely to have a diagnosis of intellectual disability (~90%), while only about one-half of females with the full mutation will have intellectual disability (Loesch et al., 2002). Females with FXS are more likely to display learning problems, especially in mathematics, and deficits in attention affecting academic performance, as well as a variety of emotional and behavioral concerns (Rinehart, Cornish, & Tonge, 2010; Bartholomay et al., 2019). As is evidenced in most people with intellectual disabilities, the gap in cognitive functioning and adaptive behavior between children with FXS and their typically developing peers is likely to widen over time (Hall et al., 2008a; Klaiman et al., 2014).

In terms of physical health, male children with FXS have been shown to have almost double the rate of obesity as typically developing children, and they engage in less physical activity (Raspa, Bailey, Bishop, Holiday, & Olmsted, 2010).

Adulthood

While the majority of FXS research focuses on early development and childhood, a growing body of research explores the lives of adults with FXS. In adulthood, most males with FXS live with family members or in a group home and have relatively low levels of employment and independence. In contrast, women with FXS show greater variation in outcomes, with approximately half living independently and having full-time employment (Hartley et al., 2011). Behavioral and mental health concerns that are prevalent in childhood persist into adulthood, with half of adults with FXS having concerns related to ADHD symptoms, 58% of women with FXS and 71% of men with FXS with co-occurring affective disorders, and 16% of women and 47% of men with FXS displaying self-injury (Hartley et al., 2011). Aggressive behaviors are likely to continue into adulthood, with some research suggesting that aggression worsens as individuals transition into adulthood (Hardiman & McGill, 2018). As people with FXS grow into adulthood, aggressive behaviors are more likely to cause damage and create extreme stress for families and other caregivers.

PREDICTORS AND MODERATORS

FXS is a genetic disorder; thus, the mutation of *FMR1* and consequent FMRP reduction is the driving force behind its core features. IQ has been linked to levels of FMRP in repeat-size or methylation-mosaic male and females with FXS, with higher levels of FMRP being associated with higher IQ (Huddleston, Visootsak, & Sherman, 2014; Tassone et al., 1999). Lower levels of FMRP have also been linked to more compulsive behaviors in females with FXS (Hall et al., 2008b). While FXS is a single-gene disorder, it is known that the cognitive and behavioral phenotype is modified by background genetic and environmental factors. Variation in the home environment and parental intelligence and psychological health are all related to child outcomes (Hessl et al., 2001; Dyer Friedman et al., 2002). A small longitudinal study of females with FXS found that fluid intelligence was related to genetic factors only, while crystallized intelligence was influenced by environmental factors (del Hoyo Soriano, Thurman, Harvey, Brown & Abbeduto, 2018).

Reiss and Dant (2003) emphasized the variability of behavioral and cognitive symptoms in FXS between males and females with the explanation of a complex interaction of genetic, environmental, and biological risk factors. Although the deficit of FMRP is the cause of FXS, variation in this protein does not appear to be significantly associated with severity of autistic symptoms, especially after adjusting for level of cognitive impairment (Hessl et al., 2001; Loesch et al., 2007). A large, in-home evaluation study (Hessl et al., 2001) showed an impact of educational and therapeutic services and parental psychopathology on problem behavior, and home environment quality was associated with the severity of autism-related behaviors.

Hessl et al. (2008) found that genotype differences in the serotonin transporter polymorphism (*5-HTTLPR*) were associated with both aggressive and stereotyped behavior in males, with FXS providing evidence of the potential impacts of secondary genetic factors in phenotype modification. Attentional and social behavior concerns have been linked to higher daily levels of cortisol, while cortisol reductions in response to a social task were associated with higher level of gaze avoidance, suggesting that gaze avoidance is a coping response to reduce the stress reaction (Hessl et al., 2002, 2006).

As with any child, the quality of the early environment is linked to later outcomes. A high-quality home environment, defined by availability of learning materials, exposure to arts, organization, positive parenting approaches, and availability of space and materials for play, was found to be linked to cognitive and behavioral outcomes in young children with FXS (Dyer-Friedman et al., 2002; Glaser et al., 2003). Maternal responsivity has also been linked to child language use at 36 months (Warren, Brady, Sterling, Fleming, & Marquis, 2010). As people with FXS tend to be highly dependent on their families, it is not surprising that family patterns continue to be associated with differing outcomes at older ages. In adolescence and adulthood, higher maternal warmth is associated with positive outcomes such as higher adaptive behavior and decreases in challenging behavior over time, while maternal criticisms were linked to increased psychopathology (Smith, Hong, Greenberg, & Mailick, 2016). It should be noted however, that this is likely a bidirectional relationship, as child challenges in turn are likely to increase parenting stress, thus creating more barriers to a warm and nurturing environment and relationship.

The co-occurrence of ASD in people with FXS is a consistent predictor of a variety of outcomes. Children with co-occurring ASD have been shown to have poorer cognitive, adaptive, and behavioral outcomes, as well as a slower rate of development than those who do not meet criteria for ASD (Roberts et al., 2008; Lewis et al., 2006; Symons et al., 2010). Children with FXS and ASD have an increased rate of CNS medical diagnoses, such as seizures, compared to children with only FXS, though the mechanism of this correlation is unknown (García-Nonell et al., 2008).

Regarding cognitive performance, one of the challenges of standardized testing, including IQ assessment in FXS, is the fact that a large proportion of individuals obtain scores at the floor of the test measurable range, limiting precision and characterization of relative strengths and weaknesses. Revised scoring, such as measurement of true deviation of performance from general population norms without floor restriction, has been used successfully to better characterize level of functioning in FXS and other causes of intellectual disability (Hessl et al., 2009, 2016; Sansone et al., 2014). The approach described in the 2009 Hessl et al. study demonstrated that a *z*-score normalization could eliminate the floor problems in the cognitive assessment with the Wechsler Intelligence Scale for Children (WISC-III), leading to normally distributed scores. In addition, the authors found correlations between cognitive performance and adaptive behavior, and between cognition and FMRP, that were improved when using these normalized scores in contrast to the usual standardized scores. A similar method was proposed and evaluated for the Stanford–Binet 5, and deviation-derived scores again ameliorated the floor effects and improved the precision of IQ measurement. Hessl et al. (2016) presented three preliminary studies utilizing the NIH Toolbox Cognitive Battery as an alternative to typical IQ measures for FXS, Down syndrome, and idiopathic intellectual disability. Results showed good to excellent feasibility and test–retest reliability, as well as evidence of concurrent validity.

TREATMENT AND INTERVENTION

While there is no cure for FXS, a multidisciplinary approach that focuses on the associated, specific behavioral, communicative, and educational difficulties is most often used. First, we review common behavioral treatments, followed by pharmacological treatments for the "associated" symptoms of FXS, though most are based on clinical expertise and/or open-label trials rather than being empirically validated in patients with FXS specifically. Then we review the most common pharmacological "targeted" treatments for FXS that have been attempted and/or that are frequently used off-label, based on preclinical successes and clinician expertise.

Behavioral Treatments

While there is limited research on behavioral treatments specific to FXS, clinicians are generally guided by behavioral interventions that have been demonstrated effective in other disorders with similar features and characteristics, including ASD. One of the strongest findings from research in other disorders associated with cognitive delays is the importance of early intervention. There are a variety of well-established and validated early intervention models for the treatment of ASD such as Treatment and Education of Autistic and Related Communication Handicapped Children (TEACCH; Mesibov, Shea,

& Schopler, 2005), pivotal response training (PRT; Koegel & Koegel, 2006), and applied behavior analysis (ABA; Peters-Scheffer, Didden, Korzilius, & Sturmey, 2011). Despite the abundance of research on the use of these interventions in children with ASD, there remains a paucity of research on interventions in FXS. Regarding early intervention, one of the only studies to examine early intervention in FXS involved training parents to implement a naturalistic behavioral intervention, the Early Start Denver Model (ESDM). While the sample size for this pilot study was small, the intervention appeared to be feasible for the children, and three out of four participants were reported to make developmental gains (Vismara, McCormick, Shields, & Hessl, 2019).

Hessl and colleagues (2019b) conducted a randomized controlled trial (RCT) of computer-based Cogmed working memory training, targeting working memory, executive function, and behavior in 100 children and adolescents with FXS. Participants were randomized to adaptive or nonadaptive (control condition) forms of Cogmed and completed 5–6 weeks of training at home supported by a parent training aide and supportive coaching by phone. While no difference was found between the adaptive and nonadaptive control conditions for most comparisons, the intervention was feasible, and the full sample demonstrated improvements in working memory and executive function objective measures, as well as parent- and teacher-reported attention and executive function. As both groups improved, further research, such as using a nonactive control condition, is needed to determine whether the executive function gains are specific to Cogmed itself, or perhaps to other aspects of the intervention.

A parent-implemented language intervention (PILI) has been assessed in FXS in several studies (McDuffie et al., 2016). In PILI, parents are coached to learn strategies for interacting with their child, which are aimed at increasing the child's spoken language. In a study of 20 male children and adolescents with FXS, after PILI treatment, mothers in the treatment group used these strategies more than those in the control group, and children spent more time involved in shared storytelling and used a wider vocabulary than those in the control group (McDuffie et al., 2018). An innovative aspect of PILI is that it is conducted in a telehealth setting, which allows for wider and easier access to the treatment. This approach is being utilized in a large-scale clinical trial of mavoglurant (an mGluR5 negative modulator) in young children with FXS. The study (NCT02920892; AFQ056 for Language Learning in Children with FXS) aims to determine whether the drug in combination with PILI can enhance language learning in comparison to placebo with PILI.

Regarding anxiety, attention, irritability, and aggression, behavioral treatments have rarely been validated in FXS specifically. An RCT (NCT03510156) is being conducted on the use of function-based behavior-analytic interventions delivered via telehealth to treat problem behaviors in males with FXS. In a pilot sample of 10 boys with FXS (ages 3–10 years) from this larger study, there was a reduction in problem behaviors of 78–95% across participants (Monlux, Pollard, Rodriguez, & Hall, 2019). Additionally, caregivers rated the treatment as effective and very reasonable on average. Further research is needed on telehealth treatment frequency and on measuring behaviors from a greater portion of daily life rather than just session behaviors.

Though not focused specifically on FXS, one study of participants with comorbid intellectual disability and anxiety found that 9 weeks of a structured mindfulness-based cognitive therapy program significantly reduced anxiety scores on the Hospital Anxiety and Depression Scale (Idusohan-Moizer, Sawicka, Dendle, & Albany, 2013). It is important to note that studies on treatment effectiveness in intellectual disability or ASD do not necessarily generalize to FXS, but these studies can provide a first step of support for behavioral treatments that may be effective in patients with FXS, as their pattern of symptoms and behavior show significant overlap. Additional data, including RCTs, are sorely needed to better demonstrate effectiveness, limitations, and potential adaptations for use in FXS patients.

Pharmacological Treatments

Associated Symptoms

Associated symptoms that are commonly treated with medications include inattention and hyperactivity, anxiety, aggression, irritability, and seizures (Raspa, Wheeler, & Riley, 2017; Berry-Kravis & Potanos, 2004). Though most of these treatments have not been empirically validated in RCTs in FXS, they are often used off-label to address these symptoms in patients with FXS based on extensive clinical experience.

Attention difficulties and hyperactivity are the most common symptoms to be treated pharmacologically in FXS (Berry-Kravis & Potanos, 2004). Standard stimulant medications such as methylphenidate and dextroamphetamine are frequently used (Hagerman et al., 2009). One FXS controlled trial on attention problems was conducted by Hagerman, Murphy, and Wittenberger (1988). In this crossover study, 15 children with severe attention difficulties were treated with a stimulant. Teacher ratings showed improvement in social skills and attention with treatment, and 10 children were identified as responders based on parent and teacher reports. Nonstimulant treatments commonly used in FXS are alpha-adrenergic receptor agonists (e.g., guanfacine), the nutritional supplement L-acetyl-carnitine, and valproic acid (Hagerman et al., 2009; Torriolo et al., 2010). Additionally, folic acid has been used for many years, based on anecdotal reports that it reduces hyperactivity, as well as reducing repetitive behaviors and improving language in FXS (Gustavson et al., 1985; Brown et al., 1984).

For anxiety, selective serotonin reuptake inhibitors (SSRIs) appear to be effective in relieving symptoms in patients with FXS, with over 50% of patients showing improvement in anxiety measures after SSRI treatment (Hagerman et al., 2009). In one case study, fluoxetine was effective at treating selective mutism in an adolescent female with FXS (Hagerman, Hills, Scharfenaker, & Lewis, 1999). Hall, Lightbody, McCarthy, Parker, and Reiss (2012) found that a single intranasal administration of oxytocin reduced certain social anxiety related symptoms and cortisol level in a study of 10 males with FXS during a structured social challenge.

Seizures in FXS are generally treated with standard anticonvulsant medications such as carbamazepine and valproic acid (Berry-Kravis et al., 2010). Some anticonvulsants can exacerbate irritability and hyperactivity, hypotonia, and/or cognitive impairment and are thus sometimes avoided in FXS (Hagerman et al., 2009).

Aggression and irritability are often treated with antipsychotics, such as risperidone and aripiprazole (Bailey, Raspa, Olmsted, & Holiday, 2008; Berry-Kravis & Potanos, 2004). In a prospective, open-label study, Erickson et al. (2011) examined aripiprazole as a treatment for irritability in FXS. Of the 12 participants, 10 were considered responders based on clinician ratings of irritability, and parent ratings of irritability also significantly improved. Finally, sleep problems are frequently reported in FXS; melatonin is often used to improve sleep (Raspa, Wheeler, & Riley, 2017).

Targeted Treatments

As described earlier, several molecular mechanisms have been identified as being impacted by the reduced FMRP that characterizes FXS; multiple promising targeted treatments have been developed from preclinical animal work aimed at these impaired neurobiological pathways (Berry-Kravis et al., 2017). Several animal models have been developed, starting with an *FMR1* knockout (KO) mouse, a KO rat, a zebrafish, and a drosophila model (Dahlhaus, 2018). FXS has thus been at the forefront of translational research for neurodevelopmental disorders. Controlled trials of targeted treatments aim to improve specific pathophysiological mechanisms and thus phenotypic symptoms as a result. Overall, these human trials have been unsuccessful; however, many experts in the field suggest that factors such as treatment translation from animals to humans, clinical trial design, and placebo response issues could be significant reasons for the failure of many of these trials (Erickson et al., 2017). Many new targeted treatment trials are currently underway, with a recent emphasis on lessons learned from trial failures (Budimirovic et al., 2017; Protic, Salcedo-Arellano, Dy, Potter, & Hagerman, 2019). Presently there is no U.S. Food and Drug Administration (FDA)-approved medication to treat FXS.

Several targeted treatments have been based on the excitatory mGluR5 pathway (Bear, Huber, & Warren, 2004; Pop et al., 2014), including mGluR5 antagonists mavoglurant, basimglurant, and fenobam (Berry-Kravis et al., 2016; Youssef et al., 2018). Gamma-aminobutyric acid (GABA) agonists, working upstream of the mGluR5 receptor, have also been assessed, including arbaclofen, acamprosate, ganaxolone, and gaboxadol (Berry-Kravis et al., 2016; NCT03697161). Despite preclinical successes, these treatments overall have had negative results on primary outcomes in clinical trials. Sertraline, which stimulates neurogenesis and increases brain-derived neurotropic factor (BDNF), has been extensively utilized in patients with FXS. Although an RCT of SSRIs targeting anxiety in patients with FXS has yet to be completed, low-dose sertraline was trialed in young children with FXS. Potential benefits were seen in secondary analyses of motor and visual perceptual abilities and social participation (Greiss Hess et al., 2016); however, there was no benefit in the primary outcome of expressive language. Minocycline, an antibiotic that lowers matrix metalloproteinase 9, has been evaluated in several FXS studies with mixed results (Leigh et al., 2013; Dziembowska et al., 2013). In the minocycline trial, event-related potentials (ERPs) were used for the first time as an outcome measure and showed some reduced auditory excitability and improved habituation in some participants (Schneider et al., 2013). Other drugs currently being tested are lovastatin (Osterweil et al., 2013; NCT02642653), cannabidiol (Heussler et al., 2019; NCT03614663), and metformin (Gantois, Popic, Khoutorsky, & Sonenberg, 2019; NCT03479476).

The largest targeted treatment trials with results available thus far were trials of mavoglurant (Phase IIb RCTs), basimglurant (Phase II RCTs), and arbaclofen (Phase III RCTs) (Berry-Kravis et al., 2016; Youssef et al., 2018; Berry-Kravis et al., 2017). The primary outcome measures were the Aberrant Behavior Checklist (ABC), the Anxiety Depression and Mood Scale, and the ABC Social Avoidance subscale, respectively. These trials had no significant difference in the treatment group improvement relative to placebo group, or had no significant improvement, on the primary outcomes. In the arbaclofen child sample, however, there was a trend toward improvement on the primary outcome in those receiving the highest dose relative to placebo. Additionally, Hessl et al. (2019a) used an infrared eye-tracking protocol to measure social gaze processing as a secondary outcome in the mavoglurant trial. They showed that the adolescents and adults with FXS treated with mavoglurant had improved gaze to the eye region of human faces and changes in pupillary response to faces relative to those treated with placebo. This result provided some evidence of target engagement despite the lack of improvement over placebo on the behavioral measure of interest in the trial.

The potential to reactivate *FMR1* and increase FMRP expression has been a new focus of investigation. For example, Liu et al. (2018) showed that targeted demethylation of CGG repeats by dCas9-Tet1 reactivates *FMR1* in induced pluripotent stem cells (iPSCs), and Haenfler et al. (2018) were able to use CRISPR/dCas9 to reactivate transcription at the site (see Yrigollen & Davidson, 2019, for a review of these important developments). It is unknown at this time whether correction of *FMR1* function postnatally or later in development can ameliorate the phenotype in humans, or whether off-target effects of these techniques might produce toxic effects.

While preclinical research targeting molecular mechanisms of FXS have been, and continue to be, successful, translation to clinical trials in humans has had repeated challenges. Several important points have been cited as lessons learned and goals for improvement in order to gain confidence in trial results (Erickson et al., 2017; Lee, Ventola, Budimirovic, Berry-Kravis, & Visootsak, 2018). These include the need for psychometrically appropriate and more objective outcome measures, better ways to mitigate and understand placebo response, and the idea of clustering outcomes together rather than measuring efficacy with a single measure. Targeted treatments for FXS remain an area of extensive and ongoing research.

CONCLUSIONS AND FUTURE DIRECTIONS

Following identification of the *FMR1* gene mutation as the cause of FXS, the field has benefited from a remarkable expansion of research to better understand the phenotype, molecular factors, gene regulatory pathways, and environmental modifiers, as well as preclinical testing of potentially disease-modifying treatments. Efforts to translate widely effective genetic or pharmacological intervention in murine and fly models to beneficial treatments in humans have been to date unsuccessful. Future research must focus on understanding the breakdown of this translation, develop additional animal or human cellular models that more closely model the human clinical condition, and identify more objective, sensitive, and clinically relevant outcome measures. The dearth of empirically validated behavioral, cognitive, and educational interventions for individuals with FXS reflect major knowledge gaps. Indeed, targeted pharmacological treatments, if effective in normalizing brain functioning in FXS, may need to be paired with learning paradigms or behavioral approaches over extended time periods to allow for the improved processing supported by medications to yield substantial gains in development and behavioral/emotional adaptation. Finally, emerging and increasingly refined technologies and techniques, such as telehealth delivery of behavioral and cognitive intervention, more ecologically valid behavioral assessment, and utilization of new biomarker and biobehavioral probes of functioning are likely to advance the field and contribute to effective treatment opportunities for patients and their families.

REFERENCES

Abbeduto, L., Murphy, M. M., Cawthon, S. W., Richmond, E. K., Weissman, M. D., Karadottir, S., & O'Brien, A. (2003). Receptive language skills of adolescents and young adults with Down or fragile X syndrome. *American Journal of Mental Retardation, 108*(3), 149–160.

Angkustsiri, K., Wirojanan, J., Deprey, L. J., Gane, L. W., & Hagerman, R. J. (2008). Fragile X syndrome with anxiety disorder and exceptional verbal intelligence. *American Journal of Medical Genetics A, 146*(3), 376–379.

Bailey, D. B., Jr., Raspa, M., Olmsted, M., & Holiday, D. B. (2008). Co-occurring conditions associated with FMR1 gene variations: Findings from a national parent survey. *American Journal of Medical Genetics A, 146*(16), 2060–2069.

Bailey, D. B., Jr., Hatton, D. D., Mesibov, G., Ament, N., & Skinner, M. (2000). Early development, temperament, and functional impairment in autism and fragile X syndrome. *Journal of Autism and Developmental Disorders, 30*(1), 49–59.

Bailey, D. B., Jr., Hatton, D. D., & Skinner, M. (1998). Early developmental trajectories of males with fragile X syndrome. *American Journal of Mental Retardation,* 103(1), 29–39.

Bailey, D. B., Jr., Raspa, M., Bishop, E., & Holiday, D. (2009a). No change in the age of diagnosis for fragile X syndrome: Findings from a national parent survey. *Pediatrics, 124*(2), 527–533.

Bakker, C. E., Verheij, C., Willemsen, R., Vanderhelm, R., Oerlemans, F., Vermey, M., . . . Willems, P. J. (1994). FMR1 knockout mice: A model to study fragile X mental retardation. *Cell, 78,* 23–33.

Ballinger, E. C., Cordeiro, L., Chavez, A. D., Hagerman, R. J., & Hessl, D. (2014). Emotion potentiated startle in fragile X syndrome. *Journal of Autism and Developmental Disorders, 44*(10), 2536–2546.

Bartholomay, K. L., Lee, C. H., Bruno, J. L., Lightbody, A. A., & Reiss, A. L. (2019). Closing the gender gap in fragile X Syndrome: Review on females with FXS and preliminary research findings. *Brain Sciences, 9*(1), Article 11.

Bassell, G. J., & Warren, S. T. (2008). Fragile X syndrome: Loss of local mRNA regulation alters synaptic development and function, *Neuron, 60*(2), 201–214.

Bear, M. F., Huber, K. M., & Warren, S. T. (2004). The mGluR theory of fragile X mental retardation. *Trends in Neurosciences, 27,* 370–377.

Belser, R. C., & Sudhalter, V. (2001). Conversational characteristics of children with fragile X syndrome: Repetitive speech. *American Journal of Mental Retardation, 106*(1), 28–38.

Bennetto, L., & Pennington, B. F. (2002). Neuropsychology. In R. J. Hagerman & P. J. Hagerman (Eds.), *Fragile X syndrome: Diagnosis, treatment, and research* (3rd ed., pp. 206–248). Baltimore: Johns Hopkins University Press.

Berry-Kravis, E., Abrams, L., Coffey, S. M., Hall, D. A., Greco, C., Gane, L. W., . . . Leehey, M. A. (2007). Fragile X-associated tremor/ataxia syndrome: Clinical features, genetics, and testing guidelines. *Movement Disorders, 22*(14), 2018–2030.

Berry-Kravis, E., Des Portes, V., Hagerman, R., Jacquemont, S., Charles, P., Visootsak, J., . . . von Raison, F. (2016). Mavoglurant in fragile X syndrome: Results of two randomized, double-blind, placebo-controlled trials. *Science Translational Medicine, 8*(321), 321ra5.

Berry-Kravis, E., Hagerman, R., Visootsak, J., Budimirovic, D., Kaufmann, W. E., Cherubini, M., . . . Carpenter, R. L. (2017). Arbaclofen in fragile X syndrome: Results of phase 3 trials. *Journal of Neurodevelopmental Disorders, 9,* Article 3.

Berry-Kravis, E., & Potanos, K. (2004). Psychopharmacology in fragile X syndrome—Present and future. *Mental Retardation and Developmental Disabilities Research Reviews, 10,* 42–48.

Berry-Kravis, E., Raspa, M., Loggin-Hester, L., Bishop, E., Holiday, D., & Bailey Jr, D. B. (2010). Seizures in fragile X syndrome: Characteristics and comorbid diagnoses. *American Journal on Intellectual and Developmental Disabilities, 115*(6), 461–472.

Brown, W. T., Jenkins, E. C., Friedman, E., Brooks, J., Cohen, I. L., Duncan, C., . . . Opitz, J. M. (1984). Folic acid therapy in the fragile X syndrome. *American Journal of Medical Genetics, 17,* 289–297.

Brown, W. T., Jenkins, E. C., Friedman, E., Brooks, J., Wisniewski, K., Raguthu, S., & French, J. (1982). Autism is associated with the fragile-X syndrome. *Journal of Autism and Developmental Disorders, 12*(3), 303–308.

Budimirovic, D. B., Berry-Kravis, E., Erickson, C. A., Hall, S. S., Hessl, D., Reiss, A. L., . . . Kaufmann, W. E. (2017). Updated report on tools to measure outcomes of clinical trials in fragile X syndrome. *Journal of Neurodevelopmental Disorders, 9,* Article 14.

Burris, J. L., Barry-Anwar, R. A., Sims, R. N., Hagerman, R. J., Tassone, F., & Rivera, S. M. (2017). Children with fragile X syndrome display threat-specific biases toward emotion. *Biological Psychiatry: Cognitive Neuroscience and Neuroimaging, 2*(6), 487–492.

Chen, X., Wang, J., Xie, H., Zhou, W., Wu, Y., Wang, J., . . . Jiang, Y. (2015). Fragile X syndrome screening in Chinese children with unknown intellectual developmental disorder. *BMC Pediatrics, 15,* Article 77.

Chernenok, M., Burris, J. L., Owen, E., & Rivera, S. M. (2019). Impaired attention orienting in young children with fragile X syndrome. *Frontiers in Psychology, 10,* Article 1567.

Ciaccio, C., Fontana, L., Milani, D., Tabano, S., Miozzo, M., & Esposito, S. (2017). Fragile X syndrome: A review of clinical and molecular diagnoses. *Italian Journal of Pediatrics, 43*(1), Article 39.

Coffey, S. M., Cook, K., Tartaglia, N., Tassone, F., Nguyen, D. V., Pan, R., . . . Hagerman, R. J. (2008). Expanded clinical phenotype of women with the FMR1 premutation. *American Journal of Medical Genetics A, 146*(8), 1009–1016.

Cohen, I. L., Fisch, G. S., Sudhalter, V., Wolf-Schein, E. G., Hanson, D., Hagerman, R. J., . . . Brown, W. T. (1988). Social gaze, social avoidance, and repetitive behavior in fragile X males: A controlled study. *American Journal on Mental Retardation, 92*(5), 436–446.

Cordeiro, L., Ballinger, E., Hagerman, R., & Hessl, D. (2011). Clinical assessment of DSM-IV anxiety disorders in fragile X syndrome: Prevalence and characterization. *Journal of Neurodevelopmental Disorders, 3*(1), 57–67.

Cornish, K. M., Kogan, C. S., Li, L., Turk, J., Jacquemont, S., & Hagerman, R. J. (2009). Lifespan changes in working memory in fragile X premutation males. *Brain and Cognition, 69*(3), 551–558.

Cornish, K. M., Kogan, C., Turk, J., Manly, T., James, N., Mills, A., & Dalton, A. (2005). The emerging fragile X premutation phenotype: Evidence from the domain of social cognition. *Brain and Cognition, 57*(1), 53–60.

Cornish, K. M., Munir, F., & Cross, G. (2001). Differential impact of the FMR-1 full mutation on memory and attention functioning: A neuropsychological perspective. *Journal of Cognitive Neuroscience, 13*(1), 144–150.

Cornish, K. M., Sudhalter, V., & Turk, J. (2004a). Attention and language in fragile X. *Mental Retardation and Developmental Disabilities Research Reviews, 10*(1), 11–16.

Cornish, K. M., Turk, J., & Levitas, A. (2007). Fragile X syndrome and autism: Common developmental pathways? *Current Pediatric Reviews, 3,* 61–68.

Cornish, K. M., Turk, J., Wilding, J., Sudhalter, V., Munir, F., Kooy, F., & Hagerman, R. J. (2004b). Annotation: Deconstructing the attention deficit in fragile X syndrome: A developmental neuropsychological approach. *Journal of Child Psychology and Psychiatry, 45*(6), 1042–1053.

Crawford, D. C, Acuña, J. M., & Sherman, S. (2001). *FMR1* and the fragile X syndrome: Human genome epidemiology review. *Genetics in Medicine, 3*(5), 359–371.

Cronister, A., Schreiner, R., Wittenberger, M., Amiri, K., Harris, K., & Hagerman, R. J. (1991). Heterozygous fragile X female: Historical, physical, cognitive, and cytogenetic features. *American Journal of Medical Genetics, 38*(2–3), 269–274.

Dahlhaus R. (2018). Of men and mice: Modeling the fragile X syndrome. *Frontiers in Molecular Neuroscience, 11,* Article 41.

Dalton, K. M., Holsen, L., Abbeduto, L., & Davidson, R. J. (2008). Brain function and gaze fixation during facial-emotional processing in fragile X and autism. *Autism Research, 1,* 231–239.

Das, D., & Turk, J. (2002, July). *The development of social and communicatory functioning in boys with fragile X syndrome.* Paper presented at the National Fragile X Conference, Chicago, IL.

del Hoyo Soriano, L., Thurman, A. J., Harvey, D. J., Brown, W. T., & Abbeduto, L. (2018). Genetic and maternal predictors of cognitive and behavioral trajectories in females with fragile X syndrome. *Journal of Neurodevelopmental Disorders, 10*(1), Article 22.

Dyer-Friedman, J., Glaser, B., Hessl, D., Johnston, C., Huffman, L. C., Taylor, A., . . . Reiss, A. L. (2002). Genetic and environmental influences on the cognitive outcomes of children with fragile X syndrome. *Journal of the American Academy of Child and Adolescent Psychiatry, 41*(3), 237–244.

Dziembowska, M., Pretto, D. I., Janusz, A., Kaczmarek, L., Leigh, M. J., Gabriel, N., . . . Tassone, F. (2013). High MMP-9 activity levels in fragile X syndrome are lowered by minocycline. *American Journal of Medical Genetics A, 161*(8), 1897–1903.

Eberhart, D. E., Malter, H. E., Feng, Y., & Warren, S. T. (1996). The fragile X mental retardation protein is a ribonucleoprotein containing both nuclear localization and nuclear export signals. *Human Molecular Genetics, 5*(8), 1083–1091.

Eliez, S., Blasey, C., Freund, L. S., Hastie, T., & Reiss, A. (2001). Brain anatomy, gender and IQ in children and adolescents with fragile X syndrome. *Brain, 124*(Pt. 8), 1610–1618.

Erickson, C. A., Stigler, K. A., Wink, L. K., Mullett, J. E., Kohn, A., Posey, D. J., & McDougle, C. J. (2011). A prospective open-label study of aripiprazole in fragile X syndrome. *Psychopharmacology, 216*, 85–90.

Erickson, C. A., Davenport, M. H., Schaefer, T. L., Wink, L. K., Pedapati, E, V., Sweeney J. A., . . . Berry-Kravis, E. (2017). Fragile X targeted pharmacotherapy: Lessons learned and future directions. *Journal of Neurodevelopmental Disorders, 9*, Article 7.

Farzin, F., & Rivera, S. M. (2010). Dynamic object representations in infants with and without fragile X syndrome. *Frontiers in Human Neuroscience, 4*, Article 12.

Farzin, F., Rivera, S. M., & Hessl, D. (2009). Brief report: Visual processing of faces in individuals with fragile X syndrome: An eye tracking study. *Journal of Autism and Developmental Disorders, 39*(6), 946–952.

Farzin, F., Whitney, D., Hagerman, R. J., & Rivera, S. M. (2008). Contrast detection in infants with fragile X syndrome. *Vision Research, 48*(13), 1471–1478.

Fisch, G. S., Simensen, R. J., & Schroer, R. J. (2002). Longitudinal changes in cognitive and adaptive behavior scores in children and adolescents with the fragile X mutation or autism. *Journal of Autism and Developmental Disorders, 32*(2), 107–114.

Fisch, G. S., Simensen, R., Tarleton, J., Chalifoux, M., Holden, J. J., Carpenter, N., . . . Maddalena, A. (1996). Longitudinal study of cognitive abilities and adaptive behavior levels in fragile X males: A prospective multicenter analysis. *American Journal of Medical Genetics, 64*(2), 356–361.

Freund, L. S., & Reiss, A. L. (1991). Cognitive profiles associated with the fra(X) syndrome in males and females. *American Journal of Medical Genetics, 38*(4), 542–547.

Gantois, I., Popic, J., Khoutorsky, A., & Sonenberg, N. (2019). Metformin for treatment of fragile X syndrome and other neurological disorders. *Annual Review of Medicine, 70*, 167–181.

Garber, K. B., Visootsak, J., & Warren, S. T. (2008). Fragile X syndrome. *European Journal of Human Genetics, 16*(6), 666–672.

García-Nonell, C., Ratera, E. R., Harris, S., Hessl, D., Ono, M. Y., Tartaglia, N., . . . Hagerman, R. J. (2008). Secondary medical diagnosis in fragile X syndrome with and without autism spectrum disorder. *American Journal of Medical Genetics A, 146*(15), 1911–1916.

Garner, C., Callias, M., & Turk, J. (1999). Executive function and theory of mind performance of boys with fragile-X syndrome. *Journal of Intellectual Disability Research, 43*(Pt. 6), 466–474.

Garrett, A. S., Menon, V., MacKenzie, K., & Reiss, A. L. (2004). Here's looking at you, kid: Neural systems underlying face and gaze processing in fragile X syndrome. *Archives of General Psychiatry, 61*(3), 281–288.

Glaser, B., Hessl, D., Dyer-Friedman, J., Johnston, C., Wisbeck, J., Taylor, A., & Reiss, A. (2003). Biological and environmental contributions to adaptive behavior in fragile X syndrome. *American Journal of Medical Genetics A, 117*(1), 21–29.

Grant, C. M., Apperly, I., & Oliver, C. (2007). Is theory of mind understanding impaired in males with fragile X syndrome? *Journal of Abnormal Child Psychology, 35*(1), 17–28.

Greiss Hess, L., Fitzpatrick, S. E., Nguyen, D. V., Chen, Y., Gaul, K. N., Schneider, A., . . . Rivera, S. (2016). A randomized, double-blind, placebo-controlled trial of low-dose sertraline in young children with fragile X syndrome. *Journal of Developmental and Behavioral Pediatrics, 37*(8), 619–628.

Grigsby, J., Brega, A. G., Leehey, M. A., Goodrich, G. K., Jacquemont, S., Loesch, D. Z., . . . Hagerman, R. J. (2007). Impairment of executive cognitive functioning in males with fragile X-associated tremor/ataxia syndrome. *Movement Disorders, 22*(5), 645–650.

Gustavson, K., Dahlbom, K., Flood, A., Holmgren, G., Blomquist, H. K., & Sanner, G. (1985). Effect of folic acid treatment in the fragile X syndrome. *Clinical Genetics, 27*, 463–467.

Haenfler, J. M., Skariah, G., Rodriguez, C. M.,

Monteiro da Rocha, A., Parent, J. M., Smith, G. D., & Todd, P. K. (2018). Targeted reactivation of *FMR1* transcription in fragile X syndrome embryonic stem cells. *Frontiers in Molecular Neuroscience, 11,* Article 282.

Hagan, C. C., Hoeft, F., Mackey, A., Mobbs, D., & Reiss, A. L. (2008). Aberrant neural function during emotion attribution in female subjects with fragile X syndrome. *Journal of the American Academy of Child and Adolescent Psychiatry, 47*(12), 1443–1354.

Hagerman, R. J. (2002). Physical and behavioral phenotype. In R. J. Hagerman & P. J. Hagerman (Eds.), *Fragile X syndrome: Diagnosis, treatment and research* (3rd ed., pp. 3–109). Baltimore: Johns Hopkins University Press.

Hagerman, R. J., Berry-Kravis, E., Kaufmann W. E., Ono, M. Y., Tartaglia, N., Lachiewicz, A.,. . . . Tranfaglia, M. (2009). Advances in the treatment of fragile X syndrome. *Pediatrics, 123*(1), 378–390.

Hagerman, R. J., Hills, J., Scharfenaker, S., & Lewis, H. (1999). Fragile X syndrome and selective mutism. *American Journal of Medical Genetics, 83*(4), 313–317.

Hagerman, R. J., Hull, C. E., Safanda, J. F., Carpenter, I., Staley, L. W., O'Connor, R. A., . . . et al. (1994). High functioning fragile X males: Demonstration of an unmethylated fully expanded FMR-1 mutation associated with protein expression. *American Journal of Medical Genetics, 51*(4), 298–308.

Hagerman, R. J., Kemper, M., & Hudson, M. (1985). Learning disabilities and attentional problems in boys with the fragile X syndrome. *American Journal of Diseases of Children, 139*(7), 674–678.

Hagerman, R. J., Leavitt, B. R., Farzin, F., Jacquemont, S., Greco, C. M., Brunberg, J. A., . . . Hagerman, P. J. (2004). Fragile-X-associated tremor/ataxia syndrome (FXTAS) in females with the FMR1 premutation. *American Journal of Human Genetics, 74*(5), 1051–1056.

Hagerman, R. J., Leehey, M., Heinrichs, W., Tassone, F., Wilson, R., Hills, J., . . . Hagerman, P. J. (2001). Intention tremor, parkinsonism, and generalized brain atrophy in male carriers of fragile X. *Neurology, 57,* 127–130.

Hagerman, R. J., & McBogg, P. M. (Eds.). (1983). *The fragile X syndrome: Diagnosis, biochemistry, and intervention.* New York: Spectra.

Hagerman, R. J., Murphy, M. A., & Wittenberger, M. D. (1988). A controlled trial of stimulant medication in children with the fragile X syndrome. *American Journal of Medical Genetics, 30,* 377–392.

Hagerman, R. J., Rivera, S. M., & Hagerman, P. J. (2008). The fragile X family of disorders: A model for autism and targeted treatments. *Current Pediatric Reviews, 4,* 40–52.

Hall, S. S., Burns, D. D., Lightbody, A. A., & Reiss, A. L. (2008a). Longitudinal changes in intellectual development in children with fragile X syndrome. *Journal of Abnormal Child Psychology, 36*(6), 927–939.

Hall, S. S., Lightbody, A. A., & Reiss, A. L. (2008b). Compulsive, self-injurious, and autistic behavior in children and adolescents with fragile X syndrome. *American Journal on Mental Retardation, 113*(1), 44–53.

Hall, S. S., Lightbody, A. A., McCarthy, B. E., Parker, K. J., & Reiss, A. L. (2012). Effects of intranasal oxytocin on social anxiety in males with fragile X syndrome. *Psychoneuroendocrinology, 37*(4), 509–518.

Hammond, L. S., Macias, M. M., Tarleton, J. C., & Shashidhar Pai, G. (1997). Fragile X syndrome and deletions in FMR1: New case and review of the literature. American *Journal of Medical Genetics, 72,* 430–434.

Hardiman, R. L., & McGill, P. (2018). How common are challenging behaviours amongst individuals with fragile X syndrome?: A systematic review. *Research in Developmental Disabilities, 76,* 99–109.

Harris, S. W., Hessl, D., Goodlin-Jones, B., Ferranti, J., Bacalman, S., Barbato, I., . . . Hagerman, R. J. (2008). Autism profiles of males with fragile X syndrome. *American Journal of Mental Retardation, 113*(6), 427–438.

Hartley, S. L., Seltzer, M. M., Raspa, M., Olmstead, M., Bishop, E., & Bailey, D. B., Jr. (2011). Exploring the adult life of men and women with fragile X syndrome: Results from a national survey. *American Journal of Intellectual and Developmental Disabilities, 116*(1), 16–35.

Hatton, D. D., Sideris, J., Skinner, M., Mankowski, J., Bailey, D. B., Jr., Roberts, J. E., & Mirrett, P. (2006). Autistic behavior in children with fragile X syndrome: Prevalence, stability, and the impact of FMRP. *American Journal of Medical Genetics A, 140*(17), 1804–1813.

Hernandez, R. N., Feinberg, R. L., Vaurio, R., Passanante, N. M., Thompson, R. E., & Kaufmann, W. E. (2009). Autism spectrum disorder in fragile X syndrome: A longitudinal evaluation. *American Journal of Medical Genetics A, 149*(6), 1125–1137.

Hessl, D., Dyer-Friedman, J., Glaser, B., Wisbeck, J., Barajas, R. G., Taylor, A., & Reiss, A. L. (2001). The influence of environmental and genetic factors on behavior problems and autistic symptoms in boys and girls with fragile X syndrome. *Pediatrics, 108*(5), Article E88.

Hessl, D., Glaser, B., Dyer-Friedman, J., Blasey, C., Hastie, T., Gunnar, M., & Reiss, A. L. (2002). Cortisol and behavior in fragile X syndrome. *Psychoneuroendocrinology, 27*(7), 855–872.

Hessl, D., Glaser, B., Dyer-Friedman, J., & Reiss, A. L. (2006). Social behavior and cortisol reactivity in children with fragile X syndrome. *Journal of Child Psychology and Psychiatry, 47*(6), 602–610.

Hessl, D., Harvey, D., Sansone, S., Crestodina, C., Chin, J., Joshi, R., . . . Berry-Kravis, E. (2019a). Effects of mavoglurant on visual attention and pupil reactivity while viewing photographs of faces in fragile X syndrome. *PLoS ONE, 14*(1), e0209984.

Hessl, D., Nguyen, D. V., Green, C., Chavez, A., Tassone, F., Hagerman, R. J., . . . Hall, S. (2009). A solution to limitations of cognitive testing in children with intellectual disabilities: The case of fragile X syndrome. *Journal of Neurodevelopmental Disorders, 1*(1), 33–45.

Hessl, D., Sansone, S. M., Berry-Kravis, E., Riley, K., Widaman, K. F., Abbeduto, L., . . . Gershon, R. C. (2016). The NIH Toolbox Cognitive Battery for intellectual disabilities: Three preliminary studies and future directions. *Journal of Neurodevelopmental Disorders, 8*(1), Article 35.

Hessl, D., Schweitzer, J. B., Nguyen, D. V., McLennan, Y. A., Johnston, C., Shickman, R., & Chen, Y. (2019b). Cognitive training for children and adolescents with fragile X syndrome: A randomized controlled trial of Cogmed. *Journal of Neurodevelopmental Disorders, 11*(1), Article 4.

Hessl, D., Tassone, F., Cordeiro, L., Koldewyn, K., McCormick, C., Green, C., . . . Hagerman, R. J. (2008). Brief report: Aggression and stereotypic behavior in males with fragile X syndrome—Moderating secondary genes in a "single gene" disorder. *Journal of Autism and Developmental Disorders, 38*(1), 184–189.

Heussler, H., Cohen, J., Silove, N., Tich, N., Bonn-Miller, M. O., Du, W., . . . Sebree, T. (2019). A phase 1/2, open-label assessment of the safety, tolerability, and efficacy of transdermal cannabidiol (ZYN002) for the treatment of pediatric fragile X syndrome. *Journal of Neurodevelopmental Disorders, 11*(1), Article 16.

Holsen, L. M., Dalton, K. M., Johnstone, T., & Davidson, R. J. (2008). Prefrontal social cognition network dysfunction underlying face encoding and social anxiety in fragile X syndrome. *NeuroImage, 43*(3), 592–604.

Hooper, S. R., Hatton, D., Sideris, J., Sullivan, K., Hammer, J., Schaaf, J., . . . Bailey, D. B., Jr. (2008). Executive functions in young males with fragile X syndrome in comparison to mental age-matched controls: Baseline findings from a longitudinal study. *Neuropsychology, 22*(1), 36–47.

Huddleston, L. B., Visootsak, J., & Sherman, S. L. (2014). Cognitive aspects of fragile X syndrome. *Wiley Interdisciplinary Reviews: Cognitive Science, 5*(4), 501–508.

Hunter, J., Rivero-Arias, O., Angelov, A., Kim, E., Fotheringham, I., & Leal, J. (2014). Epidemiology of fragile X syndrome: A systematic review and meta-analysis. *American Journal of Medical Genetics A, 164*, 1648–1658.

Idusohan-Moizer, H., Sawicka, A., Dendle, J., & Albany, M. (2013). Mindfulness-based cognitive therapy for adults with intellectual disabilities: An evaluation of the effectiveness of mindfulness in reducing symptoms of depression and anxiety. *Journal of Intellectual Disability Research, 59*(2), 93–104.

Irwin, S. A., Patel, B., Idupulapati, M., Harris, J. B., Crisostomo, R. A., Larsen, B. P., . . . Greenough, W. T. (2001). Abnormal dendritic spine characteristics in the temporal and visual cortices of patients with fragile-X syndrome: A quantitative examination. *American Journal of Medical Genetics, 98*(2), 161–167.

Jacquemont, S., Hagerman, R. J., Leehey, M. A., Hall, D. A., Levine, R. A., Brunberg, J. A., . . . Hagerman, P. J. (2004). Penetrance of the fragile X-associated tremor/ataxia syndrome in a premutation carrier population. *Journal of the American Medical Association, 291*(4), 460–469.

Kaufmann, W. E., Cortell, R., Kau, A. S., Bukelis, I., Tierney, E., Gray, R. M., . . . Stanard, P. (2004). Autism spectrum disorder in fragile X syndrome: Communication, social interaction, and specific behaviors. *American Journal of Medical Genetics A, 129*(3), 225–234.

Klaiman, C., Quintin, E. M., Jo, B., Lightbody, A. A., Hazlett, H. C., Piven, J., . . . Reiss, A. L. (2014). Longitudinal profiles of adaptive behavior in fragile X syndrome. *Pediatrics, 134*(2), 315–324.

Koegel, R. L., & Koegel, L. K. (2006). *Pivotal response treatments for autism: Communication, social, and academic development*. Baltimore: Brookes.

Kogan, C. S., Bertone, A., Cornish, K. M., Boutet, I., Der Kaloustian, V. M., Andermann, E.,

. . . Chaudhuri, A. (2004a). Integrative cortical dysfunction and pervasive motion perception deficit in fragile X syndrome. *Neurology, 63*(9), 1634–1639.

Kogan, C. S., Boutet, I., Cornish, K. M., Zangenehpour, S., Mullen, K. T., Holden, J. J., . . . Chaudhuri, A. (2004b). Differential impact of the FMR1 gene on visual processing in fragile X syndrome. *Brain, 127*(Pt. 3), 591–601.

Lee, A. W., Ventola, P., Budimirovic, D., Berry-Kravis, E., & Visootsak, J. (2018). Clinical development of targeted fragile X syndrome treatments: An industry perspective. *Brain Sciences, 8*(12), Article 214.

Leigh, M. J., Nguyen, D. V., Mu, Y., Winarni, T. I., Schneider, A., Chechi, T., . . . Hagerman, R. J. (2013). A randomized double-blind, placebo-controlled trial of minocycline in children and adolescents with fragile X syndrome. *Journal of Developmental and Behavioral Pediatrics, 34,* 147–155.

Leung, H. T. T., & Ring, H. (2013). Epilepsy in four genetically determined syndromes of intellectual disability. *Journal of Intellectual Disability Research, 57*(1), 3–20.

Lewis, P., Abbeduto, L., Murphy, M., Richmond, E., Giles, N., Bruno, L., & Schroeder, S. (2006). Cognitive, language and social-cognitive skills of individuals with fragile X syndrome with and without autism. *Journal of Intellectual Disability Research, 50*(7), 532–545.

Liu, X. S., Wu, H., Krzisch, M., Wu, X., Graef, J., Muffat, J., . . . Jaenisch, R. (2018). Rescue of fragile X syndrome neurons by DNA methylation editing of the *FMR1* gene. *Cell, 172*(5), 979–992.

Loesch, D. Z., Bui, Q. M., Dissanayake, C., Clifford, S., Gould, E., Bulhak-Paterson, D., . . . Huggins, R. M. (2007). Molecular and cognitive predictors of the continuum of autistic behaviours in fragile X. *Neuroscience and Biobehavioral Reviews, 31*(3), 315–326.

Loesch, D. Z., Huggins, R. M., Bui, Q. M., Epstein, J. L., Taylor, A. K., & Hagerman, R. J. (2002). Effect of the deficits of fragile X mental retardation protein on cognitive status of fragile X males and females assessed by robust pedigree analysis. *Journal of Developmental and Behavioral Pediatrics, 23*(6), 416–423.

Loesch, D. Z., Huggins, R. M., & Hagerman, R. J. (2004). Phenotypic variation and FMRP levels in fragile X. *Mental Retardation and Developmental Disabilities Research Reviews, 10*(1), 31–41.

Lubs, H. A. (1969). A marker X chromosome. *American Journal of Human Genetics, 21*(3), 231–244.

Maddalena, A., Richards, C. S., McGinniss, M. J., Brothman, A., Desnick, R. J., Grier, R. E., . . . Wolff, D. J. (2001). Technical standards and guidelines for fragile X: The first of a series of disease-specific supplements to the Standards and Guidelines for Clinical Genetics Laboratories of the American College of Medical Genetics. Quality Assurance Subcommittee of the Laboratory Practice Committee. *Genetics in Medicine, 3*(3), 200–205.

Martin, J. P., & Bell, J. (1943). A pedigree of mental defect showing sex linkage. *Journal of Psychiatry and Neuroscience, 6,* 154–157.

McDuffie, A., Banasik, A., Bullard, L., Nelson, S., Feigles, R. T., Hagerman, R., & Abbeduto, L. (2018). Distance delivery of a spoken language intervention for school-aged and adolescent boys with fragile X syndrome. *Developmental Neurorehabilitation, 21*(1), 48–63.

McDuffie, A., Machalicek, W., Bullard, L., Nelson, S., Mello, M., Tempero-Feigles, R., . . . Abbeduto, L. (2016). A spoken-language intervention for school-aged boys with fragile X syndrome. *American Journal on Intellectual and Developmental Disabilities, 121*(3), 236–265.

Mesibov, G. B., Shea, V., & Schopler, E. (2005). *The TEACCH approach to autism spectrum disorders.* New York: Springer Science + Business Media.

Miller, L. J., McIntosh, D. N., McGrath, J., Shyu, V., Lampe, M., Taylor, A. K., . . . Hagerman, R. J. (1999). Electrodermal responses to sensory stimuli in individuals with fragile X syndrome: A preliminary report. *American Journal of Medical Genetics, 83*(4), 268–279.

Monlux, K. D., Pollard, J. S., Bujanda Rodriguez, A. Y., & Hall, S. S. (2019). Telehealth delivery of function-based behavioral treatment for problem behaviors exhibited by boys with fragile X syndrome. *Journal of Autism and Developmental Disorders, 49,* 2461–2475.

Munir, F., Cornish, K. M., & Wilding, J. (2000). A neuropsychological profile of attention deficits in young males with fragile X syndrome. *Neuropsychologia, 38*(9), 1261–1270.

Niu, M., Han, Y., Dy, A., Du, J., Jin, H., Qin, J., . . . Hagerman, R. J. (2017). Fragile X syndrome: Prevalence, treatment, and prevention in China. *Frontiers in Neurology, 8,* Article 254.

Nolin, S. L., Glicksman, A., Ding, X., Ersalesi, N., Brown, W. T., Sherman, S. L., & Dobkin, C. (2011). Fragile X analysis of 1112 prenatal samples from 1991 to 2010. *Prenatal Diagnosis, 31,* 925–931.

Oakes, A., Kover, S. T., & Abbeduto, L. (2013).

Language comprehension profiles of young adolescents with fragile X syndrome. *American Journal of Speech–Language Pathology, 22*, 615–626.

Oberle, I., Rousseau, F., Heitz, D., Kretz, C., Devys, D., Hanauer, A., . . . Mandel, J. L. (1991). Instability of a 550-base pair DNA segment and abnormal methylation in fragile X syndrome. *Science, 252*(5010), 1097–1102.

Osterweil, E. K., Chuang, S. C., Chubykin, A. A., Sidorov, M., Bianchi, R., Wong, R. K., & Bear, M. F. (2013). Lovastatin corrects excess protein synthesis and prevents epileptogenesis in a mouse model of fragile X syndrome. *Neuron, 77*(2), 243–250.

Owens, K. M., Dohany, L., Holland, C., DaRe, J., Mann, T., Settler, C., & Longman, R. E. (2018). *FMR1* premutation frequency in a large, ethnically diverse population referred for carrier testing. *American Journal of Medical Genetics A, 176*, 1304–1308.

Pang, C. P., Poon, P. M., Chen, Q. L., Lai, K. Y., Yin, C. H., Zhao, Z., . . . Brown, W. T. (1999). Trinucleotide CGG repeat in the FMR1 gene in Chinese mentally retarded patients. *American Journal of Medical Genetics, 84*(3), 179–183.

Peprah, E. (2012). Fragile X syndrome: The FMR1 CGG repeat distribution among world populations. *Annals of Human Genetics, 76*(2), 178–191.

Peters-Scheffer, N., Didden, R., Korzilius, H., & Sturmey, P. (2011). A meta-analytic study on the effectiveness of comprehensive ABA-based early intervention programs for children with autism spectrum disorders. *Research in Autism Spectrum Disorders, 5*(1), 60–69.

Pop, A. S., Levenga, J., de Esch, C. E. F., Buijsen, R. A. M., Nieuwenhuizen, I. M., . . . Willemsen, R. (2014). Rescue of dendritic spine phenotype in *Fmr1* KO mice with the mGluR5 antagonist AFQ056/Mavoglurant. *Psychopharmacology, 231*, 1227–1235.

Protic, D., Salcedo-Arellano, M. J., Dy, J. B., Potter, L. A., & Hagerman, R. J. (2019). New targeted treatments for fragile X syndrome. *Current Pediatric Reviews, 15*, 251–258.

Qin, M., Kang, J., Burlin, T. V., Jiang, C., & Smith, C. B. (2005). Postadolescent changes in regional cerebral protein synthesis: An in vivo study in the FMR1 null mouse. *Journal of Neuroscience, 25*(20), 5087–5095.

Raspa, M., Bailey, D. B., Jr., Bishop, E., Holiday, D., & Olmsted, M. (2010). Obesity, food selectivity, and physical activity in individuals with fragile X syndrome. *American Journal on Intellectual and Developmental Disabilities, 115*(6), 482–495.

Raspa, M., Wheeler, A. C., & Riley, C. (2017). Public health literature review of fragile X syndrome. *Pediatrics, 139*(Suppl. 3), S153–S171.

Reddy, K. S. (2005). Cytogenetic abnormalities and fragile-X syndrome in autism spectrum disorder. *BMC Medical Genetics, 6*(1), Article 3.

Reiss, A. L., Abrams, M. T., Greenlaw, R., Freund, L., & Denckla, M. B. (1995a). Neurodevelopmental effects of the FMR1 full mutation in humans. *Nature Medicine, 1*(2), 159–167.

Reiss, A. L., & Dant, C. C. (2003). The behavioral neurogenetics of fragile X syndrome: Analyzing gene–brain–behavior relationships in child developmental psychopathologies. *Development and Psychopathology, 15*(4), 927–968.

Reiss, A. L., Freund, L., Vinogradov, S., Hagerman, R. J., & Cronister, A. (1989). Parental inheritance and psychological disability in fragile X females. *American Journal of Human Genetics, 45*(5), 697–705.

Reiss, A. L., Lee, J., & Freund, L. (1994). Neuroanatomy of fragile X syndrome: The temporal lobe. *Neurology, 44*(7), 1317–1324.

Reiss, A. L., Mazzocco, M. M. M., Greenlaw, R., Freund, L. S., & Ross, J. L. (1995b). Neurodevelopmental effects of X monosomy: A volumetric imaging study. *Annals of Neurology, 38*, 731–738.

Reiss, A. L., Patel, S., Kumar, A. J., & Freund, L. (1988). Preliminary communication: Neuroanatomical variations of the posterior fossa in men with the fragile X (Martin–Bell) syndrome. *American Journal of Medical Genetics, 31*(2), 407–414.

Rinehart, N. J., Cornish, K. M., & Tonge, B. J. (2010). Gender differences in neurodevelopmental disorders: Autism and fragile X syndrome. In J. C. Neill & J. Kulkarni (Eds.), *Biological basis of sex differences in psychopharmacology* (pp. 209–229). Berlin: Springer Nature.

Rivera, S. M., Menon, V., White, C. D., Glaser, B., & Reiss, A. L. (2002). Functional brain activation during arithmetic processing in females with fragile X syndrome is related to FMR1 protein expression. *Human Brain Mapping, 16*, 206–218.

Roberts, J. E., Boccia, M. L., Bailey, D. B., Hatton, D., & Skinner, M. (2001a). Cardiovascular indices of physiological arousal in boys with fragile X syndrome. *Developmental Psychobiology, 39*(2), 107–123.

Roberts, J. E., Long, S. H., Malkin, C., Barnes, E., Skinner, M., Hennon, E. A., & Anderson, K. (2005a). A comparison of phonological skills of boys with fragile X syndrome and Down syndrome. *Journal of Speech, Language, and Hearing Research, 48*(5), 980–995.

Roberts, J. E., Mankowski, J. B., Sideris, J., Goldman, B. D., Hatton, D. D., Mirrett, P. L., . . . Bailey, D. B., Jr. (2008). Trajectories and predictors of the development of very young boys with fragile X syndrome. *Journal of Pediatric Psychology, 34*(8), 827–836.

Roberts, J. E., Mirrett, P., & Burchinal, M. (2001b). Receptive and expressive communication development of young males with fragile X syndrome. *American Journal on Mental Retardation, 106*(3), 216–230.

Roberts, J. E., Schaaf, J. M., Skinner, M., Wheeler, A., Hooper, S., Hatton, D. D., & Bailey, D. B., Jr. (2005b). Academic skills of boys with fragile X syndrome: Profiles and predictors. *American Journal on Mental Retardation, 110*(2), 107–120.

Rogers, S. J., Wehner, E. A., & Hagerman, R. J. (2001). The behavioral phenotype in fragile X: Symptoms of autism in very young children with fragile X syndrome, idiopathic autism, and other developmental disorders. *Journal of Developmental and Behavioral Pediatrics, 22*(6), 409–417.

Sabaratnam, M. (2006). Fragile-X syndrome. *Psychiatry, 5*(9), 325–330.

Saldarriaga, W., Forero-Forero, J. V., González-Teshima, L. Y., Fandiño-Losada, A., Isaza, C., Tovar-Cuevas, J. R., . . . Hagerman, R. J. (2018). Genetic cluster of fragile X syndrome in a Colombian district. *Journal of Human Genetics, 63*(4), 509–516.

Sandoval, G. M., Shim, S., Hong, D. S., Garrett, A. S., Quintin, E.-M., Marzelli, M. J., . . . Reiss, A. L. (2018). Neuroanatomical abnormalities in fragile X syndrome during the adolescent and young adult years. *Journal of Psychiatry. 107*, 138–144.

Sansone, S., Schneider, A., Bickel, E., Berry-Kravis, E., Prescott, C., & Hessl, D. (2014). Improving IQ measurement in intellectual disabilities using true deviation from population norms. *Journal of Neurodevelopmental Disorders, 6*, 1–14.

Scerif, G., Cornish, K. M., Wilding, J., Driver, J., & Karmiloff-Smith, A. (2004). Visual search in typically developing toddlers and toddlers with fragile X or Williams syndrome. *Developmental Science, 7*(1), 116–130.

Scerif, G., Karmiloff-Smith, A., Campos, R., Elsabbagh, M., Driver, J., & Cornish, K. M. (2005). To look or not to look?: Typical and atypical development of oculomotor control. *Journal of Cognitive Neuroscience, 17*(4), 591–604.

Schneider, A., Leigh, M. J., Adams, P., Nanakul, R., Chechi, T., Olichney, J., . . . Hessl, D. (2013). Electrocortical changes associated with minocycline treatment in fragile X syndrome. *Journal of Psychopharmacology (Oxford, England), 27*(10), 956–963.

Sherman, S. L., Jacobs, P. A., Morton, N. E., Froster-Iskenius, U., Howard-Peebles, P. N., Nielsen, K. B., . . . Watson, M. (1985). Further segregation analysis of the fragile X syndrome with special reference to transmitting males. *Human Genetics, 69*(4), 289–299.

Shields, R. H., Kaat, A. J., McKenzie, F. J., Drayton, A., Sansone, S. M., Coleman, J., . . . Hessl, D. (2020). Validation of the NIH Toolbox Cognitive Battery in intellectual disability. *Neurology, 94*(12), e1229–e1240.

Simon, E. W., & Finucane, B. M. (1996). Facial emotion identification in males with fragile X syndrome. *American Journal of Medical Genetics, 67*(1), 77–80.

Skinner, M., Hooper, S., Hatton, D. D., Roberts, J. E., Mirrett, P., Schaaf, J., . . . Bailey, D. B., Jr. (2005). Mapping nonverbal IQ in young boys with fragile X syndrome. *American Journal of Medical Genetics A, 132*(1), 25–32.

Smith, L. E., Hong, J., Greenberg, J. S., & Mailick, M. R. (2016). Change in the behavioral phenotype of adolescents and adults with FXS: Role of the family environment. *Journal of Autism and Developmental Disorders, 46*(5), 1824–1833.

Sobesky, W. E., Pennington, B. F., Porter, D., Hull, C. E., & Hagerman, R. J. (1994). Emotional and neurocognitive deficits in fragile X. *American Journal of Medical Genetics, 51*(4), 378–385.

Sullivan, K., Hatton, D., Hammer, J., Sideris, J., Hooper, S., Ornstein, P., & Bailey, D., Jr. (2006). ADHD symptoms in children with FXS. *American Journal of Medical Genetics A, 140*(21), 2275–2288.

Sutcliffe, J. S., Nelson, D. L., Zhang, F., Pieretti, M., Caskey, C. T., Saxe, D., & Warren, S. T. (1992). DNA methylation represses FMR-1 transcription in fragile X syndrome. *Human Molecular Genetics, 1*(6), 397–400.

Symons, F. J., Byiers, B. J., Raspa, M., Bishop, E., & Bailey, D. B., Jr. (2010). Self-injurious behavior and fragile X syndrome: Findings from the National Fragile X Survey. *American Journal on Intellectual and Developmental Disabilities, 115*(6), 473–481.

Symons, F. J., Clark, R. D., Hatton, D. D., Skinner, M., & Bailey, D. B., Jr. (2003). Self-injurious behavior in young boys with fragile X syndrome. *American Journal of Medical Genetics A, 118*(2), 115–121.

Tamm, L., Menon, V., Johnston, C. K., Hessl, D.

R., & Reiss, A. L. (2002). fMRI study of cognitive interference processing in females with fragile X syndrome. *Journal of Cognitive Neuroscience, 14*(2), 160–171.

Tassone, F., Hagerman, R. J., Iklé, D. N., Dyer, P. N., Lampe, M., Willemsen, R., . . . Taylor, A. K. (1999). FMRP expression as a potential prognostic indicator in fragile X syndrome. *American Journal of Medical Genetics, 84*(3), 250–261.

Tassone, F., Hagerman, R. J., Taylor, A. K., Gane, L. W., Godfrey, T. E., & Hagerman, P. J. (2000a). Elevated levels of FMR1 mRNA in carrier males: A new mechanism of involvement in the fragile-X syndrome. *American Journal of Human Genetics, 66*(1), 6–15.

Tassone, F., Hagerman, R. J., Taylor, A. K., Mills, J. B., Harris, S. W., Gane, L. W., & Hagerman, P. J. (2000b). Clinical involvement and protein expression in individuals with the FMR1 premutation. *American Journal of Medical Genetics, 91*(2), 144–152.

Thurman, A. J., McDuffie, A., Kover, S. T., Hagerman, R. J., & Abbeduto, L. (2015a). Autism symptomatology in boys with fragile X syndrome: A cross-sectional developmental trajectories comparison with nonsyndromic autism spectrum disorder. *Journal of Autism and Developmental Disorders, 45,* 2816–2832.

Thurman, A. J., McDuffie, A., Kover, S. T., Hagerman, R. J., Channell, M. M., Mastergeorge, A., & Abbeduto, L. (2015b). Use of emotional cues for lexical learning: A comparison of autism spectrum disorder and fragile X syndrome. *Journal of Autism and Developmental Disorders, 45,* 1042–1061.

Thurman, A. J., McDuffie, A., Hagerman, R. J., Josol, C. K., & Abbeduto, L. (2017). Language skills of males with fragile X syndrome or nonsyndromic autism spectrum disorder. *Journal of Autism and Developmental Disorders, 47*(3), 728–743.

Torrioli, M., Vernacotola, S., Setini, C., Bevilacqua, F., Martinelli, D., Snape, M., . . . Neri, G. (2010). Treatment with valproic acid ameliorates ADHD symptoms in fragile X syndrome boys. *American Journal of Medical Genetics A, 152,* 1420–1427.

Tranebjaerg, L., & Orum, A. (1991). Major depressive disorder as a prominent but underestimated feature of fragile X syndrome. *Comprehensive Psychiatry, 32*(1), 83–87.

Turk, J. (1998). Fragile X syndrome and attentional deficits. *Journal of Applied Research in Intellectual Disabilities, 11,* 175–191.

Turk, J., & Cornish, K. M. (1998). Face recognition and emotion perception in boys with fragile-X syndrome. *Journal of Intellectual Disability Research, 42*(Pt. 6), 490–499.

Turk, J., & Graham, P. (1997). Fragile X syndrome, autism, and autistic features. *Autism, 1*(2), 175–197.

Turk, J., & Patton, M. (2000). Sensory impairment and head circumference in fragile X syndrome, Down syndrome and idiopathic intellectual disability. *Journal of Intellectual and Developmental Disability, 25*(1), 59–68.

Van der Molen, M. J. W., Huizinga, M., Huizenga, H. M., Ridderinkhof, K. R., Van der Molen, M. W., Hamel, B. J. C., . . . Ramakers, G. J. A. (2010). Profiling fragile X syndrome in males: Strengths and weaknesses in cognitive abilities. *Research in Developmental Disabilities, 31*(2), 426–439.

Verkerk, A. J., Pieretti, M., Sutcliffe, J. S., Fu, Y. H., Kuhl, D. P., Pizzuti, A., . . . Warren, S. T. (1991). Identification of a gene (FMR-1) containing a CGG repeat coincident with a breakpoint cluster region exhibiting length variation in fragile X syndrome. *Cell, 65*(5), 905–914.

Vismara, L. A., McCormick, C. E., Shields, R., & Hessl, D. (2019). Extending the parent-delivered Early Start Denver Model to young children with fragile X syndrome. *Journal of Autism and Developmental Disorders, 49*(3), 1250–1266.

Warren, S. F., Brady, N., Sterling, A., Fleming, K., & Marquis, J. (2010). Maternal responsivity predicts language development in young children with fragile X syndrome. *American Journal on Intellectual and Developmental Disabilities, 115*(1), 54–75.

Watson, C., Hoeft, F., Garrett, A. S., Hall, S. S., & Reiss, A. L. (2008). Aberrant brain activation during gaze processing in boys with fragile X syndrome. *Archives of General Psychiatry, 65*(11), 1315–1323.

Weiler, I. J., Irwin, S. A., Klintsova, A. Y., Spencer, C. M., Brazelton, A. D., Miyashiro, K., . . . Greenough, W. T. (1997). Fragile X mental retardation protein is translated near synapses in response to neurotransmitter activation. *Proceedings of the National Academy of Sciences USA, 94,* 5395–5400.

Wheeler, A. C., Raspa, M., Bishop, E., & Bailey, D. B., Jr. (2016). Aggression in fragile X syndrome. *Journal of Intellectual Disability Research, 60*(2), 113–125.

Wilding, J., Cornish, K., & Munir, F. (2002). Further delineation of the executive deficit in males with fragile-X syndrome. *Neuropsychologia, 40*(8), 1343–1349.

Willemsen, R., Bontekoe, C., Tamanini, F., Galjaard, H., Hoogeveen, A., & Oostra, B. (1996). Association of FMRP with ribosomal precursor particles in the nucleolus. *Biochemical and Biophysical Research Communications, 225*(1), 27–33.

Youssef, E. A., Berry-Kravis, E., Czech, C., Hagerman, R. J., Hessl, D., Wong, C. Y., . . . FragXis Study Group (2018). Effect of the mGluR5-NAM Basimglurant on behavior in adolescents and adults with fragile X syndrome in a randomized, double-blind, placebo-controlled trial: FragXis Phase 2 results. *Neuropsychopharmacology, 43*(3), 503–512.

Yrigollen, C. M., & Davidson, B. L. (2019). CRISPR to the rescue: Advances in gene editing for the *FMR1* gene. *Brain Sciences, 9*(1), Article 17.

Yrigollen, C. M., Durbin-Johnson, B., Gane, L., Nelson, D. L., Hagerman, R., Hagerman, P. J., & Tassone, F. (2012). AGG interruptions within the maternal *FMR1* gene reduce the risk of offspring with fragile X syndrome. *Genetics in Medicine, 14*(8), 729–736.

Zingerevich, C., Greiss-Hess, L., Lemons-Chitwood, K., Harris, S. W., Hessl, D., Cook, K., & Hagerman, R. J. (2009). Motor abilities of children diagnosed with fragile X syndrome with and without autism. *Journal of Intellectual Disability Research, 53*(1), 11–18.

CHAPTER 17

Williams Syndrome

Carolyn B. Mervis
Caroline Greiner de Magalhães

HISTORICAL OVERVIEW

The first detailed descriptions of individuals with Williams syndrome (WS; referred to as Williams–Beuren syndrome in Europe) were provided by cardiologists in the early 1960s (Beuren, Apitz, & Harmjanz, 1962; Williams, Barratt-Boyes, & Lowe, 1961). However, the children described in an earlier article on idiopathic infantile hypercalcemia—Fanconi type (IIH-F; Fanconi, Giardet, Schlesinger, Butler, & Black, 1952) later were shown to be a subgroup of children with WS (Martin, Snodgrass, & Cohen, 1984; Morris & Mervis, 2020). Von Armin and Engel (1964), who were not aware of the publications on WS or IIH-F but had considerable experience with children with intellectual disability (ID), provided a detailed description of a group of children who had ID, many of whom also had had infantile hypercalcemia, and concluded that "they must belong to a well-defined group suffering from a special syndrome" (p. 366). The authors noted that although these children consistently had moderate to severe ID, their intellectual level initially appeared to be much higher. This illusion regarding intellectual ability is due to "an unusual command of language" (p. 367). Von Armin and Engel also noted that although the children had difficulty interacting with other children, they were "uninhibited" (p. 369) in interacting with adults; "adult strangers are often greeted like old friends" (p. 369). Difficulty with drawing, hypersensitivity to frustration, and excessive levels of anxiety and insecurity also were identified as consistent characteristics. Although later research would temper their statements on intellectual level and language ability, von Armin and Engel's observations on social interaction, personality, and temperament were prescient.

In the next two decades, only a few studies of the psychological characteristics of individuals with WS were published. These studies focused on standardized assessment performance and/or language abilities, primarily of very small samples. The findings made clear the considerable variability—from severe intellectual disability to average intelligence—among children with WS. They also documented that (1) among children with IQs in the mild intellectual disability or higher range, verbal abilities often were stronger than visuospatial abilities (Bennett, LaVeck, & Sells, 1978; Udwin, Yule, & Martins, 1987) and (2) while children with WS performed at the same level on a variety of language assessments as did same-chronological-age (CA) children with other types of ID who had similar receptive vocabulary ability, the children with WS had considerably weaker visuospatial construction abilities (MacDonald & Roy, 1988). Other studies documented that language abilities were well below CA expectations (Kataria, Goldstein, & Kushnick, 1984; Meyerson & Frank, 1987).

These articles did not receive much attention from researchers or clinicians who were not explicitly focused on WS. In contrast, another article published at about the same time (Bellugi, Marks, Bihrle, & Sabo, 1988) returned to von Armin and Engel's (1964) theme of an unusual command of language in the face of severe ID and catapulted WS to the forefront of the debate on language modularity. In a study of three adolescents with WS, Bellugi et al. (1988) reported that despite having severe ID, still being in Piaget's preoperational period, evidencing severe difficulties with visuospatial tasks (e.g., drawing), and requiring constant parental supervision (including assistance with tasks of daily living such as dressing), these individuals had excellent vocabulary, including a variety of unusual words, and spoke in complete and grammatically complex sentences. The authors argued that these observations indicated that their language abilities were far stronger than their cognitive abilities and thus provided strong evidence of the independence of language from cognition. Bellugi et al.'s findings were quickly picked up both by pundits supporting the modularity of language and by the lay press (see description in Mervis & John, 2010a), both of whom took a much more strident tone than Bellugi et al. (1988). Researchers who were interested in the relation between language and cognition, who previously had not heard of WS, began to study individuals with this syndrome. For the next 20 or so years, psychological research on WS focused primarily on language and/or cognition. Over the last 15 or so years, increased interest in autism spectrum disorders (ASD), including descriptions of WS as seemingly the opposite of ASD, has led to a second research emphasis on social and personality characteristics.

EPIDEMIOLOGY

The prevalence of WS, established in an epidemiological study in Norway, is 1 in 7,500 live births (Strømme, Bjørnstad, & Ramstad, 2002). WS occurs at the same rate in girls and boys (Morris, Braddock, & Council on Genetics, 2020), and cases have been identified in different racial and ethnic groups across the world (Strømme et al., 2002).

ETIOLOGY, NEUROPATHOLOGY, AND NEURAL SUBSTRATES

Etiology

WS, which is caused by a submicroscopic hemideletion of 25–27 genes on chromosome 7q11.23 (Kozel et al., 2021), was shown to be a genetic disorder by Ewart et al. (1993). The deleted region is flanked by low-copy repeats that predispose it to unequal crossing over during meiosis, increasing the likelihood of deletion (WS), duplication (7q11.23 duplication syndrome), or inversion. Approximately 95% of individuals with WS have the same set of genes deleted ("classic deletion"). Most of the remaining individuals have a longer deletion, extending telomerically from the endpoint of the classic deletion.

Most cases of WS occur sporadically. However, a person who has WS has a 50% chance with each pregnancy that his or her child will have WS. The other known risk factor is the inversion of the WS region, present in ~6% of the general population (Hobart et al., 2010). Individuals with this inversion—who do not evidence any of the phenotypic characteristics of WS—have a fivefold increased likelihood of having a child with WS. However, the parents of most children with WS do not have this inversion (Hobart et al., 2010).

Neuroimaging Findings

The WS behavioral phenotype includes a cognitive profile characterized by relative strengths in concrete language, phonological processing, nonverbal reasoning, and verbal short-term memory and considerable weakness in visuospatial construction (Kozel et al., 2021; Mervis et al., 2000; Mervis & John, 2010a) and an unusual personality profile characterized by "hypersociability," including gregariousness, inappropriate social approach to strangers (social disinhibition), eagerness for attention, tenseness, and nonsocial anxiety (Klein-Tasman & Mervis, 2003). Neuroimaging results provide evidence of the brain bases for many of these characteristics. Structural imaging studies of adults with WS who have borderline to average intellectual ability have identified two relevant areas in which gray matter is significantly reduced bilaterally relative to CA-matched adults in the general population, one in the intraparietal sulcus (IPS) and one in the orbitofrontal cortex (see review in Meyer-Lindenberg, Mervis, & Berman, 2006).

The bilateral reduction in gray matter in the IPS, which has been reported for both children and adults with WS across the IQ spectrum, is the most replicated neuroimaging finding in WS (Gregory et al., 2019). Functional neuroimaging studies have indicated isolated hypoactivation in the parietal portion of the dorsal stream immediately adjacent to the region of gray matter reduction in the IPS, and path analysis demonstrated that the functional abnormalities could be attributed to impaired input from this structurally altered region (Meyer-Lindenberg et al., 2004). In a study of resting-state functional connectivity of the IPS, Gregory et al. (2019) found that for children with WS who had IQs in the borderline to average range for the general population, 95% of the voxels showing *increased* IPS connectivity were outside the IPS connectivity network of the sex- and CA-matched typically developing (TD) comparison group. Furthermore, 99.5% of the voxels with *decreased* IPS connectivity for the children with WS were within the IPS-connected network for TD children. Follow-up studies comparing IPS resting-state connectivity for adolescents and adults in the general population as a function of *LIMK1* promotor haplotype found that individuals with Haplotype 1 (associated with reduced *LIMK1* transcription rate) had decreased connectivity between the IPS and the right posterior fusiform gyrus, an area that showed reduced connectivity in the WS group. These structural and functional differences likely underlie the specific weakness in visuospatial construction found for individuals with WS and point toward the involvement of one of the deleted genes, *LIMK1*, in these changes.

For the general population, the second area of reduced gray matter for individuals with WS—the orbitofrontal cortex—is involved in regulating the amygdala. Consistent with this reduction, in a functional magnetic resonance imaging (fMRI) study involving adults with WS who had IQs in the normal range, Meyer-Lindenberg et al. (2005) found that amygdala activation was atypical: Activation was reduced to angry or fearful faces but significantly increased to threatening or scary scenes. Using path analysis, Meyer-Lindenberg et al. showed that the area of reduced gray matter was not regulating the amygdala and argued that this lack of regulation contributes to the social disinhibition, reduced reactivity to social cues, and nonsocial specific phobia that characterize children with WS. Further evidence of atypical connectivity involving social processing was reported by Gregory et al. (2019), who found that the IPS, rather than being connected to regions involved in visual processing, was strongly connected to regions that previously have been implicated in social processing, including the posterior cingulate, bilateral medial prefrontal cortex, bilateral temporoparietal junction, right orbitofrontal cortex, bilateral superior frontal gyri, and right inferior temporal gyrus.

NEUROPSYCHOLOGICAL CONSEQUENCES

General Intellectual Functioning and Academic Achievement

Intellectual Functioning

Most research groups who report Full Scale IQ scores for individuals with WS base this information on performance on one or more of the Wechsler intellectual ability tests. Mean Full Scale IQ is typically in the mild to moderate intellectual disability range, with rare individuals scoring in the average range and many at floor (see Martens, Wilson, & Reutens, 2008, for review). Although mean Verbal IQ is consistently higher than mean Performance IQ, the difference typically is small (4 or 5 points), and in the two studies that addressed the relation between Verbal IQ and Performance IQ at the individual level, the difference for most participants was not statistically significant (Howlin, Davies, & Udwin, 1998; Searcy et al., 2004). The rarity of significant differences at the individual level likely is due in part to the inclusion of both visuospatial and nonverbal reasoning subtests in the same Index. Although this confound was rectified in the fifth edition of the Wechsler Intelligence Scale for Children (WISC-V), to date no studies have been reported using that measure. Furthermore, similarly to prior versions, the WISC-V is only normed three standard deviations (*SD*s) below the general population mean. The resulting floor effect, which is especially likely for the Visual Spatial Index, makes detection of a significant difference between that Index and either the Verbal Index or the Fluid Reasoning Index difficult.

The pattern of relative strengths and weaknesses in intellectual ability is more clearly shown on the Differential Ability Scales–II (DAS-II; Elliott, 2007), which provides separate Verbal, Nonverbal Reasoning, and Spatial standard scores (SSs) based on performance on subtests that are normed four SDs below the general population mean. For 269 4- to 17-year-olds with classic WS deletions tested in our laboratory, mean General Conceptual Ability (GCA; similar to IQ), which is based on performance on the Verbal, Nonverbal Reasoning, and Spatial ability clusters, was 61.98 (*SD*: 12.94, range: 31–96). This overall score masks stark differences between performance on the Verbal cluster (M: 71.00, *SD*: 16.88, range: 30–107) and the Nonverbal Reasoning cluster (M: 75.04, *SD*: 14.76, range: 36–118) on the one hand and performance on the Spatial cluster (M: 53.16, *SD*: 13.04, range: 32–86) on the other, as shown in Figure 17.1. For 70% of the sample,

Verbal SS did not differ significantly from Nonverbal Reasoning SS. In contrast, Spatial SS was significantly lower than Verbal SS for 68% and significantly lower than Nonverbal Reasoning for 83%. For 89%, Verbal SS, Nonverbal Reasoning SS, or both were significantly higher than Spatial SS. At the other extreme, Spatial SS was significantly higher than Verbal SS for 3% and Nonverbal Reasoning SS for 0.4%. Verbal short-term memory ability (*M*: 73.10, *SD*: 16.61, range: 40–109) as measured by the Recall of Digits-Forward subtest (not included in the GCA) was consistent with Verbal cluster SS. This pattern of relative strengths in verbal and nonverbal reasoning abilities and considerable weakness in spatial ability is evident even in young toddlers (Mervis & John, 2010a).

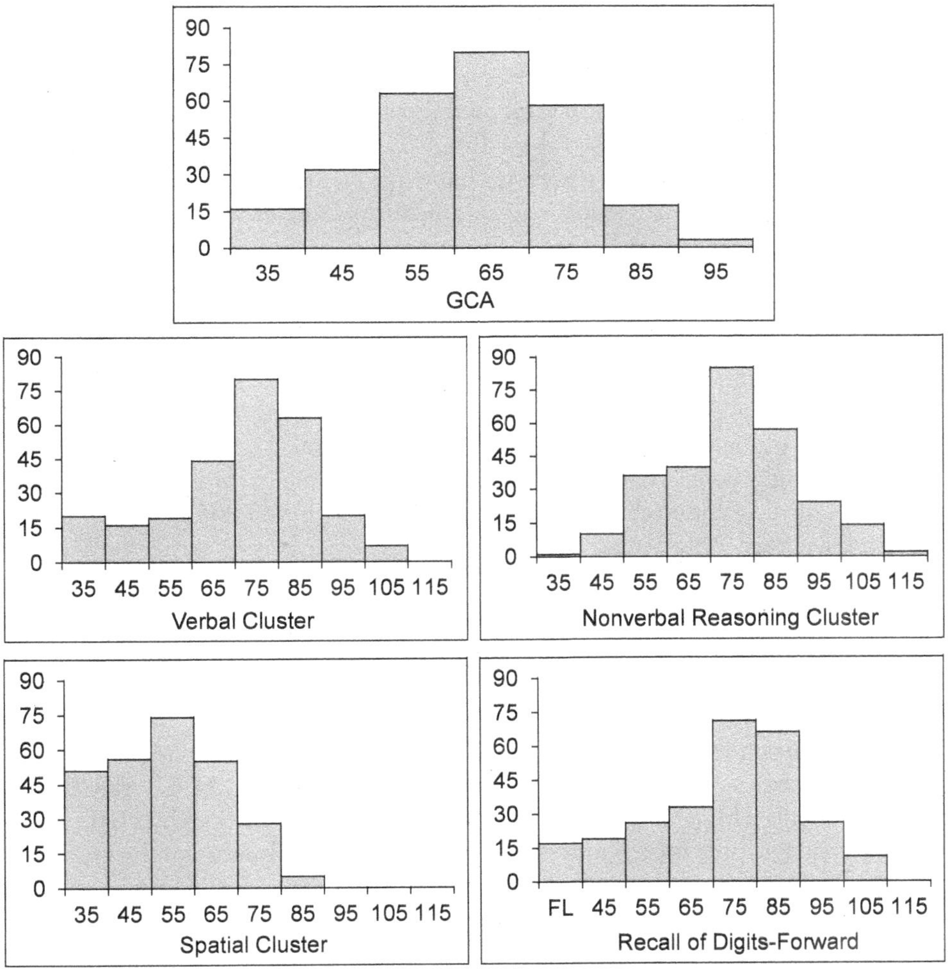

FIGURE 17.1. Histograms of Differential Ability Scales–II (DAS-II) General Conceptual Ability (GCA), Verbal Cluster, Nonverbal Reasoning Cluster, Spatial Cluster, and Recall of Digits-Forward standard scores for 269 children ages 4–17 years with classic WS deletions. Recall of Digits-Forward *T*-scores have been converted to standard scores. FL, floor (lowest possible standard score).

Academic Achievement

The first report of performance on academic achievement tests was provided by Pagon, Bennett, LaVeck, Stewart, and Johnson (1987), who presented data for nine individuals ages 10–20 years. Despite the small sample, their data showed the full range of reading ability as measured by later studies, with the oldest individual able to read only a few words and a ninth grader able to decode and comprehend at grade level. In a recent study of 30 adolescents and adults, Brawn, Kohnen, Tassabehji, and Porter (2018) found that although 93% could read at least a few words, word reading skills were at a functional literacy level for only 27%. A significant relation between phonological processing (one of the strongest abilities of individuals with WS; Miezah, Porter, Batchelor, Boulton, & Campos Veloso, 2020) and word reading has been found for individuals with WS for all languages for which this has been studied (see review in Mervis, 2009; Brawn et al., 2018), and significant relations with IQ often are reported (see review in Brawn et al., 2018). However, Mervis, Greiner de Magalhães, and Cardoso-Martins (2022), in a study of 70 9-year-olds with WS, found that word reading SSs were significantly more strongly correlated with method of reading instruction than with IQ and that children taught to read using systematic phonics instruction had significantly stronger word reading skills than children taught to read using other types of instruction, even after controlling for IQ. As word reading ability was the strongest predictor of reading comprehension ability, the benefit of systematic phonics instruction extended to reading comprehension as well. In addition to method of reading instruction, phonological processing skills and visuospatial skills contributed significant unique variance to word reading SSs (Mervis et al., 2022). As predicted by the Simple View of Reading (Gough & Tunmer, 1986) and as found repeatedly for children in the general population (Quinn & Wagner, 2018), word reading ability and listening comprehension ability made significant unique contributions to individual differences in reading comprehension SSs for children with WS (Mervis et al., 2022).

There have been only a few studies of math achievement in individuals with WS, and these studies reported age equivalents (AE) or grade equivalents (GE) rather than SSs. Given the strong relation between spatial ability and math ability, it is not surprising that math achievement is on average considerably more limited than reading achievement. Pagon et al. (1987) reported that GEs for their sample ranged from early kindergarten to late third grade. O'Hearn and Landau (2007) administered the Test of Early Mathematics Abilities-2 (Ginsburg & Baroody, 1990) to 14 adolescents and adults with WS (mean CA: 17.75 years). AE scores ranged from 5 years, 6 months to > 8 years, 11 months (the ceiling for this assessment) with a median of 7 years, 0 months. Individuals with WS have specific difficulty with magnitude representation (including conceptualization of the number line), with better performance on verbal aspects of arithmetic (see Van Herwegen & Simms, 2020, for a systematic review). This pattern is consistent with the reduction in gray matter in the IPS and previously described differences in IPS connectivity in individuals with WS.

Perceptual and Sensorimotor Skills

Motor Abilities

Most infants with WS are hypotonic and have hyperextensible joints, resulting in delayed attainment of early sensorimotor milestones (Morris & Mervis, 2020), including reaching for objects, rolling from stomach to back, sitting unsupported, and walking (Kozel et al., 2021; Masataka, 2001). Difficulties with fine (e.g., tool use, drawing, and handwriting; e.g., Bellugi, Lichtenberger, Jones, Lai, & George, 2000) and gross motor abilities (including atypical posture, trouble jumping and running, and impaired balance; Elliott & Bunn, 2004), and motor planning difficulties (Cowie, Braddick, & Atkinson, 2012) are very common.

Vision and Hearing

Vision problems are common; 50% of infants have strabismus, and 67% of children and adults have hyperopia (Morris & Mervis, 2020). Chronic otitis media also is common, affecting 50% of children, half of whom are treated surgically (Morris & Mervis, 2020). Mild to moderately severe sensorineural or mixed hearing loss in at least one ear was found in 63% of 43 school-age children; in most cases, parents had not realized their child had hearing loss (Marler, Sitcovsky, Mervis, Kistler, & Wightman, 2010). Hypersensitivity to sounds occurs in 85–95% (Morris & Mervis, 2020) and is associated with both specific phobia and fascination with certain sounds (Leyfer, Woodruff-Borden, Klein-Tasman, Fricke, & Mervis, 2006).

Sensory Modulation

Sensory integration difficulties are very common. Based on parents' responses on the Short Sensory Profile (McIntosh, Miller, Shyu, & Hagerman, 1999), 56% of 72 4- to 10-year-olds were classified as having definite overall sensory modulation issues and 34% as having probable issues. The most common areas of definite abnormality were Auditory Filtering (59.0%), Low Energy/Weak (64.1%), and Underresponsive/Seeks Sensations (62.8%). Children with severe sensory impairment had significantly poorer executive functioning, more negativity, less effortful control, and more attention-related complications and anxiety than did children with milder sensory impairment. Sensory modulation difficulties also were found on direct assessment, as were repetitive behaviors and restricted interests (Klein-Tasman, Mervis, Lord, & Phillips, 2007; Lincoln, Searcy, Jones, & Lord, 2007). Children with WS who find the sensory environment unpredictable may use repetitive behaviors to regain predictability in their world (Glod, Riby, & Rodgers, 2019).

Language

The onset of language is delayed for children with WS. Becerra and Mervis (2019) reported that at age 24 months, 79% of 47 participants scored below the 5th percentile on the MacArthur–Bates Communicative Development Inventory: Words and Sentences (Fenson et al., 2007) expressive vocabulary norms. Nevertheless, 2-year-olds with WS had significantly larger expressive vocabularies than same-age children with Down syndrome (DS; Mervis & Robinson, 2000). The language delay is not likely to be due primarily to difficulty with statistical learning (a domain-general mechanism that detects statistical regularities in the input, in this case the speech stream). Infants with WS as young as 8 months (M: 15.5 months) were able to segment the speech stream in an artificial language into words using only the statistical properties of the input (i.e., the probability of co-occurrence of specific syllable sequences, which is high within words and low between words; Cashon, Ha, Graf Estes, Saffran, & Mervis, 2016). Furthermore, toddlers with WS were able to make rapid associations between objects and their names at the same point in expressive vocabulary development as TD children (Ha, Cashon, Holt, & Mervis, 2020). However, delays in the onset of comprehension and production of communicative gestures, such as referential pointing, likely do contribute to the language delay. TD children and children with other genetic syndromes almost always begin to produce referential pointing gestures prior to beginning to produce referential language, and the onset of these gestures typically leads to changes in maternal linguistic input that are supportive of vocabulary development (see review in Becerra & Mervis, 2019). In contrast, only 4% of the participants in the Becerra and Mervis study began to produce referential pointing gestures prior to producing words referentially. Relative to the contribution of expressive vocabulary size at 24 months, age at onset of referential pointing (median: 24 months) accounted for three to seven times more unique variance in individual differences in various measures of vocabulary at 48 months (Becerra & Mervis, 2019).

WS is associated with a specific pattern of relative strength and weakness in vocabulary ability: Concrete vocabulary (names for objects, actions, and descriptors) is considerably stronger than relational vocabulary (e.g., labels for spatial, temporal, and quantitative concepts). On the Peabody Picture Vocabulary Test–4 (PPVT-4; Dunn & Dunn, 2007), an assessment of concrete vocabulary, mean SS for 129 4- to 17-year-olds was 81.84 (*SD*: 15.04, range: 40–124), with 83% earning SSs ≥ 70 and 8% earning SSs ≥ 100 (Mervis & John, 2010a). Similarly, mean Expressive Vocabulary Test–2 (EVT-2; Williams, 2007) SS was 79.43, with 83% earning SSs ≥ 70 and 6% earning SSs ≥ 100 (Mervis & John, 2010a). Relational vocabulary performance is considerably weaker, with SSs on the Test of Relational Concepts (Edmonston & Litchfield Thane, 1988) very similar to SSs on the DAS Pattern Construction subtest and ~30 points below PPVT SSs (Mervis & John, 2008). This pattern is consistent with Walsh's (2003) argument that spatial, temporal, and quantitative processing are controlled by a common magnitude system located in the IPS—a region that, as described in the Section "Neuroimaging Findings," in WS is characterized by reduced gray matter and reduced functional connectivity to dorsal stream regions.

By age 7 years, most children with WS talk in complete sentences, although they may continue to make some grammatical errors. Grammatical abilities typically are similar to those of CA- and IQ-matched individuals with ID of mixed or unknown etiology (Gosch, Städing, & Pankau, 1994; Udwin & Yule, 1990), but significantly stronger than those of CA- and ability-matched children with DS (e.g., Bellugi et al., 1988, 2000; Klein & Mervis, 1999). This latter difference likely reflects a specific weakness in grammatical abilities for individuals with DS rather than a strength for individuals with WS (Mervis, 2006). Individuals with WS have difficulty with both the form and function components of prosody (see Loveall, Hawthorne, & Gaines, 2021, for a meta-analysis).

Despite their striking drive to engage with other people, individuals with WS have considerable difficulty with the pragmatic components of language, as evidenced by both direct assessment of conversational abilities (e.g., Stojanovik, 2006) and parent ratings on the Children's Communication Checklist–2 (CCC-2; Bishop, 2003). Lane, Van Herwegen, and Freeth (2019) reported that 76% of 34 children with WS scored in the impaired range on the CCC-2 pragmatic language scales. The combination of CCC-2 structural language SS and CA accounted for 25% of the variance in CCC-2 pragmatic language SS, with higher structural language SSs and younger CA associated with higher pragmatic language SSs.

Further evidence of pragmatic communication difficulties comes from the performance of children with WS on the Autism Diagnostic Observation Schedule (ADOS; Lord, Rutter, DiLavore, & Risi, 1999), a semistructured, play-based assessment evaluating communication and reciprocal social interaction skills. Klein-Tasman and colleagues (2007) found that at least 50% of young children with WS who completed ADOS Module 1 (designed for children with very limited or no expressive language) had significant difficulties with pointing, giving, and showing objects and with appropriate use of eye contact for communication. Many also had difficulty with initiation of joint attention, response to the examiner's bids for joint attention, and integration of gaze with other behaviors. Klein-Tasman, van der Fluit, and Mervis (2018) evaluated the communication and reciprocal social interaction skills of children who produced at least phrase speech. At least 50% of the children who completed Module 2 (for children with phrase speech) had difficulties with abnormal speech associated with autism, immediate echolalia, conversation, gestures, directed facial gestures, showing, and unusually repetitive interests or stereotyped behaviors. At least 50% of the children who completed Module 3 (for children with fluent language) evidenced speech abnormalities associated with autism, difficulties with directed facial expression, expression of empathy or comments on other people's emotions, and social insight. Lower intellectual ability was associated with greater pragmatic difficulty on Modules 1 and 2 but not on Module 3.

Attention

Orienting and Disengaging

Infants and toddlers with WS ages 3–48 months demonstrate extended and intense looking at faces relative to same-CA children with other developmental delays, due at least in part to difficulty disengaging attention (Mervis et al., 2003). Devoting so much of their attention to people's faces rather than to what the person is doing or to other objects in the environment significantly reduces the opportunities of children with WS to learn about their world (Mervis et al., 2003). More general difficulties with orienting to a target (Brown et al., 2003) and disengaging from a target at one location and orienting to another target at a different location (Cornish, Scerif, & Karmiloff-Smith, 2007) further reduce these opportunities.

Selective Attention

Very young children with WS also have more difficulty with selective attention than CA- and ability-matched children with other syndromes, finding targets significantly more slowly than do matched toddlers with DS and confusing targets and distractors significantly more than do toddlers with DS or fragile X syndrome (Cornish et al., 2007). Similarly, Scerif, Cornish, Wilding, Driver, and Karmiloff-Smith (2004) found that 3- to 4-year-olds with WS had more difficulty ignoring distractors than did CA- and cognitive ability-matched children with fragile X syndrome. In contrast, Breckenridge, Braddick, Anker, Woodhouse, and Atkinson (2013) reported that the performance of 5- to

15-year-olds with WS on a visual search task did not differ from that of CA- and cognitive ability-matched children with DS, and Costanzo et al. (2013) found that performance of 10- to 34-year-olds with WS on both visual and auditory selective attention tasks did not differ significantly from that of 8- to 21-year-olds with DS matched by nonverbal ability. These differences in findings could be due to different developmental trajectories across syndromes, different tasks, and/or small sample sizes.

Sustained Attention

Findings on sustained attention also are inconsistent. Breckenridge et al. (2013) found that children with WS performed significantly worse than matched children with DS on an auditory sustained attention task but that the performance of the two groups did not differ significantly on either a visual sustained attention task or a dual sustained attention task. However, the performance of an older and smaller sample of individuals with WS did not differ significantly from that of a matched group with DS on a similar auditory sustained attention task, and the WS group performed significantly better than the DS group on cancellation tasks measuring visuospatial sustained attention (Costanzo et al., 2013). Shalev et al. (2019) compared the performance of 25 5- to 8-year-olds with WS and 18 4- to 8-year-olds with DS matched on CA and visuospatial abilities on both overall performance on a visual continuous performance task and performance on the second half of the task relative to the first. The two groups did not differ significantly on overall performance. However, the group with WS showed a significant decrement in performance over the second half of the task, indicating a selective impairment in the ability to sustain visual attention over time. This decrement over time was predictive of symptoms of attention-deficit/hyperactivity disorder (ADHD) as measured by teacher report.

Attention-Deficit/Hyperactivity Disorder

Given their difficulties with auditory filtering and both selective and sustained attention, it is not surprising that distractibility and problems with concentration have consistently been identified as major concerns for children and adolescents with WS (Morris & Mervis, 2020). On the Child Behavior Checklist (CBCL; e.g., Achenbach & Rescorla, 2001), attention problems are the most common concern reported by parents across a variety of cultures (Pérez-García, Brun-Gasca, Pérez-Jurado, & Mervis, 2017) and are uniquely associated with difficulty with inhibition as measured by the Behavior Rating Inventory of Executive Function–2 (BRIEF-2; Gioia, Isquith, Guy, & Kenworthy, 2015; Greiner de Magalhães, Pitts, & Mervis, 2022). Based on semistructured diagnostic interviews with parents of 119 4- to 16-year-olds with WS, Leyfer et al. (2006) found that 64.7% met full DSM-IV criteria for ADHD, with similar rates for boys and girls.

Memory

Short-Term and Associative Memory

Given the WS cognitive profile, individuals with WS would be expected to have a relative strength in verbal memory and a relative weakness in spatial memory. This prediction has been confirmed repeatedly for short-term memory (see Rowe & Mervis, 2006, for review). Furthermore, verbal short-term memory as measured by forward digit recall is significantly stronger for individuals with WS than for CA- and IQ-matched individuals with DS (Costanzo et al., 2013; Edgin, Pennington, & Mervis, 2010; Klein & Mervis, 1999; Wang & Bellugi, 1994) or ID of mixed etiology (Udwin & Yule, 1991). Nichols et al. (2004) found the same pattern on the first trial of a supraspan list-learning task. However, after completing several trials of a supraspan list-learning task followed by an interference trial of a different word list, the group with WS recalled significantly fewer words on the original list than the matched group with DS (Edgin et al., 2010). Individuals with WS performed worse than CA- and IQ-matched individuals with DS on short-term spatial memory, as measured by a forward Corsi span task; this difference was sometimes (Edgin et al., 2010; Wang & Bellugi, 1994) but not always (Costanzo et al., 2013) significant. Individuals with WS also performed significantly worse than matched individuals with DS on a spatial associative memory task (Edgin et al., 2010).

Working Memory

When mental manipulation is required, differences between individuals with WS and the contrast group are considerably reduced. On backward digit recall tasks, groups of individuals with WS consistently demonstrate longer spans than CA and IQ/mental age (MA) matched groups with DS (Edgin et al., 2010; Robinson, Mervis, & Robinson, 2003; Wang & Bellugi, 1994) but the between-group difference was significant in only one study (Costanzo et al., 2013). Performance on visuospatial working memory, typically measured by backward Corsi recall, does not differ significantly from that of individuals with DS matched for CA and IQ (Costanzo et al., 2013; Edgin et al., 2010).

Relations between Memory and Other Abilities

Verbal short-term memory, as measured by forward digit recall or nonword repetition, was significantly correlated with grammatical abilities for children with WS (Robinson et al., 2003). Performance on verbal working memory tasks is affected by the same semantic and phonological factors for children with WS as for TD children (Rowe & Mervis, 2006). Verbal and spatial associative and working memory were positively correlated with IQ, and verbal working memory and spatial associative memory also were positively correlated with adaptive behavior (Edgin et al., 2010).

Executive Functions

Parent Report Questionnaires

In general, children with WS show considerable evidence of deficits in tasks that involve frontal lobe dysfunction. The responses of parents of 308 children and adolescents on the BRIEF-2 indicated that 43% had potentially clinically significant or clinically significant difficulties with behavior regulation, 51% with emotion regulation, and 69% with cognitive regulation (Greiner de Magalhães et al., 2022). Performance on each of the BRIEF (Gioia, Isquith, Guy, & Kenworthy, 2000) scales was significantly worse than that of a DS group matched for CA and nonverbal reasoning ability but with more limited language ability (Camp, Karmiloff-Smith, Thomas, & Farran, 2016).

Camp et al. (2016) also reported, based on a researcher-developed parent-report questionnaire addressing practical problem solving, that the WS group was significantly less likely than the DS group to adequately solve problems that occur in either routine (e.g., getting dressed) or novel activities (e.g., finding a lost possession). For the WS group, likelihood of solving the problems was positively correlated with parental ratings of flexibility, focus, perseverance, and emotional regulation. Significant correlations were found between parent-reported performance on each of the BRIEF scales and probability of reaching a solution on the novel problems.

Inhibition

Several research groups have documented difficulties with behavioral inhibition based on direct assessment. On an antisaccade task that is performed accurately by TD 5-month-olds, Atkinson et al. (2003) found that most of the 8-month-old to 5-year-old participants with WS had considerable difficulty (see Cornish et al., 2007 for similar results). Tager-Flusberg, Sullivan, and Boshart (1997) tested 5- to 8-year-olds with WS on the day–night Stroop task and a tapping task, both of which at least 75% of same-age TD children would be expected to pass (Diamond & Taylor, 1996; Gerstadt, Hong, & Diamond, 1994). Only 25% of the WS group passed the verbal inhibition task, and only 17% passed the motoric inhibition task. Children with WS performed similarly to children with DS matched for both CA and MA on a verbal opposites task (similar to the day–night task) but significantly worse on a pointing–counterpointing task (Breckenridge et al., 2013). Carney, Brown, and Henry (2013) found that the most pervasive difficulty in executive function for school-age children with WS was inhibition, whether measured by verbal or visuospatial tasks.

Planning and Shifting

Several research groups have found impairments on spatial planning tasks. On a version of the Tower of Hanoi, children with WS performed significantly worse than younger children with ADHD matched on receptive vocabulary (Rhodes, Riby, Matthews, & Coghill, 2011). Spending more time on initial planning was related to increased inattention symptoms, as measured by parent report (Rhodes, Riby, Park, Fraser, & Campbell, 2010). On the Tower of London, children with WS performed significantly worse than matched children with DS (Costanzo et al., 2013).

Two studies have addressed verbal shifting. Costanzo et al. (2013) found that individuals with WS performed better than individuals with DS matched on nonverbal MA on an alternating category fluency task. On Balloon Sorting (an adaptation of the Wisconsin Card Sorting Test), children with WS performed similarly to CA- and MA-matched children with DS (Breckenridge et al., 2013).

Fluency

Individuals with WS perform relatively well on verbal fluency tasks. Levy and Bechar (2003) found that the performance of children with WS did not differ significantly from that of a CA- and IQ-matched group of children with ID of unknown etiology. Costanzo et al. (2013) reported that the WS group in their study performed significantly better than the DS group on the verbal fluency measure. On the Weigl Color Form Sort Test (a measure of visuospatial fluency), the performance of the group with WS did not differ significantly from that of the group with DS (Costanzo et al., 2013).

Social Cognition

Social Communication Impairments

Children and adolescents with WS are typically socially driven, with high levels of gregariousness and social disinhibition, and demonstrate more inappropriate approach to strangers than same-CA individuals with nonspecific ID (e.g., Jones et al., 2000; Klein-Tasman & Mervis, 2003). The instrument most commonly used to study social communication in WS is the Social Responsiveness Scale (SRS; Constantino & Gruber, 2005), a parent-report measure. A consistent pattern of relative strengths and weaknesses has been found: mean *T*-score in the normal range for Social Motivation (significantly better than on the remaining scales), in the mild-to-moderate social dysfunction range for Social Awareness and Social Communication (but significantly better than for Social Cognition), and in the severe social dysfunction range for Social Cognition (e.g., Klein-Tasman, Li-Barber, & Magargee, 2011; van der Fluit, Gaffrey, & Klein-Tasman, 2012). Similar findings were obtained based on teacher report (Klein-Tasman et al., 2011). In general, SRS *T*-scores were significantly correlated with performance on the Social Attribution Test, a laboratory-based measure of social cognition (van der Fluit et al., 2012). Individuals with WS classified as high-anxious based on parent report were rated as having significantly more difficulty on the Social Awareness, Social Communication, and Social Cognition scales than those classified as low-anxious (Riby et al., 2014a). The prevalence of clinically significant difficulties on the CBCL Social Problems scale is very high across a variety of cultures (Pérez-García et al., 2017).

Responsivity

Results of a study using the simulated distress procedure indicated that preschoolers with WS show significantly more empathic concern than CA- and IQ-matched children with DS or CA-matched TD children (Plesa Skwerer & Tager-Flusberg, 2016). However, in a helping scenario in the same study, the TD group received higher ratings of overall helpfulness than the WS group, and only 50% of the children with WS were helpful versus 70% of the children with DS. Whereas the TD group was consistently rated as both helpful and empathic, the WS group was rated higher on empathy than on helpfulness. Fidler, Hepburn, Most, Philofsky, and Rogers (2007), using an adaptation of the Yummy–Yucky task and a comparison group of CA- and MA-matched children with developmental disability of nonspecific etiology, reported a similar pattern of findings.

Emotion Perception

Plesa-Skwerer, Faja, Schofield, Verbalis, and Tager-Flusberg (2006) compared the performance of a group of individuals with WS to a group of CA- and IQ-matched individuals with ID of mixed etiology and a CA-matched TD group on the Faces and Paralanguage subtests of the Diagnostic Analysis of Nonverbal Accuracy Scale–2 (Nowicki & Duke, 1994), a standardized measure of emotion recognition. All three groups were close to ceiling on the happy facial expressions. In contrast, individuals with WS performed similarly to the ID group and significantly worse than the TD group on the negative emotions (sad, angry, fearful) in both visual and vocal modalities and also on the happy vocal expressions. Lacroix, Guidetti, Rogé, and Reilly (2009) found that 6- to 15-year-olds with WS could differentiate positive from negative emotions but had difficulty differentiating among the negative expressions, making significantly more errors than younger children with ASD matched on verbal MA when attempting to differentiate between fear and anger or fear and sadness (see Morel et al., 2018, for a systematic review).

Attention Bias

The dot-probe paradigm has been used by several research groups to measure attention bias to emotional faces. McGrath et al. (2016), in the study with the largest sample (46 12- to 56-year-olds), found significant effects for both IQ and parental ratings of anxiety. Individuals at or below the median Verbal IQ (77) evidenced a significant bias toward happy faces (but not angry faces) relative to neutral, whereas the opposite pattern was true for participants with higher Verbal IQ. The same pattern was found using a median split for Nonverbal IQ or parental ratings of anxiety symptoms.

Theory of Mind

Children with WS have significant difficulties with theory of mind (TOM; the ability to understand another's perspective), and these difficulties contribute to their social problems. TD children demonstrate representational understanding of beliefs by age 4 or 5 years (Gopnik & Astington, 1988) and are usually able to distinguish between ironic jokes and lies by age 5 years (Leekam, 1991). In contrast, only 30% of 57 6- to 12-year-olds with WS (M: 9.24 years) passed an unexpected contents task (John, Rowe, & Mervis, 2009) and 88% of 16 8- to 16-year-olds (M: 12.3 years) with WS misclassified jokes as lies (Sullivan, Winner, & Tager-Flusberg, 2003).

Social Referencing

Given these social communication problems, it is not surprising that there are difficulties with *social referencing*, the ability to recognize another person as a social source of information and to use this information as a method of learning about the surrounding world. Thurman and Mervis (2013) compared 20 3- to 5-year-olds (M: 4.97 years) with WS and 20 CA- and nonverbal IQ-matched children with DS with significantly lower verbal IQ on a task designed to assess the child's ability to regulate his or her own behavior toward an ambiguous stimulus in response to an adult's behavioral reaction of joy or fear. In the joyful condition, children with WS shifted their attention between the stimulus and the experimenter significantly less often than the children with DS and produced significantly fewer behaviors acknowledging the joyful display. In the fearful condition, 13 children with DS but only five with WS demonstrated any response, and only two children with WS showed the expected negative response. Results of follow-up studies indicated that the WS group was significantly less likely than the DS group either to initiate eye contact or to follow the experimenter's gaze in triadic situations.

John et al. (2009) used a more advanced social referencing task to measure the ability of 57 6- to 12-year-olds with WS (M: 9.24 years) to assess the adequacy of their interaction partner's message. When the speaker's message was inadequate, the children with WS told the speaker so less than half the time, considerably less often than 3- to 6-year-old TD children tested in the same paradigm (Abbeduto et al., 2008), demonstrating a clear difficulty with monitoring their own comprehension of the speaker's message. Even when they did indicate message inadequacy, the children with WS often did not indicate the specific problem; in some cases, they identified the wrong problem. Of the verbalizations that did not specify the problem, 54% involved a TOM error in which the child did not take into account that due to the opaque barrier between them, the experimenter was unable to see what the child could see. Both CA and TOM contributed significantly and independently to the prediction of overall likelihood that message inadequacy would be verbalized.

Autism Spectrum Disorder

These difficulties in social communication (including difficulties with pragmatic language), along with repetitive behaviors and restricted interests, belie the popular characterization of WS as the opposite of ASD (Mervis & John, 2010a; Thurman & Fisher, 2015). In a recent study, 54% of 45 6- to 18-year-olds with WS screened positive for ASD based on parental responses to the Social Communication Questionnaire (Rutter, Bailey, & Lord, 2003), in comparison to 22% of a similar age group with DS (Kirchner & Walton, 2021). Results of studies using the ADOS to provide a descriptive (rather than diagnostic) characterization of social communication by children with WS indicated that 48% of children assessed with ADOS Module 1, 35% assessed with Module 2, and 30% assessed with Module 3 met or exceeded the ADOS criterion for ASD (Klein-Tasman et al., 2007, 2018). Many of these children would not have been clinically diagnosed with ASD (Klein-Tasman et al., 2007, 2018). In the two studies that reported rate of ASD clinical diagnosis based on ADOS performance combined with clinical judgment of a licensed psychologist who had extensive experience with both children with WS and children with ASD, 20% (Lincoln et al., 2007) or 19% (Becerra & Mervis, 2019) were diagnosed with ASD.

Adaptive and Social Functioning

Adaptive Behavior

The adaptive functioning of individuals with WS is well below age expectations; overall adaptive level typically is in the mild to moderate disability range, with the full range extending from average for the general population to severe disability (see Brawn & Porter, 2018, for a systematic review). Children with WS typically evidence relative strengths in socialization and communication skills, and considerable weakness in daily living and motor skills (Brawn & Porter, 2018). This pattern of findings is consistent with expectations based on the WS cognitive and personality profiles. Difficulties with behavior and emotion regulation are related to adaptive behavior limitations (Greiner de Magalhães et al., 2022).

Personality Profile and Temperament

The first study of the temperament of children with WS included 196 participants ages 1–12 years. Findings indicated that relative to both CA and MA norms, parents on average rated their child with WS as significantly more approaching; significantly higher in intensity, distractibility, and negative mood; and significantly lower in persistence and threshold of excitability (Tomc, Williamson, & Pauli, 1990). Tomc et al. noted that in contrast to the stereotype that children with WS had an easy temperament, older children with WS, even though they were high on approach (typically associated with an easy temperament) were likely to be perceived as difficult, and parents were likely to need support.

Klein-Tasman and Mervis (2003) used the Children's Behavior Questionnaire (CBQ; Rothbart & Ahadi, 1994) and the Multidimensional Personality Questionnaire (MPQ; Tellegen, 1985) to quantify the Williams Syndrome Personality Profile of 8- to 10-year-olds with WS relative to a CA- and IQ-matched group of children with ID of mixed etiology. On the CBQ, high mean ratings on Sociability (based on reverse-coding of the Shyness scale, resulting in high ratings that indicate low shyness and high sociability) and Empathy together characterized 96% of the WS group, but only 15% of the mixed etiology group. On the MPQ, a high mean rating across items measuring gregariousness, people-orientation, tenseness, sensitivity, and visibility was characteristic of 96% of the children with WS but only 15% of the mixed etiology group. This combination of traits is consistent with Tomc et al.'s (1990) position that school-age children with WS demonstrate an unusual temperament that combines both socially approaching and difficult-to-manage traits.

Social Approach and Vulnerability

In keeping with the findings from studies of temperament, other research groups have consistently reported high levels of social approach. Studies measuring the social approach behavior of children with WS based on parental responses to the Salk Institute Sociability Questionnaire (Jones et al., 2000) have reported significantly higher levels of global sociability and a significantly greater tendency to approach strangers when compared to children with other disabilities or to TD CA- or MA-matched peers (e.g., Järvinen-Pasley et al., 2010; Jones et al., 2000; Zitzer-Comfort, Doyle, Masataka, Korenberg, & Bellugi, 2007). Porter, Coltheart, and Langdon (2007) and Little et al. (2013) argued that this indiscriminate social approach behavior is best explained by difficulties in response inhibition. Riby, Kirk, Hanley, and Riby (2014b), using video vignettes to investigate stranger danger awareness, found that only 27% of 16 8- to 17-year-olds (M: 12.1 years) showed appropriate awareness and knowledge of issues related to interaction with strangers compared to 60% of TD 5- to 12-year-olds (M: 7.75 years) matched for verbal ability.

Social Vulnerability

The combination of an intense desire to approach and engage other people, limited stranger-danger awareness, and difficulties with social cognition and social awareness leads to social vulnerability. Problems that have been identified include difficulty forming and maintaining friendships (Fisher, Moskowitz, & Hodapp, 2013), victimization related to bullying and social isolation (for reviews, see Jawaid et al., 2012; Thurman & Fisher, 2015), teasing and persuasion, and physical or sexual abuse (Fisher et al., 2013).

Anxiety Disorders

Leyfer et al. (2006) found that full DSM-IV criteria were met by 54% for specific phobia and 12% for generalized anxiety disorder (GAD), with no sex differences. Consistent with the high prevalence of auditory sensory modulation difficulties (John & Mervis, 2010), the most common specific phobia (28% of the full sample) was for loud noises. DSM-IV criteria for GAD did not capture the nature of worrying in children with WS; if the criteria reflected this type of worrying, the prevalence of GAD would be much higher (Leyfer et al., 2006). Most children with WS worry in anticipation of both events they expect to dislike and events they expect to enjoy. The worry is perseverative, manifested by repeated questions about upcoming activities, and causes significant interference in daily life (Mervis & John, 2010b). On the CBCL, parents across a variety of cultures report anxiety problems as a common concern (Pérez-García et al., 2017). Anxiety problems, as measured by the CBCL, are uniquely associated with inflexibility, as measured by the BRIEF-2 (Greiner de Magalhães et al., 2022).

Developmental Considerations

Intellectual and Adaptive Functioning

When measured by SSs (rather than AEs), the pattern of relative intellectual strengths and weaknesses for individuals with WS is stable from early toddlerhood (the youngest age at which it has been measured) through adulthood (Mervis & John, 2010a, 2010b). Findings from the two studies (Fisher, Lense, & Dykens, 2016; Mervis, Kistler, John, & Morris, 2012) that used growth curve modeling to address potential changes in IQ over time indicated that by middle childhood, Composite IQ, Verbal SS, and Nonverbal (reasoning) SS on the Kaufman Brief Intelligence Test–2 (Kaufman & Kaufman, 2004) were on average stable, although some participants evidenced considerable change (decrease or increase). DAS-II SSs over a 3-year period on average changed more for children who were < 7.5 years old at Time 1 than for those who were older, and Time 1 and Time 2 SSs were more strongly correlated for the older group (Mervis & Pitts, 2015). Although on average the GCA, Verbal SS, and Nonverbal Reasoning SS declined over this period, both increases and decreases were found for individual participants. This pattern also was found for receptive (PPVT-4) and expressive (EVT-2) vocabulary (Mervis & Pitts, 2015).

In contrast, adaptive behavior SSs declined significantly both during childhood (Mervis & Pitts, 2015) and adulthood (Fisher et al., 2016). Over the 3-year period studied, 43% of children evidenced a significant decline in overall adaptive behavior SS, and only 7% evidenced a significant increase, with SSs more stable for older than younger children (Mervis & Pitts, 2015). The area of adaptive behavior with the greatest SS decline was community living skills.

No evidence of regression to the mean was found for any of the intellectual or adaptive behavior SSs in either study. Both Mervis and Pitts (2015) and Fisher et al. (2016) noted that the declines identified, although significant and concerning, primarily represent plateauing or failure to improve skills at the rate expected given the participant's initial SS, rather than loss of skills.

Psychopathology

Although the majority of children and adolescents with WS met DSM-IV criteria for ADHD, the predominant type of ADHD changed with age. For children ages 4–6 years, the prevalence of ADHD-predominantly inattentive and ADHD-combined diagnoses is similar. In contrast, for older children, the most likely diagnosis is ADHD-predominantly inattentive (Leyfer et al., 2006). The prevalence of DSM-IV diagnoses of specific phobia declines significantly from age 6 to 16 years (Pitts, Klein-Tasman, Osborne, & Mervis, 2016), but DSM-IV diagnoses of GAD increased significantly, from 0% for 4- to 6-year-olds to 23% for 11- to 16-year-olds (Leyfer et al., 2006).

Developmental Cascades

As D'Souza and Karmiloff-Smith (2017) have noted, an early difference in a basic process is likely to have a cascading effect on later development across a variety of domains. An example of this for WS involves the well-documented sticky gaze (problems with disengaging from the person or object at which they are looking) that is characteristic of infants and toddlers. This difficulty disengaging leads to problems with both initiating triadic joint attention and responding to another person's bids for triadic joint attention. This in turn leads to a delay in language onset, which affects later vocabulary, grammatical, and pragmatic language abilities. These delays affect not only literacy but also the development of visuospatial skills such as drawing or handwriting (for which verbal scaffolding is particularly helpful for children with WS), the development of appropriate social skills, and friendship formation and maintenance, with cascading influences potentially extending to employment opportunities in adulthood.

Transition to Adulthood and Adult Outcomes

Long-term outcomes for individuals with WS who have classic deletions vary dramatically. Some adolescents and adults with WS can read only a few words, whereas others decode and comprehend at the high school level. A few individuals have passed district or state high school exit exams in both English and mathematics. These individuals have overall IQs ranging from the top of the mild ID range to the lower part of the average range (Mervis & John, 2010b).

Fisher, Josol, and Shivers (2020) reported that of a recent sample of 114 adults with WS (M: 27.99 years), 83% had completed high school and 29% had attended some type of postsecondary program. At the time of the survey, 44% were employed at least part-time in a paid position, and 17% were in a volunteer position; the remaining 38% stayed at home during the day, with no regular daytime activities. Most participants (83%) lived with parents or another family member; 11% lived in supported living arrangements including group homes, and 6% lived independently in their own apartment.

Strong family support that includes a focus, from early childhood, on taking responsibility for oneself to the extent possible contributes to the development of strong adaptive skills and the discipline to try one's best, which in turn considerably increases the likelihood of positive adult outcomes for individuals with WS (Mervis & Morris, 2007). The most successful adults with WS are not necessarily the ones with the highest IQs; the most striking characteristics of these individuals are their adaptive behavior and mastery motivation—willingness to persevere on a moderately difficult task and expression of pleasure upon mastery of the task (Mervis & John, 2010a)—which are reliably near the top of the range for individuals with WS (Mervis & John, 2010b).

PREDICTORS AND MODERATORS

Biological Factors

Because WS is caused by a microdeletion, a major predictor of outcome is the specific set of genes that is deleted. Most individuals with WS (~95%) have the same ("classic") deletion. Several of the deleted genes are transcription factors, leading to significant changes in methylation across the genome, which further contribute to the WS phenotype (Strong et al., 2015). The set of differentially methylated genes is significantly enriched for genes on pathways involved in neurodevelopment, ASD candidate genes, and imprinted genes (Strong et al., 2015). Kimura et al. (2020) reported that the oxytocin receptor gene (*OXTR*) is hypermethylated in individuals with WS, a finding the authors noted is also characteristic of individuals with ASD, providing further support for the overlaps in WS and ASD phenotypes described earlier in this chapter.

Individuals with shorter deletions that do not include *GTF2I* (the most telomeric gene in the classic deletion) have higher overall IQs, although the pattern of relative cognitive strengths and weaknesses is usually the same as for classic WS (Morris et al., 2003; see also Kozel et al., 2021), suggesting that deletion of this gene contributes to the ID associated with WS. Research on individuals with very small deletions suggests that deletion of *LIMK1* contributes to the weakness in visuospatial construction (Frangiskakis et al., 1996); this possibility is further supported by Gregory et al.'s (2019) resting-state fMRI findings from individuals in the general population who have *LIMK1* alleles associated with lower rates of transcription. Individuals with longer deletions extending in the telomeric direction that include *HIP1* (previously referred to as *HSP27*) have significantly lower overall IQs than individuals with classic deletions (Stock et al., 2003; see also Lugo et al., 2020).

Psychological and Social Factors

Adaptive behavior skills are positively associated with higher IQ (Brawn & Porter, 2018), better sensory modulation (John & Mervis, 2010), lower levels of anxiety, oppositionality, impulsivity, and inattention (John & Mervis, 2010), and better emotion regulation and behavior regulation (Greiner de Magalhães et al., 2021). Higher levels of mastery motivation and better behavior regulation (Klein-Tasman & Lee, 2017) are expected to positively impact both adaptive behavior and academic achievement (Morris & Mervis, 2020). Better behavior regulation and higher IQ independently were negatively related to having a specific phobia diagnosis (Pitts et al., 2016). Children whose mothers had completed at least a bachelor's degree (a surrogate measure for socioeconomic status) had significantly higher verbal IQs than those whose mothers had less education (Mervis et al., 2012).

Families of individuals with WS are often highly stressed (Fidler, Hodapp, & Dykens, 2000). The rate of GAD among mothers of children with WS is approximately three times higher than that of women their age in the general population, despite (based on retrospective report) having had a rate of GAD similar to that of women in the general population prior to the birth of their child with WS (Leyfer, Woodruff-Borden, & Mervis, 2009). Mothers of children and young adults with WS endorsed significantly more challenges in raising their child than mothers of children with DS or ASD, and the number of endorsed challenges was significantly correlated with maternal stress (Ashworth, Palikara, & Van Herwegen, 2019). For all three groups, the highest maternal stressor was worrying about the future because of lack of specialist services for adults (Ashworth et al., 2019).

Cross-Cultural or International Considerations

Characteristics of individuals with WS have been investigated by research groups from a variety of countries in North America, South America, Europe, Asia, and Australia, with similar patterns of findings. Two behavioral studies that included a direct comparison of children with WS from different countries have been reported. In keeping with previously identified cultural differences for TD children, maternal ratings of children with WS from Spain indicated significantly more behavior and emotional problems than did maternal ratings of children with WS from the United States (Pérez-García et al., 2017) and mothers of children with WS from Japan rated their children as less likely to approach strangers than did mothers of children with WS from the United States (Zitzer-Comfort et al., 2007). However, in both studies, the children with WS showed the same pattern of behavior relative to their same-culture TD peers: Both Spanish and U.S. children with WS were rated as having significantly more emotional and behavioral problems, and both Japanese and U.S. children with WS were rated as significantly more likely to approach strangers.

TREATMENT AND INTERVENTION

Infants and toddlers with WS should be referred to an early intervention program for assessment at the time of diagnosis, if they are not already enrolled. During this period, physical, occupational (including sensory integration if needed), and speech–language therapy are crucial (Morris et al., 2020). Most children with WS would benefit from continued speech–language therapy and occupational therapy throughout their education. Detailed suggestions for goals and approaches are provided in Mervis and John (2010a), Mervis and Velleman (2011), and Morris and Mervis (2020). Once children can talk well, they should be taught to use their language skills to provide a framework for breaking down and mastering spatial tasks (Morris & Mervis, 2020). Children with WS are much more likely to learn to read well if they are taught to read using a systematic, intensive phonics approach, rather than whole-language/balanced literacy or whole-word/sight-word approaches (for detailed suggestions, see Mervis, 2009; Mervis et al., 2022; Mervis & John, 2010a); explicit instruction focused on reading comprehension also is important (Mervis & John, 2010a; Mervis et al., 2022). Even mild unilateral hearing loss is likely to negatively impact academic progress; hearing aids should be provided if appropriate and a classroom frequency modulated (FM) system considered (Marler et al., 2010; Morris & Mervis, 2020). A classroom FM system also may be helpful for children with WS who have ADHD even if they do not have hearing loss (Morris & Mervis, 2020). For adults, vocational training, including job coaching and instruction in community living skills, is critical (Morris & Mervis, 2020; Morris et al., 2020).

Behavior

Cognitive-behavioral treatments that are adjusted for the individual's developmental level show promise for treating anxiety (Phillips & Klein-Tasman, 2009). For young children, use of strategic play-based therapies such as replays (Levine & Chedd, 2007) to treat specific phobia or emotion dysregulation also is promising. For children with moderate to severe emotion dysregulation or oppositional behavior, in-home and/or in-school ABA approaches that take into account the social nature of children with WS are recommended; parental training also is likely to be helpful (Mervis & John, 2010a). Social skills training to address gullibility and social vulnerability during both in-person and online interactions is crucial (Fisher & Morin, 2017; Lough & Fisher, 2016; Morris et al., 2020). Children with WS who also have ASD or share characteristics with children with ASD are likely to benefit from the types of treatments that have been efficacious for children with ASD who do not have WS (Mervis & John, 2010a; Klein-Tasman et al., 2018). Sleep problems are common in children with WS and contribute to behavior problems and language or learning difficulties (Greiner de Magalhães, O'Brien, & Mervis, 2020). Sleep hygiene programs should be provided as needed; detailed information regarding use of melatonin for children with WS is provided in Morris and Mervis (2020). In addition to psychological/behavioral therapy, approximately 50% of individuals with WS will require pharmacological intervention for ADHD and/or anxiety disorders (Morris et al., 2020); recommendations are provided in Morris and Mervis (2020) and Morris et al. (2020).

CONCLUSIONS AND FUTURE DIRECTIONS

Methodological Concerns

Problems with the interpretation of AE or GE scores are highlighted in the manuals for most standardized assessments, and methodological issues involved in the use of these scores in psychological research are discussed in Mervis and Robinson (2005). Most critically, these scores are not on an interval scale; furthermore, they cannot be compared across assessments or even across subtests from a single assessment. Designs that involve matching children of different CAs on MA, AE, or GE assume similar rates of development for the control and target variables across the entire CA range included in the study. If development of the control and target variables proceeds at different rates (which is commonly the case; see Figure 1 in Mervis & Robinson, 2005, and further discussion in Rowe & Mervis, 2006), then differences in CA will confound the matching design, because the differences in raw scores (and therefore AE, GE, or MA) will not be stable across CA. In such cases, one cannot predict that two groups with identical AEs or MAs on control variables but different CAs should be expected to have similar scores on the target variable. For these reasons, in this chapter, we have avoided citing papers that rely on comparisons of individuals with WS to much younger groups of MA-matched children (whether TD or with other forms of disability), studies that involved comparisons of AE or GE scores rather than SSs, and studies in which AE, GE, or MA were treated as though they were on an interval scale.

Due to the very low prevalence of WS, most studies include small samples, a very wide age range, or both. Thus, studies involving individuals with WS are almost always seriously underpowered. Multisite collaborations are likely to be necessary to address this concern.

Future Directions

WS is a genomic disorder caused by a hemideletion of 25–27 genes at chromosome 7q11.23. The reciprocal duplication syndrome (7q11.23 duplication syndrome; Dup7) was first documented 15 years ago (Somerville et al., 2005). Studies of Dup7 are just beginning (e.g., Mervis et al., 2015), and only one published study has directly compared WS and Dup7 (Strong et al., 2015). Behavioral, genetic, epigenetic, and neuroimaging studies (preferably all involving the same participants) that provide direct comparisons of individuals with classic WS and individuals with classic Dup7 and/or compare the very rare individuals with different smaller deletions or duplications of 7q11.23 offer the best opportunity to understand the genetic underpinnings of WS and how these relate to the phenotype (see Kozel et al., 2021; Osborne & Mervis, 2021).

Large-sample behavioral studies of children with classic deletions incorporating both experimental and observational paradigms, as well as standardized assessments, are crucial to better understanding the subtleties of the cognitive and personality characteristics of individuals with WS. Longitudinal studies that include a large enough sample size for complex modeling methods such as path analysis or structural equation modeling to allow for investigating developmental precursors or cascades are crucial. Theory-based models would be especially valuable and would better inform the development of targeted interventions.

Carefully designed multisite treatment studies addressing behavioral and/or psychopharmacological therapies for ADHD, emotion dysregulation, and anxiety are critical; randomized controlled trials would be ideal. Other important foci for treatment studies include methods to increase mastery motivation; methods to increase social appropriateness and decrease social vulnerability; and instructional approaches to word reading, reading comprehension, and mathematics. Findings from these types of studies have the potential both to increase scientific understanding of typical and atypical development and to make a positive impact on the lives of children with WS and their families.

ACKNOWLEDGMENTS

Preparation of this manuscript was supported by Grant No. WSA 0111 from the Williams Syndrome Association. We thank the individuals with Williams syndrome and their families from around the world who have participated in research studies. Without their commitment, progress in understanding Williams syndrome would not be possible. We are grateful to the Williams Syndrome Association for the proactive role it has taken in facilitating not only our research but also the research of many others.

REFERENCES

Abbeduto, L., Murphy, M. M., Kover, S. T., Giles, N. D., Karadottir, S., Amman, A., . . . Nollin, K. A. (2008). Signaling noncomprehension of language: A comparison of fragile X syndrome and Down syndrome. *American Journal on Mental Retardation, 113,* 214–230.

Achenbach, T. M., & Rescorla, L. A. (2001). *Manual for the ASEBA school-age forms & profiles.* Burlington: University of Vermont, Research Center for Children, Youth, and Families.

Ashworth, M., Palikara, O., & Van Herwegen, J. (2019). Comparing parental stress of children with neurodevelopmental disorders: The case of Williams syndrome, Down syndrome and autism spectrum disorders. *Journal of Applied Research in Intellectual Disabilities, 32,* 1047–1057.

Atkinson, J., Braddick, O., Anker, S., Curran, W., Andrew, R., Wattam-Bell, J., & Braddick, F. (2003). Neurobiological models of visuospatial cognition in children with Williams syndrome: Measures of dorsal-stream and frontal function. *Developmental Neuropsychology, 23,* 139–172.

Becerra, A. M., & Mervis, C. B. (2019). Age at onset of declarative gestures and 24-month expressive vocabulary predict later language and intellectual abilities in young children with Williams syndrome. *Frontiers in Psychology, 10*(2648), 1–14.

Bellugi, U., Lichtenberger, L., Jones, W., Lai, Z., & St. George, M. (2000). I. The neurocognitive profile of Williams Syndrome: A complex pattern of strengths and weaknesses. *Journal of Cognitive Neuroscience, 12*(Suppl. 1), 7–29.

Bellugi, U., Marks, S., Bihrle, A., & Sabo, H. (1988). Dissociation between language and cognitive functions in Williams syndrome. In D. Bishop & K. Mogford (Eds.), *Language development in exceptional circumstances* (pp. 177–189). London: Churchill Livingstone.

Bennett, F. C., LaVeck, B., & Sells, C. J. (1978). The Williams elfin facies syndrome: The psychological profile as an aid in syndrome identification. *Pediatrics, 61,* 303–306.

Beuren, A. J., Apitz, J., & Harmjanz, D. (1962). Supravalvular aortic stenosis in association with mental retardation and a certain facial appearance. *Circulation, 26,* 1235–1240.

Bishop, D. V. (2003). *The Children's Communication Checklist:* CCC-2. San Antonio, TX: PsychCorp.

Brawn, G., Kohnen, S., Tassabehji, M., & Porter, M. (2018). Functional basic reading skills in Williams syndrome. *Developmental Neuropsychology, 43,* 454–477.

Brawn, G., & Porter, M. (2018). Adaptive functioning in Williams syndrome: A systematic review. *International Journal of Disability, Development and Education, 65,* 123–147.

Breckenridge, K., Braddick, O., Anker, S., Woodhouse, M., & Atkinson, J. (2013). Attention in Williams syndrome and Down's syndrome: Performance on the new Early Childhood Attention Battery. *British Journal of Developmental Psychology, 31,* 257–269.

Brown, J. H., Johnson, M. H., Paterson, S. J., Gilmore, R., Longhi, E., & Karmiloff-Smith, A. (2003). Spatial representation and attention in toddlers with Williams syndrome and Down syndrome. *Neuropsychologia, 41,* 1037–1046.

Camp, J. S., Karmiloff-Smith, A., Thomas, M. S., & Farran, E. K. (2016). Cross-syndrome comparison of real-world executive functioning and problem solving using a new problem-solving questionnaire. *Research in Developmental Disabilities, 59,* 80–92.

Carney, D. P., Brown, J. H., & Henry, L. A. (2013). Executive function in Williams and Down syndromes. *Research in Developmental Disabilities, 34,* 46–55.

Cashon, C. H., Ha, O. R., Graf Estes, K., Saffran, J. R., & Mervis, C. B. (2016). Infants with Williams syndrome detect statistical regularities in continuous speech. *Cognition, 154,* 165–168.

Constantino, J. N., & Gruber, C. P. (2005). *Manual for Social Responsiveness Scale.* Los Angeles, CA: Western Psychological Services.

Cornish, K., Scerif, G., & Karmiloff-Smith, A. (2007). Tracing syndrome-specific trajectories of attention across the lifespan. *Cortex, 43,* 672–685.

Costanzo, F., Varuzza, C., Menghini, D., Addona, F., Gianesini, T., & Vicari, S. (2013). Executive functions in intellectual disabilities: A comparison between Williams syndrome and Down syndrome. *Research in Developmental Disabilities, 34,* 1770–1780.

Cowie, D., Braddick, O., & Atkinson, J. (2012). Visually guided step descent in children with Williams syndrome. *Developmental Science, 15,* 74–86.

Diamond, A., & Taylor, C. (1996). Development of an aspect of executive control: Development of the abilities to remember what I said and to "Do as I say, not as I do." *Developmental Psychobiology, 29,* 315–334.

D'Souza, H., & Karmiloff-Smith, A. (2017). Neurodevelopmental disorders. *WIREs Cognitive Science, 8,* Article e1398.

Dunn, L. E., & Dunn, D. M. (2007). *Peabody Picture Vocabulary Test–4*. Minneapolis, MN: Pearson Assessments.

Edgin, J. O., Mervis, C. B., & Pennington, B. F. (2010). Neuropsychological components of intellectual disability: The contributions of immediate, working and associative memory. *Journal of Intellectual Disability Research, 54,* 406–417.

Edmonston, N. K., & Litchfield Thane, N. (1988). *TRC: Test of Relational Concepts*. Austin, TX: Pro-Ed.

Elliott, C. D. (2007). *Differential Ability Scales–II*. San Antonio, TX: Harcourt Assessment.

Elliott, D., & Bunn, L. (2004). Motor disorders in children with intellectual disabilities. In D. Dewey & D. E. Tupper (Eds.), *Developmental motor disorders: A neuropsychological perspective* (pp. 137–151). New York: Guilford Press.

Ewart, A. K., Morris, C. A., Atkinson, D., Jin, W., Sternes, K., Spallone, P., . . . Keating, M. T. (1993). Hemizygosity at the elastin locus in a developmental disorder, Williams syndrome. *Nature Genetics, 5,* 11–16.

Fanconi, G., Girardet, P., Schlesinger, B., Butler, N., & Black, J. (1952). Chronische Hypercalcaemie kombiniert mit Osteosklerose, Hyperazotaemie, Minderwuchs, und kongenitalen Missbildungen [Chronic hypercalcemia, combined with osteosclerosis, hyperazotemia, nanism, and congenital malformations]. *Helvetica Paediatrica Acta, 7,* 314–349.

Fenson, L., Marchman, V. A., Thal, D. J., Dale, P. S., Reznick, J. S., & Bates, E. (2007). *MacArthur–Bates Communicative Development Inventories: User's guide and technical manual* (2nd ed.). Baltimore: Brookes.

Fidler, D. J., Hepburn, S. L., Most, D. E., Philofsky, A., & Rogers, S. J. (2007). Emotional responsivity in young children with Williams syndrome. *American Journal on Mental Retardation, 112,* 194–206.

Fidler, D. J., Hodapp, R. M., & Dykens, E. M. (2000). Stress in families of young children with Down syndrome, Williams syndrome, and Smith–Magenis syndrome. *Early Education and Development, 11,* 395–406.

Fisher, M. H., Josol, C. K., & Shivers, C. M. (2020). An examination of social skills, friendship quality, and loneliness for adults with Williams syndrome. *Journal of Autism and Developmental Disorders, 50,* 3649–3660.

Fisher, M. H., Lense, M. D., & Dykens, E. M. (2016). Longitudinal trajectories of intellectual and adaptive functioning in adolescents and adults with Williams syndrome. *Journal of Intellectual Disability Research, 60,* 920–932.

Fisher, M. H., & Morin, L. (2017). Addressing social skills deficits in adults with Williams syndrome. *Research in Developmental Disabilities, 71,* 77–87.

Fisher, M. H., Moskowitz, A. L., & Hodapp, R. M. (2013). Differences in social vulnerability among individuals with autism spectrum disorder, Williams syndrome, and Down syndrome. *Research in Autism Spectrum Disorders, 7,* 931–937.

Frangiskakis, J. M., Ewart, A. K., Morris, C. A., Mervis, C. B., Bertrand, J., Robinson, B. F., . . . Keating, M. T. (1996). LIM-kinase 1 hemizygosity implicated in impaired visuospatial constructive cognition. *Cell, 86,* 59–69.

Gerstadt, C. L., Hong, Y. J., & Diamond, A. (1994). The relationship between cognition and action: performance of children 3½–7 years old on a Stroop-like day–night test. *Cognition, 53,* 129–153.

Ginsburg, H., & Baroody, A (1990). *Test of Early Mathematics Ability–2*. Austin, TX: Pro-Ed.

Gioia, G. A., Isquith, P. K., Guy, S. C., & Kenworthy, L. (2015). *BRIEF-2: Behavior Rating Inventory of Executive Function: Professional Manual*. Odessa, FL: Psychological Assessment Resources.

Gioia, G. A., Isquith, P. K., Guy, S. C., & Kenworthy, L. (2000). *Behavior Rating Inventory of Executive Function (BRIEF)*. Odessa, FL: Psychological Assessment Resources.

Glod, M., Riby, D. M., & Rodgers, J. (2019). Relationships between sensory processing, repetitive behaviors, anxiety, and intolerance of uncertainty in autism spectrum disorder and Williams syndrome. *Autism Research, 12,* 759–765.

Gopnik, A., & Astington, J. (1988). Children's understanding of representational change and its relation to the understanding of false belief and the appearance–reality distinction. *Child Development, 59,* 26–37.

Gosch, A., Städing, G., & Pankau, R. (1994). Linguistic abilities in children with Williams-Beuren syndrome. *American Journal of Medical Genetics, 52,* 291–296.

Gough, P. B., & Tunmer, W. E. (1986). Decoding, reading, and reading disability. *Remedial and Special Education, 7,* 6–10.

Gregory, M. D., Mervis, C. B., Elliott, M., Kippenhan, J. S., Nash, T., Czarapata, J., . . . Berman, K. F. (2019). Williams syndrome hemideletion and *LIMK1* variation both affect dorsal stream functional connectivity. *Brain, 142,* 3963–3974.

Greiner de Magalhães, C., O'Brien, L. M., & Mervis, C. B. (2020). Sleep characteristics and problems of 2-year-olds with Williams syndrome: Relations with language and behavior. *Journal of Neurodevelopmental Disorders, 12*, Article 32.

Greiner de Magalhães, C., Pitts, C. H., & Mervis, C. B. (2022). Executive function as measured by the Behavior Rating Inventory of Executive Function–2: Children and adolescents with Williams syndrome. *Journal of Intellectual Disability Research, 66*, 94–107.

Ha, O.-R., Cashon, C. H., Holt, N. A., & Mervis, C. B. (2020). Development of rapid word–object associations in relation to expressive vocabulary: Shared commonalities in infants and toddlers with and without Williams syndrome. *Developmental Science, 23*, Article e12966.

Hobart, H. H., Morris, C. A., Mervis, C. B., Pani, A. M., Kistler, D. J., Rios, C. M., . . . Bray-Ward, P. (2010). Inversion of the Williams syndrome region is a common polymorphism found more frequently in parents of children with Williams syndrome. *American Journal of Medical Genetics C, 154*, 220–228.

Howlin, P., Davies, M., & Udwin, O. (1998). Cognitive functioning in adults with Williams syndrome. *Journal of Child Psychology and Psychiatry, 39*, 183–189.

Järvinen-Pasley, A., Adolphs, R., Yam, A., Hill, K. J., Grichanik, M., Reilly, J., . . . Bellugi, U. (2010). Affiliative behavior in Williams syndrome: Social perception and real-life social behavior. *Neuropsychologia, 48*, 2110–2119.

Jawaid, A., Riby, D. M., Owens, J., White, S. W., Tarar, T., & Schulz, P. E. (2012). "Too withdrawn" or "too friendly": Considering social vulnerability in two neuro-developmental disorders. *Journal of Intellectual Disability Research, 56*, 335–350.

John, A. E., & Mervis, C. B. (2010). Sensory modulation impairments in children with Williams syndrome. *American Journal of Medical Genetics C, 154*, 266–276.

John, A. E., Rowe, M. L., & Mervis, C. B. (2009). Referential communication skills of children with Williams syndrome: Understanding when messages are not adequate. *American Journal on Intellectual and Developmental Disabilities, 114*, 85–99.

Jones, W., Bellugi, U., Lai, Z., Chiles, M., Reilly, J., & Lincoln, A. (2000). II. Hypersociability in Williams syndrome. *Journal of Cognitive Neuroscience, 12*, 30–46.

Kataria, S., Goldstein, D. J., & Kushnick, T. (1984). Developmental delays in Williams ("elfin facies") syndrome. *Applied Research in Mental Retardation, 5*, 419–423.

Kaufman, A. S., & Kaufman, N. L. (2004). *Kaufman Brief Intelligence Test–2*. Circle Pines, MN: American Guidance Services.

Kimura, R., Tomiwa, R. I., Suzuki, S., Nakata, M., Awaya, T., Okazaki, S., . . . Hagiwara, M. (2020). Dysregulation of the oxytocin receptor gene in Williams syndrome. *Psychoneuroendocrinology, 115*, Article 104631.

Kirchner, R. M., & Walton, K. M. (2021). Symptoms of autism spectrum disorder in children with Down syndrome and Williams syndrome. *American Journal on Intellectual and Developmental Disabilities, 126*, 58–74.

Klein, B. P., & Mervis, C. B. (1999). Cognitive strengths and weaknesses of 9- and 10-year-olds with Williams syndrome or Down syndrome. *Developmental Neuropsychology, 16*, 177–196.

Klein-Tasman, B. P., & Lee, K. (2017). Problem behaviour and psychosocial functioning in young children with Williams syndrome: Parent and teacher perspectives. *Journal of Intellectual Disability Research, 61*, 853–865.

Klein-Tasman, B. P., Li-Barber, K. T., & Magargee, E. T. (2011). Honing in on the social phenotype in Williams syndrome using multiple measures and multiple raters. *Journal of Autism and Developmental Disorders, 41*, 341–351.

Klein-Tasman, B. P., & Mervis, C. B. (2003). Distinctive personality characteristics of 8-, 9-, and 10-year-old children with Williams syndrome. *Developmental Neuropsychology, 23*, 271–292.

Klein-Tasman, B. P., Mervis, C. B., Lord, C., & Phillips, K. D. (2007). Socio-communicative deficits in young children with Williams syndrome: Performance on the Autism Diagnostic Observation Schedule. *Child Neuropsychology, 13*, 444–467.

Klein-Tasman, B. P., van der Fluit, F., & Mervis, C. B. (2018). Autism spectrum symptomatology in children with Williams syndrome who have phrase speech or fluent language. *Journal of Autism and Developmental Disorders, 48*, 3037–3050.

Kozel, B. A., Barak, B., Kim, C. A., Mervis, C. B., Osborne, L. R., Porter, M., & Pober, B. R. (2021). Williams syndrome. *Nature Review Disease Primers, 7*, Article 42.

Lacroix, A., Guidetti, M., Rogé, B., & Reilly, J. (2009). Recognition of emotional and nonemotional facial expressions: A comparison between Williams syndrome and autism. *Research in Developmental Disabilities, 30*, 976–985.

Lane, C., Van Herwegen, J., & Freeth, M. (2019). Parent-reported communication abilities of children with Sotos syndrome: Evidence from the Children's Communication Checklist-2. *Journal of Autism and Developmental Disorders, 49,* 1475–1483.

Leekam, S. (1991). Jokes and lies: Children's understanding of intentional falsehood. In A. Whiten (Ed.), *Natural theories of mind* (pp. 159–174). Oxford, UK: Blackwell.

Levine, K., & Chedd, N. (2007). *Replays: Using play to enhance emotional and behavioral development for children with autism spectrum disorders.* Philadelphia: Jessica Kingsley.

Levy, Y., & Bechar, T. (2003). Cognitive, lexical and morpho-syntactic profiles of Israeli children with Williams syndrome. *Cortex, 39,* 255–271.

Leyfer, O. T., Woodruff-Borden, J., Klein-Tasman, B. P., Fricke, J. S., & Mervis, C. B. (2006). Prevalence of psychiatric disorders in 4 to 16-year-olds with Williams syndrome. *American Journal of Medical Genetics B, 141,* 615–622.

Leyfer, O., Woodruff-Borden, J., & Mervis, C. B. (2009). Anxiety disorders in children with Williams syndrome, their mothers, and their siblings: Implications for the etiology of anxiety disorders. *Journal of Neurodevelopmental Disorders, 1*(1), 4–14.

Lincoln, A. J., Searcy, Y. M., Jones, W., & Lord, C. (2007). Social interaction behaviors discriminate young children with autism and Williams syndrome. *Journal of the American Academy of Child and Adolescent Psychiatry, 46,* 323–331.

Little, K., Riby, D. M., Janes, E., Clark, F., Fleck, R., & Rodgers, J. (2013). Heterogeneity of social approach behaviour in Williams syndrome: The role of response inhibition. *Research in Developmental Disabilities, 34,* 959–967.

Lord, C., Rutter, M., DiLavore, P., & Risi, S. (1999). *Autism Diagnostic Observation Schedule (ADOS).* Los Angeles: Western Psychological Services.

Lough, E., & Fisher, M. H. (2016). Internet use and online safety in adults with Williams syndrome. *Journal of Intellectual Disability Research, 60,* 1020–1030.

Loveall, S. J., Hawthorne, K., & Gaines, M. (2021). A meta-analysis of prosody in autism, Williams syndrome, and Down syndrome. *Journal of Communication Disorders, 89,* Article 106055.

Lugo, M., Wong, Z. C., Billington, Jr., C. J., Parrish, P. C. R., Muldoon, G., Liu, D., . . . Kozel, B. A. (2020). Social, neurodevelopmental, endocrine, and head size differences associated with atypical deletions in Williams–Beuren syndrome. *American Journal of Medical Genetics A, 182,* 1008–1020.

MacDonald, G. W., & Roy, D. L. (1988). Williams syndrome: A neuropsychological profile. *Journal of Clinical and Experimental Neuropsychology, 10,* 125–131.

Marler, J. A., Sitcovsky, J. L., Mervis, C. B., Kistler, D. J., & Wightman, F. L. (2010). Auditory function and hearing loss in children and adults with Williams syndrome: Cochlear impairment in individuals with otherwise normal hearing. *American Journal of Medical Genetics C, 154,* 249–265.

Martens, M. A., Wilson, S. J., & Reutens, D. C. (2008). Research Review: Williams syndrome: A critical review of the cognitive, behavioral, and neuroanatomical phenotype. *Journal of Child Psychology and Psychiatry, 49,* 576–608.

Martin, N. D., Snodgrass, G. J., & Cohen, R. D. (1984). Idiopathic infantile hypercalcaemia—A continuing enigma. *Archives of Disease in Childhood, 59,* 605–613.

Masataka, N. (2001). Why early linguistic milestones are delayed in children with Williams syndrome: late onset of hand banging as a possible rate-limiting constraint on the emergence of canonical babbling. *Developmental Science, 4,* 158–164.

McGrath, L. M., Oates, J. M., Dai, Y. G., Dodd, H. F., Waxler, J., Clements, C. C., . . . Mullett, J. (2016). Attention bias to emotional faces varies by IQ and anxiety in Williams syndrome. *Journal of Autism and Developmental Disorders, 46,* 2174–2185.

McIntosh, D. N., Miller, L. J., Shyu, V., & Hagerman, R. J. (1999). Sensory-modulation disruption, electrodermal responses, and functional behaviors. *Developmental Medicine and Child Neurology, 41,* 608–615.

Mervis, C. B. (2006). Language abilities in Williams–Beuren syndrome. In C. A. Morris, H. M. Lenhoff, & P. P. Wang (Eds.), *Williams–Beuren syndrome: Research, evaluation, and treatment* (pp. 159–206). Baltimore: Johns Hopkins University Press.

Mervis, C. B. (2009). Language and literacy development of children with Williams syndrome. *Topics in Language Disorders, 29,* 149–169.

Mervis, C. B., Greiner de Magalhães, C., & Cardoso-Martins, C. (2022, July 3). Concurrent predictors of word reading and reading comprehension for 9-year-olds with Williams syndrome. *Reading and Writing: An Interdisciplinary Journal, 35,* 377–397.

Mervis, C. B., & John, A. E. (2008). Vocabulary abilities of children with Williams syndrome: Strengths, weaknesses, and relation to visuospatial construction ability. *Journal of Speech, Language, and Hearing Research, 51*, 967–982.

Mervis, C. B., & John, A. E. (2010a). Cognitive and behavioral characteristics of children with Williams syndrome: Implications for intervention approaches. *American Journal of Medical Genetics C, 154*, 229–248.

Mervis, C. B., & John, A. E. (2010b). Intellectual disability syndromes. In K. O. Yeates, M. D. Ris, H. G. Taylor, & B. F. Pennington (Eds.), *Pediatric neuropsychology: Research, theory, and practice* (2nd ed., pp. 447–470). New York: Guilford Press.

Mervis, C. B., Kistler, D. J., John, A. E., & Morris, C. A. (2012). Longitudinal assessment of intellectual abilities in children with Williams syndrome: Multilevel modeling of performance on the Kaufman Brief Intelligence Test–2. *American Journal on Intellectual and Developmental Disabilities, 117*, 134–155.

Mervis, C. B., Klein-Tasman, B. P., Huffman, M. J., Velleman, S. L., Pitts, C. H., Henderson, D. R., . . . Osborne, L. R. (2015). Children with 7q11.23 duplication syndrome: Psychological characteristics. *American Journal of Medical Genetics A, 167*, 1436–1450.

Mervis, C. B., & Morris, C. A. (2007). Williams syndrome. In M. M. M. Mazzocco & J. L. Ross, *Neurogenetic developmental disorders: Variation of manifestation in childhood* (pp. 199–262). Cambridge, MA: MIT Press.

Mervis, C. B., Morris, C. A., Klein-Tasman, B. P., Bertrand, J., Kwitny, S., Appelbaum, L. G., & Rice, C. E. (2003). Attentional characteristics of infants and toddlers with Williams syndrome during triadic interactions. *Developmental Neuropsychology, 23*, 245–270.

Mervis, C. B., & Pitts, C. H. (2015). Children with Williams syndrome: Developmental trajectories for intellectual abilities, vocabulary abilities, and adaptive behavior. *American Journal of Medical Genetics C, 169*, 158–171.

Mervis, C. B., & Robinson, B. F. (2000). Expressive vocabulary of toddlers with Williams syndrome or Down syndrome: A comparison. *Developmental Neuropsychology, 17*, 111–126.

Mervis, C. B., & Robinson, B. F. (2005). Designing measures for profiling and genotype/phenotype studies of individuals with genetic syndromes or developmental language disorders. *Applied Psycholinguistics, 26*, 41–64.

Mervis, C. B., Robinson, B. F., Bertrand, J., Morris, C. A., Klein-Tasman, B. P., & Armstrong, S. C. (2000). The Williams syndrome cognitive profile. *Brain and Cognition, 44*, 604–628.

Mervis, C. B., & Velleman, S. L. (2011). Children with Williams syndrome: Language, cognitive, and behavioral characteristics and their implications for intervention. *ASHA Perspectives on Language Learning and Education, 18*, 98–107.

Meyer-Lindenberg, A., Hariri, A. R., Munoz, K. E., Mervis, C. B., Mattay, V. S., Morris, C. A., & Berman, K. F. (2005). Neural correlates of genetically abnormal social cognition in Williams syndrome. *Nature Neuroscience, 8*, 991–993.

Meyer-Lindenberg, A., Kohn, P., Mervis, C. B., Kippenhan, J. S., Olsen, R., Morris, C. A., & Berman, K. F. (2004). Neural basis of genetically determined visuospatial construction deficit in Williams syndrome. *Neuron, 43*, 623–631.

Meyer-Lindenberg, A., Mervis, C. B., & Berman, K. F. (2006). Neural mechanisms in Williams syndrome: A unique window to genetic influences on cognition and behavior. *Nature Reviews: Neuroscience, 7*, 380–393.

Meyerson, M. D., & Frank, R. A. (1987). Language, speech and hearing in Williams syndrome: Intervention approaches and research needs. *Developmental Medicine and Child Neurology, 29*, 258–270.

Miezah, D., Porter, M., Batchelor, J., Boulton, K., & Campos Veloso, G. (2020). Cognitive abilities in Williams syndrome. *Research in Developmental Disabilities, 104*, Article 103701.

Morel, A., Peyroux, E., Leleu, A., Favre, E., Franck, N., & Demily, C. (2018). Overview of social cognitive dysfunctions in rare developmental syndromes with psychiatric phenotype. *Frontiers in Pediatrics, 6*(102), 1–21.

Morris, C. A., Braddock, S. R., & Council on Genetics. (2020). Health care supervision for children with Williams syndrome. *Pediatrics, 145*(2), e20193761.

Morris, C. A., & Mervis, C. B. (2020). Williams syndrome. In J. C. Carey, S. Cassidy, A. Battaglia, & D. Viskochil (Eds.), *Management of genetic syndromes* (4th ed., pp. 1021–1038). New York: Wiley.

Morris, C. A., Mervis, C. B., Hobart, H. H., Gregg, R. G., Bertrand, J., Ensing, G. J., . . . Stock, A. D. (2003). *GTF2I* hemizygosity implicated in mental retardation in Williams syndrome: Genotype–phenotype analysis of 5 families with deletions in the Williams syndrome region. *American Journal of Medical Genetics A, 123*, 45–59.

Nichols, S., Jones, W., Roman, M. J., Wulfeck, B.,

Delis, D. C., Reilly, J., & Bellugi, U. (2004). Mechanisms of verbal memory impairment in four neurodevelopmental disorders. *Brain and Language, 88,* 180–189.

Nowicki, S., Jr., & Duke, M. P. (1994). Individual differences in the nonverbal communication of affect: The Diagnostic Analysis of Nonverbal Accuracy Scale. *Journal of Nonverbal Behavior, 18,* 9–35.

O'Hearn, K., & Landau, B. (2007). Mathematical skill in individuals with Williams syndrome: Evidence from a standardized mathematics battery. *Brain and Cognition, 64,* 238–246.

Osborne, L. R., & Mervis, C. B. (2021). 7q11.23 deletion and duplication. *Current Opinion in Genetics and Development, 68,* 41–48.

Pagon, R. A., Bennett, F. C., LaVeck, B., Stewart, K. B., & Johnson, J. (1987). Williams syndrome: Features in late childhood and adolescence. *Pediatrics, 80,* 85–91.

Pérez-García, D., Brun-Gasca, C., Pérez-Jurado, L. A., & Mervis, C. B. (2017). Behavioral profiles of children with Williams syndrome from Spain and the United States: Cross-cultural similarities and differences. *American Journal on Intellectual and Developmental Disabilities, 122,* 156–172.

Phillips, K. D., & Klein-Tasman, B. P. (2009). Mental health concerns in Williams syndrome: Intervention considerations and illustrations from case examples. *Journal of Mental Health Research in Intellectual Disabilities, 2,* 110–133.

Pitts, C. H., Klein-Tasman, B. P., Osborne, J. W., & Mervis, C. B. (2016). Predictors of specific phobia in children with Williams syndrome. *Journal of Intellectual Disability Research, 60,* 1031–1042.

Plesa-Skwerer, D., Faja, S., Schofield, C., Verbalis, A., & Tager-Flusberg, H. (2006). Perceiving facial and vocal expressions of emotion in individuals with Williams syndrome. *American Journal on Mental Retardation, 111,* 15–26.

Plesa Skwerer, D., & Tager-Flusberg, H. (2016). Empathic responsiveness and helping behaviours in young children with Williams syndrome. *Journal of Intellectual Disability Research, 60,* 1010–1019.

Porter, M. A., Coltheart, M., & Langdon, R. (2007). The neuropsychological basis of hypersociability in Williams and Down syndrome. *Neuropsychologia, 45,* 2839–2849.

Quinn, J. M., & Wagner, R. K. (2018). Using meta-analytic structural equation modeling to study developmental change in relations between language and literacy. *Child Development, 89,* 1956–1969.

Rhodes, S. M., Riby, D. M., Matthews, K., & Coghill, D. R. (2011). Attention-deficit/hyperactivity disorder and Williams syndrome: Shared behavioral and neuropsychological profiles. *Journal of Clinical and Experimental Neuropsychology, 33,* 147–156.

Rhodes, S. M., Riby, D. M., Park, J., Fraser, E., & Campbell, L. E. (2010). Executive neuropsychological functioning in individuals with Williams syndrome. *Neuropsychologia, 48,* 1216–1226.

Riby, D. M., Hanley, M., Kirk, H., Clark, F., Little, K., Fleck, R., . . . Allday, M. H. (2014a). The interplay between anxiety and social functioning in Williams syndrome. *Journal of Autism and Developmental Disorders, 44,* 1220–1229.

Riby, D. M., Kirk, H., Hanley, M., & Riby, L. M. (2014b). Stranger danger awareness in Williams syndrome. *Journal of Intellectual Disability Research, 58,* 572–582.

Robinson, B. F., Mervis, C. B., & Robinson, B. W. (2003). The roles of verbal short-term memory and working memory in the acquisition of grammar by children with Williams syndrome. *Developmental Neuropsychology, 23,* 13–31.

Rothbart, M. K., & Ahadi, S. A. (1994). Temperament and the development of personality. *Journal of Abnormal Psychology, 103,* 55–66.

Rowe, M. L., & Mervis, C. B. (2006). Working memory in Williams syndrome. In T. P. Alloway & S. E. Gathercole (Eds.), *Working memory and neurodevelopmental conditions* (pp. 267–293). Hove, UK: Psychology Press.

Rutter, M., Bailey, A., & Lord, C. (2003). *The Social Communication Questionnaire.* Los Angeles: Western Psychological Services.

Scerif, G., Cornish, K., Wilding, J., Driver, J., & Karmiloff-Smith, A. (2004). Visual search in typically developing toddlers and toddlers with fragile X or Williams syndrome. *Developmental Science, 7,* 116–130.

Searcy, Y. M., Lincoln, A. J., Rose, F. E., Klima, E. S., Bavar, N., & Korenberg, J. R. (2004). The relationship between age and IQ in adults with Williams syndrome. *American Journal on Mental Retardation, 109,* 231–236.

Shalev, N., Steele, A., Nobre, A. C., Karmiloff-Smith, A., Cornish, K., & Scerif, G. (2019). Dynamic sustained attention markers differentiate atypical development: The case of Williams syndrome and Down's syndrome. *Neuropsychologia, 132*(107148), 1–9.

Somerville, M. J., Mervis, C. B., Young, E. J., Seo, E.-J., del Campo, M., Bamforth, S., . . . Osborne, L. R. (2005). Severe expressive language delay related to duplication of the Williams–Beuren locus. *New England Journal of Medicine, 353,* 1694–1701.

Stock, A. D., Spallone, P. A., Dennis, T. R., Netski, D., Morris, C. A., Mervis, C. B., & Hobart, H. H. (2003). Heat shock protein 27 gene: Chromosomal and molecular location and relationship to Williams syndrome. *American Journal of Medical Genetics A, 120,* 320–325.

Stojanovik, V. (2006). Social interaction deficits and conversational inadequacy in Williams syndrome. *Journal of Neurolinguistics, 19,* 157–173.

Strømme, P., Bjørnstad, P. G., & Ramstad, K. (2002). Prevalence estimation of Williams syndrome. *Journal of Child Neurology, 17,* 269–271.

Strong, E., Butcher, D. T., Singhania, R., Mervis, C. B., Morris, C. A., De Carvalho, D., . . . Osborne, L. R. (2015). Symmetrical dose-dependent DNA methylation profiles in children with deletion or duplication of chromosome 7q11.23. *American Journal of Human Genetics, 97,* 216–227.

Sullivan, K., Winner, E., & Tager-Flusberg, H. (2003). Can adolescents with Williams syndrome tell the difference between lies and jokes? *Developmental Neuropsychology, 23,* 85–103.

Tager-Flusberg, H., Sullivan, K., & Boshart, J. (1997). Executive functions and performance on false belief tasks. *Developmental Neuropsychology, 13,* 487–493.

Tellegen, A. (1985). Structures of mood and personality and their relevance to assessing anxiety, with an emphasis on self-report. In A. H. Tuma & J. D. Maser (Eds.), *Anxiety and the anxiety disorders* (pp. 681–716). Hillsdale, NJ: Erlbaum.

Thurman, A. J., & Fisher, M. H. (2015). The Williams syndrome social phenotype: Disentangling the contributions of social interest and social difficulties. *International Review of Research in Developmental Disabilities, 49,* 191–227.

Thurman, A. J., & Mervis, C. B. (2013). The regulatory function of social referencing in preschoolers with Down syndrome or Williams syndrome. *Journal of Neurodevelopmental Disorders, 5*(2), 1–20.

Tomc, S. A., Williamson, N. K., & Pauli, R. M. (1990). Temperament in Williams syndrome. *American Journal of Medical Genetics, 36,* 345–352.

Udwin, O., & Yule, W. (1990). Expressive language of children with Williams syndrome. *American Journal of Medical Genetics Supplement, 6,* 108–114.

Udwin, O., & Yule, W. (1991). A cognitive and behavioural phenotype in Williams syndrome. *Journal of Clinical and Experimental Neuropsychology, 13,* 232–244.

Udwin, O., Yule, W., & Martin, N. (1987). Cognitive abilities and behavioural characteristics of children with idiopathic infantile hypercalcaemia. *Journal of Child Psychology and Psychiatry, 28,* 297–309.

van der Fluit, F., Gaffrey, M. S., & Klein-Tasman, B. P. (2012). Social cognition in Williams syndrome: Relations between performance on the social attribution task and cognitive and behavioral characteristics. *Frontiers in Psychology,* 3(197), 1–11.

Van Herwegen, J., & Simms, V. (2020). Mathematical development in Williams syndrome: A systematic review. *Research in Developmental Disabilities, 106,* Article 103746.

Von Arnim, G., & Engel, P. (1964). Mental retardation related to hypercalcaemia. *Developmental Medicine and Child Neurology, 6,* 366–377.

Walsh, V. (2003). A theory of magnitude: Common cortical metrics of time, space and quantity. *Trends in Cognitive Sciences, 7,* 483–488.

Wang, P. P., & Bellugi, U. (1994). Evidence from two genetic syndromes for a dissociation between verbal and visual-spatial short-term memory. *Journal of Clinical and Experimental Neuropsychology, 16,* 317–322.

Williams, J. C. P., Barratt-Boyes, B. G., & Lowe, J. B. (1961). Supravalvular aortic stenosis. *Circulation, 24,* 1311–1318.

Williams, K. T. (2007). *Expressive Vocabulary Test–2.* Minneapolis, MN: Pearson Assessments.

Zitzer-Comfort, C., Doyle, T., Masataka, N., Korenberg, J., & Bellugi, U. (2007). Nature and nurture: Williams syndrome across cultures. *Developmental Science, 10,* 755–762.

CHAPTER 18

22q11.2 Deletion Syndrome

Renée Lajiness-O'Neill
Casey E. Swick

HISTORICAL OVERVIEW

The 22q11.2 deletion syndrome (22q11.2DS) is the most common survivable human genetic deletion disorder (Jensen et al., 2018) caused by a 1.5 to 3 megabase (Mb; 1,000,000 bases) microdeletion and rare copy number variant (CNV), resulting in a chromosomal microdeletion of ~50 protein-coding contiguous genes on the q arm of chromosome 22. Microdeletions or duplications of chromosomal regions (i.e., CNVs) are causally involved in a range of genomic and developmental brain disorders (Bassett et al., 2017). However, 22q11.2DS is characterized by common clinical features such as velar and palatal abnormalities, congenital heart defects, immune deficiencies, and hypocalcemia (McDonald-McGinn, Emanuel, & Zackai, 2013). Approximately 93% of probands have a de novo deletion (new mutation), while about 7% have inherited the 22q11.2 deletion in an autosomal dominant manner (McDonald-McGinn et al., 2013). Offspring of affected individuals have a 50% chance of inheriting the deletion. Penetrance is complete in those with 22q11.2DS, but with significant variability in clinical manifestations. The haploinsufficiency of the ~50 genes results in a multisystem disorder. Given that phenotypic expression is highly variable, some individuals experience life-threatening conditions, while others have only a few associated features. 22q11.2DS is of substantial relevance to pediatric neuropsychologists given that the phenotype includes neurodevelopmental, neurocognitive, and neuropsychiatric disorders.

During the 1980s, visible cytogenic deletions of chromosome 22q11.2 were identified in ~25% of patients with DiGeorge syndrome, an unbalanced translocation involving chromosome 22q11.2. In the 1990s, with the advent of fluorescent *in situ* hybridization (FISH), it became evident that the majority of patients with DiGeorge syndrome had a submicroscopic deletion of 22q11.2. Thereafter, the list of associated features was expanded to include dysmorphic craniofacial features, palatal anomalies, laryngotracheoesophogeal abnormalities, and speech and language impairment. Concurrently, there was recognition that other, previously described diagnoses and syndromes actually had a 22q11.2 deletion, including patients with velocardiofacial syndrome, Shprintzen syndrome (Shprintzen, 2008), conotruncal anomaly face syndrome, some cases of autosomal dominant Opitz G/BBB syndrome, and Cayler cardiofacial syndrome (Swillen & McDonald-McGinn, 2015).

The diagnosis, with its extremely broad phenotypic expression, is now referred to by the cytogenetic abnormality, 22q11.2DS.

EPIDEMIOLOGY

Prevalence

Estimated prevalence figures have varied, ranging predominately from 1 in 2,000 to 1 in 4,000 (Devriendt, Fryns, & Mortier, 1998; Girirajan, Campbell, & Eichler, 2011). The reported rates are extrapolations of limited populations using FISH. A population-based study in the United States by the Centers for Disease Control and Prevention reported an overall prevalence of appropriately 1 in 6,000 in Whites, Blacks, or African Americans and Asians, and 1 in 3,800 in Hispanics (Botto et al., 2003). Given the significant variability in expression, the prevalence is believed to be higher than previously thought. The increased use of chromosomal microarray analysis has revealed a high incidence of familial deletions in those with smaller, atypical "nested" deletions. Many adults will therefore go undetected until the deletion is diagnosed in a more seriously affected child.

Gender and Racial Distribution

Males and females are equally affected, and there is no strong evidence that the deletion is more frequently associated with any particular ethnic background. Non-Whites may be less likely to receive an early diagnosis, possibly due to less readily recognized dysmorphic features. Sex differences in the rates of psychiatric disorders are generally comparable to those reported in the general population (Swillen & McDonald-McGinn, 2015); however, the male predominance of autism spectrum disorder (ASD) and psychotic disorders in the general population has not been observed in 22q11.2DS.

ETIOLOGY, NEUROPATHOLOGY, AND NEURAL SUBSTRATES

The inheritance of 22q11.2DS is considered autosomal dominant because a single deletion in one copy of chromosome 22 is sufficient to cause this condition. However, as noted, about 90–94% of cases of 22q11.2DS are not inherited. Affected individuals typically have no history of the disorder in their family, although they can pass the condition to their offspring. In about 7–10% of cases, an individual with this condition inherits the deletion in chromosome 22 from a parent.

22q11.2DS is caused by a microdeletion within the q11.2 region of chromosome 22, that is flanked by low copy repeats (LCRs). The majority of affected individuals (~85%) have the 3 Mb deletion while the remaining (~15%) individuals have smaller, 1.5 Mb atypical deletion. The deletion is caused by a nonallelic meiotic recombination event during spermatogenesis or oogenesis resulting in either a 22q11.2 deletion or duplication. Four discrete blocks labeled LCR A–D (see Figure 18.1) are located in the region, and each block comprises multiple repeats. These blocks define the breakpoints and are used to describe the size of the deletion/duplication. The most common deletion present in 85% of those with 22q11.2DS extends from LCR A–D. The other 15% of affected individuals

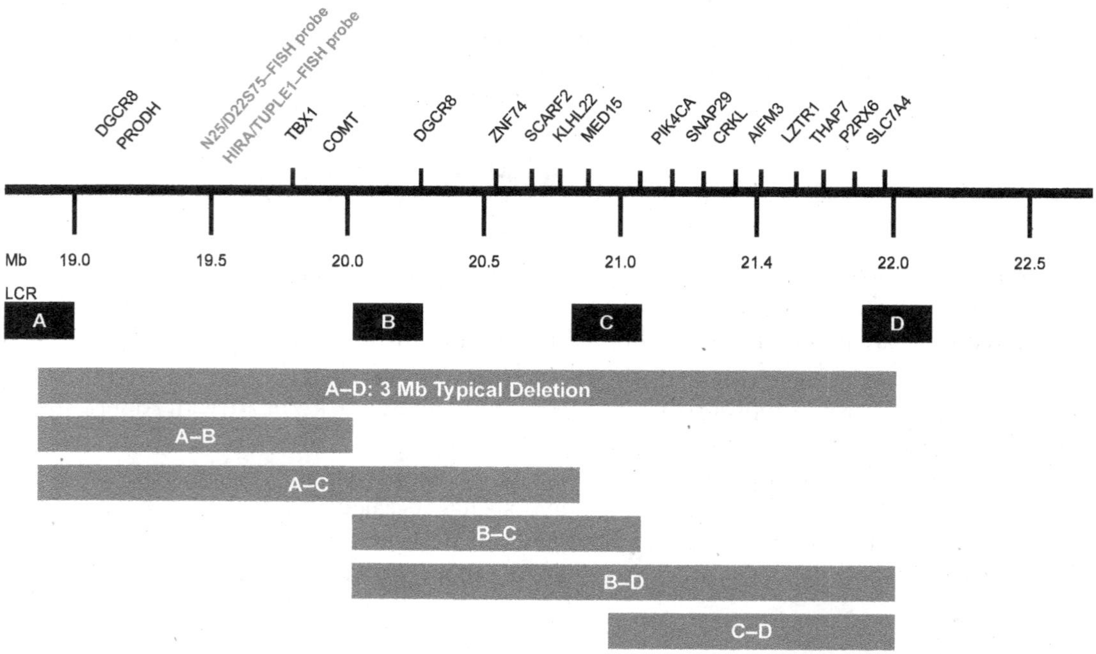

FIGURE 18.1. Low-copy repeats, represented here as A, B, C, and D, bracket the 22q11.2 deletion and define the breakpoints, with the standard 3Mb 22q11.2 deletion extending from A to D. Atypical nested deletions include A–B, A–C, B–C, B–D, and C–D. Notable genes within the deleted regions of chromosome 22q11.2 include *PRODH, TBX1,* and *COMT* within A–B, and *SNAP 29* and *CRKL1* within C–D. Note that FISH probes D22S75 (N25) and HIRA (TUPLE1) are located within A–B and would be present in those patients with nested deletions excluding the A–B region. Reprinted from Swillen and McDonald-McGinn (2015) with permission from Wiley Periodical, Inc.

have the less common, nested deletions. These atypical deletions include A–B, A–C, B–C, B–D, or C–D deletions. The 22q11.2 deletion affects neural crest cell migration of the third and fourth pharyngeal pouches, resulting in thymic hypoplasia and subsequent immunodeficiency, hypoplasia of the parathyroid glands leading to hypocalcemia, and the structural abnormalities of the outflow tract of the heart, resulting in the conotruncal cardiac defects (Swillen & McDonald-McGinn, 2015).

Molecular Genetic Testing/Cytogenetic Testing

Historically, the diagnosis of the submicroscopic deletion on chromosome 22 was made by FISH. More recently, genomewide methods such as multiplex ligation-dependent probe amplification (MLPA) and high-resolution single-nucleotide polymorphism (SNP) chromosomal microarray (CMA) have become the clinical standard due to their increased sensitivity and ability to size the deletion (Sørensen et al., 2010). CMA technologies are the most appropriate test to identify the 22q11.2DS in an individual, because the phenotype is highly variable, with children often evaluated due to developmental delay or intellectual disability.

Little is known about which genes within the 22q11.2 region contribute to clinical features of the disorder and whether there are combinatorial effects or reduced dosage of multiple genes acting in combination to modulate the phenotypic presentation. Clinical features are not completely penetrant, and there is significant phenotypic variability between patients, suggesting the involvement of variants elsewhere in the genome (Jensen et al., 2018). *TBX1*, a gene located within the A–B region, is responsible for the conotruncal cardiac anomalies (Zweier, Sticht, Aydin-Yaylagül, Campbell, & Rauch, 2007). Interactions between fibroblast growth factor genes and 22q11.2 genes have been suggested to contribute to the palatal abnormalities (Widdershoven et al., 2013). Additional large rare CNVs (> 200 Kb in size) are significantly higher in individuals with 22q11.2DS with intellectual disability. Several of the ~50 genes in the deleted region of 22q11 are involved in neurotransmission (e.g., catechol-O-methyltransferase [COMT] and proline dehydrogenase) and myelination (e.g., phosphatidylinositol 4-kinase).

Clinical/Medical Features

The pediatric neuropsychologist should consider 22q11.2DS in individuals who present with any of the following clinical features, either singularly or in combination: congenital heart disease, palatal abnormalities, hypocalcemia, immune deficiency, learning disorders, characteristic facial features such as auricular and nasal abnormalities, hooded eyelids, hypertelorism, and cleft lip and/or palate. Psychiatric conditions, particularly attention-deficit/hyperactivity disorder (ADHD), ASD, mood and anxiety disorders, and schizophrenia (in adulthood) in combination with the previously mentioned features should heighten suspicion of 22q11.2DS. Although less common, severe dysphagia, growth hormone deficiency, autoimmune disease (thrombocytopenia, juvenile rheumatoid arthritis, Graves disease, vitiligo, neutropenia, hemolytic anemia), and hearing loss should also alert a clinician to consider 22q11.2DS (McDonald-McGinn & Sullivan, 2011).

Studies have identified 22q11.2DS in a subset of patients primarily with conotruncal heart malformations including tetralogy of Fallot (TOF) (20%), truncus arteriosus (TA), ventricular septal defect (VSD; 14%), and interrupted aortic arch (IAA; 13%) (Peyvandi et al., 2013). Patients with this subset of conotruncal defects are also more likely to have a 22q11.2 deletion in the presence of a concurrent aortic arch anomaly (AAA; Peyvandi et al., 2013). The association of AAAs with deletion status underscores the role of the fourth pharyngeal arch development in 22q11.2DS. McDonald-McGinn et al. (2013) summarized the clinical findings of 250 individuals with 22q11.2DS (48% males), revealing that *congenital heart defects* are the major cause of mortality (> 90% of all deaths), with lower mortality in childhood (~5%).

Nearly 70% of individuals with 22q11.2DS have *palatal abnormalities* (McDonald-McGinn & Sullivan, 2011). In addition to velopharyngeal insufficiency, they can display structural palatal problems such as short palate, as well as functional problems, including hypotonia of the velopharyngeal musculature. Submucosal cleft palate and/or a bifid uvula are common, while overt cleft palate and cleft lip/palate are less common. Upwards of 11% of individuals with a seemingly isolated cleft palate may have 22q11.2DS, suggesting that this is the most common genetic disorder associated with cleft palate, and submucosal cleft. 22q11.2DS is also the most common genetic cause of congenital velopharyngeal insufficiency. More than one-third of children with 22q11.2DS have significant *feeding difficulties*, frequently severe dysphagia requiring nasogastric tube feedings and/or gastrostomy tube placement.

The rates of *hypocalcemia* range from 17 to 60% (McDonald-McGinn et al., 2013; Ryan et al., 1997). Hypocalcemia is due to hypoparathyroidism caused by aplasia or hypoplasia of the parathyroid gland. Hypocalcemia is most severe during the neonatal period, enters latency in later childhood, and manifests again in adolescence. Calcium homeostasis typically normalizes with age. When seizures are observed in those with 22q11.2DS, it is most often associated with hypocalcemia.

Immunodeficiency occurs due to thymic hypoplasia (McDonald-McGinn et al., 2013). Impaired T cell production is the primary defect due to the role of the thymus to support T cell maturation. Children often experience frequent sinusitis or otitis media and lower respiratory infections. Autoimmune disease is common in children with 22q11.2DS. Juvenile rheumatoid arthritis and autoimmune cytopenias are the most common disorders and may occur 20–100 times more frequently than in the general population (McDonald-McGinn et al., 2013). The rate of immune thrombocytopenia has been reported to be 200 times more frequent than that in the general population in those with 22q11.2DS.

A significant number of *craniofacial findings* are reported, including auricular and nasal abnormalities, hooded eyelids, ocular hypertelorism, cleft lip and palate, craniosynostosis, and asymmetric crying faces (McDonald-McGinn et al., 2013). Elongated faces and malar flatness are also variably present. Ear abnormalities include cupped, microtic, and protuberant ears, overfolded or squared helices, preauricular tags and pits, and narrow external auditory meatus. Individuals with 22q11.2DS often have a prominent nasal root, bulbous nasal tip, hypoplastic alae nasi, and/or nasal dimple/bifid nasal tip.

Central Nervous System/Neuroimaging Features

Qualitative Abnormalities

Central nervous system (CNS) developmental anomalies that affect midline brain structures such as cavum vergae or cavum septum pellucidum occur in 30–45% of patient samples (Tan, Arnone, McIntosh, & Ebmeier, 2009). Variable rates of microcephaly are reported (Kobrynski & Sullivan, 2007; McDonald-McGinn et al., 2013), and polymicrogyria is noted in a small number of individuals (Tan et al., 2009). White matter hyperintensities on T2-weighted magnetic resonance imaging (MRI) and perisylvian dysplasia are also reported (Bingham et al., 1997).

Structural/Volumetric Findings

Widespread cortical changes are noted in children and adolescents with 22q11.2DS, including enlarged ventricles and a decrease in total brain volume, with white matter affected more than gray matter (Kates et al., 2001). Reductions in cortical thickness, surface area, gyral complexity, and alterations in white matter microstructure are similar to those found in cases of idiopathic schizophrenia (Roalf et al., 2017).

A meta-analysis of volumetric MRI studies reported an increase in the size of the corpus callosum, but global brain volumetric reductions in all major lobar regions (i.e., frontal, temporal, parietal, and occipital), as well as decreased volume of the hippocampus and cerebellum (Tan et al., 2009). However, there may be a relative sparing of frontal lobe volumes in children, who appear to demonstrate greater reductions in posterior regions. More significant white matter loss is noted in left occipital and parietal regions (Barnea-Goraly et al., 2003; Kates et al., 2001), and greater volumetric reductions are noted in the cerebellum, caudate, thalamus, fusiform gyrus, and in the posterior relative to anterior corpus callosum (Campbell et al., 2006; Tan et al., 2009). However, larger right caudal volumes have also been noted (Campbell et al., 2006). Studies of cortical thickness in children with 22q11.2DS reveal lateral cortical thinning of the parieto–occipital, occipital, and inferior prefrontal regions, and medial cortical thinning in the anterior and posterior cingulate, medial frontal gyrus, subgenual prefrontal cortex, cuneus, and lingual gyrus (Bearden et al., 2009).

The Enhancing Neuroimaging Genetics through Meta-Analysis (ENIGMA) 22q11.2 Working Group, has examined 474 subjects (age = 18.2+/- 8.6; 46.9% female) with 22q11.2DS from 10 centers worldwide and 315 typically developing matched controls (Sun et al., 2020). Compared to controls, individuals with 22q11.2DS have (1) thicker cortical gray matter overall but with focal thickness reductions in temporal, cingulate, and parahippocampal cortices, as well as (2) widespread reductions in cortical surface area. The reductions in surface area appear to be most prominent in parieto–occipital regions and anterior cingulate. When cortical structures of individuals with 22q11.2DS with psychosis were compared to individuals with idiopathic schizophrenia, significant convergence in affected cortical regions was reported, specifically in frontotemporal brain regions (Sun et al., 2020).

Structural connectivity in 22q11.2DS has been examined primarily with voxel-based diffusion tensor imaging (DTI) measures and more recently with tractography or graph theoretical matrices (see review by Scariati, Padula, Schaer, & Eliez, 2016). Most of the voxel-based studies used whole-brain approaches, which have revealed equivocal findings. Both reduced and increased fractional anisotropy (a metric of white matter integrity) has been reported in frontal, temporal, and parietal cortices. Alterations are noted in long association tracts, including the inferior and superior longitudinal fasciculi (ILF and SLF, respectively) and the inferior fronto-occipital fasciculus (IFOF), uncinate fasciculus, arcuate fasciculus, and cingulum bundle. Consistent reductions in fractional anisotropy have been noted in the ILF, uncinate, and frontoparietal course of the arcuate. Discordant results are noted in the SLF and cingulum bundle, with reports of both increased and decreased fractional anisotropy. Studies reporting on axial diffusivity (a metric of axonal integrity) reveal a more consistent reduction in axial diffusivity in individuals with 22q11.2DS, specifically in the SLF, ILF, IFOF, and cingulum (Jalbrzikowski et al., 2014; Scariati et al., 2016).

Functional Connectivity

Only recently has functional connectivity been examined in adolescents and adults with 22q11.2DS (Scariati et al., 2016). Using resting-state fMRI (rs-fMRI) Scariati and colleagues (2014) reported a predominance of frontal dysconnectivity and an impairment of visuospatial networks including parietal, occipital, and right inferior temporal connectivity. Alterations in sensorimotor networks and decreased connectivity between anterior and posterior nodes of the default mode network are also reported (Padula et al., 2015).

NEUROPSYCHOLOGICAL CONSEQUENCES

General Intellectual Functioning

The majority of investigations of intellectual functioning in this population have involved children and adolescents. Less is known about the intellectual ability of adults with 22q11.2DS (Green et al., 2009). Intellectual functioning is children and adolescents is highly variable and follows a normal distribution centered about 2 standard deviations (30 points) below the normative mean. Mean Full Scale IQ (FSIQ) tends to be in the mid-70s (70–75). About 55% of individuals have borderline to average intelligence (FSIQ > 70), with the majority of scores falling in the borderline range (FSIQ 70–84) (Antshel, Fremont, & Kates, 2008; Schneider et al., 2014). About 35–45% have mild (to moderate) intellectual disability (FSIQ 55–70). More severe intellectual disability is uncommon in children but is more frequent in adults (Swillen & McDonald-McGinn, 2015). Familial deletions have been associated with lower IQ scores compared to de novo deletions. Verbal reasoning skills are better developed than visuospatial reasoning, especially earlier in childhood, although there is some question as to whether this gap persists over time (Moberg et al., 2018). A possible basis for this discrepancy is that individuals with 22q11.2DS are more impaired in skills related to fluid as opposed to crystallized intelligence. While fund of knowledge tends to remain intact, these individuals may have more difficulty in higher-level integration of skills and complex reasoning.

Sensorimotor, Perceptual–Motor, and Visuospatial Skills

Individuals with 22q11.2DS demonstrate difficulties with motor coordination and visual perception. These difficulties are not closely related to IQ and the presence of more severe psychopathology such as schizophrenia but are associated with ASD, ADHD, and anxiety (Cunningham et al., 2019). Developmental coordination disorder (DCD) is prevalent in this population, though more common in boys. ADHD, especially the inattentive type, is often accompanied by motor and coordination difficulties (Cunningham et al., 2018). Because 22q11.2DS is associated with movement disorders later in life, inclusion of motor assessment as part of clinical standards for childhood management of the disorder could also help in early identification of motor impairment.

Poorer visuomotor and visuospatial skills are consistently reported in individuals with 22q11.2DS, including deficits in motor speed, form coherence, and perceptual-motor and spatial reasoning skills. Although the cortical and pathophysiological mechanisms for these deficits are an active area of investigation, a generalized impairment in complex visual processing has also been proposed to account for these deficits (McCabe, Rich, Loughland, Schall, & Campbell, 2011). Numerous studies have suggested that there are disruptions in the early stages of sensory processing that may precede and contribute to the often reported higher-order perceptual deficits. Deficits on tasks involving both dorsal (*motion coherence*) and ventral stream (*form coherence*) processing have been reported (Howley, Prasad, Pender, & Murphy, 2012; Lajiness-O'Neill et al., 2005), with some evidence that deficits in the dorsal stream may be specific to the 22q11.2DS genotype (Piccini et al., 2017). A more general breakdown in higher-order fluid reasoning and integration of skills has also been proposed to explain these deficits (Jacobson et al., 2010).

Speech and Language

Around 60% of children and 30% of adults with 22q11.2DS have hearing impairment, most often involving conductive loss but in some cases involving sensorineural or mixed types of impairment (Persson, Friman, Oskarsdottir, & Jonsson, 2012). Speech is marked by high rates of velopharyngeal impairment, disordered articulation, and reduced intelligibility. Speech motor deficits are characteristic of 22q11.2DS, at least in younger children (Baylis & Shriberg, 2018). Though physical limitations and articulation difficulties contribute to language impairments, speech–language difficulties exist regardless of health status, indicating that these difficulties are part of the 22q11.2DS phenotype.

Early language development is delayed, with difficulties in both receptive and expressive language (Glaser et al., 2002; Solot et al., 2001). Early investigators reported slightly better receptive compared to expressive language development prior to school age (< 6 years) (Golding-Kushner, Weller, & Shprintzen, 1985). Additional studies have failed to find significant differences in receptive and expressive language by school age (Gerdes, Solot, Wang, McDonald-McGinn, & Zackai, 2001; Moss et al., 1999). In contrast, language comprehension problems are well documented (Van Den Heuvel, Manders, Swillen, & Zink, 2018). During school years, deficits in reading comprehension also become evident. Reports have suggested that comprehension difficulties are the most pronounced in processing word meanings within sentences (Persson et al., 2006). School-age children with 22q11.2DS demonstrate difficulties with language at the sentence level, even when compared to peers with similar IQ (Van Den Heuvel et al., 2018). When compared to children with idiopathic intellectual disability (IID), who make progress in comprehending instructions over time, children with 22q11.2DS only improve in understanding simple phrases. Despite evidence that language skills may be an area of relative strength (Solot et al., 2001), these children may thus have weaknesses in receptive language and may be especially challenged by more complex, abstract, and deductive language processes.

Attention

Attentional difficulties, particularly in attentional shifting, are a well-recognized feature of the cognitive phenotype of 22q11.2DS. Deficits with sustained attention or vigilance are variably reported, although poor vigilance is considered a key predictor of psychosis in 22q11.2DS (Kates et al., 2015). Sobin et al. (2004, 2005) used the NEPSY (a developmental NEuroPSYchological assessment) and Attention Network Test to investigate attention in youth with 22q11.2DS. Below-average ability was noted on both visual and auditory attention tasks. Individuals with 22q11.2DS display a particular deficit in orientation of attention in space, specifically, shifting attention from one location and reorienting to another target location (Bish, Chiodo, Mattei, & Simon, 2007; Simon et al., 2005). Problems with higher-order attentional tasks that involve planning persist into adulthood.

ADHD is common in 22q11.2DS, with a prevalence rate of 30–40% (Antshel et al., 2014); however, the higher prevalence of ADHD in males reported in the general population is not observed in individuals with 22q11.2DS. Longitudinal research reveals that upwards of 65% of children with 22q11.2DS continue to exhibit symptoms of ADHD in adolescence (Antshel et al., 2014), and that childhood factors associated with persistence include higher rates of familial ADHD and depression, higher levels of hyperactivity, and intrusion errors on a verbal list learning test (California Verbal Learning Test—Children's Version [CVLT-C]). Given the high base rate of psychosis and schizophrenia in 22q11.2DS, this condition serves as a genetic model for the development of symptoms of thought disorder in other psychopathologies. ADHD symptoms, particularly inattention, may be related to the onset of psychosis and could even serve as a marker of a prodromal period (Kates et al., 2015; Niarchou et al., 2018).

Memory and Learning

The memory profile of children with 22q11.2DS mirrors that of their intellectual profile, with better verbal compared to visual memory abilities (Furniss, Biswas, Gumber, & Singh, 2011; Lajiness-O'Neill et al., 2005). The magnitude of difference between verbal and visuospatial memory does not appear to be related to FSIQ (Bearden, Woodin, Wang, & Moss, 2001). General memory composites are typically low average (80–89), while rote verbal learning is average (90–109). With respect to memory processes, encoding seems to be relatively intact for individuals with 22q11.2DS, while retrieval is more difficult. Memory performance may be similar to that observed in association with schizophrenia. Individuals with 22q11.2DS do not appear to benefit from contextual cues for retrieval (Debbané, Glaser, & Eliez, 2008). Consistent with other studies that report preservation of verbal list learning with impaired memory for sentences (Van Den Heuvel et al., 2018), this pattern suggests an ineffectual use of context to retrieve meaningful information. This finding also raises the possibility that the superiority of verbal relative to visual memory may only apply to tasks requiring less complex information processing.

The cognitive factors contributing to memory impairment are unclear. In a study by Lajiness-O'Neill et al. (2005) that included siblings of participants with 22q11.2DS, as well as an additional IQ control group, children with 22q11.2DS *and* their siblings demonstrated significantly better verbal than visual memory performance compared to controls. This finding suggests that the discrepancy between verbal and visual memory may reflect genetic risk factors related to but not a direct result of the 22q1.2 deletion. Additionally, children with 22q11.2DS perform poorly and more similarly to children with ASD on facial memory, another reported weakness. The superiority of verbal memory may be a core feature of 22q11.2DS, although further investigations are warranted to examine memory development (Jacobson et al., 2010).

Another characteristic of the neuropsychological profile of 22q11.2DS is the presence of *learning difficulties* in school-age children, particularly with math. Stronger reading decoding and spelling abilities compared to math are universally reported (Antshel et al., 2008). Individuals with 22q11.2DS experience difficulty with numerical operations and mathematical reasoning, as well as reading comprehension (Jacobson et al., 2010). Other specific deficits in math are with tasks involving number and object magnitude comparisons, time perception, and serial order (Furniss et al., 2011). Simon and colleagues (2002) suggest that math deficits may be related to visuospatial memory difficulties. Simple arithmetical operations, such as judging the relative magnitude of two values, may be impaired because they entail spatial representations of the quantities. A review by De Smedt, Swillen, Verschaffel, and Ghesqui (2009) indicates that individuals with 22q11.2DS have specific difficulty determining quantities and deriving numerical meaning from symbols, but are able to perform as well as control children on number reading, counting backwards, dot counting, single-digit multiplication, and single-digit addition and subtraction not involving borrowing. Children with 22q11.2DS also can solve problems as quickly as controls using a retrieval strategy but are slow in applying calculation strategies. This pattern of ability suggests that these children may have less difficulty with the verbal subsystem involved in number processing (and integrity of the angular gyrus) than with the quantity subsystem (and integrity of the intraparietal sulcus) (De Smedt et al., 2009; Simon et al., 2005). Poor math performance and procedural math difficulties appear unrelated to problems accessing rote information from long-term storage. Instead, math difficulties appear to reflect a breakdown in basic visuospatial and attentional abilities believed to be foundational to later math skills learning. Frontoparietal dysfunction is postulated to be a potential neural mechanism underlying disordered math learning in 22q11.2DS.

Executive Functions

Executive functioning is variably affected in individuals with 22q11.2DS, with deficits in cognitive flexibility, set shifting, working memory, planning, and developing organizational strategies to complete problem-solving tasks (Campbell et al., 2010). For example, individuals with 22q11.2DS experience difficulty on Trails B (Woodin et al., 2001) and display a tendency toward perseverative errors on the Wisconsin Card Sorting Test (Lajiness-O'Neill et al., 2006). The verbal–visual split often seen in IQ and some aspects of attention and memory is not consistently observed in working memory profiles in 22q11.2DS. These individuals are also at risk for weaknesses in verbal working memory (Lajiness-O'Neill et al., 2005). However, investigators have not reported specific problems with inhibitory control on measures such as the Test of Variables of Attention (TOVA) or go/no-go paradigms (Gothelf et al., 2007; Lajiness-O'Neill et al., 2006).

Executive functioning changes may also indicate risk for development of psychotic symptoms in late adolescence and early adulthood. When compared with healthy controls, individuals with 22q11.2DS with psychotic symptoms completed fewer categories and made more errors on a modified card sort task, and their errors were positively related to clinician-rated symptoms of psychosis (Rockers et al., 2009).

Social Cognition

Impaired social cognition is common in individuals with 22q11.2DS, as documented on tasks assessing emotion processing, social perception, attribution bias, and theory of mind (ToM). Eye-tracking technology has also been used to examine face exploration during emotion processing (Norkett, Lincoln, Gonzalez-Heydrich, & Angelo, 2017). Accumulating evidence of social-cognitive deficits in periods before the onset of psychosis suggests that these problems may be useful predictors of psychiatric disorder and thus a worthwhile target for treatment (Norkett et al., 2017).

Individuals with 22q11.2DS display impaired emotion processing and ToM, although other neurocognitive and intellectual deficits may partially account for these difficulties. Emotion recognition or identification, as well as emotion differentiation (i.e., distinguishing between levels of emotional intensity), has been assessed in 22q11.2DS across a variety of facial and vocal affect stimuli (Leleu et al., 2016). Emotion recognition impairment for basic emotions (happy, sad, anger, fear) may be more evident on facial compared to vocal affect recognition tasks (Shashi et al., 2011). Individuals with 22q11.2DS also may take longer or require more intense facial cues to recognize emotions (Franchini et al., 2016; Leleu et al., 2016). Eye-tracking technology reveals that these individuals have a tendency to display poor visual exploration patterns of faces and a lack of attention to salient facial features. ToM has been examined with tools such as the The Awareness of Social Inference Test (TASIT) and false-belief tasks. Results reveal that individuals with 22q11.2DS demonstrate impaired ToM compared to controls, though deficits in higher-order processing or executive functioning may be contributory (Campbell, McCabe, Melville, Strutt, & Schall, 2015). Research is needed on the early development of social-cognitive abilities in this population to characterize how and when such deficits surface and their relationship to psychiatric comorbidity. There is some evidence that social-cognitive deficits and related difficulties in social interactions increase risks for developing positive and negative symptoms of psychosis (Biswas & Furniss, 2016).

Adaptive and Social Functioning

Longitudinal research suggests that parent-reported executive functioning abilities in childhood predict adaptive functioning in young adulthood (Albert, Abu-Ramadan, Kates, Fremont, & Antshel, 2018). According to the 22q11.2DS International Consortium (Schneider et al., 2014), anxiety disorders in children with 22q11.2DS are more closely related to adaptive functioning than IQ. In contrast, both lower intellectual functioning and schizophrenia predict poorer adaptive functioning in adulthood, though employability and activities of daily living are considered relative strengths in adults with this disorder (Butcher et al., 2012).

Few investigations have examined potential mechanisms underlying the social disruption in individuals with 22q11.2DS. Anxiety, ADHD, ASD, schizophrenia, and psychosis are psychopathologies accompanied by deficits in social functioning. Individual with 22q11.2DS are at increased risk for one or more of these disorders and are thus particularly vulnerable to social impairment. Weaknesses in social cognition, such as having a poor understanding of the intent of others or difficulty identifying emotional states likely further contribute to the socialization deficits (Norkett et al., 2017; Olszewski et al., 2017). Lower intellectual functioning and accompanying executive deficits also likely contribute to social problems, though they may not fully account for the degree of social impairment (Campbell et al., 2015). An investigation examining social trajectories in children with 22q11.2DS and IID revealed that they were more likely to exhibit increased social problems over time compared to their IQ-matched peers (Van Den Heuvel et al., 2018). Efforts to facilitate socialization in children with 22q11.2DS may thus enhance functional outcomes later in life (Campbell et al., 2015).

Emotional and Behavioral Adjustment

The most prevalent disorders in children and adolescents with 22q11.2DS are ADHD (30–40%), oppositional defiant disorder (8–43%), specific and social phobias (23–61%), generalized anxiety disorder (17–29%), separation anxiety disorder (16–21%), obsessive-compulsive disorder (4–33%), and autism spectrum disorders (14–45%), while, as noted earlier, 25–30% of adult cases develop schizophrenia (Gothelf et al., 2005; Jacobson et al., 2010). Anxiety disorders are more prevalent than mood disorders at all ages, especially in children (Schneider et al., 2014), and about one-third qualify for multiple anxiety disorders. Mood disorders emerge in young adults, possibly related to difficulties with social integration and independence, though earlier reports of elevated rates of bipolar disorder have not been confirmed. Early-onset psychosis is relatively common in individuals with 22q11.2DS, with results from the International Consortium on Brain Behavior in 22q11.2 DS reporting that 10% of the adolescents studied qualified for a diagnosis of psychotic disorder. Rates of psychotic disorder "not otherwise specified" are significantly more prevalent in children with 22q11.2DS, while schizophrenia spectrum disorders increase significantly in adolescence and young adulthood (Schneider et al., 2014) (see Plate 18.1 in the color insert).

Symptoms of psychosis can be evident as early as 6 years of age, even in individuals not diagnosed with psychosis. In addition, there is some indication that childhood trauma (e.g., sexual abuse, negative home environment) may be specifically implicated in the development of positive symptoms of psychosis, particularly hallucinations (Varese, Barkus, & Bentall, 2012).

Brain–Behavior Relationships

A number of investigators have examined both cross-sectional and longitudinal relationships between neuroanatomical findings and the cognitive and psychiatric phenotype of 22q11.2DS. Dufour and colleagues (2008) examined subgroups of individuals diagnosed with 22q11.2DS with and without symptoms of psychosis, and with high and low executive functioning (> 9 years). Reductions in right cingulate volumes were noted in those with lower executive functioning and with symptoms of psychoses. In a cohort of adolescents with 22q11.2DS, Perlstein et al. (2014) reported a negative relationship between positive prodromal symptoms on the Scale of Prodromal Symptoms (SOPS) and measures of radial diffusivity in the white matter tracts of the uncinate fasciculus and anterior limb of the internal capsule. Jalbrzikowski et al. (2014) reported that for both individuals with 22q11.2DS and controls, reduced axial diffusivity in the IFOF was related to more symptoms of psychopathology as assessed on the SOPS, while higher axial diffusivity in the IFOF was associated with better social cognition (Jalbrzikowski et al., 2013, 2014). Kates and colleagues (2011) obtained measures of regional brain volumes, IQ, and psychiatric status at mean age 11.9 years and completed the SOPS at mean age 15.1 years. Higher SOPS Positive Symptom scores were associated with white matter volume reductions and in temporal lobe gray matter.

Neuroimaging studies in children, adolescents, and young adults with 22q11.2DS further illustrate a pattern of cortical abnormalities that likely underlie the perceptual–motor and visuospatial deficits observed in 22q11.2DS. This pattern includes decreased cortical thickness over superior parietal and parieto-occipital regions (Franchini et al., 2016), alterations in parietal and occipital gray and white matter (Campbell et al., 2006; Eliez et al., 2001; Kates et al., 2001), atypical trajectory in cortical gyrification of parietal regions, and reduced functional connectivity in parietal, temporal, and occipital regions (Scariati et al., 2014), with specific alterations noted in frontoparietal connectivity (Barnea-Goraly et al., 2003). Reductions in cortical thickness in bilateral ventromedial occipitotemporal cortices (Bearden et al., 2009), as well as volumetric reduction in bilateral inferior temporal cortices (Jalbrzikowski et al., 2013), further support altered cortical development and functioning as a major contributor to deficits visual perception and complex visuospatial processing.

DEVELOPMENTAL CONSIDERATIONS

Genetic Counseling

Prenatal testing for pregnancies at increased risk based on family history may be warranted if the diagnosis has been confirmed in an affected family member. Many patients are now being diagnosed prenatally by fetal ultrasound/echocardiography, often as a result of evaluations for congenital cardiac disease. Additional prenatal conditions that may justify testing including polyhydramnios, cleft lip and/or palate, polydactyly, clubfoot, renal anomalies, diaphragmatic hernia, spina bifida, and craniosynostosis (McDonald-McGinn et al., 2013).

Early Development/Preschool

Limited data are available on developmental outcome during infancy and early childhood (0–4 years), though the majority of individuals with 22q11.2DS have a history of hypotonia in infancy. Gross and fine motor difficulties and speech problems and language delay predominate in infancy and toddlerhood (Gerdes et al., 2001; Solot et al., 2001; Swillen et al., 1999). In a sample of 88 children with 22q11.2DS examined retrospectively, gross motor functioning and expressive language were more delayed than other areas of development (Roizen et al., 2007). The average age for walking unsupported is about 18 months of age. In an early investigation by Swillen et al. (1997) of children ages 6–30 months, higher functioning children (IQ > 70) spoke their first words at ~18 months of age and their first sentences at ~36 months old. In contrast, children with lower IQs (IQ < 70) spoke their first words at ~32 months and used sentences at ~60 months. Many children are nonverbal at 2–3 years of age.

While early developmental assessment often reveals delayed cognitive and motor skills, early delays are not always predictive of later intellectual impairment (Antshel et al., 2008). Some studies report that early receptive language delays predict later intellectual functioning. In a study of toddlers who underwent developmental assessment, mental development was average in about one-fifth of the group, mildly delayed in about one-third, and significantly delayed in nearly one-half (McDonald-McGinn et al., 2013). Motor development was average or mildly delayed in about 20% of the sample and significantly delayed in nearly 80%. Despite their early learning difficulties, preschoolers with this condition function at a somewhat higher IQ level than infants and toddlers. A cross-sectional investigation of preschoolers using the Wechsler Preschool and Primary Scale of Intelligence (WPPSI-R) revealed similar proportions of children functioning within the average range (IQ > 85), the mildly delayed range (IQ 70–85), and delayed range (IQ < 75). The mean FSIQ and PIQs were 78 and mean VIQ was 82 (Antshel et al., 2008; Gerdes et al., 2001).

Childhood

IQ scores may be somewhat unstable in children with 22q11.2DS, and the discrepancy between verbal and visuospatial skills is less evident with advancing age. Both cross-sectional (Green et al., 2009) and longitudinal investigations (Antshel et al., 2010; Duijff, Klaassen, Beemer, Sinnema, & Vorstman, 2013) suggest declines in IQ with age, primarily due to reductions in VIQ. Although declines in IQ starting in early childhood may be partially explained as the result of children "growing into" their deficits, a subgroup of children exhibit an absolute loss of cognitive ability measured over 2- and 6-year follow-ups (Duijff et al., 2013).

With respect to the developmental progression of behavioral features, children with 22q11.2DS display more externalizing features (e.g., oppositionality, impulsivity) in early childhood and more internalizing features (e.g., anxiety, depression, withdrawal) in adolescence (Swillen et al., 1999). Social impairment has been documented across development for those with and without psychiatric diagnoses.

Adolescence and Adulthood

Recent investigations of developmental trajectories in IQ in youth with 22q11.2DS indicate continued functioning within the borderline to very low range from childhood into adolescence (Duijff et al., 2013; Swillen & McDonald-McGinn, 2015), with a lessening of the discrepancy between visuospatial and language abilities (Moberg et al., 2018). A decline in verbal reasoning skills is steeper for children who subsequently develop psychotic symptoms (Evers et al., 2014). Longitudinal investigations demonstrate that from primary/elementary school, several divergent trajectories are apparent: (1) a relatively stable IQ trajectory; (2) a decrease in IQ that reflects insufficient cognitive development to maintain pace with peers; and (3) an absolute decline in intellect, revealed by lower subtest raw scores on at least two subtests. There is some suggestion that the latter trajectory may represent children at risk for schizophrenia. The International 22q11.2 Brain Behavior Consortium reports that children with 22q11.2DS demonstrate an average decline of 7 FSIQ points (~1/2 *SD*) or 9 VIQ points (Swillen & McDonald-McGinn, 2015; Vorstman et al., 2015). In a subgroup that developed psychotic symptoms, this decline was steeper. The precise mechanism of this cognitive decline has yet to be elucidated. About 60% of adults have a psychiatric disorder, including schizophrenia in about 25–30% and high rates of anxiety and mood disorders (Bassett et al., 2011). Premature death has also been reported in adults (Bassett et al., 2009).

PREDICTORS AND MODERATORS

The neurodevelopmental outcome of 22q11.2DS is contingent on the interaction of multiple risk and protective factors that can be categorized as (1) person-specific, (2) family and environmental, and (3) time and age dependent (Swillen, Moss, & Duijff, 2018). Both genetic and environmental factors play an essential role in cognitive development over time and throughout the lifespan. Several factors help to explain the wide variability in intellectual and cognitive outcome in patients with 22q11.2DS, including origin of the deletion (familial vs. de novo), genetic variation within the 22q11.2 region, parental and sibling IQ, and environmental factors such as socioeconomic status. A steeper early cognitive decline is a risk factor for the development of psychosis. VIQ, visual memory, and executive functioning are also related to mental health outcomes (Biswas & Furniss, 2016).

Biological Factors

A more severe cognitive phenotype is found in inherited cases, but outcomes are also related to socioeconomic factors, heritable components contributed by the unaffected parent, variants in the genes on the intact 22q11.2, variation within the 22q11.2 region, prematurity and untreated hypocalcemia, seizures, and undiagnosed or untreated thyroid disease. One of the genes mapping to the region of chromosome 22 deleted in this disorder codes for COMT, an enzyme critical in the metabolism of dopamine in the prefrontal cortex (Van, Boot, & Bassett, 2017). A functional polymorphism involving a valine/methionine substitution is associated with lower or higher COMT activity, and evidence implicates *COMT* as a possible risk factor for psychiatric symptomatology (Bearden et al., 2005). Much less is known about other possible risk factors contributing to outcome, such as the size of the deletion, additional genes within the region (e.g., *PRODH*, *TBX1*, *CRKL1*) and other genetic effects, the negative impact of associated medical problems (e.g., severity and type of congenital heart disease (CHD), medical stress, temperament, level of stress sensitivity and anxiety, and the additive or interacting effects of comorbid ID, additional neurodevelopmental disorders (e.g., ADHD, ASD) and psychiatric disorders. Given the high but incomplete penetrance of the 22q11.2 deletion for schizophrenia, it is vital to identify additional genetic factors that increase the probability of an individual developing this illness. Research from the International 22q11.2 Brain and Behavior Consortium suggests that additional rare CNVs overlapping one or more protein-coding genes outside of the 22q11.2 region contribute to the schizophrenia risk, supporting a multigenic hypothesis for schizophrenia (Bassett et al., 2017).

Psychological and Social Factors

Cross-sectional and longitudinal studies have identified a decline in VIQ as a risk factor for the development of psychotic disorder (Antshel et al., 2010; Green et al., 2009). Antshel et al. (2010) followed 70 youth, age 15 years, who were originally assessed at 11.9 years. While no participants met diagnostic criteria for schizophrenia at follow-up, the best predictors of the overall score from the SOPS were baseline VIQ, visual memory ability, processing speed, executive functioning, and parent-reported atypical and anxious behaviors. Selective deficits in VIQ performance are evident by 11 years of age for children at risk for a psychotic disorder (Vorstman et al., 2015). Recent investigations have also identified social-perceptual and social-cognitive abilities as correlates of emotional problems and symptoms of psychosis. Performance on TOM tasks predicts the severity of positive symptoms, while processing speed is the best predictor of negative symptoms (Jalbrzikowski et al., 2012).

Research has identified family and environmental factors related to social-behavioral and psychiatric outcomes in children with 22q11.2DS, including socioeconomic status (Allen et al., 2014; De Smedt et al., 2007), parental and sibling IQ (Olszewski et al., 2017) and family organization (Allen et al., 2014; Kates et al., 2015). Later prodromal/overt psychosis is least likely in children with low avoidant-anxiety, stronger verbal learning, and higher visual vigilance, but more likely in individuals with low dysregulation and low family organization. Many potential risk factors remain understudied, such as negative parent–child interactions or ineffective parenting styles, parental stress, and limited quality of life and social network/supports.

Cross-Cultural and International Considerations

Most studies of individuals with 22q11.2DS have focused on those of European descent. Research on diverse populations has been more challenging (Kruszka et al., 2017; Liu et al., 2014; McDonald-McGinn et al., 2005). Craniofacial dysmorphisms in African Americans are different than those reported in Caucasians. Characteristic facial features that would suggest a possible diagnosis of 22q11.2DS are often not detected in Chinese adults (Liu et al., 2014). A large study of individuals with 22q11.2DS from 11 countries (average age 11.7) grouped participants into the categories African descent (African), Asian, and Latin American using clinical and facial analysis technology to examine the phenotype across populations. CHD and learning problems were found in more than 50% of the participants, but the researchers found limited similarity between groups based on specific clinical features. More consistency was evident when Africans were removed from the analysis, suggesting difficulties in classification of the clinical features of individuals in this category.

Recently, the largest study of lifetime psychiatric diagnoses in 22q11.2DS (N = 1,402; ages 6–68 years) examined data from cohorts from 22 international sites (Schneider et al., 2014) and reported similar prevalence and developmental trends across countries. ADHD, ASD, and anxiety disorders were the most common diagnoses in childhood, while rates of psychosis and mood disorders increased substantially in adolescence and young adulthood. Generalized anxiety disorder and specific and social phobia were most frequently reported during childhood and adolescence.

TREATMENT AND INTERVENTION

Given the clinical complexity of 22q11.2DS, a multidisciplinary team approach is warranted. The team may include any of the following subspecialties depending on the child's clinical characteristics: audiology, cardiology, psychology/neuropsychology, dental, endocrine, feeding specialist, gastroenterology, general pediatrics, surgery, immunology, clinical genetics, neurology/neurosurgery, ophthalmology, orthopedics, otolaryngology, psychiatry, pulmonary, rheumatology, speech and language pathology, and urology. The International 22q11.2 Consortium developed practice guidelines for managing patients with 22q11.2DS that emphasizes this complexity and the multisystem nature of the condition and includes recommendations for assessment by age and at diagnosis (Bassett et al., 2011).

Medical Treatment

Surgical and medical treatments and monitoring are required for individuals affected with CHD and/or palatal and/or cleft anomalies. Calcium supplementation and thyroid monitoring by endocrinology is warranted for individuals with hypocalcemia. Regular blood examinations are critical for early diagnosis and treatment of hypocalcemia. Immune deficiency requires close monitoring and treatment of infections. A feeding specialist may be indicated to address gastroesophageal reflux and gastrointestinal dysmotility. Endocrinology can be consulted to treat the child's growth hormone deficiency and small stature.

Developmental Intervention

Early intervention by developmental and allied health specialists (i.e., psychology, occupational, physical, and speech therapy) is recommended to monitor development, minimize long-term effects of delays, and foster development. Speech therapy including the initiation of sign language is vital when the diagnosis is made early in development. In school-age children, intervention should focus on the diagnosis and management of ADHD and learning disorders, particularly math impairment. Standard management options are suggested for ADHD including behavioral and pharmacological treatment. Stimulants are effective and have been recently reported to be relatively well tolerated by children with 22q11.2DS (Schneider et al., 2014), though monitoring of cardiovascular status during treatment is recommended. As social deficits can negatively impact adjustment, treatments to improve social functioning are warranted. Approaches to consider are adapting social demands to ensure positive interactions with others, evidence-based social-cognitive remediation programs, and cognitive-behavioral interventions to improve social skills.

Psychiatric and Neuropsychological Treatment

Despite the high prevalence of psychiatric disorders in children with 22q11.2DS, only approximately 30–40% who have a psychiatric disorder receive psychosocial or pharmacological treatment (Armando, Lin, Pontillo, & Vicari, 2017; Tang et al., 2014). Given the markedly high risk for developing schizophrenia, these children need to be closely monitored for prodromal or overt symptoms. Negative symptoms such as social withdrawal and poverty of speech are highly prevalent in adolescents with 22q11.2DS. Screening for anxiety and depression is advised across childhood and adolescence, as successful management of these problems may reduce the severity of psychiatric disorders or prevent or delay their onset. A systematic review failed to find studies on the efficacy and/or feasibility of nonpharmacological treatments targeting common psychiatric disorders in individuals with 22q11.2DS (Buijs & Boot, 2018), revealing an area requiring ongoing investigation.

Preliminary studies have examined computer-based or group interventions to improve the neuropsychological deficits that may be associated with psychiatric disorders (Harrell et al., 2008; Mariano, Tang, Kurtz, & Kates, 2015). Although the sample sizes were small, findings document the feasibility of these interventions and report improvements in the neuropsychological domains of working memory, attention, cognitive flexibility, and social cognition.

Surveillance

Surveillance of the child's medical, developmental, and psychiatric care is contingent on presenting conditions. Routine assessment of serum ionized calcium and thyroid studies, ongoing evaluation of immunological status, ophthalmological and audiology evaluations are advised prior to school entry. Once the child enters school, serial neuropsychological and educational assessments are indicated to monitor development and guide ongoing interventions. Given the changing cognitive phenotype and possible declines in skills or increased behavior problems with age, anticipatory guidance including regular follow-up assessments, screening for anxiety and mood disorders, and monitoring for prodromal and overt symptoms of psychosis are also indicated.

CONCLUSIONS AND FUTURE DIRECTIONS

Clinical molecular testing for 22q11.2DS has been available for more than two decades; however, the disorder continues to be underrecognized, and delays in the diagnosis persist. Features such as palatal and cardiac anomalies are associated with shorter times to diagnosis, but identification of developmental delay and ID fails to consistently result in referral for a molecular diagnosis. Clinicians also need to be sensitive to the fact that non-European ethnicity may mask behavioral features of the disorder. A recent investigation suggested that patients were seen in about seven different specialty clinics prior to a molecular diagnosis (Palmer et al., 2019).

A prenatal or postnatal diagnosis of TOF, TA, IAA type B, or conoventricular VSD should prompt an assessment for 22q11.2DS. Early identification of a child with 22q11.2DS in individuals with cardiac or craniofacial anomalies allows for timely intervention of the associated features including hypocalcemia, feeding issues, developmental delay, learning problems, speech and language deficits, and psychiatric illness. Newborn screening would likely maximize early detection and optimize opportunities to enhance outcome. From a developmental perspective, there is need for early, comprehensive screening of milestone attainment and tracking of long-term trajectories (Lajiness-O'Neill et al., 2018). A further goal is to better understand the mechanisms underlying variability in outcome in relation to age, severity of associated physical illness, and resultant medical procedures, and the genetic variant and deletion type of 22q11.2DS. Attempts to isolate specific genotypes and their cognitive correlates have been generally unsuccessful, though some deletion types have worse intellectual outcomes (Franconi et al., 2016; Zhao et al., 2018). The absence of the more typical male predominance in diagnoses of ASD and psychosis is unexplained, but it raises the possibility of a unique genetic basis for these disorders in children with 22q11.2DS.

Further studies are warranted to better characterize the social and attentional deficits of individuals with 22q11.2DS and their association with the onset of psychosis. Ongoing and multisite imaging studies that focus on illuminating brain–behavior relationships through both structural and functional imaging across the lifespan are clearly needed. An additional need is to investigate environmental risk and protective factors that contribute to the variable medical, neurocognitive, and neuropsychiatric phenotypes of 22q11.2DS. More longitudinal studies will help to characterize the nature of age-related cognitive changes in youth with 22q11.2DS in domains other than IQ. More large-scale prospective investigations focused on the interaction among the genetic, clinical, cognitive, psychiatric, and environmental factors are warranted to clarify the variable outcomes in 22q11.2DS. Awareness of the cognitive, behavioral, and physical features of 22q11.2DS by pediatricians, clinicians, and teachers is lower than for other genetic syndromes, and it will be vital for neuropsychologists to aid in educating fellow practitioners and educators about this disorder.

REFERENCES

Albert, A. B., Abu-Ramadan, T., Kates, W. R., Fremont, W., & Antshel, K. M. (2018). Childhood executive functioning predicts outcomes in 22q11 deletion syndrome. *Journal of the International Neuropsychological Society, 24*(9), 905–916.

Allen, T. M., Hersch, J., Schoch, K., Curtiss, K., Hooper, S. R., & Shashi, V. (2014). Association of the family environment with behavioural and cognitive outcomes in children with chromosome 22q11.2 deletion syndrome. *Journal of Intellectual Disability Research, 58*(1), 31–47.

Antshel, K. M., Fremont, W., & Kates, W. R. (2008). The neurocognitive phenotype in velo-cardio-facial syndrome: A developmental perspective. *Developmental Disabilities Research Reviews, 14*(1), 43–51.

Antshel, K. M., Hendricks, K., Shprintzen, R., Fremont, W., Higgins, A. M., Faraone, S. V., & Kates, W. R. (2014). The longitudinal course of ADHD in velo-cardio-facial syndrome. *Journal of Pediatrics, 163*(1), 187–193.

Antshel, K. M., Shprintzen, R. J., Fremont, W. P., Higgins, A. M., Faraone, S. V., & Kates, W. R. (2010). Cognitive and psychiatric predictors to psychosis in velocardiofacial syndrome: A 3-year follow-up study. *Journal of American Academy Child and Adolescent Psychiatry, 49*(4), 333–344.

Armando, M., Lin, A., Pontillo, M., & Vicari, S. (2017). Prevalence and treatment of psychiatric disorders other than psychosis in children and adolescents with 22q11DS: Examining associations with social and role functioning. *Psychiatry Research, 254*, 238–243.

Barnea-Goraly, N., Menon, V., Krasnow, B., Ko, A., Reiss, A., & Eliez, S. (2003). Investigation of white matter structure in velocardiofacial syndrome: A diffusion tensor imaging study. *American Journal of Psychiatry, 160*(10), 1863–1869.

Bassett, A. S., Chow, E. W. C., Husted, J., Hodgkinson, K. A., Oechslin, E., Harris, L., & Silversides, C. (2009). Premature death in adults with 22q11.2 deletion syndrome. *Journal of Medical Genetics, 46*(5), 324–330.

Bassett, A. S., Lowther, C., Merico, D., Costain, G., Chow, E. W. C., van Amelsvoort, T., . . . Swillen, A. (2017). Rare genome-wide copy number variation and expression of schizophrenia in 22q11.2 deletion syndrome. *American Journal of Psychiatry, 174*(11), 1054–1063.

Bassett, A. S., McDonald-McGinn, D. M., Devriendt, K., Digilio, M. C., Goldenberg, P., Habel, A., . . . Zackai, E. H. (2011). Practical guidelines for managing patients with 22q11.2 deletion syndrome. *Journal of Pediatrics, 159*(2), 332–339.

Baylis, A. L., & Shriberg, L. D. (2018). Estimates of the prevalence of speech and motor speech disorders in youth with 22q11.2 deletion syndrome. *American Journal of Speech–Language Pathology, 28*(1), 53–82.

Bearden, C. E., Jawad, A. F., Lynch, D. R., Monterossso, J. R., Sokol, S., McDonald-McGinn, D. M., . . . Simon, T. J. (2005). Effects of COMT genotype on behavioral symptomatology in the 22q11.2 deletion syndrome. *Child Neuropsychology, 11*(1), 109–117.

Bearden, C. E., Van Erp, T. G. M., Dutton, R. A., Lee, A. D., Simon, T. J., Cannon, T. D., . . . Thompson, P. M. (2009). Alterations in midline cortical thickness and gyrification patterns mapped in children with 22q11.2 deletions. *Cerebral Cortex, 19*(1), 115–126.

Bearden, C. E., Woodin, M. F., Wang, P. P., & Moss, E. (2001). The neurocognitive phenotype of the 22q11.2 deletion syndrome: Selective deficit in visual-spatial memory. *Journal of Clinical and Experimental Neuropsychology, 23*(4), 447–464.

Bingham, P. M., Zimmerman, R. A., McDonald-McGinn, D., Driscoll, D., Emanuel, B. S., & Zackai, E. (1997). Enlarged Sylvian fissures in infants with interstitial deletion of chromosome 22q11. *American Journal of Medical Genetics, 74*(5), 538–543.

Bish, J. P., Chiodo, R., Mattei, V., & Simon, T. J. (2007). Domain specific attentional impairments in children with chromosome 22q11.2 deletion syndrome. *Brain and Cognition, 64*(3), 265–273.

Biswas, A. B., & Furniss, F. (2016). Cognitive phenotype and psychiatric disorder in 22q11.2 deletion syndrome: A review. *Research in Developmental Disabilities, 54*(53–54), 242–257.

Botto, L. D., May, K., Fernhoff, P. M., Correa, A., Coleman, K., Rasmussen, S. A., . . . Campbell, R. M. (2003). A population-based study of the 22q11.2 deletion: Phenotype, incidence, and contribution to major birth defects in the population. *Pediatrics, 112*(1), 101–107.

Buijs, P. C. M., & Boot, E. (2018). Non-pharmacological treatment of psychiatric disorders in individuals with 22q11.2 deletion syndrome: A systematic review. *American Journal of Medical Genetics A, 176*, 1742–1747.

Butcher, N. J., Chow, E. W. C., Costain, G., Karas, D., Ho, A., & Bassett, A. S. (2012). Functional outcomes of adults with 22q11.2 deletion syndrome. *Genetics in Medicine, 14*(10), 836–843.

Campbell, L. E., Azuma, R., Amery, F., Stevens, A., Smith, A., Morris, R. G., . . . Murphy, K. C. (2010). Executive functions and memory abilities in children with 22q11.2 deletion syndrome. *Royal Australian and New Zealand College of Psychiatrists, 44*, 364–371.

Campbell, L. E., Daly, E., Toal, F., Stevens, A., Azuma, R., Catani, M., . . . Murphy, K. C. (2006). Brain and behaviour in children with 22q11.2 deletion syndrome: A volumetric and voxel-based morphometry MRI study. *Brain, 129*(5), 1218–1228.

Campbell, L. E., McCabe, K. L., Melville, J. L., Strutt, P. A., & Schall, U. (2015). Social cognition dysfunction in adolescents with 22q11.2 deletion syndrome (velo-cardio-facial syndrome): Relationship with executive functioning and social competence/functioning. *Journal of Intellectual Disability Research, 59*(9), 845–859.

Cunningham, A. C., Delport, S., Cumines, W., Busse, M., Linden, D. E. J., Hall, J., . . . Bree, M. B. M. Van Den. (2018). Developmental coordination disorder, psychopathology and IQ in 22q11.2 deletion syndrome. *British Journal of Psychiatry, 212*, 27–33.

Cunningham, A. C., Hill, L., Mon-williams, M., Peall, K. J., Linden, D. E. J., Hall, J., . . . Van Den Bree, M. B. M. (2019). Using kinematic analyses to explore sensorimotor control impairments in children with 22q11.2 deletion syndrome. *Journal of Neurodevelopmental Disorders, 11*(8), 1–8.

De Smedt, B., Devriendt, K., Fryns, J. P., Vogels, A., Gewillig, M., & Swillen, A. (2007). Intellectual abilities in a large sample of children with velo-cardio-facial syndrome: An update. *Journal of Intellectual Disability Research, 51*(9), 666–670.

De Smedt, B., Swillen, A., Verschaffel, L., & Ghesqui, P. (2009). Mathematical learning disabilities in children with 22q11.2 deletion syndrome: A review. *Developmental Disabilities Research Reviews, 15*, 4–10.

Debbané, M., Glaser, B., & Eliez, S. (2008). Encoding and retrieval processes in velo-cardio-facial syndrome (VCFS). *Neuropsychology, 22*(2), 226–234.

Devriendt, K., Fryns, J., & Mortier, G. (1998). The annual incidence of DiGeorge/velocardiofacial syndrome. *Journal of Medical Genetics, 35*(9), 789–790.

Dufour, F., Schaer, M., Debbané, M., Farhoumand, R., Glaser, B., & Eliez, S. (2008). Cingulate gyral reductions are related to low executive functioning and psychotic symptoms in 22q11.2 deletion syndrome. *Neuropsychologia, 46*(12), 2986–2992.

Duijff, S. N., Klaassen, P. W. J., Beemer, F. A., Sinnema, G., & Vorstman, J. A. S. (2013). Research in developmental disabilities cognitive and behavioral trajectories in 22q11DS from childhood into adolescence?: A prospective 6-year follow-up study. *Research in Developmental Disabilities, 34*, 2937–2945.

Eliez, S., Blasey, C. M., Menon, V., White, C. D., Schmitt, J. E., & Reiss, A. L. (2001). Functional brain imaging study of mathematical reasoning abilities in velocardiofacial syndrome (del22q11.2). *Genetics in Medicine, 3*(1), 49–55.

Evers, L. J. M., van Amelsvoort, T. A. M. J., Candel, M. J. J. M., Boer, H., Engelen, J. J. M., & Curfs, L. M. G. (2014). Psychopathology in adults with 22q11 deletion syndrome and moderate and severe intellectual disability. *Journal of Intellectual Disability Research, 58*(10), 915–925.

Franchini, M., Schaer, M., Glaser, B., Kott-Radecka, M., Debanne, M., Schneider, M., . . . Eliez, S. (2016). Visual processing of emotional dynamic faces in 22q11.2 deletion syndrome. *Journal of Intellectual Disability Research, 60*(4), 308–321.

Franconi, C. P., McDonald-McGinn, D., Zackai, E. H., McNamara, M. A., Salmons, H., Moss, E., . . . Emanuel, B. S. (2016). IQ and hemizygosity for the Val158Met functional polymorphism of

COMT in 22q11DS. *American Journal of Medical Genetics B, 171*(8), 1112–1115.

Furniss, F., Biswas, A. B., Gumber, R., & Singh, N. (2011). Cognitive phenotype of velocardiofacial syndrome: A review. *Research in Developmental Disabilities, 32*(6), 2206–2213.

Gerdes, M., Solot, C., Wang, P. P., McDonald-McGinn, D. M., & Zackai, E. H. (2001). Taking advantage of early diagnosis: Preschool children with the 22q11.2 deletion. *Genetics in Medicine, 3*(1), 40–44.

Girirajan, S., Campbell, C. D., & Eichler, E. E. (2011). Human copy number variation and complex genetic disease. *Annual Review of Genetics, 45*(1), 203–226.

Glaser, B., Mumme, D. L., Blasey, C., Morris, M. A., Dahoun, S. P., Antonarakis, S. E., . . . Eliez, S. (2002). Language skills in children with velocardiofacial syndrome (deletion 22q11.2). *Journal of Pediatrics, 140*(6), 753–758.

Golding-Kushner, K. J., Weller, G., & Shprintzen, R. J. (1985). Velo-cardio-facial syndrome: Language and psychological profiles. *Journal of Craniofacial Genetics and Developmental Biology, 5*(3), 259–266.

Gothelf, D., Eliez, S., Thompson, T., Hinard, C., Penniman, L., Feinstein, C., . . . Reiss, A. L. (2005). COMT genotype predicts longitudinal cognitive decline and psychosis in 22q11.2 deletion syndrome. *Nature Neuroscience, 8*(11), 1500–1502.

Gothelf, D., Hoeft, F., Hinard, C., Hallmayer, J., Van Dover Stoecker, J., Antonarakis, S. E., . . . Reiss, A. L. (2007). Abnormal cortical activation during response inhibition in 22q11.2 deletion syndrome. *Human Brain Mapping, 28*(6), 533–542.

Green, T., Gothelf, D., Glaser, B., Debbane, M., Frisch, A., Kotler, M., . . . Eliez, S. (2009). Psychiatric disorders and intellectual functioning throughout development in velocardiofacial (22q11.2 deletion) syndrome. *Journal of the American Academy of Child and Adolescent Psychiatry, 48*(11), 1060–1068.

Harrell, W., Eack, S., Hooper, S. R., Keshavan, M., Bonner, M. S., Schock, K., & Shashi, V. (2008). Feasibility and preliminary efficacy data from a computerized cognitive intervention in children with chromosome 22q11.2 deletion syndrome. *Research in Developmental Disabilities, 34*(9), 2606–2613.

Howley, S. A., Prasad, S. E., Pender, N. P., & Murphy, K. C. (2012). Relationship between reaction time, fine motor control, and visual-spatial perception on vigilance and visual-motor tasks in 22q11.2 deletion syndrome. *Research in Developmental Disabilities, 33*(5), 1495–1502.

Jacobson, C., Shearer, J., Habel, A., Kane, F., Tsakanikos, E., & Kravariti, E. (2010). Core neuropsychological characteristics of children and adolescents with 22q11.2 deletion. *Journal of Intellectual Disability Research, 54*(8), 701–713.

Jalbrzikowski, M., Carter, C., Senturk, D., Chow, C., Hopkins, J. M., Green, M. F., . . . Beardoen, C., E. (2012). Social cognition in 22q11.2 microdeletion syndrome: Relevance to psychosis. *Schizophrenia Research, 142*(0), 99–107.

Jalbrzikowski, M., Jonas, R., Senturk, D., Patel, A., Chow, C., Green, M. F., & Bearden, C. E. (2013). Structural abnormalities in cortical volume, thickness, and surface area in 22q11.2 microdeletion syndrome: Relationship with psychotic symptoms. *NeuroImage: Clinical, 3*, 405–415.

Jalbrzikowski, M., Villalon-Reina, J. E., Karlsgodt, K. H., Senturk, D., Chow, C., Thompson, P. M., & Bearden, C. E. (2014). Altered white matter microstructure is associated with social cognition and psychotic symptoms in 22q11.2 microdeletion syndrome. *Frontiers in Behavioral Neuroscience, 8*, 1–18.

Jensen, M., Kooy, R. F., Simon, T. J., Reyniers, E., Girirajan, S., & Tassone, F. (2018). A higher rare CNV burden in the genetic background potentially contributes to intellectual disability phenotypes in 22q11.2 deletion syndrome. *European Journal of Medical Genetics, 61*, 209–212.

Kates, W. R., Bansal, R., Fremone, W., Antshel, K. M., Hao, X., Higgins, A. M., . . . Peterson, B. S. (2011). Mapping cortical morphology in youth with velo-cardio-facial (22q11.2 deletion) syndrome. *Journal of American Academy Child and Adolescent Psychiatry, 50*(3), 272–282.

Kates, W. R., Burnette, C. P., Jabs, E. W., Rutberg, J., Murphy, A. M., Grados, M., . . . Pearlson, G. D. (2001). Regional cortical white matter reductions in velocardiofacial syndrome: A volumetric MRI analysis. *Biological Psychiatry, 49*(8), 677–684.

Kates, W. R, Russo, N., Wood, W. M., Antshel, K. M., Faraone, S. V, & Fremont, W. P. (2015). Neurocognitive and familial moderators of psychiatric risk in velocardiofacial (22q11.2 deletion) syndrome: A longitudinal study. *Psychological Medicine, 45*, 1629–1639.

Kobrynski, L. J., & Sullivan, K. E. (2007). Velocardiofacial syndrome: diGeorge syndrome: The chromosome 22q11.2 deletion syndromes. *Lancet, 370*(9596), 1443–1452.

Kruszka, P., Addissie, Y. A., McGinn, D. E., Porras, A. R., Biggs, E., Share, M., . . . Muenke, M. (2017). 22q11.2 deletion syndrome in diverse populations. *American Journal of Medical Genetics A, 173*, 879–888.

Lajiness-O'Neill, R., Beaulieu, I., Asamoah, A., Titus, J. B., Bawle, E., Ahmad, S., . . . Pollack, R. (2006). The neuropsychological phenotype of velocardiofacial syndrome (VCFS): Relationship to psychopathology. *Archives of Clinical Neuropsychology, 21*(2), 175–184.

Lajiness-O'Neill, R., Beaulieu, I., Titus, J. B., Bigler, E. D., Bawle, E. V, & Pollack, R. (2005). Memory and learning in children with 22q11.22 deletion syndrome: Evidence for ventral and dorsal stream disruption? *Child Neuropsychology, 11*(1), 55–71.

Lajiness-O'Neill, R., Brooks, J., Lukomski, A., Schilling, S., Huth-Bocks, A., Warschausky, S., . . . Lyddy, J. E. (2018). Development and validation of PediaTrac™: A web-based tool to track developing infants. *Infant Behavior and Development, 50*, 224–237.

Leleu, A., Saucourt, G., Rigard, C., Chesnoy, G., Baudouin, J. Y., Rossi, M., . . . Demily, C. (2016). Facial emotion perception by intensity in children and adolescents with 22q11.2 deletion syndrome. *European Child and Adolescent Psychiatry, 25*(3), 297–310.

Liu, A. P. Y., Pak-Cheong, C., Lee, P. P., Mok, G. T. K., Tang, W.-F., Lau, E. T., . . . Chung, B. H. Y. (2014). Under-recognition of 22q11.2 deletion in adult Chinese patients with conotruncal anomalies: Implications in transitional care. *European Journal of Medical Genetics, 57*(6), 306–3011.

Mariano, M. A., Tang, K., Kurtz, M., & Kates, W. R. (2015). Cognitive remediation for adolescents with 22q11 deletion syndrome (22q11DS): A preliminary study examining effectiveness, feasibility, and fidelity of a hybrid strategy, remote and computer-based intervention. *Schizophrenia Research, 166*(1–3), 283–289.

McCabe, K., Rich, D., Loughland, C. M., Schall, U., & Campbell, L. E. (2011). Visual scanpath abnormalities in 22q11.2 deletion syndrome: Is this a face specific deficit? *Psychiatry Research, 189*(2), 292–298.

McDonald-McGinn, D. M., Emanuel, B. S., & Zackai, E. H. (2013). 22q11.2 deletion syndrome summary. *GeneReviews*. Retrieved from *www.ncbi.nlm.nih.gov/books/nbk1523*.

McDonald-McGinn, D. M., Minugh-Purvis, N., Kirschner, R. E., Tonnesen, M. K., Catanzaro, J. R., Goldmuntz, E., . . . Zackai, E. H. (2005). The 22q11.2 deletion in African-American patients: An underdiagnosed population? *American Journal of Medical Genetics, 134*(3), 242–246.

McDonald-McGinn, D. M., & Sullivan, K. E. (2011). Chromosome 22q11.2 deletion syndrome (DiGeorge syndrome/velocardiofacial syndrome). *Medicine (Baltimore), 90*(1), 1–18.

Moberg, P. J., Richman, M. J., Roalf, D. R., Morse, C. L., Graefe, A. C., Brennan, L., . . . Gur, R. E. (2018). Neurocognitive functioning in patients with 22q11.2 deletion syndrome: A Meta-analytic review. *Behavior Genetics, 48*(4), 259–270.

Moss, E. M., Batshaw, M. L., Solot, C. B., Gerdes, M., Mcdonald-Mcginn, D. M., Wang, P. P., et al. (1999). Psychoeducational profile of the 22q.2 microdeletion: A complex pattern. *The Journal of Pediatrics, 134*, 193–198.

Niarchou, M., Calkins, M. E., Moore, T. M., Tang, X., McDonald-McGinn, D. M., Zackai, E. H., . . . Gur, R. E. (2018). Attention deficit hyperactivity disorder symptoms and psychosis in 22q11.2 deletion syndrome. *Schizophrenia Bulletin, 44*(4), 824–833.

Norkett, E. M., Lincoln, S. H., Gonzalez-Heydrich, J., & Angelo, E. J. D. (2017). Social cognitive impairment in 22q11 deletion syndrome: A review. *Psychiatry Research, 253*, 99–106.

Olszewski, A. K., Kikinis, Z., Gonzalez, C. S., Coman, I. L., Makris, N., Gong, X., . . . Kates, W. R. (2017). The social brain network in 22q11.2 deletion syndrome: A diffusion tensor imaging study. *Behavioral and Brain Functions, 13*, Article 4.

Padula, M. C., Schaer, M., Scariati, E., Schneider, M., Van De Ville, D., Debbané, M., & Eliez, S. (2015). Structural and functional connectivity in the default mode network in 22q11.2 deletion syndrome. *Journal of Neurodevelopmental Disorders, 7*(1), 1–13.

Palmer, L., Butcher, N. J., Boot, E., Hodgkinson, K. A., Heung, T., Chow, E. W. C., . . . McDonald-McGinn, D. M. (2019). Elucidating the diagnostic odyssey of 22q11.2 deletion syndrome. *American Journal of Medical Genetics A, 176*(4), 936–944.

Perlstein, M. D., Chohan, M. R., Coman, I. L., Antshe, K. M., Fremont, W. P., Gnirke, M. H., . . . Kates, W. R. (2014). White matter abnormalities in 22q11.2 deletion syndrome: Preliminary associations with the Nogo-66 receptor gene and symptoms of psychosis. *Schizophrenia Research, 152*(1), 117–123.

Persson, C., Friman, V., Oskarsdottir, S., & Jonsson, R. (2012). Speech and hearing in adults with 22q11.2 deletion syndrome. *American Journal of Medical Genetics A, 158*(12), 3017–3079.

Persson, C., Niklasson, L., Oskarsdóttir, S., Johansson, S., Jonsson, R., & Soderpalm, E. (2006). Language skills in 5–8-year-old children with 22q11 deletion syndrome. *International Journal of Language and Communication Disorders, 41*(3), 313–333.

Peyvandi, S., Lupo, P., Garbarini, J., Woycleichowki, S., Edman, S., Emanuel, B. S., . . . Goldmuntz, E. (2013). 22q11.2 deletions in patients with conotruncal defects: Data from 1,610 consecutive cases. *Pediatric Cardiology, 34*(7), 1687–1694.

Piccini, G., Menghini, D., Andrea, A. D., Caciolo, C., Pontillo, M., Armando, M., . . . Salerni, A. (2017). Visual perception skills: a comparison between patients with Noonan syndrome and 22q11.2 deletion syndrome. *Genes, Genomes, Genetics, 16*, 627–634.

Roalf, D. R., Schmitt, J. E., Vandekar, S. N., Satterthwaite, T. D., Shinohara, R. T., Ruparel, K., . . . Gur, R. E. (2017). White matter microstructural deficits in 22q11.2 deletion syndrome. *Psychiatry Research, 30*(268), 35–44.

Rockers, K., Ousley, O., Sutton, T., Schoenberg, E., Coleman, K., Walker, E., & Cubells, J. F. (2009). Performance on the Modified Card Sorting Test and its relation to psychopathology in adolescents and young adults with 22q11.2 deletion syndrome. *Journal of Intellectual Disability Research, 53*, 665–676.

Roizen, N. J., Antshel, K. M., Fremont, W. P., AbdulSabur, N., Higgens, A. M., Shprintzen, R. J., & Kates, W. R. (2007). 22q11.2DS Deletion Syndrome: Developmental Milestones in Infants and Toddlers. *Journal of Developmental and Behavioral Pediatrics, 28*(2), 119–125.

Ryan, A. K., Goodship, J. A., Wilson, D. I., Philip, N., Levy, A., Seidel, H., Schuffenhauer, S., . . . Scamber, P. J. (1997). Spectrum of clinical features associated with interstitial chromosome 22q11 deletions: A European collaborative study. *Journal of Medical Genetics, 34*, 798–804.

Scariati, E., Padula, M. C., Schaer, M., & Eliez, S. (2016). Long-range dysconnectivity in frontal and midline structures is associated to psychosis in 22q11.2 deletion syndrome. *Journal of Neural Transmission, 123*(8), 823–839.

Scariati, E., Schaer, M., Richiardi, J., Schneider, M., Debbané, M., Van De Ville, D., & Eliez, S. (2014). Identifying 22q11.2 deletion syndrome and psychosis using resting-state connectivity patterns. *Brain Topography, 27*(6), 808–821.

Schneider, M., Debbané, M., Bassett, A. S., Chow, E. W. C., Fung, W. L. A., Van Den Bree, M. B. M., . . . for the International Consortium on Brain and Behavior in 22q11.2 Deletion Syndrome. (2014). Psychiatric disorders from childhood to adulthood in 22q11.2 deletion syndrome: Results From the International Consortium on Brain and Behavior in 22q11.2 Deletion Syndrome. *American Journal of Psychiatry, 171*(6), 627–639.

Shashi, V., Veerapandiyan, A., Schoch, K., Kwapil, T., Keshavan, M., Ip, E., & Hooper, S. (2011). Social skills and associated psychopathology in children with chromosome 22q11.2 deletion syndrome: Implications for interventions. *Journal of Intellectual Disability Research, 56*(9), 865–878.

Shprintzen, R. J. (2008). Velo-cardio-facial syndrome: 30 years of study. *Developmental Disabilities Research Reviews, 14*(1), 3–10.

Simon, T. J., Bearden, C. E., Moss, E. M., McDonald-McGinn, D. M., Zackai, E. H., & Wang, P. P. (2002). Cognitive development in VCFS. *Progress in Pediatric Cardiology, 15*(2), 109–117.

Simon, T. J., Bish, J. P., Bearden, C. E., Ding, L., Ferrante, S., Nguyen, V., . . . Emanuel, B. S. (2005). A multilevel analysis of cognitive dysfunction and psychopathology associated with chromosome 22q11.2 deletion syndrome in children. *Developmental Psychopathology, 17*(3), 753–784.

Sobin, C., Kiley-Brabeck, K., Daniels, S., Blundell, M., Anyane-Yeboa, K., & Karayiorgou, M. (2004). Networks of attention in children with 22q11 Deletion Syndrome. *Developmental Neuropsychology, 26*(2), 611–626.

Sobin, C., Kiley-Brabeck, K., Daniels, S., Khuri, J., Taylor, L., Blundell, M., . . . Karayiorgou, M. (2005). Neuropsychological characteristics of children with the 22q11 deletion syndrome: A descriptive analysis. *Child Neuropsychology, 11*(1), 39–53.

Solot, C. B., Gerdes, M., Kirschner, R. E., McDonald-McGinn, D. M., Moss, E., Woodin, M., . . . Wang, P. P. (2001). Communication issues in 22q11.2 deletion syndrome: Children at risk. *Genetics in Medicine, 3*(1), 67–71.

Sørensen, K. M., Agergaard, P., Olesen, C., Andersen, P. S., Larsen, L. A., Østergaard, J. R., . . . Christiansen, M. (2010). Detecting 22q11.2 deletions by use of multiplex ligation-dependent probe amplification on DNA from neonatal dried blood spot samples. *Journal of Molecular Diagnostics, 12*(2), 147–151.

Sun, D., Ching, C. R. K., Lin, A., Jennifer, K., Kushan, L., Vajdi, A., . . . Jonas, R. K. (2020). Large-scale mapping of cortical alterations in 22q11.2 deletion syndrome: Convergence with idiopathic psychosis and effects of deletion size. *Molecular Psychiatry, 25,* 1822–1834.

Swillen, A., Devriendt, K., Legius, E., Eyskens, B., Dumoulin, M., Gewillig, M., . . . Fryns, J. P. (1997). Intelligence and psychosocial adjustment in velo-cardio-facial syndrome: A study of 37 children and adolescents with VCFS. *Genetic Counseling, 8*(3), 260–261.

Swillen, A., & McDonald-McGinn, D. (2015). Developmental trajectories in 22q11.2 deletion. *American Journal of Medical Genetics C, 169,* 172–181.

Swillen, A., Moss, E., & Duijff, S. (2018). Neurodevelopmental outcome in 22q11.2 deletion syndrome and management. *American Journal of Medical Genetics A, 176*(10), 2160–2166.

Swillen, A., Vandeputte, L., Cracco, J., Maes, B., Ghesquière, P., Devriendt, K., & Fryns, J.-P. (1999). Neuropsychological, learning and psychosocial profile of primary school aged children with the velo-cardio-facial syndrome (22q11 deletion): Evidence for a nonverbal learning disability? *Child Neuropsychology, 5*(4), 230–241.

Tan, G. M., Arnone, D., McIntosh, A. M., & Ebmeier, K. P. (2009). Meta-analysis of magnetic resonance imaging studies in chromosome 22q11.2 deletion syndrome (velocardiofacial syndrome). *Schizophrenia Research, 115*(2–3), 173–181.

Tang, S. X., Yi, J. J., Moore, T. M., Calkins, M. E., Kohler, C. G., Whinna, D. A., . . . Gur, R. E. (2014). Subthreshold psychotic symptoms in 22q11.2 deletion syndrome. *Journal of the American Academy of Child and Adolescent Psychiatry, 53*(9), 991–1000.

Van, L., Boot, E., & Bassett, A. S. (2017). Update on the 22q11.2 deletion syndrome and its relevance to schizophrenia. *Current Opinion in Psychiatry, 30*(3), 191–196.

Van Amelsvoort, T., Henry, J., Morris, R., Owen, M., Linszen, D., Murphy, K., & Murphy, D. (2004). Cognitive deficits associated with schizophrenia in velo-cardio-facial syndrome. *Schizophrenia Research, 70*(2–3), 223–232.

Van Den Heuvel, E., Jonkers, E., Rombouts, E., Manders, E., Zink, I., & Swillen, A. (2018). Exploratory study on cognitive abilities and social responsiveness in children with 22q11.2 deletion syndrome (22q11DS) and children with idiopathic intellectual disability (IID). *Research in Developmental Disabilities, 81,* 89–102.

Van Den Heuvel, E., Manders, E., Swillen, A., & Zink, I. (2018). Atypical language characteristics and trajectories in children with 22q11.2 deletion syndrome. *Journal of Communication Disorders, 75,* 37–56.

Varese, F., Barkus, E., & Bentall, R. P. (2012). Dissociation mediates the relationship between childhood trauma and hallucination-proneness. *Psychological Medicine, 42*(5), 1025–1036.

Vorstman, J. A. S., Breetvelt, E. J., Duijff, S. N., Eliez, S., Schneider, M., Jalbrzikowski, M., . . . Pontillo, M. (2015). Cognitive decline preceding the onset of psychosis in patients with 22q11.2 deletion syndrome. *JAMA Psychiatry, 72*(4), 377–385.

Widdershoven, J., Bowser, M., Sheridan, M. B., McDonald-McGinn, D. M., Zackai, E. H., Solot, C. B., . . . Emanuel, B. S. (2013). A candidate gene approach to identify modifiers of the palatal phenotype in 22q11.2 deletion syndrome patients. *International Journal of Otorhinolaryngology, 77*(1), 123–127.

Woodin, M., Wang, P. P., Aleman, D., McDonald-McGinn, D., Zackai, E., & Moss, E. (2001). Neuropsychological profile of children and adolescents with the 22q11.2 microdeletion. *Genetics in Medicine, 3*(1), 34–39.

Zhao, Y., Guo, T., Fiksinski, A., Breetvelt, E., Terrence, D. M. M., Alexander, B. C., . . . Morrow, B. E. (2018). Variance of IQ is partially dependent on deletion type among 1,427 22q11.2 deletion syndrome subjects. *American Journal of Medical Genetics A, 176,* 2172–2181.

Zweier, C., Sticht, H., Aydin-Yaylagül, I., Campbell, C. E., & Rauch, A. (2007). Human TBX1 missense mutations cause gain of function resulting in the same phenotype as 22q11.2 deletions. *American Journal of Human Genetics, 80*(3), 510–517.

CHAPTER 19

Down Syndrome

Nancy Raitano Lee
Catherine Stephan
Rebecca I. LaQuaglia

HISTORICAL OVERVIEW

Down syndrome (DS), the most common genetic cause of intellectual disability (ID), was first systematically described in the medical literature over 150 years ago by Langon Down (1866). A physician in England, Down observed a likeness in the physical appearance of a group of patients living at an asylum (Wright, 2011). These patients, who would today receive a diagnosis of DS, were described by Down as "Mongols," due to certain facial features, such as a flatter facial appearance and narrow palpebral fissures. Thus, early accounts of DS refer to it as Mongolism. It was not until 1961, almost 100 years later, that there was a movement among scientists to refrain from the use of the term *Mongolism*. Instead, the term *Down syndrome* was proposed and adopted (Wright, 2011). This change in terminology occurred a few years after the genetic origin of DS was discovered by Jerome Lejeune, whose cytogenetic research revealed that individuals with DS have three rather than two copies of a chromosome that would later be referred to as the 21st chromosome (Lejeune, Gauthier, & Turpin, 1959; Gautier & Harper, 2009). Hence, DS is also referred to as *trisomy 21*.

Reviewing the history of DS is important for not only understanding changes in diagnostic terminology but also recognizing that life expectancy has changed dramatically. As will be reviewed in later sections, DS is associated with numerous medical comorbidities that were historically associated with greatly shortened life expectancy. In 1929, the average life expectancy of a person with DS was 9 years (Penrose, 1949); in 1983, it was 25 years (American Academy of Pediatrics & American College of Obstetricians, 1983). The 21st century has witnessed a remarkable increase in life expectancy for those with DS, with a report from 2007 indicating that average life expectancy is approximately 60 years (Bittles, Bower, Hussain, & Glasson, 2007). Given this increase, research on adult physical, cognitive, and emotional well-being has increased. There is also a greater urgency for pediatric researchers to identify more effective methods to support the development of those with DS in order to promote independence and quality of life in adulthood.

EPIDEMIOLOGY

Globally, DS is estimated to occur at a rate of approximately 1 in 1,000 to 1 in 1,100 live births (World Health Organization, 2011), making it the most commonly identified genetic form of ID. In the United States, the birth prevalence of DS is 1 in 691 live births (Parker et al., 2010), while the population prevalence is estimated to be 1 in 1,209 (Presson et al., 2013). Differences in prevalence exist among nationalities and racial/ethnic groups. For example, in 2012, the prevalence of DS was 22 of every 100,000 live births in Iceland (World Health Organization, 2019), while in 2013, the prevalence in the United States was approximately 132 of every 100,000 live births (de Graaf, Buckley, & Skotko, 2015). Differences in prevalence based on nationalities and racial/ethnic prevalence may be attributable to differences in maternal age, variations in prenatal care and diagnosis, and selective termination (Sherman, Allen, Bean, & Freeman, 2007).

Advanced maternal age is the most significant risk factor for DS, as it increases the risk for nondisjunction errors in the oocyte (Sherman, Freeman, Allen, & Lamb, 2005). Advanced maternal age exponentially increases the chance of having a child with DS until plateauing in the mid-40s (Morris, Mutton, & Alberman, 2002). In 2005, advanced maternal age accounted for more than 50% of DS pregnancies (Resta, 2005). Improvements in technology, as well as increases in the availability of prenatal screening techniques for DS, are also impacting the live birth rate of the disorder (De Groot-van der Mooren, Tamminga, Oepkes, Weijerman, & Cornel, 2018; Natoli, Ackerman, McDermott, & Edwards, 2012; Sherman et al., 2007).

ETIOLOGY, NEUROPATHOLOGY, AND NEURAL SUBSTRATES

Etiology

As reviewed in Comparetto and Borruto (2009), DS, or trisomy 21, is due in most cases (~95%) to nondisjunction during meiosis (parental gamete cell division), which results in the presence of three rather than two copies of chromosome 21 in the zygote. Most cases of DS are nonfamilial (i.e., the syndrome does not run in families). However, a very small proportion of cases is familial and caused by *translocation*. In the case of translocation, one parent may have a "rearrangement" of genetic material involving chromosome 21 and another chromosome (National Library of Medicine, 2019). In the parent, this is likely to be a "balanced" translocation, meaning that they have no extra genetic material, just a rearrangement of chromosomes. However, their offspring may inherit an unbalanced translocation, a situation in which they have extra genetic material from chromosome 21, resulting in DS. Last, a third cause of DS, which accounts for a small number of cases, is mosaicism, which results from an error in mitosis (somatic cell division). Individuals with mosaic DS have some cells in their body with three copies of chromosome 21 and others with two copies.

Trisomy 21, translocation, and mosaic DS all result in gene expression imbalances. The imbalance in genetic expression is not limited to genes on chromosome 21, which are thought to number 200 to 300 alone (National Library of Medicine, 2019). Rather, genes on other chromosomes are also impacted and may be under- or overexpressed. Thus, the pathway from the genetic etiology of DS to the developing brain to the cognitive-behavioral phenotype is not a simple one, and the consequences of having a supernumerary 21st chromosome (in all or some cells of the body) are widespread. In addition, the effects of DS are not limited to the developing neural system. DS is a multisystem disorder characterized by atypical development of multiple body systems, causing those with the disorder to experience numerous medical comorbidities (Pikora et al., 2014).

Neuropathology and Neural Substrates

Postmortem investigations of fetuses with DS have documented abnormalities in both subcortical and cortical structures. Specifically, abnormal cell number has been reported in the hippocampus (Guidi et al., 2008) and the cerebellum (Guidi, Ciani, Bonasoni, Santini, & Bartesaghi, 2011). Additionally, atypical and delayed cortical lamination has been reported in the prenatal period (Golden & Hyman, 1994). In the first several months of postnatal life, differences in brain morphometry, including decreased fronto-occipital length and a narrowed superior temporal gyrus, have also been noted (Schmidt-Sidor, Wisniewski, Shepard, & Sersen, 1990). Moreover, an overall reduction in neuron number and density, particularly in layers II and IV of the cortex, as well as atypical synaptic density and length, have been reported (Wisniewski, 1990).

The findings from the prenatal and early postnatal period converge with the small structural neuroimaging literature on the developing brain in children, adolescents, and young adults with DS. Across pediatric structural neuroimaging studies, there is a good deal of consistency in findings. For example, as reviewed by Hamner, Udhnani, Osipowicz and Lee (2018), all studies that have described total brain volume in DS have reported that it is reduced relative to same-age peers. There is also fairly consistent support for reduced total gray matter and white matter volumes relative to typical peers.

Turning to regional brain differences, reductions in the following structures (relative to same-age peers) have been reported: the hippocampus (Pinter et al., 2001a), cerebellum (Pinter et al., 2001b; Jernigan & Bellugi, 1990), and the cerebral cortex (Kates, Folley, Lanham, Capone, & Kaufmann, 2002; Lee et al., 2016; Pinter et al., 2001b). Within the cerebral cortex, reduced volume of all lobes has been reported in the literature, though whether this reduction is in gray matter, white matter, or both varies across investigations (Kates et al., 2002; Lee et al., 2016). More recent research examining the cortex in DS in greater detail has documented large-scale reductions in cortical surface area, with prominent reductions in much of the frontal lobes (particularly the medial surface) and lateral surface of the temporal lobes (Lee et al., 2016).

There are very few functional neuroimaging investigations of DS. However, the small existing literature has identified atypical activation patterns both at rest (as measured during resting-state functional connectivity studies) and during the completion of different cognitive tasks. For example, two studies that examined resting-state functional connectivity in DS (Anderson et al., 2013; Vega, Hohman, Pryweller, Dykens, & Thornton-Wells, 2015) reported atypically *increased* brain synchrony *between networks* in youth with DS relative to typically developing controls, perhaps suggesting a less mature or functionally specialized neural architecture. Complementing these findings are those that have examined the neural correlates of story listening in DS and reported regionally atypical activation patterns relative to what was observed in typical controls. For example, in one study (Jacola et al., 2014), typical controls showed activation in expected lateral temporal regions previously associated with language functioning, while participants with DS showed activation in the frontal and parietal lobes, as well as regions of the cingulate cortex. Again, these findings suggest that the brain in DS may be characterized by atypical functional organization, which is likely to be one of several factors underlying atypical cognition for this group.

NEUROPSYCHOLOGICAL CONSEQUENCES

In this section, we review what is known about the DS cognitive-behavioral phenotype, starting with global intellectual functioning, then focusing on specific cognitive domains. Table 19.1 summarizes this content, as well as the research reviewed in other chapter sections.

General Intellectual Functioning

Probably the most commonly recognized feature of the DS neuropsychological phenotype or profile is ID. According to the fifth edition of the *Diagnostic and Statistical Manual of Mental Disorders* (DSM-5; American Psychiatric Association, 2013), ID is characterized by marked weaknesses in general intellectual functioning and adaptive functioning, both of which are apparent in the "developmental period." The severity of ID in individuals with DS falls across a spectrum. Currently, the DSM-5 uses adaptive function levels to characterize the degree of ID experienced by an individual. However, most descriptions of the severity of ID in the DS literature utilize definitions from DSM-IV (American Psychiatric Association, 1994) and earlier. In these instances, severity of ID was classified by intellectual ability (or IQ) level instead. Using this older classification system, prior research has indicated that ID levels range from mild to severe (e.g., Määttä, Tervo-Määttä, Taanila, Kaski, & Iivanainen, 2006), with the average level falling in the moderate range (Mégarbané et al., 2013). There have also been some reported cases with general intellectual functioning in the average range (Epstein, 1989). However, these cases are exceptional and do not represent typical intellectual functioning for those with DS.

In the sections that follow, we review the research literature on specific domains of cognitive functioning. Before doing so, it is important to note that unlike research on disorders characterized by average or close to average intellectual abilities, in which a chronological-age-matched comparison group of typical peers is generally included, most studies of DS include a comparison group of children who are matched on *mental* age or overall developmental level. Thus, we describe relative strengths and weaknesses on different cognitive tasks relative to overall developmental level rather than chronological age–expectations (unless otherwise noted). This is the case for several reasons. First, because of the global learning challenges that characterize DS, it is presumed that typically developing, same-age peers would outperform those with DS on most, if not all cognitive tasks administered. Second, it is often the case that neuropsychological assessments designed for children of a particular chronological age are too difficult for individuals with DS. Third, in order to identify relative strengths and weaknesses, researchers have generally compared performance on specific cognitive tasks relative to general developmental- or mental-age expectations. As such, studies have tended to identify younger

TABLE 19.1. Summary of Major Findings Stemming from the DS Literature

Etiology, epidemiology, and neural substrates	
Etiology	Due to three rather than two complete or partial copies of chromosome 21
Epidemiology	~1/700 live births; ~1/1,200 individuals impacted in the United States
Neuroimaging findings	↓ total brain volume; ↓ cortical volume (especially frontal and temporal volumes); ↓ volume of hippocampus and cerebellum (even after accounting for ↓ total brain volume); atypical functional connectivity at rest; atypical activation patterns found during completion of language comprehension tasks
Neuropsychological consequences	
General intellectual functioning	Intellectual disability in most (but not all) cases, but heterogeneity in intellectual functioning (and other aspects of cognitive functioning)
Cognitive functioning	In general, children with DS perform less well than same-age peers on most cognitive tests; thus, researchers often compare performance to MA-matched peers, as summarized below
Perceptual and sensorimotor	Visuospatial findings are mixed; studies report performance that is similar to or below MA, depending on the nature of the task; general motor delays are noted; most studies suggest fine motor abilities below MA
Language	Hallmark area of challenge for DS; syntax and phonological processing are areas of greater challenge; receptive vocabulary abilities closer to MA expectations
Attention	Area of significant challenge relative to MA expectations
Memory	Significant impairments (below MA) are noted on verbal short-term memory tasks, as well as both verbal and nonverbal long-term memory tasks; findings for nonverbal short-term memory are mixed, with performance closer to MA
Executive function	Varied profile; significant weaknesses in working memory (in lab and according to parent report); consistent challenges on lab-based cognitive flexibility tasks; evidence for planning difficulties (in lab and according to parent report)
Social, adaptive, and emotional functioning	During childhood, social and emotional functioning are often considered areas of relative strength
Social cognition	Uneven profile; social motivation generally at or above MA expectations; evidence mixed for other aspects of social cognition
Adaptive and social functioning	Adaptive behavior below chronological age expectations; significant impairments in communication and daily living skills; social skills often found to be relative strength
Emotional and behavioral adjustment	Common comorbidities include autism spectrum disorder and attention-deficit/hyperactivity disorder; in childhood, DS found to have fewer psychiatric comorbidities than other neurodevelopmental disorders; in adolescence, higher rates of psychosis and depression noted

(continued)

TABLE 19.1. *(continued)*

Developmental considerations and moderators of outcomes	
Developmental	Intelligence test standard scores decrease over childhood and plateau in early adulthood (not loss of skills but slower development resulting in greater deviation from peers); individuals with DS at heightened risk for early onset Alzheimer's dementia
Moderators	Both psychiatric and medical comorbidities, especially sleep problems, associated with poorer outcomes; limited research suggests background genetic factors may also moderate outcomes
Education and treatment	
Early intervention	Infants and young children with DS eligible for federally funded early intervention
Primary school intervention	In public schools, services often provided via an IEP; goal is least restrictive environment but many children with DS spend time in both mainstream and special education classrooms
Behavioral intervention	ABA can be effective to address behavioral challenges
Syndrome-specific intervention	Tailored speech–language therapy interventions are being developed, but syndrome-specific, empirically supported interventions not yet readily available

Note. ABA, applied behavior analysis; IEP, individualized education program; MA, mental age.

typically developing children with an overall developmental level that is similar to the DS group and include these children as the comparison group. This approach is not without its limitations, as the choice of mental-age-matched controls can influence study findings (i.e., results may vary based on whether a researcher matches on overall mental age, verbal mental age, or nonverbal mental age). This is a problem for the field of ID research, not just DS research. Thus, we must acknowledge this limitation prior to describing the existing research literature below.

Perceptual and Sensorimotor Skills

Visual-perceptual abilities, specifically visuospatial abilities, had been characterized in early research as a relative strength for individuals with DS (e.g., Wang & Bellugi, 1994). However, a careful review of the literature from several years ago brought this into question. Specifically, Yang, Conners, and Merrill (2014) argued that the existing literature provides evidence for an asymmetrical profile of visuospatial abilities in DS, in which some abilities are similar to mental age levels and some fall below expectations for overall mental age. Moreover, they noted that there does *not* appear to be evidence that visuospatial abilities exceed overall cognitive level or represent a relative strength for those with DS.

Significant deficits in motor skills within the DS population are noted in the literature. Specifically, gross (e.g., walking) and fine (e.g., grasping) motor skills are reported to develop at a slower rate than in typically developing peers; in addition, the completion of motor actions is slower and less coordinated (de Campos, Rocha, & Savelsbergh, 2010; Latash, 2007; Palisano et al., 2001). Furthermore, most relevant studies have found that individuals with DS perform worse on fine motor skill assessments than mental-age-matched typically developing controls (Clements & Barrett, 1994; Vimercati et al., 2015), although some studies report no significant differences (e.g., Fidler, Hepburn, & Rogers, 2006). Thus, while there are some inconsistencies in the literature, at least some aspects of fine motor functioning appear to fall below mental age expectations and represent a relative weakness for those with DS.

Language

Language impairment has been described as a hallmark of DS (e.g., Abbeduto, Warren, & Conners, 2007). Although children with DS typically meet early language milestones, such as babbling, within an age-expected range (Smith & Oller, 1981; Oller & Siebert, 1988), language capabilities of children with DS fall behind those of their typically developing peers as the demand for advanced language (e.g., multiword phrases) increases (Oliver & Buckley, 1994). School-age children with DS exhibit significant impairments in expressive language, with greatest deficits in phonological processing, including speech intelligibility, and syntax (Chapman, Seung, Schwartz, & Kay-Raining Bird, 1998; Chapman, Hesketh, & Kistler, 2002). Syntactic abilities generally fall below both mental age expectations and vocabulary abilities, creating challenges in verbal expression and comprehension for individuals with DS (Abbeduto et al., 2003; Chapman, Schwartz, & Bird, 1991).

Attention

Children with DS are markedly impacted in the many domains of attention (e.g., selective attention, sustained attention, and attention control) beyond what is expected for their mental age (Trezise, Gray, & Sheppard, 2008; Lanfranchi, Jerman, Dal Pont, Alberti, & Vianello, 2010; Costanzo et al., 2013). Regarding selective attention, it has been demonstrated that individuals with DS perform worse than peers with other forms of ID on standardized assessments (Cornish, Scerif, & Karmiloff-Smith, 2007; Wilding, Munir, & Cornish, 2001). Similarly, sustained attention is an area of challenge for children with DS; however, some studies suggest that there may be an improvement in sustained attention as children with DS age (Cornish et al., 2007).

Memory

DS is well known for its impairments in explicit retrospective memory (Edgin, Pennington, & Mervis, 2010; Pennington, Moon, Edgin, Stedron, & Nadel, 2003). The most consistent evidence for these deficits comes from studies of *verbal short-term memory*, or the ability to recall small amounts of verbal information verbatim, revealing a profound weakness for individuals with DS. Research indicates that verbal short-term memory abilities fall not only below mental-age-matched typically developing peers but also peers with other forms of ID (Bower & Hayes, 1994; Carney et al., 2013; Jarrold, Baddeley, & Phillips, 2002; Marcell & Weeks, 1988; Pennington et al., 2003; Wang & Bellugi, 1994). In contrast, findings for nonverbal short-term memory are mixed in DS. Some research has reported stronger spatial short-term memory performance by children with DS relative to typically developing controls matched on mental age (e.g., Frenkel & Bourdin, 2009), others have reported similar performance (e.g., Jarrold & Baddeley, 1997; Visu-Petra, Benga, Ţincaş, & Miclea, 2007), and still others have reported poorer performance on nonverbal short-term memory tasks, such as picture recognition, spatial span, visual pattern memory, and imitation (Frenkel & Bourdin, 2009; Vicari, Bellucci, & Carlesimo, 2000).

Long-term memory is an area of active research inquiry for DS, likely due to the high prevalence of early-onset Alzheimer's disease in adults (Zigman, Schupf, Urv, Zigman, & Silverman, 2002). Although findings in very young children are mixed (Roberts & Richmond, 2015; Milojevich & Lukowski, 2016), significant impairments in verbal and nonverbal long-term memory have been reported by the school-age years and continue into adolescence and adulthood. For example, deficits relative to mental-age-matched typically developing children and other groups with ID have been noted on supraspan verbal long-term memory tasks (Pennington et al., 2003; Carlesimo, Marotta, & Vicari, 1997). Moreover, impairments are noted on visual associative memory tasks, picture recognition tasks, and visuospatial long-term memory tasks in excess of global learning challenges associated with the syndrome (Pennington et al., 2003; Visu-Petra et al., 2007).

Executive Function

Executive function is defined as a multifaceted and complex set of cognitive processes that is essential for the cognitive control of behaviors, including but not limited to inhibition, working memory, planning, and set shifting (Lezak, 1995; Alvarez & Emory, 2006). A review of research on executive function skills in youth with DS reveals a varied profile of skills, both when measured in the laboratory and when using parent report of everyday executive function.

Studies focused on inhibition abilities in children and adolescents with DS have produced mixed results, with some finding significant impairment in abilities relative to mental age expectations (e.g., Borella, Carett, & Lanfranchi, 2013; Cornish et al., 2007; Lanfranchi et al., 2010) and others failing to find a significant difference (Carney et al., 2013; Pennington et al., 2003). The majority of studies examining working memory suggest performance below mental age in both verbal and nonverbal working memory (e.g., Carney et al., 2013; Costanzo et al., 2013; Lanfranchi, Baddeley, Gathercole, & Vianello, 2012; Lanfranchi et al., 2009); however, impairments are more consistently reported for verbal working memory. Everyday impairments in working memory in excess of mental age expectations as measured by parent report measures are also prominent (Daunhauer et al., 2014; Lee et al., 2011).

Another area of significant impairment in executive function for youth with DS is cognitive flexibility (i.e., the ability to flexibility shift between mental sets or behaviors in response to changing cognitive or environmental demands). Most studies of cognitive flexibility have reported performance below mental age on both nonverbal (Costanzo et al., 2013; Lanfranchi et al., 2010) and verbal tasks (Costanzo et al., 2013). Furthermore, impairments relative to mental age have been noted in both laboratory-based investigations (e.g., Fidler, Hepburn, Mankin, & Rogers, 2005; Lanfranchi et al., 2010; Visu-Petra et al., 2007) and parent-report studies (Lee et al., 2011; Daunhauer et al., 2014) of planning and organization.

Social Cognition

Social cognition is broadly defined as the decoding of social stimuli—the ability to understand other people and respond in an appropriate manner (Kunda, 1999). Although there is research to suggest that early social orienting and engagement (two aspects of social cognition) are areas of relative strength for young children with DS (Fidler, Most, Booth-LaForce, & Kelly, 2008), the social-cognitive phenotype in DS is nuanced and characterized by atypical development in several ways. For example, infants with DS have been reported to spend a prolonged period of time gazing at their mothers relative to what is observed in typically developing babies (Carvajal & Iglesias, 2000). Other research has suggested an increased preference for social interactions in children with DS, as illustrated by their maintenance of eye contact with caregivers over toys that were simultaneously presented to them (Landry & Chapieski, 1990). Findings on joint attention skills are mixed, but a recent meta-analysis suggests that these abilities are likely to be consistent with overall developmental level (Hahn, Loveall, Savoy, Neumann, & Ikuta, 2018).

Adaptive and Social Functioning

As a disorder characterized by ID, adaptive functioning is impacted in children with DS, as these skills follow a slowed developmental trajectory (Dykens, Hodapp, & Evans, 1994). Compared to typically developing peers of a similar chronological age and peers with other forms of ID, infants and young children with DS are impacted significantly across all domains of adaptive functioning (Will, Caravella, Hahn, Fidler, & Roberts, 2018). In childhood and adulthood, adaptive impairments persist, and research suggests that communication skills are a relative weakness (Dykens et al., 1994; Tomaszewski, Fidler, Talapatra, & Riley, 2018), consistent with performance-based assessments of language functioning (Abbeduto et al., 2007).

Social functioning is noted to be a relative strength for children with DS (Fidler et al., 2008). Individuals with DS are observed by others to be sociable and affectionate, with prominent personality traits including kindness and forgiveness (Dykens, 2007; Fidler et al., 2008). Preference for social interaction serves as a strong motivator for children with DS; however, social distraction behaviors have been noted to be used by children with DS to prevent completion of unwanted tasks (Kasari & Freeman, 2001).

Emotional or Behavioral Adjustment

Children with DS have been found to have lower prevalence of significant emotional or behavioral disturbances in comparison to children with other forms of ID (Dykens, 2007). However, in comparison to typically developing peers, children with DS have higher rates of externalizing behaviors, especially in early childhood and in school-age years (Grieco, Pulsifier, Seligsohn, Skotko, & Schwartz, 2015). Parents, family members, educators, and therapists report higher rates of hyperactivity, impulsivity, repetitive movements, and agitation (Dykens & Kasari, 1997; Capone, Goyal, Ares, & Lannigan, 2006; Siegel & Smith, 2010), some of which may be the result of weak communication abilities (Skotko, Davidson, & Weintraub, 2013).

Psychiatric disorders such as attention-deficit/hyperactivity disorder (ADHD) and autism spectrum disorder are two of the more commonly co-occurring conditions, with prevalence rates estimated to be ~44% (Oxelgren et al., 2017) and 16% (Richards, Jones, Groves, Moss, & Oliver, 2015), respectively. As children with DS grow into adolescence and young adulthood, an increase in social withdrawal, depression, and anxiety can be observed (Dykens, 2007; Siegel & Smith, 2010). In addition, research has suggested that adolescents with DS have significantly higher rates of depression with psychotic features and psychosis not otherwise specified compared to peers with other forms of ID (Dykens et al., 2015).

DEVELOPMENTAL CONSIDERATIONS

As a neurodevelopmental disorder, it should come as no surprise that the trajectory of intellectual development in DS is atypical in childhood and adolescence. Specifically, research suggests that standard scores on measures of intellectual ability undergo a period of gradual decline during both infancy and childhood. This decline in IQ standard scores does not represent a loss of skills; rather, the mental age of individuals with DS does not keep pace with their chronological age (Carr, 2005; Couzens, Hayes, & Cuskelly, 2012). Thus, children and adolescents deviate further from their same-age peers on standardized testing as they age (i.e., their growth in raw cognitive abilities is flatter than that observed in typical children), resulting in declining standard scores on IQ tests but not declining raw scores. This decline in general intellectual functioning subsides and stabilizes beginning in young adulthood (Carr, 2005).

In contrast to the decline in IQ standard scores described earlier, an actual regression or loss of language, social, motor, or adaptive functioning skills has been reported in the literature for a small subset of individuals with DS during childhood or late adolescence/young adulthood. Unfortunately, systematic research on this is sparse. However, the limited available research suggests that the majority of cases of such regression are associated with co-occurring autism spectrum disorder (O'Neill & Capone, 2017). There are also reports in the literature of a regression in functioning in adolescents and young adults with DS, including instances of reduced language production (which may manifest in mutism), a reduction in or total loss of independence in the completion of daily living skills, and a loss of previously mastered academic skills. In addition, the onset of psychiatric symptoms, including mood disorders, catatonia, or a slowing of motor functioning, and the presence of the stereotypies, has been noted among those with a regression in functioning in adolescence (Mircher et al., 2017). In all cases reviewed, a significant psychosocial stressor was noted to precede the regression and may have served as a trigger. Although such significant regressions are not commonplace for young people with DS, the occurrence of these skills losses is obviously of great concern and may bring a child or young adult to a neuropsychologist for an evaluation.

Last, it is also important to note that DS is a disorder characterized by heightened rates of precocious-onset Alzheimer's disease. Although research suggests that virtually all adults with DS will harbor the plaques and tangles associated with Alzheimer's dementia by age 45 (Wisniewski, Wisniewski, & Wen, 1985), very few individuals will present with symptoms of dementia by that age. Rather, approximately 9% of people with DS present with dementia by age 45 (Zigman et al., 2002). However, this number is quite elevated compared to the rate of 0.003% in the general population (Lambert et al., 2014). By age 72, this number increases to ~67% in DS (compared to ~5% in the general population; Plassman et al., 2007; Zigman et al., 2002). Individual differences in the presentation of dementia symptoms in the face of almost universal neuropathology is an area of active research inquiry and a powerful example of cognitive resilience. Given the increased rates of precocious-onset Alzheimer's disease but variability in the occurrence of this comorbidity across individuals, pediatric neuropsychologists may be faced with questions about risk of dementia by concerned parents of adolescents and young adults with DS. Thus, knowledge of the risk for Alzheimer's disease is crucial even for neuropsychologists who work with adolescents and young adults.

PREDICTORS AND MODERATORS

One increasingly recognized characteristic of DS is the syndrome's heterogeneity, both in terms of medical comorbidities and cognitive functioning. Specifically, while certain medical comorbidities occur at higher rates in DS, they are not universal (Pikora et al., 2014). Similarly, cognitive outcomes vary widely; as a result, there has been a call among researchers for increased attention to individual differences in DS and an examination of factors that moderate outcomes (Karmiloff-Smith et al., 2016). This is the focus of the sections that follow.

Biological Factors

Variation in *background genetics* (i.e., genetic variation unrelated to the triplication of the 21st chromosome) and the co-occurrence of different medical comorbidities are two possible sources of variation in outcomes. However, research on how cognitive ability varies as a function of these biological factors is limited. With regard to background genetics, allelic variation of at least two classes of genes—dopamine and apolipoprotein genes—has been examined in relation to cognitive outcomes. For example, variations in the dopamine receptor D4 (*DRD4*; located on chromosome 11) and dopamine transporter (*DAT1*; located on chromosome 5) genes have been associated with individual differences in executive function and adaptive behavior in DS (Del Hoyo et al., 2016; Mason, Spanó, & Edgin, 2015). Similarly, variations in the apolipoprotein E (*APOE*; located on chromosome 19) gene, especially the *APOE4* genotype, have been examined in relation to Alzheimer's risk in DS. In a review of 10 studies from the literature, Rohn, McCarty, Love, and Head (2014) concluded that although findings in the literature are somewhat mixed, the preponderance of data supports an increased risk of Alzheimer's disease in those with DS with the *APOE4* genotype.

With regard to medical comorbidities, two have been studied in relation to cognitive outcomes in particular—the co-occurrence of congenital heart defects and sleep disturbance. Although the exact prevalence varies from study to study, congenital heart defects (e.g., ventricular septal and atrial septal defects) occur in approximately 50% of infants with DS (Bergström et al., 2016; Freeman et al., 1998). Early research by Visootsak, Hess, Bakeman, and Adamson (2013) in a small sample of toddlers with DS suggested that the presence of congenital heart defects was associated with poorer communication skills. More recently, a large chart review study of over 1,000 children with DS from birth to age 18 years (Alsaied et al., 2016) confirmed the increased risk for language difficulties (and also reported poorer visuomotor skills) in preschoolers with DS. However, at school age, group differences were not observed in those with and without congenital heart defects on measures of language, intellectual functioning, academic achievement, ADHD, executive function, and emotional–behavioral difficulties. These findings highlight the importance of examining not only medical comorbidities and their relation to cognition in DS but also *the developmental periods* in which these relations are examined.

Sleep difficulties, including obstructive sleep apnea, are exceptionally common in DS, and there is research to suggest that the occurrence of these difficulties increases with age (Edgin, Breslin, Spano, Bootzin, & Nadel, 2012). Numerous adverse cognitive outcomes have been associated with poor sleep in DS. These include reduced verbal abilities (Breslin et al., 2014; Edgin et al., 2015), higher rates of executive dysfunction (Breslin et al., 2014; Esbensen & Hoffman, 2018; Lukowski & Milojevich, 2017), poorer academic achievement (Brooks et al., 2015), lower daily living skills (Churchill, Kieckhefer, Bjornson, & Herting, 2015), and more behavior problems (Esbensen, Hoffman, Beebe, Byars, & Epstein, 2018). The nature of existing research makes it difficult to know the directionality of the relationship between poor sleep and suboptimal cognitive outcomes—we cannot say whether poor sleep is causing these suboptimal outcomes or whether some other factor may put these children at risk for both poor sleep and poorer cognitive outcomes. However, research does suggest that poor sleep may be a red flag for poorer outcomes, and thus is an important aspect of medical well-being to be evaluated in children with DS.

Psychological Factors

As reviewed earlier, youth with DS present with higher rates of disorders such as ADHD (Oxelgren et al., 2017) and autism spectrum disorder (Richards et al., 2015). However, limited research is available on how the cognitive outcomes of children with these comorbidities compare to same-age peers with DS without these comorbidities. Two exceptions to this are as follows. First, comorbid autism spectrum disorder is associated with greater overall intellectual impairment (DiGuiseppi et al., 2010; Hamner et al., 2020). Similarly, research utilizing parent report has noted greater executive dysfunction for this group and for youth with DS and comorbid disruptive behavior disorders (Pritchard, Kalback, McCurdy, & Capone, 2015). Thus, neuropsychological evaluations of young people with DS should include an assessment of psychiatric functioning, including a screening for autism spectrum disorder, as these children may need more support than those with DS without these comorbidities.

Social Factors

We provide a very brief review of social factors that may moderate cognitive and behavioral outcomes in DS. In particular, we focus on (1) relations between psychosocial stressors and behavior, and (2) parenting behaviors and cognition in DS. With regard to psychosocial stressors, as one would expect, research suggests that negative life events in adolescents and adults with DS are adversely related to mood and behavior (Mircher et al., 2017; Nevill & Benson, 2018). Thus, just as would be the case in evaluations of individuals without ID syndromes, a thorough review of psychosocial stressors and supports may provide insights into emotional and behavioral problems experienced by individuals with DS who present for a neuropsychological evaluation.

With regard to parenting, Schworer, Fidler, Lunkenheimer, and Daunhauer (2019) found that parenting behaviors were related to executive function skills in school-age children with DS. Specifically, during the completion of a laboratory-based challenge task, parents who engaged in more teaching behavior and less directive behavior had children who performed better on laboratory executive function measures. Of course, we cannot assume that the direction of this relationship is causal from parenting behavior to child behavior; however, these findings suggest that differences in parenting behaviors are meaningfully related to child outcomes and thus could be a target of intervention in future research.

Cross-Cultural or International Considerations

A criticism of the DS research literature is that it has focused on a select subset of the population that is largely White and living in Western industrialized nations (Cuskelly, Hauser-Cram, & Van Riper, 2008). Yet investigations into cross-cultural familial experiences indicate that are there are significant differences for families with a child with DS across nations and cultures (Van Riper, Knafl, & Knafl, 2019), suggesting that more cross-cultural research is needed. For example, Blacher and McIntyre (2006) found that in the United States, Latina mothers of individuals with ID, including DS, reported higher levels of depressive symptoms and lower morale than did Anglo mothers of children with ID; however, Latina mothers reported a greater positive impact of having a child with special needs than did Anglo mothers. Furthermore, research suggests international differences in parents' rating of how they manage the care of their child with DS. For example, it has been reported that caregivers from Ireland, Italy, Korea, and Thailand perceived the management of DS (e.g., how they manage their child's condition, how much their child's disability impacts family life, how they perceive the child's condition impacting the family's future) as more challenging than did caregivers from Portugal, Spain, and the United States, while caregivers in Brazil, the Netherlands, and the United Kingdom reported varied management experiences across domains (Van Riper et al., 2019). Last, it is likely that social determinants of health, including societal attitudes toward disability, religion, and national approaches to prenatal screening, play a role in the experience of DS across cultures (Cuskelly et al., 2008; Van Riper et al., 2019), highlighting the need for further research in this area.

TREATMENT AND INTERVENTION

Treatments for DS tend to look to improve an individual's quality of life by targeting adaptive skills and reducing associated problems rather than addressing the core underlying cognitive deficits associated with the syndrome (Hartley, Horrell, & Maclean, 2007). However, this is slowly changing, as is evident from recent intervention research studies targeting language and cognition in DS. We describe these studies in the sections that follow, but first we provide a background on practices for educating children with DS and disabilities more generally. We begin with a brief introduction to international efforts focused on the educational needs of students with disabilities, including DS. We then focus on more specific practices, with an emphasis on the U.S. public school system.

International Perspectives on Educating Children with Special Needs

According to the United Nations Educational, Scientific and Cultural Organization (UNESCO, 2017), children with disabilities comprise a particularly vulnerable group that has often been excluded from receiving high-quality education. International efforts such as the UN Convention on the Rights of Persons with Disabilities, the World Banks's Education for All initiative, and UNESCO's Global Education 2030 Agenda, promote inclusion for students with disabilities. Although inclusive educational practices are desired widely, policies and practices vary from country to country (UNESCO, 2017). Variation in practices includes educating children with special needs in separate schools, providing primary instruction in special classrooms in mainstream schools, or including children with special needs in mainstream classrooms. Ultimately, while a fully inclusive education may be the goal for many countries, funds, resources, and teacher training may limit actual practices (Frankel, Gold, & Ajodhia-Andrews, 2010). In the sections that follow, we summarize practices in the United States, beginning with early intervention for children with DS.

Early Intervention

Within the United States, youth with DS are eligible for federally mandated, no-cost early intervention services through the age of 5 (Individuals with Disabilities Education Act [IDEA], 2004). Early intervention aims to teach specific strategies and techniques that can be learned and continually implemented as development continues (Capone, 2004). Treatment is intended to be flexible and adaptive, with specific goals created in response to family needs (Van Hooste & Maes, 2003). Early intervention consists of three major features—resource support, social support, and provision of information and services—that work to support an individual's intellectual and adaptive functioning while fostering growth at a family systems level (Spiker, Hebbeler, & Mallik, 2005; Van Hooste & Maes, 2003). Early intervention aims to promote independence and competence in caregivers, provide access to both formal and informal supports, and coordinate care across the health, educational, and social services domains (Van Hooste & Maes, 2003).

Caregivers play a large role in the early intervention team, as active caregiver involvement has been identified as a key factor in the effectiveness of interventions in populations with DS. Specifically, intervention techniques that incorporate higher degrees of parent involvement have been shown to be more effective than those with little or no parent participation (Shonkoff & Hauser-Cram, 1987). Van Hooste and Maes (2003) posit that by working together during treatment, the parent–child dyad is strengthened, while parents learn from the treatment team how to react sensitively and responsively.

Educational Supports for School-Age Children

The inclusion of youth with DS in mainstream academic settings varies widely by nation (Gilmore, Campbell, & Cuskelly, 2003; Fidler, Hodapp, & Dykens, 2002; Pappas, Papoutsi, & Drigas, 2018). Within the United States, the IDEA (2004) declares that states must put in place procedures that ensure to the maximum extent appropriate that children with disabilities are educated in the least restrictive environment possible, and are removed from the regular education environment only when deemed necessary. In practice, the majority of students with DS in the United States are being educated in mainstream or partially integrated settings (Fidler et al., 2002).

In the academic setting, students with DS benefit from a variety of services, with approximately 90% of students surveyed in one study receiving speech–language services, a little less than one-fourth receiving reading, writing, and math services, and one-fifth of the sample receiving one-on-one aides and physical therapy (Fidler et al., 2002). However, caregivers of these students reported a desire for more services, with over half of the caregiver sample reporting that their child would benefit from additional time with speech, occupational, reading, and writing services (Fidler et al., 2002). It should be noted that these data are from a study conducted two decades ago. Thus, rates of these different services may currently be higher; however, there was not a more current resource available that covered this topic.

Speech–Language Therapy

Though impairments in communication abilities are frequently documented in populations with DS, there is currently a dearth of empirically supported interventions targeting these deficits (Abbeduto et al., 2003; Finestack & Abbeduto, 2010). A few exceptions to this are emerging in the literature. First, research has provided support that treatments focused on *speech recasts* (i.e., repeating back the linguistically appropriate version of a child's utterance) may be a promising intervention for improving speech comprehensibility and sentence length in children with DS (Camarata, Yoder, & Camarata, 2006). For children with general developmental delays, including DS, milieu communication treatment (MCT) has been used to target expressive language development in early childhood using a three-prompt procedure (i.e., model, mand [i.e., prompt for a response], and time delay). MCT targets parent responsivity and prelinguistic, nonverbal communication techniques prior to intervening on lexical targets (Fey, Yoder, Warren, & Bredin-Oja, 2013). While findings regarding MCT's efficacy in populations with DS are mixed (Yoder & Warren, 2002; Fey et al., 2006), outcomes may be impacted by treatment dosage, such that higher doses are associated with better outcomes (Yoder, Woynaroski, Fey, & Warren, 2014).

In addition, preliminary research shows promise for speech–language interventions that incorporate a social communication component to improving prelinguistic and linguistic communication in young children with DS. Wright, Kaiser, Reikowsky, and Roberts (2013) reported increases in nonverbal communication after receipt of an intervention that blended elements of MCT with components of the social communication intervention, JASPER (Joint Attention, Symbolic Play, Engagement, and Regulation). Additional studies using social interaction as a core element of intervention found increases in both verbal imitation and requesting behaviors in children with DS (Feeley, Jones, Blackburn, & Bauer, 2011; Bauer & Jones 2015). Although these studies demonstrate possible future directions for speech–language interventions in DS, further research is necessary.

Behavioral Health Interventions

Applied behavior analysis (ABA) is a frequently used treatment technique targeting challenging behaviors in individuals with DS. For individuals with ID, ABA has been shown to be an effective means of reducing various challenging behaviors (for review, see Heyvaert, Maes, & Onghena, 2010; Hassiotis et al., 2009). Within DS populations, emphasis has been placed on using ABA to address avoidance behaviors seen early in development and leading to downstream effects due to missed learning opportunities (Feeley & Jones, 2006). In addition, ABA has been identified as an effective treatment for several other forms of challenging behaviors seen in populations with DS, including self-injury, aggression, and behaviors that result in social isolation (Feeley & Jones, 2006). However, further research is needed to investigate the effectiveness of these treatment techniques in populations with DS specifically.

CONCLUSION AND FUTURE DIRECTIONS

In summary, DS is a multisystem neurogenetic disorder that impacts not only neural development but also numerous body systems. As a result, the etiological underpinnings of the DS cognitive-behavioral phenotype are complex. With increasing life expectancy for individuals with DS, there is a greater need than ever before to develop systems of support to optimize cognitive, adaptive, and social outcomes. Like many other complex medical disorders, future research on DS would benefit from an even greater emphasis on multidisciplinary collaborations that permit scientists to examine relations between different aspects of the phenotype that extend beyond the expertise of any one scientific discipline. One powerful example of such a collaboration is the LonDownS Consortium, in which psychologists and psychiatrists, human and mouse geneticists, and cellular scientists are working together to study the link between DS and Alzheimer's disease.

Scientists studying other developmental disorders, such as reading and language disorders (e.g., Pennington, 2006), have utilized causal models to organize research and theory across different levels of analysis (behavior, cognition, biology). These models provide a framework for testing hypotheses about the causes of learning difficulties in a particular disorder and a structure to organize studies of the relations between different levels of analysis. These models have been less commonly utilized for DS (but see Moore & George, 2011), perhaps due to the complexity of the cognitive-behavioral phenotype and genetic etiology of the disorder. However, we introduce a simplified causal model here (Figure 19.1) in order to organize our discussion of gaps in the research literature and directions for future research.

When reviewing existing DS research within the context of this framework, we would like to first emphasize the relative dearth of knowledge about the DS neural phenotype. Relative to other neurodevelopmental disorders (e.g., autism spectrum disorder), research on the brain in DS is much more limited. For example, a Web of Science search

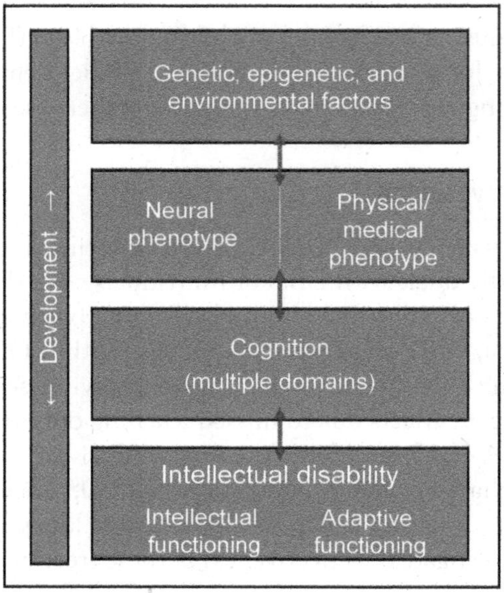

FIGURE 19.1. An example of a simplified causal model that could be used to test hypotheses about the underpinnings of ID in DS.

(completed August 3, 2019) using the topic "magnetic resonance imaging" or MRI and the terms "autism" or "Down syndrome" in the title yielded 1,255 entries for autism spectrum disorder and 139 for DS. Moreover, as reviewed by Hamner et al. (2018), there are no longitudinal MRI studies of children and adolescents with DS. This contrasts with autism spectrum disorder, in which there are longitudinal studies of both infants at risk for the disorder (e.g., Hazlett et al., 2017) and adolescents studied over time (e.g., Wallace et al., 2015).

Thus, we first suggest that a priority for future research is an increase in neuroimaging investigations of the DS neural phenotype, how it develops over time, and how individual differences in the brain relate to individual differences in cognition and behavior. Such research may benefit from the use of newer neuroimaging technologies, such as functional near-infrared spectroscopy, which is more patient-friendly than other imaging modalities that can be difficult for children to tolerate (Casey & De Haan, 2002).

Second, a greater focus on heterogeneity in outcomes in individuals with DS is recommended. For a thoughtful discussion of this, see Karmiloff-Smith et al. (2016). Sources of heterogeneity in DS include background genetic factors, the co-occurrence of medical and psychiatric comorbidities, parenting behaviors, school placement, and differences in treatment, to name a few. Examining heterogeneity will provide a richer description of the differing needs of individuals with DS, thus permitting more tailored service provision and greater insight into factors that may be important to target in future intervention research.

Third, more developmentally focused, longitudinal research would greatly improve our understanding of the unfolding of the DS cognitive-behavioral and neural phenotypes over time. As argued by Karmiloff-Smith (2018), studies of developmental disorders such as DS should focus on studying *development* rather than providing snapshots of how children with DS differ from typical peers at one point in time. This is especially important for DS given the slowing of cognitive development reported for those with the disorder in childhood and the heightened risk for early-onset Alzheimer's dementia in adulthood. Longitudinal research may help researchers to understand points at which developmental trajectories for individuals with DS converge or diverge from typical peers, thus possibly providing clues to points in development where interventions may be maximally advantageous (or alternatively, contraindicated).

Fourth, more treatment research is needed to help develop interventions that target the cognitive underpinnings of the complex learning difficulties experienced by children and adults with DS. In addition, it has been suggested that personalized, precision treatments to address not only phenotype-specific challenges but also individual weaknesses are needed (McDaniel & Yoder, 2016). Last, with the increase in pharmacological approaches to augment cognition in DS (Stagni, Giacomini, Guidi, Ciani, & Bartesaghi, 2015), future research may benefit from investigations of combined pharmacological–behavioral interventions, with the goal of maximizing each intervention's effectiveness. It is hoped that these varied lines of research will converge to improve developmental outcomes for individuals with DS and support greater quality of life for those with DS and their families.

REFERENCES

Abbeduto, L., Murphy, M. M., Cawthon, S. W., Richmond, E. K., Weissman, M. D., Karadottir, S., & O'Brien, A. (2003). Receptive language skills of adolescents and young adults with Down syndrome or fragile X syndrome. *American Journal on Mental Retardation, 108,* 149–160.

Abbeduto, L., Warren, S., & Conners, F. (2007). Language development in Down syndrome: From the prelinguistic period to the acquisition of literacy. *Mental Retardation and Developmental Disabilities Research Reviews, 13*(3), 247–261.

Alsaied, T., Marino, B. S., Esbensen, A. J., Anixt, J. S., Epstein, J. N., & Cnota, J. F. (2016). Does congenital heart disease affect neurodevelopmental outcomes in children with Down syndrome? *Congenital Heart Disease, 11*(1), 26–33.

Alvarez, J. A., & Emory, E. (2006). Executive function and the frontal lobes: A meta-analytic review. *Neuropsychological Review, 16,* 17–42.

American Academy of Pediatrics & American College of Obstetricians and Gynecologists. (1983). *Guidelines for perinatal care.* Elk Grove Village, IL: American Academy of Pediatrics.

American Psychiatric Association. (1994). *Diagnostic and statistical manual of mental disorders* (4th ed.). Washington, DC: Author.

American Psychiatric Association. (2013). *Diagnostic and statistical manual of mental disorders* (5th ed.). Arlington, VA: Author.

Anderson, J. S., Nielsen, J. A., Ferguson, M. A., Burback, M. C., Cox, E. T., Dai, L., . . . Korenberg, J. R. (2013). Abnormal brain synchrony in Down syndrome. *NeuroImage: Clinical, 2,* 703–715.

Bauer, S. M., & Jones, E. A. (2015). Requesting and verbal imitation intervention for infants with Down syndrome: Generalization, intelligibility, and problem solving. *Journal of Developmental and Physical Disabilities, 27*(1), 37–66.

Bergström, S., Carr, H., Petersson, G., Stephansson, O., Bonamy, A. K. E., Dahlström, A., . . . Johansson, S. (2016). Trends in congenital heart defects in infants with Down syndrome. *Pediatrics, 138*(1), e20160123.

Bittles, A. H., Bower, C., Hussain, R., & Glasson, E. J. (2007). The four ages of Down syndrome. *European Journal of Public Health, 17*(2), 221–225.

Blacher, J., & McIntyre, L. L. (2006). Syndrome specificity and behavioural disorders in young adults with intellectual disability: Cultural differences in family impact. *Journal of Intellectual Disability Research, 50*(3), 184–198.

Borella, E., Carett, B., & Lanfranchi, S. (2013). Inhibitory mechanisms in Down syndrome: Is there a specific or general deficit? *Research in Developmental Disabilities, 34*(1), 65–71.

Bower, A., & Hayes, A. (1994). Short-term memory deficits and Down syndrome: A comparative study. *Down Syndrome: Research and Practice, 2*(2), 47–50.

Breslin, J., Spano, G., Bootzin, R., Anand, P.,

Nadel, L., & Edgin, J. (2014). Obstructive sleep apnea syndrome and cognition in Down syndrome. *Developmental Medicine and Child Neurology, 56*(7), 657–664.

Brooks, L. J., Olsen, M. N., Bacevice, A. M., Beebe, A., Konstantinopoulou, S., & Taylor, H. G. (2015). Relationship between sleep, sleep apnea, and neuropsychological function in children with Down syndrome. *Sleep and Breathing, 19*(1), 197–204.

Camarata, S., Yoder, P., & Camarata, M. (2006). Simultaneous treatment of grammatical and speech-comprehensibility deficits in children with Down syndrome. *Down Syndrome: Research and Practice, 11*(1), 9–17.

Capone, G., Goyal, P., Ares, W., & Lannigan, E. (2006). Neurobehavioral disorders in children, adolescents, and young adults with Down syndrome. *American Journal of Medical Genetics C, 142*(3), 158–172.

Capone, G. T. (2004). Down syndrome: Genetic insights and thoughts on early intervention. *Infants and Young Children,17*(1), 45–58.

Carlesimo, G. A., Marotta, L., & Vicari, S. (1997). Long-term memory in mental retardation: Evidence for a specific impairment in subjects with Down's syndrome. *Neuropsychologia, 35*(1), 71–79.

Carney, D. P., Brown, J. H., & Henry, L. A. (2013). Executive function in Williams and Down syndromes. *Research in Developmental Disabilities, 34*(1), 46–55.

Carney, D. P. J., Henry, L. A., Messer, D. J., Danielsson, H., Brown, J. H., & Rönnberg, J. (2013b). Using developmental trajectories to examine verbal and visuospatial short-term memory development in children and adolescents with Williams and Down syndromes. *Research in Developmental Disabilities, 34*(10), 3421–3432.

Carr, J. (2005). Stability and change in cognitive ability over the life span: A comparison of populations with and without Down's syndrome. *Journal of Intellect Disabilities Research, 49*(12), 915–928.

Carvajal, F., & Iglesias, J. (2000). Looking behavior and smiling in Down syndrome infants. *Journal of Nonverbal Behavior, 24*, 225–236.

Casey, B. J., & De Haan, M. (2002). Introduction: New methods in developmental science. *Developmental Science, 5*(3), 265–267.

Chapman, R., Hesketh, L., & Kistler, D. (2002). Predicting longitudinal change in language production and comprehension in individuals with Down syndrome: Hierarchical modeling. *Journal of Speech, Language, and Hearing Research, 45*(5), 902–915.

Chapman, R. S., Schwartz, S. E., & Bird, E. K. (1991). Language-skills of children and adolescents with Down syndrome: 1. Comprehension. *Journal of Speech and Hearing Research, 34*(5), 1106–1120.

Chapman, R. S., Seung, H. K., Schwartz, S. E., & Kay-Raining Bird, E. (1998). Language skills of children and adolescents with Down syndrome: II. Production deficits. *Journal of Speech, Language, and Hearing Research, 41*(4), 861–873.

Churchill, S. S., Kieckhefer, G. M., Bjornson, K. F., & Herting, J. R. (2015). Relationship between sleep disturbance and functional outcomes in daily life habits of children with Down syndrome. *Sleep, 38*(1), 61–71.

Comparetto, C., & Borruto, F. (2009). Down syndrome: Genetics, screening, and health. In D. Jelinek & G. Dvorak (Eds.), *Handbook of Down syndrome research* (pp. 1–54). Hauppauge, NY: Nova Science.

Clements, W., & Barrett, M. (1994). The drawings of children and young people with Down's syndrome: A case of delay or difference? *British Journal of Educational Psychology, 64*(3), 441–452.

Cornish, K., Scerif, G., & Karmiloff-Smith, A. (2007). Tracing syndrome-specific trajectories of attention across the lifespan. *Cortex, 43*(6), 672–685.

Costanzo, F., Varuzza, C., Menghini, D., Addona, F., Gianesini, T., & Vicari, S. (2013). Executive functions in intellectual disabilities: A comparison between Williams syndrome and Down syndrome. *Research in Developmental Disabilities, 34*(5),1770–1780.

Couzens, D., Hayes, M., & Cuskelly, M. (2012). Individual and environmental characteristics associated with cognitive development in Down syndrome: A longitudinal study. *Journal of Applied Research in Intellectual Disabilities, 25*(5), 396–413.

Cuskelly, M., Hauser-Cram, P., & Van Riper, M. (2008). Families of children with Down syndrome: What we know and what we need to know. *Down Syndrome Research and Practice, 12*(3), 105–113.

Daunhauer, L. A., Fidler, D. J., Hahn, L., Will, E., Lee, N. R., & Hepburn, S. (2014). Profiles of everyday executive functioning in young children with Down syndrome. *American Journal on Intellectual and Developmental Disabilities, 119*(4), 303–318.

de Campos, A. C., Rocha, N. A. C. F., & Savelsbergh, G. J. (2010). Development of reaching and grasping skills in infants with Down syndrome. *Research in Developmental Disabilities, 31*(1), 70–80.

de Graaf, G., Buckley, F., & Skotko, B. G. (2015). Estimates of the live births, natural losses, and elective terminations with Down syndrome in the United States. *American Journal of Medical Genetics A, 167*(4), 756–767.

De Groot-van der Mooren, M. D., Tamminga, S., Oepkes, D., Weijerman, M. E., & Cornel, M. C. (2018). Older mothers and increased impact of prenatal screening: Stable livebirth prevalence of trisomy 21 in the Netherlands for the period 2000–2013. *European Journal of Human Genetics, 26*(2), 157–165.

Del Hoyo, L., Xicota, L., Langohr, K., Sánchez-Benavides, G., de Sola Llopis, S., Cuenca Royo, A., . . . TESDAD Study Group. (2016). VNTR-DAT1 and COMTVal158Met genotypes modulate mental flexibility and adaptive behavior skills in Down syndrome. *Frontiers in Behavioral Neuroscience, 10*, Article 193.

DiGuiseppi, C., Hepburn, S., Davis, J. M., Fidler, D. J., Hartway, S., Lee, N. R., . . . Robinson, C. (2010). Screening for autism spectrum disorders in children with Down syndrome: Population prevalence and screening test characteristics. *Journal of Developmental and Behavioral Pediatrics, 31*(3), 181–191.

Down, J. L. H. (1866). Observations on an ethnic classification of idiots. *London Hospital Clinical Lectures and Reports, 3*, 259–262.

Dykens, E. M. (2007). Psychiatric and behavioral disorders in persons with Down syndrome. *Mental Retardation and Developmental Disabilities Research Reviews, 13*(3), 272–278.

Dykens, E. M., Hodapp, R. M., & Evans, D. W. (1994). Profiles and development of adaptive behavior in children with Down syndrome. *American Journal on Mental Retardation, 98*, 580–587.

Dykens, E. M., & Kasari, C. (1997). Maladaptive behavior in children with Prader–Willi syndrome, Down syndrome and non-specific mental retardation. *American Journal on Mental Retardation, 102*(3), 228–237.

Dykens, E., Shah, B., Davis, B., Baker, C., Fife, T., & Fitzpatrick, J. (2015). Psychiatric disorders in adolescents and young adults with Down syndrome and other intellectual disabilities. *Journal of Neurodevelopmental Disorders, 7*(1), Article 9.

Edgin, J. O., Breslin, J. H., Spano, G., Bootzin, R., & Nadel, L. (2012). Sleep disturbance in children with Down syndrome increases with age. In *Sleep* (Vol. 35, pp. A19–A20). Westchester, IL: American Academy of Sleep Medicine.

Edgin, J. O., Pennington, B. F., & Mervis, C. B. (2010). Neuropsychological components of intellectual disability: The contributions of immediate, working, and associative memory. *Journal of Intellectual Disability Research, 54*(5), 406–417.

Edgin, J. O., Tooley, U., Demara, B., Nyhuis, C., Anand, P., & Spano, G. (2015). Sleep disturbance and expressive language development in preschool-age children with Down syndrome. *Child Development, 86*(6), 1984–1998.

Epstein, C. J. (1989). Down syndrome. In C. R. Scriver, A. L. Beaudet, W. S. Sly, & P. Valle (Eds.), *The metabolic basis of inherited disease* (pp. 291-396). New York: McGraw-Hill.

Esbensen, A. J., & Hoffman, E. K. (2018). Impact of sleep on executive functioning in school-age children with Down syndrome. *Journal of Intellectual Disability Research, 62*(6), 569–580.

Esbensen, A. J., Hoffman, E. K., Beebe, D. W., Byars, K. C., & Epstein, J. (2018). Links between sleep and daytime behaviour problems in children with Down syndrome. *Journal of Intellectual Disability Research, 62*(2), 115–125.

Feeley, K., & Jones, E. (2006). Addressing challenging behaviour in children with Down syndrome: The use of applied behaviour analysis for assessment and intervention. *Down Syndrome Research and Practice, 11*(2), 64–77.

Feeley, K. M., Jones, E. A., Blackburn, C., & Bauer, S. (2011). Advancing imitation and requesting skills in toddlers with Down syndrome. *Research in Developmental Disabilities, 32*(6), 2415–2430.

Fey, M. E., Warren, S. F., Brady, N., Finestack, L. H., Bredin-Oja, S. L., Fairchild, M., . . . Yoder, P. J. (2006). Early effects of responsivity education/prelinguistic milieu teaching for children with developmental delays and their parents. *Journal of Speech, Language, and Hearing Research, 49*(3), 526–547.

Fey, M. E., Yoder, P. J., Warren, S. F., & Bredin-Oja, S. L. (2013). Is more better?: Milieu communication teaching in toddlers with intellectual disabilities. *Journal of Speech, Language, and Hearing Research, 56*(2), 679–693.

Fidler, D. J., Hepburn, S. L., Mankin, G., & Rogers, S. J. (2005a). Praxis skills in young children with Down syndrome, other developmental disabilities, and typically developing children. *American Journal of Occupational Therapy, 59*(2), 129–138.

Fidler, D., Hepburn, S., & Rogers, S. (2006). Early learning and adaptive behaviour in toddlers with Down syndrome: Evidence for an emerging behavioural phenotype? *Down Syndrome Research and Practice, 9*(3), 37–44.

Fidler, D. J., Hodapp, R. M., & Dykens, E. M. (2002). Behavioral phenotypes and special education: Parent report of educational issues for children with Down syndrome, Prader–Willi syndrome, and Williams syndrome. *Journal of Special Education, 36*(2), 80–88.

Fidler, D. J., Most, D. E., Booth-LaForce, C., & Kelly, J. F. (2008). Emerging social strengths in young children with Down syndrome. *Infants and Young Children, 21,* 207–220.

Finestack, L. H., & Abbeduto, L. (2010). Expressive language profiles of verbally expressive adolescents and young adults with Down syndrome or fragile X syndrome. *Journal of Speech, Language, and Hearing Research, 53*(5), 1334–1348.

Frankel, E. B., Gold, S., & Ajodhia-Andrews, A. (2010). International preschool inclusion: Bridging the gap between vision and practices. *Young Exceptional Children, 13*(5), 2–16.

Freeman, S. B., Taft, L. F., Dooley, K. J., Allran, K., Sherman, S. L., Hassold, T. J., . . . Saker, D. M. (1998). Population-based study of congenital heart defects in Down syndrome. *American Journal of Medical Genetics, 80*(3), 213–217.

Frenkel, S., & Bourdin, B. (2009). Verbal, visual, and spatio-sequential short-term memory: Assessment of the storage capacities of children and teenagers with Down's syndrome. *Journal of Intellectual Disability Research, 53*(2), 152–160.

Gautier, M., & Harper, P. S. (2009). Fiftieth anniversary of trisomy 21: Returning to a discovery. *Human Genetics, 126*(2), 317–324.

Gilmore, L., Campbell, J., & Cuskelly, M. (2003). Developmental expectations, personality stereotypes, and attitudes towards inclusive education: Community and teacher views of Down syndrome. *International Journal of Disability, Development and Education, 50*(1), 65–76.

Golden, J. A., & Hyman, B. T. (1994). Development of the superior temporal neocortex is anomalous in trisomy 21. *Journal of Neuropathology and Experimental Neurology, 53*(5), 513–520.

Grieco, J., Pulsifer, M., Seligsohn, K., Skotko, B., & Schwartz, A. (2015). Down syndrome: Cognitive and behavioral functioning across the lifespan. *American Journal of Medical Genetics C, 169*(2), 135–149.

Guidi, S., Bonasoni, P., Ceccarelli, C., Santini, D., Gualtieri, F., Ciani, E., & Bartesaghi, R. (2008). Neurogenesis impairment and increased cell death reduce total neuron number in the hippocampal region of fetuses with Down syndrome. *Brain Pathology, 18*(2), 180–197.

Guidi, S., Ciani, E., Bonasoni, P., Santini, D., & Bartesaghi, R. (2011). Widespread proliferation impairment and hypocellularity in the cerebellum of fetuses with Down syndrome. *Brain Pathology, 21*(4), 361–373.

Hahn, L. J., Loveall, S. J., Savoy, M. T., Neumann, A. M., & Ikuta, T. (2018). Joint attention in Down syndrome: A meta-analysis. *Research in Developmental Disabilities, 78,* 89–102.

Hamner, T., Hepburn, S., Zhang, F., Fidler, D., Rosenberg, C. R., Robins, D. L., & Lee, N. R. (2020). Cognitive profiles and autism symptoms in comorbid Down syndrome and autism spectrum disorder. *Journal of Developmental & Behavioral Pediatrics, 41*(3), 172–179.

Hamner, T., Udhnani, M. D., Osipowicz, K. Z., & Lee, N. R. (2018). Pediatric brain development in Down syndrome: A field in its infancy. *Journal of the International Neuropsychological Society, 24*(9), 966–976.

Hartley, S. L., Horrell, S. V., & Maclean, W. E. (2007) Science to practice in intellectual disability. In J. W. Jacobson, J. A. Mulick, & J. Rojahn (Eds.), *Handbook of intellectual and developmental disabilities* (pp. 425–444). Boston: Springer.

Hassiotis, A., Robotham, D., Canagasabey, A., Romeo, R., Langridge, D., Blizard, R., . . . King, M. (2009). Randomized, single-blind, controlled trial of a specialist behavior therapy team for challenging behavior in adults with intellectual disabilities. *American Journal of Psychiatry, 166*(11), 1278–1285.

Hazlett, H. C., Gu, H., Munsell, B. C., Kim, S. H., Styner, M., Wolff, J. J., . . . Zwaigenbaum, L. (2017). Early brain development in infants at high risk for autism spectrum disorder. *Nature, 542*(7641), 348–351.

Heyvaert, M., Maes, B., & Onghena, P. (2010). A meta-analysis of intervention effects on challenging behaviour among persons with intellectual disabilities. *Journal of Intellectual Disability Research, 54*(7), 634–649.

Individuals with Disabilities Education Act, 20 U.S.C. § 1400 (2004).

Jacola, L. M., Byars, A. W., Hickey, F., Vannest, J., Holland, S. K., & Schapiro, M. B. (2014). Functional magnetic resonance imaging of story listening in adolescents and young adults with Down syndrome: Evidence for atypical neurodevelopment. *Journal of Intellectual Disability Research, 58*(10), 892–902.

Jarrold, C., & Baddeley, A. D. (1997). Short-term

memory for verbal and visuospatial information in Down's syndrome. *Cognitive Neuropsychiatry, 2*, 101–122.

Jarrold, C., Baddeley, A. D., & Phillips, C. E. (2002). Verbal short-term memory in Down syndrome: A problem of memory, audition, or speech? *Journal of Speech, Language, and Hearing Research, 45*(3), 531–544.

Jernigan, T. L., & Bellugi, U. (1990). Anomalous brain morphology on magnetic resonance images in Williams syndrome and Down syndrome. *Archives of Neurology, 47*(5), 529–533.

Karmiloff-Smith, A. (2018). Development itself is the key to understanding developmental disorders. In A. Karmiloff-Smith, M. S. C. Thomas, & M. H. Johnson (Eds.), *Thinking developmentally from constructivism to neuroconstructivism* (pp. 97–117). New York: Routledge.

Karmiloff-Smith, A., Al-Janabi, T., D'Souza, H., Groet, J., Massand, E., Mok, K., . . . Strydom, A. (2016). The importance of understanding individual differences in Down syndrome. *F1000 Research, 5*, 389.

Kasari, C., & Freeman, S. F. N. (2001). Task-related social behavior in children with Down syndrome. *American Journal on Mental Retardation, 106*(3), 253–264.

Kates, W. R., Folley, B. S., Lanham, D. C., Capone, G. T., & Kaufmann, W. E. (2002). Cerebral growth in fragile X syndrome: Review and comparison with Down syndrome. *Microscopy Research and Technique, 57*(3), 159–167.

Kunda, Z. (1999). *Social cognition: Making sense of people*. Cambridge, MA: MIT Press.

Lambert, M. A., Bickel, H., Prince, M., Fratiglioni, L., Von Strauss, E., Frydecka, D., . . . Reynish, E. L. (2014). Estimating the burden of early onset dementia: Systematic review of disease prevalence. *European Journal of Neurology, 21*(4), 563-569.

Landry, S. H., & Chapieski, M. L. (1990). Joint attention of six-month-old Down syndrome and preterm infants: I. Attention to toys and mother. *American Journal on Mental Retardation, 94*(5), 488–498.

Lanfranchi, S., Baddeley, A., Gathercole, S., & Vianello, R. (2012). Working memory in Down syndrome: Is there a dual task deficit? *Journal of Intellectual Disability Research, 56*(2), 157–166.

Lanfranchi, S., Jerman, O., Dal Pont, E., Alberti, A., & Vianello, R. (2010). Executive function in adolescents with Down syndrome. *Journal of Intellectual Disability Research, 54*(4), 308–319.

Latash, M. (2007). Learning motor synergies by persons with Down syndrome. *Journal of Intellectual Disability Research, 51*(12), 962–971.

Lee, N. R., Adeyemi, E. I., Lin, A., Clasen, L. S., Lalonde, F. M., Condon, E., . . . Giedd, J. N. (2016). Dissociations in cortical morphometry in youth with Down syndrome: Evidence for reduced surface area but increased thickness. *Cerebral Cortex, 26*(7), 2982–2990.

Lee, N. R., Fidler, D. J., Blakeley-Smith,, A., Daunhauer, L., Robinson, C., & Hepburn, S. (2011). Caregiver-report of executive functioning in a population-based sample of young children with Down syndrome. *American Journal on Intellectual and Developmental Disabilities, 116*(4), 290–304.

Lejeune, J., Gauthier, M., & Turpin, R. (1959). Human chromosomes in tissue cultures. *Comptes Rendus Hebdomadaires Des Seances De l'Academie Des Sciences, 248*(4), 602–603.

Lezak, M. (1995). *Neuropsychological testing*. Oxford, UK: Oxford University Press.

Lukowski, A. F., & Milojevich, H. M. (2017). Sleep problems and temperament in young children with Down syndrome and typically developing controls. *Journal of Intellectual Disability Research, 61*(3), 221–232.

Määttä, T., Tervo-Määttä, T., Taanila, A., Kaski, M., & Iivanainen, M. (2006). Mental health, behaviour and intellectual abilities of people with Down syndrome. *Down Syndrome Research and Practice, 11*(1), 37–43.

Marcell, M. M., & Weeks, S. L. (1988). Short-term memory difficulties and Down's syndrome. *Journal of Mental Deficiency Research, 32*(2), 153–162.

Mason, G. M., Spanó, G., & Edgin, J. (2015). Symptoms of attention-deficit/hyperactivity disorder in Down syndrome: effects of the dopamine receptor D4 gene. *American Journal on Intellectual and Developmental Disabilities, 120*(1), 58–71.

McDaniel, J., & Yoder, P. J. (2016). Pursuing precision speech–language therapy services for children with Down syndrome. *Seminars in Speech and Language, 37*(4), 239–251.

Mégarbané, A., Noguier, F., Stora, S., Manchon, L., Mircher, C., Bruno, R., . . . Ravel, A. (2013). The intellectual disability of trisomy 21: Differences in gene expression in a case series of patients with lower and higher IQ. *European Journal of Human Genetics, 21*(11), 1253–1259.

Milojevich, H., & Lukowski, A. (2016). Recall memory in children with Down syndrome and typically developing peers matched on developmental age. *Journal of Intellectual Disability Research, 60*(1), 89–100.

Mircher, C., Cieuta-Walti, C., Marey, I., Rebillat, A. S., Cretu, L., Milenko, E., . . . Ravel, A. (2017). Acute regression in young people with Down syndrome. *Brain Sciences, 7*(6), Article 57.

Moore, D. G., & George, R. (2011). ACORNS: A tool for the visualisation and modelling of atypical development. *Journal of Intellectual Disability Research, 55*(10), 956–972.

Morris, J. K., Mutton, D. E., & Alberman, E. (2002). Revised estimates of the maternal age specific live birth prevalence of Down's syndrome. *Journal of Medical Screening, 9*(1), 2–6.

National Library of Medicine. (2019, July). Chromosome 21. Genetics Home Reference [Internet]. Retrieved August 6, 2019, from *https://ghr.nlm.nih.gov/chromosomè/21.*

Natoli, J. L., Ackerman, D. L., McDermott, S., & Edwards, J. G. (2012). Prenatal diagnosis of Down syndrome: A systematic review of termination rates (1995–2011). *Prenatal Diagnosis, 32*(2), 142–153.

Nevill, R. E., & Benson, B. A. (2018). Risk factors for challenging behaviour and psychopathology in adults with Down syndrome. *Journal of Intellectual Disability Research, 62*(11), 941–951.

Oliver, B., & Buckley, S. (1994). The language development of children with Down's syndrome: First words to two-word phrases. *Down Syndrome Research and Practice, 2*(2), 71–75.

Oller, K., & Siebert, J. M. (1988). Babbling in prelinguistic retarded children. *American Journal of Mental Retardation, 92*(4), 369–375.

O'Neill, M., & Capone, G. (2017). Estimated prevalence of developmental regression among children referred to a Down syndrome clinic. *Annals of Neurology, 82*, S268–S269.

Oxelgren, U. W., Myrelid, Å., Annerén, G., Ekstam, B., Göransson, C., Holmbom, A, . . . Fernell, E. (2017). Prevalence of autism and attention-deficit–hyperactivity disorder in Down syndrome: A population-based study. *Developmental Medicine and Child Neurology, 59*(3), 276–283.

Palisano, R. J., Walter, S. D., Russell, D. J., Rosenbaum, P. L., Gémus, M., Galuppi, B. E., & Cunningham, L. (2001). Gross motor function of children with Down syndrome: Creation of motor growth curves. *Archives of Physical Medicine and Rehabilitation, 82*(4), 494–500.

Pappas, M., Papoutsi, C., & Drigas, A. (2018). Policies, practices, and attitudes toward inclusive education: The case of Greece. *Social Sciences,* 7(6), Article 90.

Parker, S. E., Mai, C. T., Canfield, M. A., Rickard, R., Wang, Y., Meyer, R. E., . . . Correa, A. (2010). Updated national birth prevalence estimates for selected birth defects in the United States, 2004–2006. *Birth Defects Research A: Clinical and Molecular Teratology, 88*(12), 1008–1016.

Pennington, B. F. (2006). From single to multiple deficit models of developmental disorders. *Cognition, 101*, 385–413.

Pennington, B. F., Moon, J., Edgin, J., Stedron, J., & Nadel, L. (2003). The neuropsychology of Down syndrome: Evidence for hippocampal dysfunction. *Child Development, 74*(1), 75–93.

Penrose, L. S. (1949). The incidence of mongolism in the general population. *Journal of Mental Science, 95*, 685–688.

Pikora, T. J., Bourke, J., Bathgate, K., Foley, K. R., Lennox, N., & Leonard, H. (2014). Health conditions and their impact among adolescents and young adults with Down syndrome. *PLoS ONE, 9*(5), e96868.

Pinter, J. D., Brown, W. E., Eliez, S., Schmitt, J. E., Capone, G. T., & Reiss, A. L. (2001a). Amygdala and hippocampal volumes in children with Down syndrome: A high-resolution MRI study. *Neurology, 56*(7), 972–974.

Pinter, J. D., Eliez, S., Schmitt, J. E., Capone, G. T., & Reiss, A. L. (2001b). Neuroanatomy of Down's syndrome: A high-resolution MRI study. *American Journal of Psychiatry, 158*(10), 1659–1665.

Plassman, B. L., Langa, K. M., Fisher, G. G., Heeringa, S. G., Weir, D. R., Ofstedal, M. B., . . . Steffens, D. C. (2007). Prevalence of dementia in the United States: The aging, demographics, and memory study. *Neuroepidemiology, 29*(1–2), 125–132.

Pritchard, A. E., Kalback, S., McCurdy, M., & Capone, G. T. (2015). Executive functions among youth with Down Syndrome and coexisting neurobehavioural disorders. *Journal of Intellectual Disability Research, 59*(12), 1130–1141.

Presson, A. P., Partyka, G., Jensen, K. M., Devine, O. J., Rasmussen, S. A., McCabe, L. L., & McCabe, E. R. (2013). Current estimate of Down syndrome population prevalence in the United States. *Journal of Pediatrics, 163*(4), 1163–1168.

Resta, R. G. (2005). Changing demographics of advanced maternal age (AMA) and the impact of the predicted incidence of Down syndrome in the United States: Implications for prenatal screening and genetic counseling. *American Journal of Medical Genetics A, 133*, 31–36.

Richards, C., Jones, C., Groves, L., Moss, J., & Oliver, C. (2015). Prevalence of autism spectrum disorder phenomenology in genetic disorders: A systematic review and meta-analysis. *Lancet Psychiatry, 2*(10), 909–916.

Roberts, L. V., & Richmond, J. L. (2015). Preschoolers with Down syndrome do not yet show the learning and memory impairments seen in adults with Down syndrome. *Developmental Science, 18*(3), 404–419.

Rohn, T. T., McCarty, K. L., Love, J. E., & Head, E. (2014). Is apolipoprotein E4 an important risk factor for dementia in persons with Down syndrome? *Journal of Parkinson's Disease and Alzheimer's Disease, 1*(1), 369–380.

Schmidt-Sidor, B., Wisniewski, K. E., Shepard, T. H., & Sersen, E. A. (1990). Brain growth in Down syndrome subjects 15 to 22 weeks of gestational age and birth to 60 months. *Clinical Neuropathology, 9*(4), 181–190.

Schworer, E., Fidler, D. J., Lunkenheimer, E., & Daunhauer, L. A. (2019). Parenting behaviour and executive function in children with Down syndrome. *Journal of Intellectual Disability Research, 63*(4), 298–312.

Sherman, S. L., Allen, E. G., Bean, L. H., & Freeman, S. B. (2007). Epidemiology of Down syndrome. *Mental Retardation and Developmental Disabilities Research Reviews, 13*(3), 221–227.

Sherman, S. L., Freeman, S. B., Allen, E. G., & Lamb, N. E. (2005). Risk factors for nondisjunction of trisomy 21. *Cytogenetic and Genome Research, 111*(3–4), 273–280.

Shonkoff, J. P., & Hauser-Cram, P. (1987). Early intervention for disabled infants and their families: A quantitative analysis. *Pediatrics, 80*(5), 650–658.

Siegel, M. S., & Smith, W. E. (2010). Psychiatric features in children with genetic syndromes: Toward functional phenotypes. *Child and Adolescent Psychiatric Clinics of North America, 19*(2), 229–261.

Skotko, B. G., Davidson, E. J., & Weintraub, G. S. (2013). Contributions of a specialty clinic for children and adolescents with Down syndrome. *American Journal of Medical Genetics A, 161*(3), 430–437.

Smith, B. L., & Oller, D. K. (1981). A comparative study of pre-meaningful vocalizations produced by normally developing and Down's syndrome infants. *Journal of Speech and Hearing Disorders, 46*(1), 46–51.

Spiker, D., Hebbeler, K., & Mallik, S. (2005). Developing and implementing early intervention programs for children with established disabilities. In M. J. Guralnick (Ed.), *The developmental systems approach to early intervention* (pp. 305–349). Baltimore: Brookes.

Stagni, F., Giacomini, A., Guidi, S., Ciani, E., & Bartesaghi, R. (2015). Timing of therapies for Down syndrome: The sooner, the better. *Frontiers in Behavioral Neuroscience, 9*, Article 265.

Tomaszewski, B., Fidler, D., Talapatra, D., & Riley, K. (2018). Adaptive behaviour, executive function and employment in adults with Down syndrome. *Journal of Intellectual Disability Research, 62*(1), 41–52.

Trezise, K. L., Gray, K. M., & Sheppard, D. M. (2008). Attention and vigilance in children with Down syndrome. *Journal of Applied Research in Intellectual Disabilities, 21*(6), 502–508.

United Nations Educational, Scientific and Cultural Organization (UNESCO). (2017). *A guide for ensuring inclusion and equity in education*. Paris: Author.

Van Hooste, A., & Maes, B. (2003). Family factors in the early development of children with Down syndrome. *Journal of Early Intervention, 25*(4), 296–309.

Van Riper, M. L., Knafl, G., & Knafl, K. (2019). Family management of Down syndrome: Cross-cultural perspectives. *Nursing Outlook, 67*(1), Article 116.

Vega, J. N., Hohman, T. J., Pryweller, J. R., Dykens, E. M., & Thornton-Wells, T. A. (2015). Resting-state functional connectivity in individuals with Down syndrome and Williams syndrome compared with typically developing controls. *Brain Connectivity, 5*(8), 461–475.

Vicari, S., Bellucci, S., & Carlesimo, G. A. (2000). Implicit and explicit memory: A functional dissociation in persons with Down syndrome. *Neuropsychologia, 38*(3), 240–251.

Vimercati, S., Galli, M., Stella, G., Caiazzo, G., Ancillao, A., & Albertini, G. (2015). Clumsiness in fine motor tasks: Evidence from the quantitative drawing evaluation of children with Down syndrome. *Journal of Intellectual Disability Research, 59*(3), 248–256.

Visootsak, J., Hess, B., Bakeman, R., & Adamson, L. B. (2013). Effect of congenital heart defects on language development in toddlers with Down syndrome. *Journal of Intellectual Disability Research, 57*(9), 887–892.

Visu-Petra, L., Benga, O., Ţincaş, I., & Miclea, M. (2007). Visual-spatial processing in children and adolescents with Down's syndrome: A computerized assessment of memory skills. *Journal of Intellectual Disability Research, 51*(12), 942–952.

Wallace, G. L., Eisenberg, I. W., Robustelli, B., Dankner, N., Kenworthy, L., Giedd, J. N., & Martin, A. (2015). Longitudinal cortical development during adolescence and young adulthood in autism spectrum disorder: Increased cortical thinning but comparable surface area changes. *Journal of the American Academy of Child and Adolescent Psychiatry, 54*(6), 464–469.

Wang, P. P., & Bellugi, U. (1994). Evidence from two genetic syndromes for a dissociation between verbal and visual-spatial short-term memory. *Journal of Clinical and Experimental Neuropsychology, 16*(2), 317–322.

Wilding, J., Munir, F., & Cornish, K. (2001). The nature of attentional differences between groups of children differentiated by teacher ratings of attention and hyperactivity. *British Journal of Psychology, 92*, 357–371.

Will, E. A., Caravella, K. E., Hahn, L. J., Fidler, D. J., & Roberts, J. E. (2018). Adaptive behavior in infants and toddlers with Down syndrome and fragile X syndrome. *American Journal of Medical Genetics B, 177*(3), 358–368.

Wisniewski, K. E. (1990). Down syndrome children often have brain with maturation delay, retardation of growth, and cortical dysgenesis. *American Journal of Medical Genetics, 37*(Suppl. 7), 274–281.

Wisniewski, K. E., Wisniewski, H. M., & Wen, G. Y. (1985). Occurrence of neuropathological changes and dementia of Alzheimer's disease in Down's syndrome. *Annals of Neurology, 17*(3), 278–282.

World Health Organization. (2011). Genomics. Retrieved from *www.who.int/news-room/questions-and-answers/item/genomics*.

World Health Organization. (2019). Births with Down's syndrome per 100 000 live births. Retrieved from *https://gateway.euro.who.int/en/indicators/hfa_603-7120-births-with-downs-syndrome-per-100-000-live-births/visualizations/#id=21649*.

Wright, C. A., Kaiser, A. P., Reikowsky, D. I., & Roberts, M. Y. (2013). Effects of a naturalistic sign intervention on expressive language of toddlers with Down syndrome. *Journal of Speech, Language, and Hearing Research, 56*(3), 994–1008.

Wright, D. (2011). *Downs: The history of a disability.* Oxford, UK: Oxford University Press.

Yang, Y., Conners, F. A., & Merrill, E. C. (2014). Visuo-spatial ability in individuals with Down syndrome: Is it really a strength? *Research in Developmental Disabilities, 35*(7), 1473–1500.

Yoder, P., Woynaroski, T., Fey, M., & Warren, S. (2014). Effects of dose frequency of early communication intervention in young children with and without Down syndrome. *American Journal on Intellectual and Developmental Disabilities, 119*(1), 17–32.

Yoder, P. J., & Warren, S. F. (2002). Effects of prelinguistic milieu teaching and parent responsivity education on dyads involving children with intellectual disabilities. *Journal of Speech, Language, and Hearing Research, 45*(6), 1158–1174.

Zigman, W. B., Schupf, N., Urv, T., Zigman, A., & Silverman, W. (2002). Incidence and temporal patterns of adaptive behavior change in adults with mental retardation. *American Journal on Mental Retardation, 107*(3), 161–174.

PART V

EMERGENT AND CONTROVERSIAL CONDITIONS

CHAPTER 20

Nonverbal Learning Disabilities

Margaret Semrud-Clikeman

HISTORICAL OVERVIEW

Nonverbal learning disabilities (NVLD) have not been identified by the *Diagnostic and Statistical Manual of Mental Disorders* (DSM-5: American Psychiatric Association, 2013) or ICD-10 (World Health Organization, 2019) as a recognized diagnosis. They have been clinically recognized as difficulties with processing of pragmatic language as well as visuospatial deficits. Some researchers have additionally identified difficulties in the areas of fine motor functioning, social deficits, mathematics, and in visuomotor integration, which, they argue, form a reliable collection of deficits referred to under the NVLD banner. Turner syndrome, velocardiofacial syndrome, and agenesis of the corpus callosum have been found to share characteristics with NVLD that are not the result of a medical condition. Limited research is available to evaluate the neurological, neuroimaging, and/or neuropsychological underpinnings supporting the existence of this disorder. This chapter seeks to explore empirical findings in this disorder, controversies surrounding this disorder, and possible pathways for a better understanding of NVLD. Figure 20.1 shows aspects of NVLD that have been identified in the literature.

The term *nonverbal learning disability* was originally coined by Johnson and Myklebust (1967) and included difficulties with social understanding and problems with social cues. Byron Rourke (1989) theorized NVLD to be a combination of symptoms that stem from difficulty with integrating visual, spatial, and motor skills, which in turn results in social deficits, attentional problems, and mathematical deficits (Rourke, 1995). Additional models of NVLD emphasize executive functioning and the social deficits seen in these children (Denckla, 2000; Semrud-Clikeman, 2003) with some similarity to children with high-functioning autism (HFA) or, formerly, Asperger syndrome (AS; Schultz, Romanski, & Tsatsanis, 2000; Volkmar & Klin, 2000).

The NVLD Debate

There is controversy whether NVLD is a real syndrome or a milder form of autism spectrum disorder (ASD; Ris & Nortz, 2008; Semrud-Clikeman, 2007). Differences in neonatal and postnatal brain development may underlie the social imperception difficulties seen in ASD and NVLD. It has been hypothesized that early limbic system dysfunction

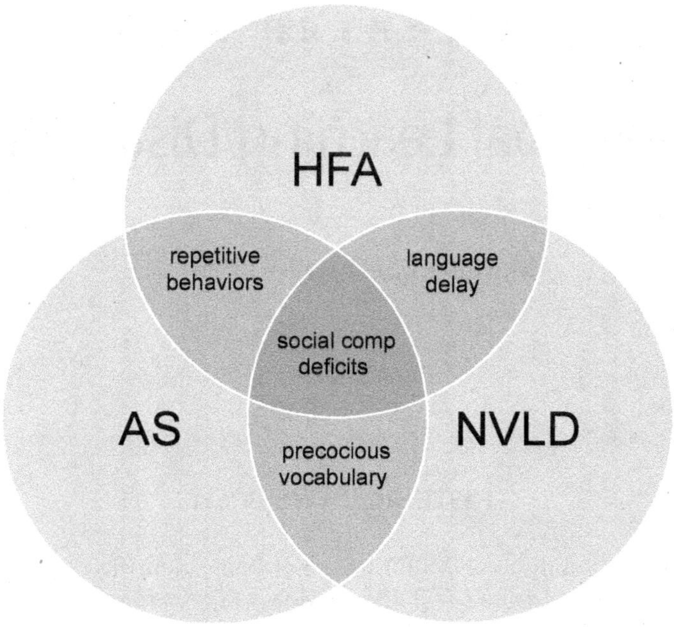

FIGURE 20.1. Similarities and differences in children with AS, HFA, and NVLD. *Note.* social comp deficits, social competence deficits.

prevents the connection between human face recognition and emotional experience (Schulz et al., 2000). Empirical studies have isolated mirror neurons that are activated when a person watches another person do something. These neurons have been thought to be the seat of empathy (Ramachandran & Oberman, 2006). If connections between the amygdala and frontal lobe are disrupted, then the child experiences reality in a distorted fashion (salience landscape theory). Because the child misperceives the environment, a small incident can set off an extreme emotional response. One may wonder, however, if the disruption is not as pronounced as is seen in ASD, would the misperceptions that occur result in a similar difficulty with visuospatial and social perception as is seen in NVLD? If facial expressions and misperception of environmental occurrences are disrupted or do not occur, then the development of empathy, emotions that match the situation, and difficulty interpreting social intent likely interferes with the development of connections between the amygdala and prefrontal cortex.

The diagnosis of NVLD remains controversial partly because it is based mostly on clinical reports. Very few empirical studies have actually been conducted with the NVLD population. Previous literature reviews (Ris et al., 2007; Fine, Semrud-Clikeman, Bledsoe, & Musielak, 2011; Mammarella & Cornoldi, 2014) have found fewer than 30 empirical studies of NVLD with various methodological challenges present. There is little agreement on diagnosis of NVLD in the literature, so study findings are difficult to interpret given varying methods of defining the sample. While data as to the prevalence of NVLD are not clear, some estimate that 5% of children show many of the characteristics of this disorder, including nonverbal, visuospatial, and social difficulties (Mammarella & Cornoldi, 2014; Yalof, 2006).

Early characteristics of NVLD are advanced verbal development and initially good motor skills. Deficits in more fine motor skills are seen around age 2 to 3 years. At that time, difficulties are noted in completion of puzzles, block building, and social development, but not to the extent seen in children with ASD (Fine, Semrud-Clikeman, Bledsoe, & Musielak, 2011). In addition, at a young age, children show significantly reduced participation in social activities, which may be related to deficits in visuospatial skills and social skills, both of which are important skills during early development (Rosenblum & Piran, 2018). These children are often not diagnosed until later, when difficulties are found academically and socially (Mammarella & Cornoldi, 2014). Because this diagnosis is generally delayed, there are additional emotional characteristics that can cloud the diagnostic picture (Davis & Broitman, 2011; Hagai, 2005).

Going forward it will be important to develop consistent diagnostic strategies. The following section summarizes various attempts at defining the diagnosis of NVLD. The measures typically used to sample behaviors from relevant areas of functioning are also presented.

Diagnostic Criteria

The most frequently used definition of NVLD comes from Rourke (1988). Table 20.1 shows comparisons between children with NVLD and those with learning disabilities in reading (RD). It is important to discuss possible differences with RD, as the initial NVLD diagnosis was based on math difficulties in the face of intact reading recognition skills.

Difficulties with pragmatic language, cause–effect reasoning, and using figurative and idiomatic language are present for children with NVLD but also for those with ASD (Forrest, 2007; Semrud-Clikeman & Glass, 2010). Difficulties with social conversation, including relational reciprocity, also can affect a child's ability to enter into peer relations, a skill that becomes more important with adolescence. Difficulty in understanding how children talk and play with each other affect children with ASD and NVLD and their adjustment. Their social difficulties may be related to difficulties with visuospatial development (Rourke & Tsatsanis, 2000); others suggest that significant perceptual problems interfere with social development (Guli, Wilkinson, & Semrud-Clikeman, 2008; Pennington, 2008).

TABLE 20.1. A Comparison of NVLD and RD

NVLD	RD
Excellent single-word reading and spelling	Phonological processing deficits
Mathematics deficits (problems aligning columns, regrouping, complex problem solving)	Difficulty with word problems due to reading difficulties
Difficulty with novel learning; good rote learning	Problem-solving skills generally intact
Deficits in fine and gross motor skills—problems learning to tie shoes, skip, print	No significant difficulties with fine and gross motor skills

A discrepancy of 10 points between verbal and performance scores on the earlier versions of the Wechsler Intelligence Scale for Children–5 (WISC-5; Wechsler, 2014) was initially used by Rourke (2000) as one of the criteria for a diagnosis of NVLD. As specified in the WISC-5 manual, a difference of 10 points magnitude is within normal limits and not uncommon. To this day, some clinicians continue to use this criterion as their main method of diagnosing NVLD even though it does not apply to the WISC-5.

The early models for diagnosing NVLD that continue to be used provide a sample of several symptoms and, depending on the domain, a certain number of symptoms is required for a diagnosis. Rourke used three to five symptoms, with the motor symptoms being primary. The literature is not helpful in determining what symptoms are primary—some indicate that, at the very least, children with NVLD need to show problems with visuospatial deficits, which were the first deficits identified by Rourke. From that point, the diagnosis becomes fuzzy, with continued questions arising as to whether all children should show mathematics learning disabilities, social imperceptions, or stronger verbal than performance skills. Studies are needed to evaluate which of the symptoms in this disorder are primary and which are secondary in order to further understanding of what NVLD is and how to diagnosis the disorder. Figure 20.2 shows the most commonly recognized aspects of NVLD.

Subtypes of NVLD

In addition to diagnostic issues, some theorists have suggested that there are subtypes of NVLD. Again, the bulk of this work comes from clinical rather than empirical evidence and has yet to be validated. Up to four subtypes have been suggested (Davis &

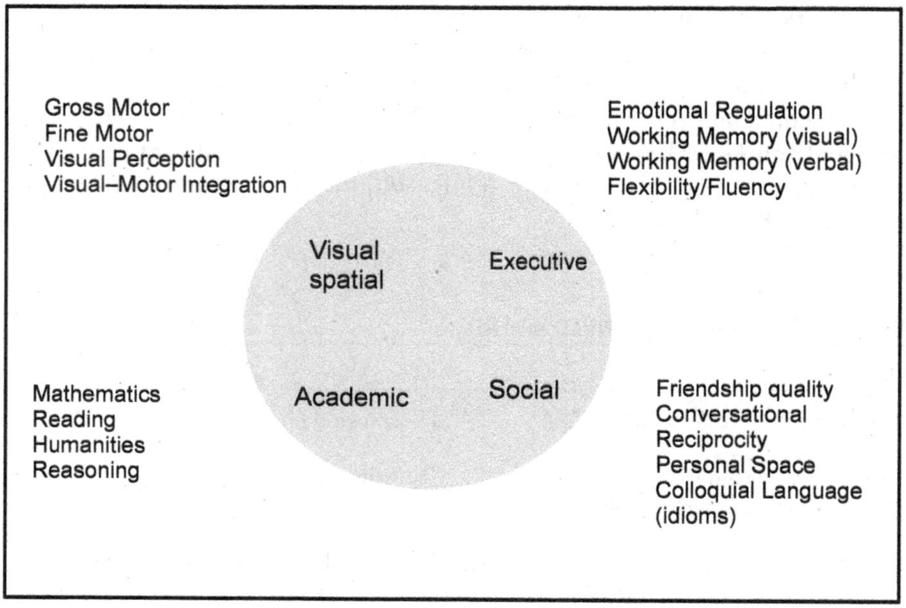

FIGURE 20.2. Typical cognitive and executive functioning deficits seen in children with NVLD.

Broitman, 2011; Palombo, 2006): Subtype 1 with visuospatial processing and social impairment problems; Subtype 2 with similar problems as Subtype 1, as well as attention and executive functioning problems; Subtype 3 including children with more emotional disturbance coupled with visuospatial difficulty and more severe social impairment; and, finally, a combination of Subtypes 2 and 3 in children who show a more severe form of the disorder (Davis & Broitman, 2008; Palombo, 2006). Difficulties with this subtype analysis include not only the lack of empirical validity but also the overarching problem that NVLD itself is already fairly poorly defined and relatively uncommon compared to RD and ASD.

Associated Neuropsychological Deficits

Attention is compromised in many children with NVLD (Brown, 2000; Prior, Smart, Sanson, & Oberlaid, 1999; Voeller, 1995). A study comparing children with NVLD, AS, and neurotypicals found the majority of children with NVLD to also have attention-deficit/hyperactivity disorder (ADHD) (Semrud-Clikeman, Walkowiak, Wilkinson, & Christopher, 2010b). Some have suggested that right-hemispheric white matter may be disrupted in NVLD and result in attentional deficits (Prior et al., 1999; Rourke, 1995). To support this hypothesis, recent studies indicate atypical asymmetry in frontal neuronal activity, with asymmetry of activity in the right frontal region for incorrect trials on attentional tasks (Ellis, Kinzel, Salgari, & Loo, 2017). In addition, this frontal asymmetry predicted more errors throughout the inhibition task. Some have also suggested that poor attention is the result of preference for auditory modalities to the general exclusion of visual perception (Fine & Semrud-Clikeman, 2011).

Difficulty in mathematics has also been found to frequently co-occur with attentional problems (Auerbach, Gross-Tsur, Manor, & Shalev, 2008). While the children in this study were not diagnosed with NVLD, they were reported to have more social problems, as well as attentional deficits, compared to children without dyscalculia. These difficulties were found to persist throughout the 6-year period of the study and particularly for boys, with fewer problems found for girls. In an additional study, approximately one-fourth of the sample of children with mathematics learning disabilities showed significant social problems. In addition, reviews of the NVLD literature have found difficulty in mathematics to be a consistent finding in most studies (Fine et al., 2011; Mammarella & Cornoldi, 2014). For example, the incidence of mathematics difficulty in children with NVLD ranges from 72% (Forrest, 2004) to 86% (Tsatsanis & Rourke, 2008).

Social and emotional issues are another area of comorbidity that has been related to the diagnosis of NVLD. Children and adolescents with NVLD show higher rates of sadness, anxiety, and social withdrawal compared to neurotypical children (Rourke, Young, & Leenaars, 1989). The isolation adolescents may feel during a time when they naturally migrate to valuing peer relations more than other relationships likely increases the likelihood of anxiety and depression in children with NVLD. Internalizing disorders have not been consistently evaluated in children with NVLD and various findings of the presence or absence of these disorders is unclear at this point and certainly require more examination (Forrest, 2007; Pelletier, Ahmad, & Rourke, 2001). The clinician, however, should be alert to the possibility that a child with NVLD can also experience significant emotional difficulties that require treatment.

Difficulties with social perception may fuel the increase seen in anxiety and depression in children with NVLD (Nangle, Erdley, Newman, Mason, & Carpenter, 2003). Misperception of social cues, nonverbal cues, and humor can result in difficulties in peer relationships (Semrud-Clikeman & Glass, 2010; Semrud-Clikeman et al., 2010b; Semrud-Clikeman, Walkowiak, Wilkinson, & Minne, 2010c). Younger children with NVLD have shown more difficulty recognizing basic emotions on faces (happy, sad). Children with NVLD at all ages showed poorer ability to regulate their emotions to the situation compared to controls (Metsala, Galway, Ishaik, & Barton, 2017). In addition, Metsala et al. found that all children enrolled in their study with NVLD were more likely to exhibit difficulties with internalizing problems, attention, and social problems. The authors hypothesized that the social skill deficits seen in these children were related to the presence of anxiety and/or depression.

Finally, difficulty with language pragmatics (understanding nuances, idioms, etc.) has been found consistently in children with NVLD as well as those with AS (Strothers & Cardy, 2012). In fact, the excellent vocabulary seen in many children with NVLD may mask the lack of understanding of higher-order language and pragmatics, which in turn explains their difficulty in understanding humor. Reviews of diagnostic criteria for NVLD have indicated that there *is a likelihood of a profile* including poor social ability, difficulty with math, and poor visuospatial integration (Fine et al., 2011; Mammarella & Cornoldi, 2014). The combination of language strengths in contrast to poorer nonverbal skills with social, spatial, and mathematics difficulties may warrant a diagnosis of NVLD.

NEUROLOGICAL BASES OF NVLD

There is a dearth of hard empirical evidence for the neurological basis of NVLD. Up to this point the neurological bases for NVLD have been inferred from clinical evidence in the form of case studies, symptoms, and test results. Beginning with a study by Goldberg and Costa (1981) it was hypothesized that the neurological markers of NVLD are located in the right hemisphere (Gross-Tsur, Shaley, Manor, & Amir, 1995; Semrud-Clikeman, Fine, & Zhu, 2011; Voeller, 1995). White matter dysfunction in the right hemisphere could be due to functional differences in the right hemisphere or, importantly, in connections to the right hemisphere. Right-hemisphere functioning is believed to be deficient in NVLD because it contains more long, myelinated neurons that are specialized for simultaneous processing of large amounts of information, a function generally needed for social understanding and new learning. Skills such as learning novel tasks have been found to be present in the activation of the right hemisphere, as well as spatial attention, abstract mathematics and reading comprehension, and the processing of emotion and affect (Ross, 2000; Shaywitz, Mody, & Shaywitz, 2006). In contrast, the left hemisphere has more short myelinated fibers that are specialized for both sequential processing and automatic processing of previously learned material (Semrud-Clikeman & Ellison, 2009). Thus, the left hemisphere is specialized for words and grammar, while the right hemisphere is adept at understanding the paralinguistic features of language.

Researchers have begun to study the neuroanatomical bases of NVLD. One method has been to contrast structural magnetic resonance imaging (MRI) findings in children with NVLD and AS, and in neurotypicals. Findings using structural MRI indicated that children with AS showed larger hippocampal and amygdala volumes compared to the other two groups (Semrud-Clikeman, Fine, Bledsoe, & Zhu, 2013). Children with AS or NVLD showed smaller anterior cingulate cortices (ACCs) compared to neurotypicals, and those with NVLD showed smaller caudate volumes compared to the other two groups. There was no difference in gray matter or white matter between the groups. The smaller volume of the ACC and caudate have been associated with difficulty modulating attention across tasks (Semrud-Clikeman et al., 2010b). Evaluation of the corpus callosum revealed that children with NVLD had significantly smaller splenial area compared to those with ADHD (inattentive type, combined type) or AS. In addition, the volume of this structure was strongly related to lower scores on visuospatial tasks (Fine, Musielak, Bledsoe, & Semrud-Clikeman, 2014). These findings suggest that the deficits seen in children with NVLD may be more related to posterior functional deficits than solely to right-hemispheric deficits. In addition to findings suggesting volumetric differences in the brain, children with NVLD appear to have more benign brain cysts compared to those with AS or controls (Semrud-Clikeman & Fine, 2011).

Functional MRI (fMRI) scans show brain activity while a child is performing a task. In an fMRI study, children with NVLD, AS, and controls were asked to view vignettes of children interacting with each other (Fine, Zhu, Bledsoe, & Semrud-Clikeman, submitted). The videos had positive and negative valence. Findings revealed that brain activations in children with NVLD and AS were similar to each other, but different than those observed in controls. Reduced activation was found in the NVLD participants in the visual processing areas and in the fusiform gyrus. The fusiform gyrus is responsible for the processing of facial expressions. Children with AS had more activation in the left-hemispheric auditory regions and more activation to negative than to positive videos. Thus, children with AS were found to prefer auditory input, while those with NVLD had more difficulty with visual processing of information. Success at understanding the emotions portrayed in the videos was strongly related to strengths in integrating cross-model information. Relying solely on visual or auditory processing resulted in poorer performance. Plate 20.1 (in the color insert) shows activation differences in these groups; as can be seen, the children with NVLD showed less activation to both positive and negative videos compared to the children with AS or controls.

A resting-state fMRI study evaluated connectivity in children with NVLD, ASD, and controls (Margolis, Pagliaccio, Thomas, Banker, & Marsh, 2019). Two networks were compared, the salience and default mode networks, which have been implicated in social processing (Li, Mai, & Liu, 2014; Menon, 2015). The salience network is activated during the interpretation of social norms and emotional awareness (Gu, Hof, Friston, & Fan, 2013; Xiang, Lohrenz, & Montague, 2013). The default mode network is associated with social cognition abilities and active during tasks that require mental analysis of a situation (Li et al., 2014; Mar, 2011). Children with ASD have reduced default mode connectivity, which is associated with symptom severity (Hull et al., 2017) and with altered functioning found in the ACC during social processing tasks (Di Martino, Ross, Uddin, Castellanos, & Milliam, 2009).

Margolis et al. (2019) found reduced connectivity between salience network regions in children with NVLD, while those with ASD showed greater connectivity in these regions.

These findings were also related to higher parent ratings of social problems. While both groups showed social processing deficits, this study suggests that these deficits arise from different neural substrates within the salience networks. This finding is similar to that of Semrud-Clikeman et al. (2013) where volumetric differences were found between the two groups, also suggesting a different substrate for social deficits seen in NVLD compared to ASD. These findings suggest that while the social processing deficits may appear similar behaviorally, neural differences underlie these areas of difficulty.

Neuropsychological Assessment

While the neurological evidence for NVLD is emerging at this time, assessment of NVLD has been ongoing over the past few decades. Comparison of findings across studies can be difficult with differences in how NVLD is diagnosed. Some researchers use a Verbal IQ (VIQ) > Performance IQ (PIQ) split, mathematics skills poorer than word reading, and difficulties in tactile, motor, and visuoconstructive skills (Casey, Rourke, & Picard, 1991; Rourke & Tsatsanis, 2000), while others use an approach of 3 out of 5 symptoms or 5 out of 7 symptoms (Mammarella, & Cornold, 2014; Poletti, 2017). While this controversy has not been resolved as of this point, it is important to note that ongoing research is now suggesting that the presence of visuospatial deficits is a crucial first criterion for diagnosis, with other skills being presented in an "or" fashion (i.e., mathematics difficulties, good reading decoding, spatial working memory deficits, emotional and social difficulties) (Spreen, 2011). General guidelines for a good NVLD assessment can be based on clinical reports of the functioning of children diagnosed with NVLD.

Several published reviews (Fine et al., 2011; Mammarella & Cornoldi, 2014; Ris & Nortz, 2008) report evidence for NVLD, with consistent findings of difficulty with visuospatial skills, visuomotor skills, and mathematics as primary symptoms. Secondary symptoms appear to include attentional difficulty, executive functioning problems, particularly in cognitive flexibility, and problems with social functioning. These difficulties are separate from those seen in children with ASD, as their difficulties are more pronounced in social-perceptual deficits with lesser difficulties present with visuospatial difficulty. It is also important to note that various empirical studies, as well as reviews, suggest that the difficulty with visuospatial reasoning often seen with a significant verbal comprehension–perceptual organization split is related to difficulties with social functioning (Fine et al., 2011; Mammarella & Cornoldi, 2014).

To diagnose NVLD, a comprehensive neuropsychological evaluation aids in providing a template for the individual child's strengths and weaknesses. The first step in any comprehensive neuropsychological assessment is to gather a good developmental history. Documenting attainment and evolution of milestones, such as language, and gross and fine motor skills during early childhood is particularly important for children suspected of having NVLD; a combination of strong verbal skills with weaker visuospatial and visuomotor skills is often seen in the histories of children with NVLD (Fine & Semrud-Clikeman, 2011). Older children frequently experience more difficulty with reading comprehension after succeeding with early reading skills, with writing (particularly in letter formation and spacing), and with mathematics.

The question remains as to what constitutes a reasonable diagnosis of NVLD. Guided by the empirical literature as well as clinical practice, our approach to diagnosing NVLD emphasizes three key elements:

1. Significant differences between verbal and nonverbal abilities.
2. Good reading decoding matched with significantly impaired performance on mathematics calculation.
3. Poor visuospatial and visuomotor skills.

These deficits appear to be primary, with secondary difficulties reflected in higher number of attention symptoms, difficulty with social perception and competence, and problems with mental flexibility. Perhaps the label of NVLD is a misnomer, as these children have no difficulty expressing themselves verbally, so they are not nonverbal! A better description may be that they have visuospatial deficits or a conceptualization of this difficulty as a visuospatial learning disability (Cornoldi, Venneri, Marconato, Molin, & Montinari, 2003).

Associated Neuropsychological Deficits in NVLD

Academics and Language

Children with NVLD may show good vocabulary and language comprehension at early ages. What is most often compromised is pragmatic language, as well as higher-order abstract language skills (Fine & Semrud-Clikeman, 2013). Difficulties are most pronounced in the child's ability to understand humor, idioms, and sarcasm (Semrud-Clikeman & Glass, 2010).

READING

Often children with NVLD begin as strong readers, with strengths in decoding and literal understanding of stories. As children age, reading becomes more about abstraction and prediction, and those with NVLD experience more difficulty assembling these details into a coherent whole. Reading comprehension is an area that may be a struggle for these children and requires in-depth evaluation during a neuropsychological examination. Often, informal data gathered from teachers and parents indicate the child has difficulty understanding the main idea. Reading comprehension skills can be directly tested through many well regarded reading measures.

WRITING AND FINE MOTOR SKILLS

An area that is frequently overlooked is written language. During early grades, difficulties are observed in letter formation, spacing, and word spacing in writing.

Fine motor and visuospatial tasks are also important in evaluating children for possible NVLD. The use of pegboards and copying tasks should be part of this assessment. It is often helpful to contrast different copying tasks. For example, the Developmental

Test of Visual–Motor Integration has grid lines for the child and the page is formatted for copying. In contrast, the Bender Gestalt is less structured, and the child needs to organize the drawings across the paper. The Rey–Osterrieth also allows for an opportunity to evaluate how the child organizes complex figures and is able to copy these. The strategy used is important on this measure; whether the child sees the configuration as a whole or tries to make the details fit the picture can be important for understanding how the child perceives complex visual information. Findings from reviews of NVLD literature find visuospatial skills to be the most compromised in children with NVLD (Fine et al., 2011; Mammarella & Cornoldi, 2014).

MATHEMATICS

Some have argued that in order for a child to have an NVLD, he or she must have a learning disability (Cornoldi & Vecchi, 2003). The learning disability most commonly seen in children with NVLD is in mathematics, particularly in the visuospatial aspects of arithmetic (lining up columns, reading charts, graphs, maps). The sensitivity of mathematics tests in identifying NVLD has been found to show large effect sizes (Mammarella & Cornoldi, 2014), possibly indicating that this index may be one of the most powerful methods of identifying children with NVLD.

Executive Functions and Attention

Executive function refers to a broadly defined set of cognitive processes related to planning, organization, and emotional regulation, in addition to attention. It also includes working memory, a skill important for reading comprehension and mathematics. Some children with NVLD have difficulty with planning and organization, as well as with attention (Semrud-Clikeman et al., 2010b). Difficulty with cognitive flexibility, particularly in children with NVLD and AS, likely translates into problems with social perception. One study found a strong relation between number of inattention symptoms and poor social perception (Fine, Semrud-Clikeman, Butcher, & Walkowiak, 2008). Similarly, it was found that fewer attentional symptoms were related to better emotional recognition of nonverbal cues. The relation of executive functioning, attention, and social perception deficits is an area that is just beginning to be explored.

Social and Emotional Functioning

Children with NVLD are hypothesized to have difficulty with social functioning and are especially susceptible to anxiety and depression. There is controversy as to whether social-perceptual deficits are a primary indicator for NVLD or a secondary result of difficulty with visuospatial processing, as well as inattention. As cited earlier, there are findings that inattention is related to poorer social perception. Specific difficulty with identifying nonverbal cues (Petti, Voelker, Shore, & Hayman-Abello, 2002) and understanding emotional content (Woods, Weinborn, Ball, Tiller-Nevin, & Pickett, 2000) has been linked to NVLD. A history of being excluded from social interactions due to misunderstanding of these cues has led to a finding of increased feelings of sadness and withdrawal (Rourke & Tsatsanis, 2000; Semrud-Clikeman et al., 2010a).

MEDICAL DISORDERS WITH NVLD CHARACTERISTICS

NVLD can appear in several childhood neurological disorders and may not be recognized by medical personnel. Both the history and the medical examination need to be sensitive to this possibility, and findings of difficulty with pencil control, writing, fine motor and gross motor delays at early ages, and difficulties with learning numbers and understanding quantity are early markers for a possible additional diagnosis of NVLD that can necessitate school supports. Some of the disorders that have been linked to NVLD are Turner syndrome, velocardiofacial syndrome, neurofibromatosis, and nephropathic cystinosis.

Turner Syndrome

Turner syndrome is a result of a partial or complete absence of one X chromosome in girls. It is estimated to affect approximately 1 in 2,500 girls. Physically, these girls are short, have a webbed neck, and a short hairline. Most girls with Turner syndrome have an average to above average VIQ, paired with a relatively lower perceptual organizational score particularly on visuoconstructive tasks, such as Block Design. Arithmetic calculation is often an area that is compromised, while word reading skills are within the expected range for the child's age (Murphy, Mazzocco, Gerner, & Hendry, 2006). Most girls with Turner syndrome show significant deficits also in visuospatial skills that worsen with age. Difficulties with handwriting and eventually with written language are present (Rovet, 2004). Neuroimaging findings in Turner syndrome have found impaired white matter integrity, with smaller volumes of white matter particularly in the parietal lobes. This volume decreases with age, suggesting that intervention for these children is best provided at an early age (Brown et al., 2002). The parietal lobes are very important for visuospatial reasoning and are affected in Turner syndrome, likely resulting in a similar pattern of deficits seen in children with NVLD.

22q11 Deletion Syndrome (Velocardiofacial Syndrome, DiGeorge Syndrome, Shprintzen Syndrome)

This common genetic disorder with an estimated prevalence of 1 in 2,000 children (Beaton et al., 2010) involves the deletion of the long arm of chromosome 22. These children often are short, have heart disease, cleft palate, and dysmorphic facial features (Robin & Sphrintzen, 2005). Many of these children also show intellectual disability, ASD, and attentional deficits. Alongside the difficulties in global intelligence, these children frequently show difficulty with visuospatial skills, mathematics, executive functioning, and attention. MRI studies have found a small overall brain volume with larger lateral ventricles, as well as differences in the gyri of the frontal and parietal lobes (Barnea-Gorly et al., 2003; Eliez, Schmitt, White, Hu, & Reiss, 2002).

Neurofibromatosis Type 1

Neurofibromatosis type 1 (NF1) is a relatively common neurocutaneous disorder. It is autosomal dominant and involves chromosome 17q11.2. The incidence of NF1 is estimated to be 1 in 3,000 children (Isenberg, Templer, Gao, Titus, & Gutmann, 2013).

A sizable minority of children with NF1 show a learning disability and/or attentional deficits, as well as significant deficits in visuospatial functioning (Coutinho et al., 2016; Isenberg et al., 2013). While children with NF1 are more likely to show dyslexia than dyscalculia, approximately 20% of these children do show difficulty with mathematics (Orraca-Castillo, Estevez-Perez, & Reigosa-Crespo, 2014). White matter lesions have been found in many children with NF1, but variability in lesion location may underlie why some children with NF1 show a profile similar to that of NVLD, while other are more similar to children with dyslexia (Bawden et al., 1996).

Nephropathic Cystinosis

In this rare autosomal recessive disorder, the body accumulates the amino acid cysteine within the cells, which builds up to the point of negatively affecting many organs. The gene is found on chromosome 17p13, which is responsible for transporting the protein. The incidence of cystinosis is estimated at approximately 1 in 100,000 individuals worldwide, and there is a higher incidence of carriers (Semrud-Clikeman & Trauner, 2018). Children with cystinosis show neurological and cognitive deficits despite average intelligence, with significant difficulty in visuospatial skills, spatial memory, visuomotor coordination, mathematics, and social perception deficits. Carriers of the cystinosis gene also appear to have similar difficulties in visuospatial skills, and the carrier frequency is 1 in 158 (Ballantyne, Spilkin, & Trauner, 2013). Thus, carriers of this gene may be undiagnosed with cystinosis while appearing to have NVLD.

CONCLUSION

There appears to be some empirical evidence and ongoing clinical interest to further consider the inclusion of NVLD in official psychiatric, neurological, and/or educational nomenclatures. Primary deficits are difficulty with visuospatial skills, mathematics deficits, and visuoconstructive difficulty, with secondary deficits seen in attention and mental flexibility, as well as moderate difficulties with social perception. While these children also have stronger language than perceptual organizational skills, abstract and pragmatic language appears to be compromised, particularly at older ages. While there is an overlap in the deficits with those seen in AS (or the current diagnosis of HFA), there are also differences in neuropsychological functioning, as well as neuroanatomical changes. Further research into the underlying substrates of NVLD is needed, as well as evaluating carefully how NVLD is diagnosed. The simple procedure of diagnosing NVLD based on a verbal comprehension–perceptual organizational split of 10 standard score points is not appropriate and a more substantial difference between these skills is required. Attention and social-perceptual deficits have also been found to go hand in hand for these children but differ from the social difficulties seen in children with ADHD. Children with ADHD show adequate social perception in the face of impulsive responding, which results in difficulty with social functioning. For children with NVLD, difficulty is seen in understanding of emotional and nonverbal cues, not in impulsivity.

It is also becoming more evident that there are medical conditions that show neuropsychological profiles that are similar to NVLD. It is important for clinicians, as well as medical personnel, to recognize that children with NF1, velocardiofacial syndrome, nephropathic cystinosis, and Turner syndrome may be at risk for NVLD and require additional education support and evaluation.

In addition to the difficulty with developing diagnostic criteria, the name NVLD is a misnomer. These children do not have difficulty being "nonverbal." Rather they have visuospatial deficits that lay the foundation for difficulty with mathematics, social perception, and handwriting. A task force is being led by Prudence Fisher from Columbia University to look at appropriate diagnostic criteria, as well as the name of this disorder. One of the charges of this task force is to petition DSM for inclusion of visuospatial deficit (NVLD) as a diagnostic category. ICD-10 already has such a diagnosis.

What is most needed at this time is carefully conducted research on this population, including clarifying diagnostic criteria, mapping the neural and genetic correlates, and developing effective interventions to help children and families adjust to this unique profile.

REFERENCES

American Psychiatric Association. (2013). *Diagnostic and statistical manual of mental disorders* (5th ed.). Arlington, VA: Author.

Auerbach, J. G., Gross-Tsur, V., Manor, O., & Shalev, R. S. (2008). Emotional and behavioral characteristics over a six-year period in youths with persistent and nonpersistent dyscalculia. *Journal of Learning Disabilities, 41*, 263–273.

Ballantyne, A. O., Spilkin, A. M., & Trauner, D. A. (2013). Executive function in nephropathic cystinosis. *Cognitive and Behavioral Neurology, 26*, 14–22.

Barnea-Gorly, N., Menon, V., Krasnow, B., Ko, A., Reiss, A. L., & Eliez, S. (2003). Investigation of white matter structure in velocardiofacial syndrome: A diffusion tensor imaging study. *American Journal of Psychiatry, 160*, 1863–1869.

Bawden, H., Dooley, J., Buckley, D., Camfield, P., Gordon, K., Riding, M., & Llewellyn, G. (1996). MRI and nonverbal cognitive deficits in children with neurofibromatosis 1. *Journal of Clinical and Experimental Neuropsychology, 18*(6), 784–792.

Beaton, E. A., Stoddard, J., Lai, S., Lackey, J., Shi, J., Ross, J. L., & Simon, T. J. (2010). Atypical functional brain activation during a multiple object tracking task in girls with Turner syndrome: Neurocorrelates of reduced spatiotemporal resolution. *American Journal of Intellectual Developmental Disabilities, 115*, 140–156.

Brown, T. E. (2000). Emerging understandings of attention-deficit disorders and comorbidities. In T. E. Brown (Ed.), *Attention-deficit disorders and comorbidities in children, adolescents, and adults* (pp. 3–56). Washington, DC: American Psychiatric Press.

Brown, W. E., Kesler, S. R., Eliez, S., Warsofsky, I. S., Haberecht, M., Patwardhan, A., . . . Reiss, A. L. (2002). Brain development in Turner syndrome: A magnetic resonance imaging study. *Psychiatry Research: Neuroimaging, 116*, 187–196.

Casey, J. E., Rourke, B. P., & Picard, E. M. (1991). Syndrome of nonverbal learning disabilities: Age differences in neuropsychological, academic, and socioemotional functioning. *Development and Psychopathology, 3*(3), 329–345.

Cornoldi, C., & Vecchi, T. (2003). *Visual–spatial working memory and individual differences*. Hove, UK: Psychology Press.

Cornoldi, C., Venneri, A., Marconato, F., Molin, A., & Montinari, C. (2003). A rapid screening measure for teacher identification of visuospatial learning disabilities. *Journal of Learning Disabilities, 36*, 299–306.

Coutinho, V., Kemlin, I., Dorison, N., de Villemeur, T. B., Rodriguez, D., & Dellatolas, G. (2016). Neuropsychological evaluation and parent assessment of behavioral and motor difficulties in children with neurofibromatosis type 1. *Research in Developmental Disabilities, 48*, 220–230.

Davis, J., & Broitman, J. (2008). *Nonverbal learning disabiities: diagnosis and history*. Paper presented at the International Neuropsychological Society, Kona, HI.

Davis, J. M., & Broitman, J. (2011). *Nonverbal learning disabilities in children: Bridging the gap between science and practice*. Boston: Springer.

Denckla, M. B. (2000). Learning disabilities and attention-deficit/hyperactivity disorder in adults: Overlap with executive dysfunction. In

T. E. Brown (Ed.), *Attention-deficit disorders and comorbidities in children, adolescents, and adults* (pp. 297–318). Washington, DC: American Psychiatric Press.

Di Martino, A., Ross, K., Uddin, L. Q., Castellanos, F. X., & Milliam, M. P. (2009). Functional brain correlates of social and nonsocial processes in autism spectrum disorders: An activation likelihood estimation meta-analysis. *Biological Psychiatry, 65*, 63–74.

Eliez, S., Schmitt, J. E., White, C. D., Hu, D., & Reiss, A. L. (2002). Velocardiofacial syndrome: Are structural changes in the temporal and mesial temporal regions related to schizophrenia? *American Journal of Psychiatry, 159*, 447–453.

Ellis, A., Kinzel, C., Salgari, G. C., & Loo, S. K. (2017). Frontal alpha asymmetry predicts inhibitory processing in youth with attention defict/hyperactivity disorder. *Neuropsychologia, 102*, 45–51.

Fine, J. G., Musielak, K., Bledsoe, J., & Semrud-Clikeman, M. (2014). Corpus callosal findings in children with developmental disorders. *Child Neuropsychology, 20*, 641–661.

Fine, J. G., & Semrud-Clikeman, M. (2011). Nonverbal learning disabilities. In A. Davis (Ed.), *Handbook of pediatric neuropsychology* (pp. 721–734). New York: Springer.

Fine, J. G., & Semrud-Clikeman, M. (2013). Psychopathology of nonverbal learning disabilities. In A. Davis (Ed.), *Psychopathology of childhood and adolescence: A neuropsychological approach* (pp. 163–180). New York: Springer.

Fine, J. G., Semrud-Clikeman, M., Bledsoe, J., & Musielak, K. (2011). A critical review of the NLD literature as a developmental disorder. *Child Neuropsychology, 17*, 418–443.

Fine, J. G., Semrud-Clikeman, M., Butcher, B., & Walkowiak, J. (2008). Brief report: Attention effect on a measure of social perception *Journal of Autism and Developmental Disorders, 38*, 1797–1802.

Fine, J. G., Zhu, D. C., Bledsoe, J., & Semrud-Clikeman, M. (submitted). fMRI differences in children with social deficits: A video vignette study.

Forrest, B. (2004). The utility of math difficulties, internalized psychopathology, and visual–spatial deficits to identify children with the nonverbal learning disability syndrome: Evidence for a visual spatial disability. *Child Neuropsychology, 10*(2), 129–146.

Forrest, B. (2007). Diagnosing and treating right hemisphere disorders. In S. J. Hunter & J. Donders (Eds.), *Pediatric neuropsychological intervention* (pp. 175–192). Cambridge, UK: Cambridge University Press.

Goldberg, E., & Costa, L. D. (1981). Hemisphere differences in the acquisition and use of descriptive systems. *Brain and Language, 14*, 144–173.

Gross-Tsur, V., Shaley, R. S., Manor, O., & Amir, N. (1995). Developmental right-hemisphere syndrome: Clinical spectrum of the nonverbal learning disability. *Journal of Learning Disabilities, 28*, 80–86.

Gu, X., Hof, P. R., Friston, K. J., & Fan, J. (2013). Anterior insula cortex and emotional awareness. *Journal of Comparative Neurology, 521*, 3371–3388.

Guli, L. A., Wilkinson, A., & Semrud-Clikeman, M. (2008). *Social Competence Intervention Program*. Champaign, IL: Research Press.

Hagai, I. (2005). *My special child*. Jerusalem: Modan.

Hull, J. V., Dokovna, L. B., Jacokes, Z. J., Torgeson, C. M., Irimia, A., & Van Horn, J. D. (2017). Resting-state functional connectivity in autism spectrum disorders: A review. *Frontiers in Psychiatry, 7*, Article 205.

Isenberg, J. C., Templer, A., Gao, F., Titus, J. B., & Gutmann, D. H. (2013). Attention skills in children with neurofibromatosis type 1. *Journal of Child Neurology, 28*, 45–49.

Johnson, D. J., & Myklebust, H. R. (1967). *Learning disabilities: Educational principles and practices*. New York: Grune & Stratton.

Li, W., Mai, X., & Liu, C. H. (2014). The default network and social understanding of others: What do brain connectivity studies tell us. *Frontiers in Human Neuroscience, 8*, Article 74.

Mammarella, I., & Cornoldi, C. (2014). An analysis of the criteria used to diagnose children with nonverbal learning disorder (NLD). *Child Neuropsychology, 20*, 255–280.

Mar, R. A. (2011). The neural basis of social cognition and story comprehension. *Annual Review of Psychology, 62*, 103–104.

Margolis, A. E., Pagliaccio, D., Thomas, L., Banker, S., & Marsh, R. (2019). Salience network connectivity and social processing in children with nonverbal learning disability or autism spectrum disorder. *Neuropsychology, 33*, 135–143.

Menon, V. (2015). Salience network. In A. W. Toga (Ed.), *Brain mapping: An encyclopedic reference* (pp. 597–611). Cambridge, MA: Academic Press.

Metsala, J. L., Galway, T. M., Ishaik, G., & Barton, V. E. (2017). Emotion knowledge, emotion regulation, and psychosocial adjustment in children with nonverbal learning disabilities. *Child Neuropsychology, 23*, 609–629.

Murphy, M. M., Mazzocco, M. M. M., Gerner, G., & Hendry, A. E. (2006). Mathematics learning disability in girls with Turner syndrome or fragile X syndrome. *Brain and Cognition, 61*, 195–210.

Nangle, D. W., Erdley, C. A., Newman, J. E., Mason, C. A., & Carpenter, E. M. (2003). Popularity, friendship quantity, and friendship quality: Interactive influences on children's loneliness and depression. *Journal of Clinical Child and Adolescent Psychology, 32*, 546–555.

Orraca-Castillo, M., Estevez-Perez, N., & Reigosa-Crespo, V. (2014). Neurocognitive profiles of learning disabled children with neurofribromatosis type 1. *Frontiers in Human Neuroscience, 8*, Article 386.

Palombo, J. (2006). *Nonverbal learning disabilities: A clinical perspective*. New York: Norton.

Pelletier, P. M., Ahmad, S. A., & Rourke, B. P. (2001). Classification rules for basic phonological processing disabilities and nonverbal learning disabilities: Formulation and external validity. *Child Neuropsychology, 7*(2), 84–98.

Pennington, B. F. (2008). *Diagnosing learning disabilities*. New York: Guilford Press.

Petti, V. L., Voelker, S. L., Shore, D. L., & Hayman-Abello, S. E. (2002). Perception of nonverbal emotional cues by children with nonverbal learning disabilities. *Journal of Developmental and Physical Disabilities, 15*(1), 23–36.

Poletti, M. (2017). Definition of a visuospatial dimension as a step forward in the diagnostic puzzle of nonverbal learning disability. *Applied Neuropsychology: Child, 6*, 106–109.

Prior, M., Smart, D., Sanson, A., & Oberlaid, F. (1999). Relationships between learning difficulties and psychological problems in preadolescent children from a longitudinal sample. *Journal of the American Academy of Child and Adolescent Psychiatry, 38*, 429–436.

Ramachandran, V. S., & Oberman, L. M. (2006). Broken mirrors. *Scientific American, 295*, 62–69.

Ris, D. M., Ammerman, R. T., Waller, N., Walz, N. C., Oppenheimer, S., Brown, T. M., . . . Yeates, K. O. (2007). Taxonicity of nonverbal learning disabilities. *Journal of the International Neuropsychological Society, 13*, 50–58.

Ris, D. M., & Nortz, M. J. (2008). Nonverbal learning disorder. In J. E. Morgan & J. H. Ricker (Eds.), *Textbook of clinical neuropsychology: Studies on neuropsychology, neurology, and cognition* (pp. 346–359). New York: Elsevier/Psychology Press.

Robin, N. H., & Sphrintzen, R. J. (2005). Defining the clinical spectrum of deletion 22q11.2. *Journal of Pediatrics, 147*, 90–96.

Rosenblum, S., & Piran, M. (2018). Normative or heavy clouds?: Early indicators of nonverbal learning disabilities based on mothers' reports. *Open Journal of Occupational Therapy, 6*.

Ross, E. D. (2000). Affective prosody and the aprosodias. In M. M. Mesulam (Ed.), *Principles of behavioral and cognitive neurology* (2nd ed.). Oxford, UK: Oxford University Press.

Rourke, B. P. (1988). The syndrome of nonverbal learning disabilities: Developmental manifestations in neurological disease and dysfunction. *Clinical Neuropsychologist, 4*, 293–330.

Rourke, B. P. (1989). *Nonverbal learning disabilities: The syndrome and the model*. New York: Guilford Press.

Rourke, B. P. (1995). The NVLD syndrome and the white matter model. In B. P. Rourke (Ed.), *Syndrome of nonverbal learning disabilities: Neurodevelopmental manifestations* (pp. 1–26). New York: Guilford Press.

Rourke, B. P. (2000). Neuropsychological and psychosocial subtyping: A review of investigations within the University of Windsor laboratory. *Canadian Psychology, 41*(1), 34–51.

Rourke, B. P., & Tsatsanis, K. D. (2000). Nonverbal learning disabilities and Asperger syndrome. In A. Klin, F. R. Volkmar, & S. S. Sparrow (Eds.), *Asperger syndrome* (pp. 231–253). New York: Guilford Press.

Rourke, B. P., Young, G. C., & Leenaars, A. A. (1989). A childhood learning disability that predisposes those afflicted to adolescent and adult depression and suicide risk. *Journal of Learning Disabilities, 22*(3), 169–175.

Rovet, J. (2004). Turner syndrome: Genetic and hormonal factors contributing to a specific learning disability profile. *Learning Disabilities Research and Practice, 19*, 133–145.

Schultz, R. T., Romanski, L. M., & Tsatsanis, K. D. (2000). Neurofunctional models of autistic disorder and Asperger syndrome: Clues from neuroimaging. In A. Klin, F. R. Volkmar & S. S. Sparrow (Eds.), *Asperger syndrome* (pp. 172–209). New York: Guilford Press.

Semrud-Clikeman, M. (2003). Executive functions and social communication disorders. *Perspectives, 29*, 20–22.

Semrud-Clikeman, M. (2007). *Social competence in children*. New York: Springer.

Semrud-Clikeman, M., & Ellison, P. A. T. (2009). *Child neuropsychology: Assessment and intervention*. New York: Springer.

Semrud-Clikeman, M., & Fine, J. G. (2011). Presence of cysts on magnetic resonance images

(MRIs) in children with Asperger disorder and nonverbal learning disabilities. *Journal of Child Neurology, 26*, 471–475.

Semrud-Clikeman, M., Fine, J. G., & Bledsoe, J. (2008a). *Meta-analysis of empirical literature on NVLD*. Paper presented at the International Neuropsychological Society.

Semrud-Clikeman, M., Fine, J. G., & Bledsoe, J. (2008b). *Meta-analysis of empirical research in assessment and diagnosis in NVLD*. Paper presented at the International Neuropsychological Association.

Semrud-Clikeman, M., Fine, J., Bledsoe, J., & Zhu, D. (2013). Volumetric differences among children with Asperger disorder, nonverbal learning disabilities, and controls on MRI. *Journal of Clinical and Experimental Neuropsychology, 5*, 540–550.

Semrud-Clikeman, M., Fine, J. G., & Zhu, D. C. (2011). The role of the right hemisphere for processing of social interactions in normal adults using functional magnetic resonance imaging. *Neuropsychobiology, 64*, 47–51.

Semrud-Clikeman, M., & Glass, K. (2010). The relation of humor and child development: Social, adaptive, and emotional aspects. *Journal of Child Neurology, 25*, 1248–1260.

Semrud-Clikeman, M., & Trauner, D. (2018). Nonverbal learning disabilities and associated disorders. In K. Swaiman, S. Ashwal, D. M. Ferriero, N. F. Schor, R. S. Finkel, A. L. Gropman, P. L. Pearl, & M. I Shevell (Eds.), *Swaiman's pediatric neurology* (6th ed., pp. 437–441). New York: Elsevier.

Semrud-Clikeman, M., Walkowiak, J., Wilkinson, A., & Butcher, B. (2010a). Executive functioning in children with Asperger's syndrome, ADHD-combined type, ADHD-predominately inattentive type, and controls. *Journal of Autism and Developmental Disorders, 40*, 1017–1027.

Semrud-Clikeman, M., Walkowiak, J., Wilkinson, A., & Christopher, G. (2010b). Neuropsychological findings in nonverbal learning disabilities. *Developmental Neuropsychology, 35*, 582–600.

Semrud-Clikeman, M., Walkowiak, J., Wilkinson, A., & Minne, E. (2010c). Behavior and social perception in children with Asperger's disorder, nonverbal learning disability, or ADHD. *Journal of Abnormal Child Psychology, 38*, 509–519.

Shaywitz, S. E., Mody, M., & Shaywitz, B. A. (2006). Neural mechanisms in dyslexia. *Current Directions in Psychological Science, 15*(6), 278–281.

Spreen, O. (2011). Nonverbal learning disabilities: A critical review. *Child Neuropsychology, 17*, 418–443.

Strothers, M. E., & Cardy, J. O. (2012). Oral language impairments in developmental disorders characterized by language strengths: A comparison of Asperger syndrome and nonverbal learning disorders. *Research in Autism Spectrum Disorders, 6*, 519–534.

Tsatsanis, K. D., & Rourke, B. P. (2008). Syndrome of nonverbal learning disabilities in adults. In L. Wolf, H. Schreiber, & J. Wasserstein (Eds.), *Adult learning disorders* (pp. 159–190). New York: Taylor & Francis.

Voeller, K. K. (1995). Clinical neurological aspects of the right hemisphere deficit syndrome. *Journal of Child Neurology, 10*, 16–22.

Volkmar, F. R., & Klin, A. (2000). Diagnostic issues in Asperger syndrome. In A. Klin, F. R. Volkmar & S. S. Sparrow (Eds.), *Asperger syndrome* (pp. 25–71). New York: Guilford Press.

Wechsler, D. (2014). *Wechsler Intelligence Scale for Children V.* San Antonio, TX: Psychological Corporation.

Woods, S. P., Weinborn, M, Ball, J. D., Tiller-Nevin, S., & Pickett, T. C. (2000). Periventricular leukomalacia (PVL): An identical twin case study illustration of white matter dysfunction and nonverbal learning disability (NLD). *Child Neuropsychology, 6*, 274–285.

World Health Organization. (2019). *International Classification of Diseases–10 Revision, Clinical Modification*. Geneva, Switzerland: Author.

Xiang, T., Lohrenz, T., & Montague, P. R. (2013). Computations substrates of norms and their violations during social exchange. *Journal of Neuroscience, 33*, 1099–1108.

Yalof, J. (2006). Case illustration of a boy with nonverbal learning disorder and Asperger's features: Neuropsychological and personality assessment. *Journal of Personality Assessment, 87*, 15–34.

CHAPTER 21

Dysexecutive Syndrome

Gerard A. Gioia
Peter K. Isquith
Robert M. Roth

OVERVIEW

This chapter considers the "dysexecutive syndrome," that is, a collection of executive function symptoms that define a specific clinical "dysexecutive" condition. The common understanding of a syndrome is that it captures a group of signs and symptoms that occur together and characterize a particular abnormality or condition, or a set of concurrent things, such as emotions or actions that usually form an identifiable pattern (Page, 2002). The very term *syndrome* focuses largely on a singular abnormality or condition. The question for this chapter is thus whether disruption of the executive control system results in a singular, identifiable condition or pattern of behavior. We argue that the nature and expression of the executive control processes that we call "executive functions" are not amenable to such a narrow and restrictive definition. In order for a singular condition or set of symptoms and signs related to executive dysfunction to exist, there would need to be a single, unitary executive.

Executive function has long been argued, however, to have both a unity and a diversity (Teuber, 1972), and different executive functions are at least characteristics if not indicative of a number of different syndromes. In 2000, when the literature on executive function in children was only about 15 years old and barely 200 peer-reviewed publications involving children or adolescents listed *executive function* or a similar term as a subject, we took the stance that "it is important to acknowledge and emphasize that there is no singular, core disorder of executive function" (Gioia, Isquith, & Guy, 2001, p. 324). Since then, there has been an explosion of research investigating executive functions in many different childhood disorders and diseases, with thousands of studies in the academic literature. We now have the benefit of this rich database that supports the argument against a singular "dysexecutive syndrome."

In this chapter, we begin by clarifying the meaning of *executive function* and presenting a common model of separate but related executive functions that operate within an overarching self-regulatory, supervisory system. Then we review performance measures and behavior rating measures of executive function relevant to working with children and adolescents to examine whether these suggest a single dysexecutive syndrome. With an understanding of the strengths and weaknesses of these approaches to evaluating executive functions, we turn to how problems with executive functions present in selected common developmental and acquired conditions in children, again to examine whether the presentations in these conditions constitute a dysexecutive syndrome or are disparate in their executive function characteristics. Finally, we review intervention approaches, again with an eye toward a unitary syndrome versus different executive function responses to intervention.

DEFINING EXECUTIVE FUNCTIONS

Many publications on executive functions begin by lamenting our inability to agree on a common definition of the construct, and simply list different definitions found in the literature without attempting to analyze their similarities and differences (e.g., Goldstein & Naglieri, 2014). A less cursory and more rigorous consideration of the seemingly myriad definitions reveals agreement on the fundamental construct: The executive functions are a domain-general, supervisory set of functions or processes that direct goal-oriented behavior, cognition, and emotion, overseeing and interacting with domain-specific functions such as language, spatial comprehension, new learning and remembering, motor skills, and emotional experience. Executive *function* is the overarching orchestration of thought, feeling, and action toward goal-oriented problem solving. Executive *functions* refer to the specific but interrelated control processes that contribute to that orchestration, most commonly including inhibition, flexibility, initiation, working memory, planning, organization, and self-monitoring.

Although authors vary on which functions are considered executive functions, good consensus exists as to the overarching concept of a central self-regulatory or *supervisory* system that guides, directs, and manages behavioral, emotional, and cognitive functions, particularly during active, goal-directed, novel problem solving. Most authors include at least inhibition of impulses not compatible with one's goal, ability to flexibly shift set or change behavior as needed, and ability to hold information and actively develop plans in working memory (Miyake et al., 2000; Packwood, Hodgetts, & Tremblay, 2011). Beyond these three executive functions, most authors also include the ability to plan by anticipating future events, setting goals, and developing a series of steps to achieve those goals; ability to organize complex novel information and behavioral output toward achieving a goal; and monitoring progress toward a goal in the social context and in problem solving. Initiation, an essential component of motivation to select and get started on achieving goals, has also been included in some models (e.g., Gioia, Isquith, Guy, & Kenworthy, 2000; Stuss & Benson, 1986). Importantly, executive functions are not exclusive to cognition; emotional control is relevant to effective problem-solving activity and is now considered important in many definitions of executive function (Gioia et al., 2000). In our own model, we describe each of these executive functions in terms of observed behaviors in children and adolescents (see Table 21.1).

TABLE 21.1. Executive Functions in Terms of Observed Behaviors in Children and Adolescents

Executive function	Behavioral description
Inhibition	Inhibit, resist, or not act on an impulse; stop own behavior at the proper time.
Flexibility/shifting	Move freely from one activity, situation, or aspect of a problem to another as the situation demands; solve problems flexibly.
Self-monitoring	Be aware of the effect of own behavior on others; check own actions during or shortly after finishing a task to ensure appropriate attainment of a goal.
Emotional control	Modulate emotional responses appropriately.
Initiation	Begin an activity or task; independently generate ideas.
Working memory	Hold information in mind for the purpose of completing a task.
Planning	Anticipate future events, set goals, and develop appropriate steps ahead of time to carry out a task or action.
Organization	Establish and maintain order within an activity or carry out a task in a systematic manner; strategically organize information.

MODELING EXECUTIVE FUNCTIONS

While discussion once concerned whether there is a single supervisory system, or just executive *function*, or whether that supervisory system could be "fractionated" into a few or several components (Shallice & Burgess, 1996), the general consensus by 2000 was that there is both an overarching executive function and, within that, separate but related executive functions from neuroanatomical (Owen, Schneider, & Duncan, 2000), neurobehavioral (Stuss & Alexander, 2000), cognitive (Miyake et al., 2000), and behavioral (Gioia et al., 2000) perspectives; that is, two levels or components of executive function exist: (1) an overarching supervisory system responsible for regulating our cognition, behavior, and emotions in the service of goal-directed problem solving and (2) a secondary system or collection of more specific functions such as starting (initiating), stopping (inhibiting), shifting (adapting), planning, organizing, and monitoring our behavior toward a goal.

This bilevel model, which reflects the unity and diversity of executive function, has considerable support. In one of the most widely cited articles on executive function, Miyake and colleagues (2000) modeled the relationships between cognitive measures designed to tap three specific executive functions: inhibitory control, working memory, and flexibility/shifting set. They found support for both a unity, or a singular higher-level executive function, and a diversity, or three specific factors reflecting inhibition, working memory, and flexibility. In a large-scale study, Cirino and colleagues (2018) tested models of executive function based on more than 30 standard executive function performance measures and behavior ratings in more than 800 children. They also found that a bifactor model best explained the data, with a large global executive function factor (the unity) distinct from several specific executive functions (the diversity). Duncan and colleagues (Duncan and Miller, 2002; Duncan & Owen, 2000) observed evidence of related but separable activation in frontal lobe regions reflecting distinct but related responses to executive function demands. As Stuss and Alexander (2000, p. 296) noted in their review of executive functions and the frontal lobe, "The central supervisory system is the sum of the processes recruited at any moment, for any given task." Bernstein and Waber (2018) argued, however, that executive functions are domain-general processes and are not as conducive to a modular approach as we might presume; that is, they are less fractionable or separable than we might like to think from a clinical assessment and intervention perspective. Thus, it may be tidier to think of inhibition as distinct from working memory in formulating an assessment and developing an intervention plan, yet the two are inextricably linked; inhibiting impulses and distractions enables the holding of information in working memory, while working memory allows for delay between thought and action, in turn facilitating inhibitory control.

How one defines and models the executive system depends on the general framework or model. Suchy (2009) discusses several approaches to describing executive functions, including neuroanatomical models that posit them as "what the frontal lobes do," syndrome-based models that describe what happens when there is damage to the frontal systems, neurocognitive process models that define executive functions by what putative executive function tests measure, and behavioral models that rely on everyday observed behaviors referred to as "complex skills." The complex skills model defines a set of interrelated yet separable functions that are observable in everyday behavior, including the integrated processes of holding goals and plans in working memory; inhibiting impulses; modulating emotions; flexibly shifting cognitive set or behavior; initiating activity; and planning, organizing, and monitoring progress toward a goal. Suchy suggests that this complex skills definition is the most common approach clinically, because it is the easiest to observe, measure, and communicate to others. In other words, it is more direct, practical, and useful to observe a child's inhibitory control (i.e., impulsivity) in his or her everyday behavior and discuss and develop interventions with a team than it is to hypothesize about the integrity of his or her frontal lobe or frontal systems, the possibility of a frontal lobe syndrome, or even administer a series of putative executive function tests.

It is also important to recognize that the executive functions do not stand alone. Although we may talk about a child's inhibitory control, planning, or organization in isolation, the reality is that these regulatory functions only exist in their relationship to other cognitive, behavioral, or emotional functions; that is, we cannot see or measure executive functions in isolation, but always do so through another domain-specific function such as attention, language, or motor function. For example, a child might exhibit disorganized language in defining a word on a vocabulary measure, wandering and weaving about in his or her explanation. We might question the child's organization, but because we are seeing it through language output, we must also question the child's language system. Thus, evaluating both the domain-general executive component (e.g., organization) and the domain-specific function (e.g., language) is important. It may indeed be that the problem is a central organization deficit, but it might also be that the problem is a language-specific deficit. This leads to two fundamental concepts in measuring executive function problems: We must first make sure that the specific function is intact (e.g., language), and if so and we suspect a central problem of organization, then we should look for organization problems in other specific domains (e.g., visuospatial problem solving, behavior). Because executive functions are central, overarching control processes, deficits or strengths should be seen in more than one if not multiple domains. At the same time, a deficit in one specific domain (e.g., language, motor function) can disrupt the executive control of that system in isolation.

A "conductor of the orchestra" metaphor can help illustrate the bidirectional relationship between domain general executive functions and domain-specific functions as they work together to meet an external demand situation (e.g., solve a problem). In this metaphor, the external demand situation (e.g., audience waiting for a good concert) is met by the orchestra that makes sound that is regulated and coordinated by the conductor, and music is the outcome. Each of the orchestra sections serves a separate function that is necessary to produce music. The conductor is necessary to regulate the music, telling the specific sections to begin playing (initiate), continue (sustain), change from one thing to the next (shift), and stop playing (inhibit). The conductor holds the plan in working memory while organizing and directing the specific sections and monitoring the outcome for progress toward a goal. In this model, the sections must have a conductor; otherwise, they produce chaos. At the same time, the conductor produces nothing on his or her own; there is no music without the players. Thus, the outcome (music) results from the interaction between each of the sections that serve a specific function (e.g., strings, horns, percussion) and the conductor that directs the sections to initiate, sustain, shift, and stop while organizing and planning the outcome and monitoring the progress toward the goal of making good music. In similar fashion, the domain-specific cognitive functions (e.g., language, attention, sensory, motor, learning, memory) perform their functions but the executive serves the conductor role of starting, sustaining, shifting, and stopping the sections to produce goal-directed behavior while holding a plan in working memory and monitoring progress toward that goal. In assessing why a child is not producing the expected "music," we must examine both the child's domain-specific players and the domain-general conductor to understand where the problems originate and how to improve the musical outcome. Poor music can be the result of poor domain-specific musicians or it could be the result of poor direction and supervision by the conductor. Both must be examined and understood, as their interdependency necessitates that one not be considered without the other. Clinical problems (e.g., poor social or academic functioning) associated with the domain-general supervisory executive control processes (e.g., inhibitory control, planning, working memory) must take into account their domain-specific partners (e.g., social cognition, emotion, language) and the interaction between the two in context (e.g., at home, in school, under stress) to produce a clinical diagnostic outcome (e.g., attention-deficit/hyperactivity disorder [ADHD], learning disability).

ASSESSING EXECUTIVE FUNCTIONS

Executive functions were historically measured through clinician-administered performance tasks (i.e., "tests"). Limitations of this test-based approach, however, necessitated the development of a complementary approach in assessing everyday behavioral manifestations. While some argue that performance measures are the "gold standard" of executive function assessment, and others argue that rating scales of everyday behavior provide the better estimate of self-regulation, in practice, and in research, these two approaches are most commonly used together. Performance measures attempt to tap specific executive functions in a controlled setting, while behavior ratings capture the implementation of executive functions in the everyday environment. We consider each approach separately, then look at the evolving standard found in the literature of integrating findings from both approaches.

Performance Measures

Performance measures (i.e., tests) have been the staple of clinical neuropsychological assessment since its inception. Numerous tasks have been developed or adapted for clinical use to help assess key domains of executive functioning across the age span. There are several advantages to assessing executive functions with performance measures. They offer increased specificity of the executive control processes, increased task control, and decades of research on the behavior of tests. We can sit with a child and observe his or her approach to tasks, providing rich information about the process and success of the child's ability to orchestrate his or her goal-oriented problem solving. At the same time, performance measures have well-known limitations (Goldberg & Podell, 2000; Bernstein & Waber, 1990; Pennington & Ozonoff, 1996). Tests are necessarily molar, tapping several elements of executive functions together with domain-specific nonexecutive functions. For example, while a simple digit span task might be viewed as a working memory measure, the task also requires that the child be able to inhibit motor activity (e.g., fidgeting) and inhibit attention to other stimuli (e.g., distractibility). The child must understand the task demands, regulate emotions during the task, capture auditory information, and initiate oral output (e.g., repeat the information). Individual differences in cognitive ability can affect test performance regardless of executive function demands; for example, a child with a language impairment might have greater difficulty with a digit span task because of the linguistic demands rather than an executive deficit. Sensitivity and specificity are typically limited with performance measures, in that individuals who should have executive function deficits (e.g., children with ADHD) often do well on these tests, while children who should not have executive function deficits (e.g., typically developing children) can, in some cases, do poorly on them.

One of the more common concerns with relying solely on performance measures of executive function is that the very requirements of standardized assessment for clinic-administered performance measures restricts the ability to apply assessment findings in the real world (Turkstra, Coelho, & Ylvisaker, 2005); that is, because standardized performance measures must typically be administered in the quiet, nondistracting, clinical setting in the same way each time, they fall short of capturing deficits that are present in the everyday, real-world environment. In such contexts, the evaluator provides structure by planning, organizing, and guiding the flow of the interaction to promote optimal performance, thus effectively serving as the child's executive functions (Kaplan, 1988; Stuss & Benson, 1986).

Reliance solely on clinic-based performance measures may yield a limited view of children's everyday self-regulation (Barkley, 2012; Gioia & Isquith, 2004; Silver, 2000,

2014). Performance-based measures tap limited components of the executive function system over a short time frame and not the integrated, multidimensional, relativistic, priority-based decision making that is often demanded in real-world situations (Goldberg & Podell, 2000). Barkley (2012) argues against a strict reliance on performance-based assessment methods:

> Dogmatic adherence to the psychometric tradition of understanding and assessing EF [executive function] at its most basic cognitive level is grossly inadequate. It provides only a superficial evaluation of even the conventional phenotypic view of EF. It fails to capture entirely the multilevel, concentrically arranged, affectively/motivationally charged, socially important and culturally facilitated nature of the extended phenotype of EF/SR [executive functions/self-regulation] in everyday human activities. (p. 190)

Rating Scales of Everyday Behavior

Recognizing the challenges involved in translating performance test findings to children's everyday environments, Gioia and colleagues (2000) developed the first parent–teacher rating scale to capture the everyday behaviors associated with executive function strengths and weaknesses in children, the Behavior Rating Inventory of Executive Function (BRIEF; Gioia et al., 2000). This work grew from a developmental neuropsychological assessment model that posited executive function as a broad umbrella construct within which a set of interrelated subdomains could be defined via behavioral manifestations (Bernstein & Waber, 1990). At the time, only a handful of articles concerned executive function in children and adolescents (Bernstein & Waber, 2007), few performance measures of executive function were available for this age range, and no standardized rating scales of executive function existed for any age. The BRIEF was intended as a complement to traditional performance measures, in part to serve as an index of generalizability for clinic findings, but it has been recognized as a useful measure of everyday executive function in its own right.

Assessment methods that rely on self- and/or informant reports also have their limitations. At the outset, the evaluator has limited control of environmental influences that may affect ratings on behavioral scales. Teachers may see greater executive difficulties when a student is in a demanding or less structured class than in a simpler or more structured class. Parents who provide more structure in their home environment may see fewer difficulties in their children than they would in less structured settings. Parsing deficits in specific executive functions via reported behaviors in these everyday contexts is also more difficult than via more narrowly focused performance measures. Executive functions operate in an integrative manner in the everyday context, such as allowing a child to inhibit distraction (e.g., another student's whispering to him or her), thus protecting his or her working memory to allow holding information (e.g., instructions for a writing assignment and a writing prompt) and a goal (e.g., complete the writing assignment in a timely fashion) in mind, in turn enabling planning (e.g., an approach to the assignment) and organization (e.g., the thesis, three points, and conclusion) of a task while monitoring output (e.g., checking grammar and spelling while writing). Finally, rater perspective must be considered when interpreting rating scales. An individual's emotional state or personality characteristics, or even simply whether or not he or she likes or dislikes the individual, may influence the ratings. For example, one teacher may dislike a child or, as is sometimes the case, simply dislike completing rating scales, while another teacher may enjoy the same child and value the opportunity to provide input into the evaluation process.

Performance Measures and/or Rating Scales?

Practitioners who evaluate children's executive functioning have several choices in their toolkit, including both performance measures and rating scales. While the question once was whether tests *or* scales were more accurate or useful in measure of executive functions, the question now is how best to integrate information from both tests *and* scales. An increasing body of research relies on both performance measures and rating scales to assess executive functions in children and adolescents (e.g., Cassidy, White, DeMaso, Newburger, & Bellinger, 2015; Gerst, Cirino, Fletcher, & Yoshida, 2017; Toplak, Bucciarelli, Jain, & Tannock, 2008). Researchers and practitioners who use both assessment methods are often faced with conflicting results: One measure suggests problems, while another measure suggests intact functioning in the same area. This has spawned arguments about whether one assessment approach should take precedence over the other (Barkley, 2012; Goldberg & Podell, 2000; McAuley, Chen, Goos, Schachar, & Crosbie, 2010).

A consistent observation about performance and rating scale measures of executive function is that they do not consistently correlate with each other, leading to questions about whether the two types of tools are measuring different aspects of executive function or even the same construct at all (Silver, 2000, 2014; Soto et al., 2020). Possible explanations include that one or the other type of measure is not actually tapping executive function, that performance measures assess "skills," while rating scales assess application of those skills (Faridi et al., 2015), that performance measures lack ecological validity (Goldberg & Podell, 2000), and that rating scales measure a large component of nonexecutive behaviors and are nonspecific (McAuley et al., 2010).

Despite the inconsistent relationship between performance-based tests and rating scales, several lines of evidence support using them together. First, several clinical groups show unique patterns of executive functioning on tests and on rating scales, consistent with what might be expected given the clinical disorder (e.g., Toplak et al., 2008). Second, both approaches show expected correlations with biological markers (e.g., Faridi et al., 2015). Third, a growing body of evidence shows logical concurrent and predictive relationships between executive function measures and real-world functioning such as academic skills (e.g., Gerst et al., 2017; Waber, Gerber, Turcios, Wagner, & Forbes, 2006). Fourth, both scales and tests show some sensitivity to change in executive functions over time or with treatment (Isquith, Roth, Kenworthy, & Gioia, 2014). Finally, correlations do exist between the two types of measures (Cassidy et al., 2015; Gerst et al., 2017; McAuley et al., 2010; Waber et al., 2006; Faridi et al., 2015).

We are left, then, with evidence that both performance measures and rating scales capture meaningful aspects of executive function, are related to the neurological substrate, have evidence of association with real-world functioning, and both contribute to an understanding of an individual's functioning. While some argue for an approach that relies most heavily, if not exclusively, on performance measures and others argue that rating scales should be the primary, if not sole, approach, most would agree that both approaches have merits and are best used in conjunction.

CLINICAL PROFILES OF EXECUTIVE DYSFUNCTION

Given the increasingly accepted model of the executive as a diversity of *functions* within a unity of *function*, there is little support for a singular "dysexecutive syndrome." In our earlier work on this topic (Gioia et al., 2001, p. 325), we concluded that "there is no singular disorder of executive function, but rather a variety of presentations that involve one or more aspects of executive function, including a number of common syndromes that reflect different patterns of executive dysfunction. These syndromes may be developmental in origin, such as autism spectrum disorders (ASD), Tourette syndrome, or ADHD, or acquired such as traumatic brain injury (TBI) or cranial radiation as treatment for leukemia." The body of empirical evidence since that time suggests that while executive function deficits are ubiquitous across many disorders or conditions, their presentation varies within and between those disorders. For example, while deficits in inhibitory control may be the central executive feature in ADHD-combined type, deficits in flexibility are the central feature in ASD, and working memory deficits are seen in multiple disorders such as ADHD-inattentive type and long-term outcomes of TBI. In this section, we review three clinical conditions (ADHD, ASD, TBI) that have characteristic deficits in executive functions.

Attention-Deficit/Hyperactivity Disorder

Numerous studies have examined the diagnostic relevance of executive functions in children with ADHD. In the largest meta-analysis of executive function performance measures in ADHD, Willcutt, Doyle, Nigg, Faraone, and Pennington (2005) included 83 studies with over 3,700 children with ADHD and nearly 3,000 typically developing children. They observed significant differences between the two groups, with moderate effect sizes. The greatest effect sizes, and most consistent group differences, across studies were seen for stop-signal reaction time (82% of studies), continuous performance test omission errors (77% of studies), and tower tasks (59% of studies). Group differences were also identified for working memory using span tasks in a smaller number of studies (55% of studies). Notably, they also found that less than half of children with ADHD exhibited significant impairment on any specific executive function task. Taken together, these findings indicate that some aspects of executive functions are more commonly impaired than others on performance-based tests in ADHD.

In their seminal review of executive function in ADHD, Tourette syndrome, autism, and oppositional defiant disorder, Pennington and Ozonoff (1996) found that the majority (67%) of executive function tasks revealed significantly worse performance in ADHD than control groups. They also observed that the patterns and extent of deficits were different in form and degree between their diagnostic groups, with greater problems on working memory and shifting tasks in the autism studies and no problems on executive function tasks in the Oppositional Defiant Disorder or Tourette syndrome groups unless there was also a diagnosis of ADHD. This important early analysis suggested that executive function performance measures had some sensitivity to the presence of expected deficits, that there was some specificity for ruling out executive function deficits, and that there were distinct patterns of executive function strengths and weaknesses between clinical groups.

From a behavioral perspective, our early work (Gioia & Isquith, 2001), demonstrated that ratings on the BRIEF Working Memory scale predicted the presence of ADHD with approximately 80% accuracy via parent or teacher ratings, and that ratings on the BRIEF Inhibit scale differentiated between the inattentive and combined subtypes of ADHD with over 70% accuracy. A recent study by Jacobson, Pritchard, Koriakin, Jones, and Mahone (2020) examined scale profiles on the BRIEF2 in nearly 2,000 children with either ADHD–inattentive (ADHD-I), ADHD–hyperactive/impulsive (ADHD-HI), or ADHD–combined (ADHD-C) presentations versus all other clinically referred children. They found distinctive profiles across the BRIEF2 scales for each group, with the ADHD-I group defined by substantial elevation on the Working Memory scale, the ADHD-HI group defined by substantial elevation on the Inhibit scale, and the ADHD-C group defined by elevations on both Working Memory and Inhibit scales. Meanwhile, the non-ADHD group of children seen for clinical evaluation showed much lower scores across scales. Classification accuracy was 87% for using the Working Memory scale to distinguish between children with any type of ADHD versus those with other, non-ADHD, clinical conditions, and was 87% for using the Inhibit scale to distinguish between children with ADHD-I and those with ADHD-C.

Some studies have relied on both performance tasks and rating scales in children with ADHD in an attempt to integrate findings for a more comprehensive assessment. Toplak and colleagues (2008) found differences between ADHD and control groups for stop-signal response time, verbal and spatial working memory span, planning on a tower task, and shifting set on a trail making task. Similarly, they noted differences between groups in ratings on the BRIEF across all scales. The authors then examined the relative contributions of performance measures and the BRIEF scales to predicting ADHD versus control group membership. While performance measures were helpful in predicting group membership, BRIEF ratings were substantially better. For example, stop-signal reaction time accuracy was approximately 60%, while parent and teacher ratings on the BRIEF Inhibit scale were 86–91% accurate. This improved, however, when both ratings and performance test scores were included, with accuracy increasing to over 90%. Overall, the findings provide support for integrating both behavior ratings and performance on tasks in evaluating executive functions in children with ADHD.

Autism Spectrum Disorders

Executive dysfunction is commonly reported in children with ASD (Hill, 2004; Pennington & Ozonoff, 1996). In a meta-analysis, Demetriou and colleagues (2018) reviewed 235 studies that included over 6,000 children with ASD and over 7,000 typically developing controls. They found moderate overall effect sizes for reduced executive functioning, though only a small number of executive function measures showed adequate clinical sensitivity. Their findings confirmed not only the presence of a broad executive dysfunction in children with ASD that was stable over development, but also that it was difficult to separate more global executive dysfunction into individual subdomains using performance measures.

Numerous studies have examined rating scales of executive function in children with ASD versus typically developing individuals. The majority have found that children with ASD exhibit deficits in one or more domains measured on the BRIEF (Gioia,

Isquith, Kenworthy, & Barton, 2002; Gilotty, Kenworthy, Sirian, Black, & Wagner, 2002; Kenworthy et al., 2005; Mackinlay, Charman, & Karmiloff-Smith, 2006). In one of the earliest comparisons of children with ASD versus typically developing children and those with other conditions on the BRIEF, Gioia et al. (2002) found a distinctive profile characterized by a deficit on the shift scale, reflecting limited flexibility, and distinguishing children with ASD from those with reading disorders, ADHD, or brain injuries.

In an example of an integrated assessment of executive function in children with ASD using both rating scales and performance measures, Troyb and colleagues (2014) compared typically developing children with those with high functioning ASD and children who were once diagnosed with ASD but had achieved "optimal outcomes." They found that the three groups demonstrated average overall executive functioning on performance measures including the Delis–Kaplan Executive Functioning System (D-KEFS) Color–Word Interference Test, verbal fluency, and a tower test. Children with optimal outcomes were rated as having greater deficits in flexibility and working memory than the typically developing children, and children with high-functioning ASD were rated as having greater difficulties across all executive domains on the BRIEF.

Traumatic Brain Injury

Studies of executive dysfunction in TBI have been distributed over a wide range of time postinjury, from the first year (Maillard-Wermelinger et al., 2009; Sesma, Slomine, Ding, McCarthy, & Children's Health after Trauma Study, 2008), through 1–5 years (Chapman et al., 2010; Conklin, Salorio, & Slomine, 2008; Donders, DenBraber, & Vos, 2010); and from 5–10 years postinjury (Kurowski et al., 2011; Mangeot, Armstrong, Colvin, Yeates, & Taylor, 2002; Muscara, Catroppa, & Anderson, 2008) and together suggest that executive dysfunction is a common outcome of TBI in children. A meta-analysis conducted by Babikian and Asarnow (2009) found a dose–response effect of injury severity on neuropsychological performance measures in general, including robust deficits in aspects of executive functioning (e.g., problem solving). A short-term longitudinal study observed worse working memory and shifting, but not inhibition, in children with mild TBI (Loher, Fatzer, & Roebers, 2014).

A review of ecologically valid assessment of cognition in TBI found that caregiver ratings demonstrated important utility in measuring the executive functions in children and adolescents with acquired brain injury (Chevignard, Soo, Galvin, Catroppa, & Eren, 2012). All studies using behavior ratings on the BRIEF found deficits in at least one aspect of executive function. Deficits in working memory were particularly evident in children with TBI compared to control samples as rated by parents and teachers. As a whole, these studies indicate executive dysfunction on performance tests, as well as particular deficits on ratings of everyday behavior.

Taken together, this substantial library of studies across a variety of child populations provides strong support for the role of multiple and varied profiles of executive dysfunction. These diverse findings of differing profiles of dysfunction in executive processes provide a strong argument against a singular "dysexecutive syndrome." Instead, the literature provides substantial support for the variety of ways that disruption of the supervisory processes (e.g., working memory, planning and organization, inhibitory control, flexibility) produce unique clinical diagnostic patterns or profiles.

INTERVENING WITH THE EXECUTIVE FUNCTIONS

With a deeper understanding of the unique and varied ways that the supervisory processes contribute to our clinical understanding of the child, and armed with a set of assessment tools to assist in their measurement, the scene is set for intervention. A singular syndrome approach would suggest a single intervention to address this specific problem. In contrast, as we have just reviewed, the literature over the past 30 years has documented a variety of profiles of executive dysfunction. The approach to treatment then necessarily requires an understanding of the specific profile of executive dysfunction and its domain-specific partner as the target of intervention. A range of interventions have been proposed and studied for various types of executive function-related problems in different clinical disorders.

The foundation of the intervention process is a solid working knowledge of the executive supervisory processes and the types of clinical profiles that may present in a child. Targeting the specific profile of executive dysfunction (e.g., working memory, flexibility, inhibitory control) is, therefore, the essential first step. The work of Mark Ylvisaker and Tim Feeney (1998, 2008, 2009) has informed the general principles of an intervention model in advocating for an ongoing contextualized (i.e., taking place in the person's real world), collaborative (i.e., with the student, parents, teachers, and peers working together), and hypothesis-testing (i.e., generating and implementing testable methods) approach. The ultimate goal of executive function interventions is to establish regular behavioral and cognitive routines to maximize independent, supervisory, goal-oriented problem solving and performance. Ylvisaker and Feeney pioneered a collaborative, everyday model of intervention in the real world demonstrated in Project Learnet (*www.projectlearnet.org*). They articulate the importance of accommodating executive function impairments so that the individual can experience success while learning new executive function skills through extensive modeling, scaffolding, guided practice, and then, once learned, fading supports. The model of everyday collaborative problem-solving routines has influenced a number of interventions, including Dawson and Guare's executive coaching model (2010, 2012), Cooper-Kahn and Dietzel's intervention model in *Late, Lost and Unprepared* (2008), and Kenworthy and colleagues' (2014) *Unstuck and On Target!* intervention program. The overarching model involves setting a goal and thinking through plans, considering the likelihood of success, implementing the plans, and reviewing afterward.

The varied clinical profiles of executive dysfunction described earlier have become an increasing focus of intervention. For example, medications have been studied as tools to treat aspects of executive dysfunction such as inhibitory control and working memory in ADHD (Biederman et al., 2011; Yang et al., 2011), Tourette's syndrome (Cummings, Singer, Krieger, Miller, & Mahone, 2002), TBI (Beers, Skold, Dixon, & Adelson, 2005), and hepatitis C virus (Rodrigue et al., 2011). The executive functions have also been a focus of intervention outcome following corticosteroid treatment in children with inflammatory bowel disease (Mrakostsky et al., 2013) and family-based intervention in TBI (Wade, Wolfe, Brown, & Pestian, 2005). Cognitive remediation approaches have also focused on the executive functions, emphasizing processes such as working memory, planning, organization, and problem solving in ADHD (Beck, Hanson, Puffenberger, Benninger, & Benninger, 2010; Hahn-Markowitz, Manor, & Maeir, 2011) and TBI (Chan & Fong 2011; Toglia, Johnston, Goverover, & Dain, 2010). A study of preadolescents with TBI showed improvements in several aspects of parent-rated executive functioning following a social mediation, cooperative learning, and metacognitive learning intervention program (Braga, Rossi, Moretto, da Silva, & Cole, 2012).

Interventions for children with ASD have been developed and validated by Kenworthy and colleagues (2014), adapting the Ylvisaker and Feeney model. Their intervention, "Unstuck and On Target!" is an executive function intervention for children with ASD targeting flexibility, insistence on sameness, goal setting, and planning through a cognitive-behavioral program of self-regulatory scripts, guided/faded practice, and visual/verbal cueing. The treatment is contextually based through its school and home-based implementation, critical contexts in which a child applies his or her executive function processes. The effectiveness of the Unstuck and On Target! treatment was compared to a social skills intervention in third to fifth graders with ASD delivered by school staff in small group sessions. Children with ASD exhibited greater improvements with the program than the social skills intervention in their problem solving, flexibility, and planning/organizing. The program also promoted greater improvements in the classroom in following rules, making transitions, and flexibility. This program demonstrates the effectiveness of the contextually based executive function intervention for children with ASD in a mainstream educational setting.

SUMMARY AND CONCLUSIONS

Clinicians and researchers alike have been interested in the nature and role of the executive functions now for many decades. While debate continues around specific details of definition, assessment, and treatment, a broad consensus has emerged that the executive functions serve a unique role as domain general supervisory control processes that work in concert with subordinate domain-specific functions. Importantly, over the past 20 years, a burgeoning literature has strongly bolstered the argument that representing executive dysfunction as a singular condition, a "dysexecutive syndrome," seriously limits the important ways that the executive control processes guide, direct, and manage cognition, behavior, and emotion in human beings. Rather, evidence supports a common integrative "diversity within unity" model that posits distinct but related specific elements, such as inhibitory control, working memory, and flexibility that comprise the overarching supervisory conductor that serves goal-oriented problem solving. Assessment tools, both performance measures and behavior ratings, that measure these functions and find different profiles in various clinical conditions also argue strongly against a singular dysexecutive syndrome. Instead, we find a host of clinical profiles reflecting dysfunction in specific executive functions as they manifest in, or characterize, disorders such as ADHD, ASD, and TBI. A narrow, singular dysexecutive syndrome would not do justice to the nature of these clinical conditions. The emerging intervention literature further supports the rejection of "one size fits all" as interventions target different aspects of the executive control processes such as working memory, inhibition, or flexible problem solving as they present in a variety of conditions.

Thus, we recommend conceptualizing the manifestations of dysfunctional executive control processes as variations in clinical profiles. The unity and diversity of executive function that Teuber (1972) described fits the theoretical and clinical footprint of this supervisory system, and most authors since 2000 agree with this model from neuroanatomical (Owen et al., 2000), neurobehavioral (Stuss & Alexander, 2000), cognitive (Miyake et al., 2000), and behavioral (Gioia et al., 2000) perspectives. This integrated set of executive control functions can be rendered dysfunctional by a variety of developmental and acquired neurological diagnoses to produce a number of different profiles of executive dysfunction rather than a singular dysexecutive syndrome.

REFERENCES

Babikian, T., & Asarnow, R. (2009). Neurocognitive outcomes and recovery after pediatric TBI: Meta-analytic review of the literature. *Neuropsychology, 23*(3), 283–296.

Barkley, R. A. (2012). *Executive functions: What they are, how they work and why they evolved*. New York: Guilford Press.

Beck, S. J., Hanson, C. A., Puffenberger, S. S., Benninger, K. L., & Benninger, W. B. (2010). A controlled trial of working memory training for children and adolescents with ADHD. *Journal of Clinical Child and Adolescent Psychology, 39*(6), 825–836.

Beers, S. R., Skold, A., Dixon, C. E., & Adelson, P. D. (2005). Neurobehavioral effects of amantadine after pediatric traumatic brain injury: A preliminary report. *Journal of Head Trauma Rehabilitation, 20*(5), 450–463.

Bernstein, J. H., & Waber, D. P. (1990). Developmental neuropsychological assessment: The systemic approach. In A. A. Boulton, G. B. Baker, & M. Hiscock (Eds.), *Neuromethods: Vol. 17. Neuropsychology* (pp. 311–371). Clifton, NJ: Humana.

Bernstein, J. H., & Waber, D. P. (2007). Executive capacities from a developmental perspective. In L. Meltzer (Ed.), *Executive function in education: From theory to practice* (pp. 77–105). New York: Guilford Press.

Bernstein, J. H., & Waber, D. P. (2018). Executive capacities from a developmental perspective. In L. Meltzer (Ed.), *Executive function in education: From theory to practice* (2nd ed., pp. 57–81). New York: Guilford Press.

Biederman, J., Mick, E., Fried, R., Wilner, N., Spencer, T. J., & Faraone, S. V. (2011). Are stimulants effective in the treatment of executive function deficits?: Results from a randomized double blind study of OROS-methylphenidate in adults with ADHD. *European Neuropsychopharmacology, 21*(7), 508–515.

Braga, L. W., Rossi, L., Moretto, A. L. L., da Silva, J. M., & Cole, M. (2012). Empowering preadolescents with ABI through metacognition: Preliminary results of a randomized clinical trial. *NeuroRehabilitation, 30*(3), 205–212.

Cassidy, A. R., White, M. T., DeMaso, D. R., Newburger, J. W., & Bellinger, D. C. (2015). Executive function in children and adolescents with critical cyanotic congenital heart disease. *Journal of the International Neuropsychological Society, 21*(1), 34–49.

Chapman, L. A., Wade, S. L., Walz, N. C., Taylor, H. G., Stancin, T., & Yeates, K. O. (2010). Clinically significant behavior problems during the initial 18 months following early childhood traumatic brain injury. *Rehabilitation Psychology, 55*(1), 48–57.

Chan, D. Y. K., & Fong, K. N. K. (2011). The effects of problem-solving skills training based on metacognitive principles for children with acquired brain injury attending mainstream schools: A controlled clinical trial. *Disability and Rehabilitation, 33*(21–22), 2023–2032.

Chevignard, M. P., Soo, C., Galvin, J., Catroppa, C., & Eren, S. (2012). Ecological assessment of cognitive functions in children with acquired brain injury: A systematic review. *Brain Injury, 26*(9), 1033–1057.

Cirino, P. T., Ahmed, Y., Miciak, J., Taylor, W. P., Gerst, E. H., & Barnes, M. A. (2018). A framework for executive function in the late elementary years. *Neuropsychology, 32*(2), 176.

Conklin, H. M., Salorio, C. F., & Slomine, B. S. (2008). Working memory performance following paediatric traumatic brain injury. *Brain Injury, 22*(11), 847–857.

Cooper-Kahn, J., & Dietzel, L. (2008). *Late, lost, and unprepared: A parent's guide to helping children with executive functioning*. Bethesda, MD: Woodbine House.

Cummings, D. D., Singer, H. S., Krieger, M., Miller, T. L., & Mahone, E. M. (2002). Neuropsychiatric effects of guanfacine in children with mild Tourette syndrome: A pilot study. *Clinical Neuropharmacology, 25*, 325–332.

Dawson, P., & Guare, R. (2010). *Executive skills in*

children and adolescents: A practical guide to assessment and intervention (2nd ed.). New York: Guilford Press.

Dawson, P., & Guare, R. (2012). *Coaching students with executive skills deficits.* New York: Guilford Press.

Demetriou, E. A., Lampit, A., Quintana, D. S., Naismith, S. L., Song, Y. J. C., Pye, J. E., . . . Guastella, A. J. (2018). Autism spectrum disorders: A meta-analysis of executive function. *Molecular Psychiatry, 23*(5), 1198–1204.

Donders, J., DenBraber, D., & Vos, L. (2010). Construct and criterion validity of the Behaviour Rating Inventory of Executive Function (BRIEF) in children referred for neuropsychological assessment after paediatric traumatic brain injury. *Journal of Neuropsychology, 4*(Pt. 2), 197–209.

Duncan, J., & Miller, E. K. (2002). Cognitive focus through adaptive neural coding in the primate prefrontal cortex. In D. T. Stuss & R. T. Knight (Eds.), *Principles of frontal lobe function* (pp. 278–291). New York: Oxford University Press.

Duncan, J., & Owen, A. M. (2000). Common regions of the human frontal lobe recruited by diverse cognitive demands. *Trends in Neurosciences, 23*(10), 475–483.

Faridi, N., Karama, S., Burgaleta, M., White, M. T., Evans, A. C., Fonov, V., . . . Waber, D. P. (2015). Neuroanatomical correlates of behavioral rating versus performance measures of working memory in typically developing children and adolescents. *Neuropsychology, 29*(1), 82–91.

Gerst, E. H., Cirino, P. T., Fletcher, J. M., & Yoshida, H. (2017). Cognitive and behavioral rating measures of executive function as predictors of academic outcomes in children. *Child Neuropsychology, 23*(4), 381–407.

Gioia, G. A., & Isquith, P. K. (2001). Executive function and ADHD: Exploration through children's everyday behaviors. *Clinical Neuropsychological Assessment, 2*, 61–84.

Gioia, G. A., & Isquith, P. K. (2004). Ecological assessment of executive function in traumatic brain injury. *Developmental Neuropsychology, 25*, 135–158.

Gioia, G. A., Isquith, P. K., & Guy, S. C. (2001). Assessment of executive function in children with neurological impairments. In R. Simeonsson & S. Rosenthal (Eds.), *Psychological and developmental assessment* (pp. 317–356). New York: Guilford Press.

Gioia, G. A., Isquith, P. K., Guy, S. C., & Kenworthy, L. K. (2000). *The Behavior Rating Inventory of Executive Function.* Lutz, FL: Psychological Assessment Resources.

Gioia, G. A., Isquith, P. K., Guy, S. C., & Kenworthy, L. K. (2015). *The Behavior Rating Inventory of Executive Function* (2nd ed.). Lutz, FL: Psychological Assessment Resources.

Gioia, G. A., Isquith, P. K., Kenworthy, L., & Barton, R. M. (2002). Profiles of everyday executive function in acquired and developmental disorders. *Child Neuropsychology*, 8(2), 121–137.

Gilotty, L., Kenworthy, L., Sirian, L., Black, D. O., & Wagner, A. E. (2002). Adaptive skills and executive function in autism spectrum disorders. *Child Neuropsychology, 8*(4), 241–248.

Goldberg, E., & Podell, K. (2000). Adaptive decision making, ecological validity, and the frontal lobes. *Journal of Clinical and Experimental Neuropsychology, 22*, 56–68.

Goldstein, S., & Naglieri, J. A. (2014). *Handbook of executive functioning.* New York: Springer.

Hahn-Markowitz, J., Manor, I., & Maeir, A. (2011). Effectiveness of cognitive-functional (Cog-Fun) intervention with children with attention deficit hyperactivity disorder: A pilot study. *American Journal of Occupational Therapy, 65*(4), 384–392.

Hill, E. L. (2004). Executive dysfunction in autism. *Trends in Cognitive Sciences, 8*, 26–32.

Isquith, P. K., Roth, R. M., Kenworthy, L., & Gioia, G. (2014). Contribution of rating scales to intervention for executive dysfunction. *Applied Neuropsychology: Child, 3*(3), 197–204.

Jacobson, L. A., Pritchard, A. E., Koriakin, T. A., Jones, K. E., & Mahone, E. M. (2020). Initial examination of the BRIEF2 in clinically referred children with and without ADHD symptoms. *Journal of Attention Disorders, 24*, 1775–1784.

Kaplan, E. (1988). The process approach to neuropsychological assessment. *Aphasiology*, 2(3–4), 309–311.

Kenworthy, L., Anthony, L. G., Alexander, K. C., Werner, M. A., Cannon, L., & Greenman, L. (2014). *Solving executive functioning challenges: Simple ways to get kids with autism unstuck and on target.* Baltimore: Brookes.

Kenworthy, L. E., Black, D. O., Wallace, G. L., Ahluvalia, T., Wagner, A. E., & Sirian, L. M. (2005). Disorganization: The forgotten executive dysfunction in high-functioning autism (HFA) spectrum disorders. *Developmental Neuropsychology, 28*(3), 809–827.

Kurowski, B. G., Taylor, H. G., Yeates, K. O., Walz, N. C., Stancin, T., & Wade, S. L. (2011). Caregiver ratings of long-term executive dysfunction and attention problems after early childhood traumatic brain injury: Family functioning is important. *Physical Medicine and Rehabilitation, 3*(9), 836–845.

Loher, S., Fatzer, S. T., & Roebers, C. M. (2014). Executive functions after pediatric mild traumatic brain injury: A prospective short-term longitudinal study. *Applied Neuropsychology: Child, 3*(2), 103–114.

Mackinlay, R., Charman, T., & Karmiloff-Smith, A. (2006). High functioning children with autism spectrum disorder: A novel test of multitasking. *Brain and Cognition, 61*(1), 14–24.

McAuley, T., Chen, S., Goos, L., Schachar, R., & Crosbie, J. (2010). Is the behavior rating inventory of executive function more strongly associated with measures of impairment or executive function? *Journal of the International Neuropsychological Society, 16*(3), 495–505.

Maillard-Wermelinger, A., Yeates, K. O., Gerry Taylor, H., Rusin, J., Bangert, B., Dietrich, A., . . . Wright, M. (2009). Mild traumatic brain injury and executive functions in school-aged children. *Developmental Neurorehabilitation, 12*(5), 330–341.

Mangeot, S., Armstrong, K., Colvin, A. N., Yeates, K. O., & Taylor, H. G. (2002). Long-term executive function deficits in children with traumatic brain injuries: Assessment using the Behavior Rating Inventory of Executive Function (BRIEF). *Child Neuropsychology, 8*(4), 271–284.

Miyake, A., Friedman, N. P., Emerson, M. J., Witzki, A. H., Howerter, A., & Wager, T. D. (2000). The unity and diversity of executive functions and their contributions to complex "frontal lobe" tasks: A latent variable analysis. *Cognitive Psychology, 41*(1), 49–100.

Mrakotsky, C., Forbes, P. W., Bernstein, J. H., Grand, R. J., Bousvaros, A., Szigethy, E., & Waber, D. P. (2013). Acute cognitive and behavioral effects of systemic corticosteroids in children treated for inflammatory bowel disease. *Journal of the International Neuropsychological Society, 19*(1), 96–109.

Muscara, F., Catroppa, C., & Anderson, V. (2008). Social problem-solving skills as a mediator between executive function and long-term social outcome following paediatric traumatic brain injury. *Journal of Neuropsychology, 2*(2), 445–461.

Owen, A. M., Schneider, W. X., & Duncan, J. (2000). *Executive control and the frontal lobe: Current issues*. Berlin: Springer.

Packwood, S., Hodgetts, H. M., & Tremblay, S. (2011). A multiperspective approach to the conceptualization of executive functions. *Journal of Clinical and Experimental Neuropsychology, 33*(4), 456–470.

Page, M. (2002). *The British Medical Association illustrated medical dictionary*. London: Dorling Kindersley.

Pennington, B. F., & Ozonoff, S. (1996). Executive functions and developmental psychopathology. *Journal of Child Psychology and Psychiatry, 37*(1), 51–87.

Rodrigue, J. R., Balistreri, W., Haber, B., Jonas, M. M., Mohan, P., Molleston, J. P., . . . Gonzalez-Peralta, R. P. (2011). Peginterferon with or without ribavirin has minimal effect on quality of life, behavioral/emotional, and cognitive outcomes in children. *Hepatology, 53*(5), 1468–1475.

Sesma, H. W., Slomine, B. S., Ding, R., McCarthy, M. L., & Children's Health after Trauma Study Group. (2008). Executive functioning in the first year after pediatric traumatic brain injury. *Pediatrics, 121*(6), e1686–e1695.

Shallice, T., & Burgess, P. (1996). The domain of supervisory processes and temporal organization of behaviour. *Philosophical Transactions of the Royal Society of London B: Biological Sciences, 351*(1346), 1405–1412.

Silver, C. (2000). Ecological validity in neuropsychological assessment in childhood traumatic brain injury. *Journal of Head Trauma Rehabilitation, 15*(4), 973–988.

Silver, C. H. (2014). Sources of data about children's executive functioning: Review and commentary. *Child Neuropsychology, 20*(1), 1–13.

Soto, E. F., Kofler, M. J., Singh, L. J., Wells, E. L., Irwin, L. N., Groves, N. B., & Miller, C. E. (2020). Executive functioning rating scales: Ecologically valid or construct valid? *Neuropsychology, 34*(6), 605–619.

Stuss, D. T., & Alexander, M. P. (2000). Executive functions and the frontal lobes: A conceptual view. *Psychological Research, 63*(3–4), 289–298.

Stuss, D. T., & Benson, D. F. (1986). *The frontal lobes*. New York: Raven.

Suchy, Y. (2009). Executive functioning: Overview, assessment, and research issues for non-neuropsychologists. *Annals of Behavioral Medicine, 37*, 106–116.

Teuber, H. L. (1972). Unity and diversity of frontal lobe functions. *Acta Neurobiologiae Experimentalis, 32*, 615–656.

Toglia, J., Johnston, M. V., Goverover, Y., & Dain, B. (2010). A multicontext approach to promoting transfer of strategy use and self regulation after brain injury: An exploratory study. *Brain Injury, 24*, 664–677.

Toplak, M. E., Bucciarelli, S. M., Jain, U., & Tannock, R. (2008). Executive functions: Performance-based measures and the behavior rating inventory of executive function (BRIEF) in adolescents with attention deficit/hyperactivity disorder (ADHD). *Child Neuropsychology, 15*(1), 53–72.

Turkstra, L. S., Coelho, C., & Ylvisaker, M. (2005). The use of standardized tests for individuals with cognitive-communication disorders. *Seminars in Speech and Language, 26*(4), 215–222.

Troyb, E., Rosenthal, M., Eigsti, I. M., Kelley, E., Tyson, K., Orinstein, A., . . . Fein, D. (2014). Executive functioning in individuals with a history of ASDs who have achieved optimal outcomes. *Child Neuropsychology, 20*(4), 378–397.

Waber, D. P., Gerber, E. B., Turcios, V. Y., Wagner, E. R., & Forbes, P. W. (2006). Executive functions and performance on high-stakes testing in children from urban schools. *Developmental Neuropsychology, 29*, 459–477.

Wade, S. L., Wolfe, C., Brown, T. M., & Pestian, J. P. (2005). Putting the pieces together: Preliminary efficacy of a web-based family intervention for children with traumatic brain injury. *Journal of Pediatric Psychology, 30*(5), 437–442.

Wade, S. L., Wolfe, C. R., & Pestian, J. P. (2004). A web-based family problem-solving intervention for families of children with traumatic brain injury. *Behavior Research Methods, instruments, and Computers, 36*(2), 261–269.

Willcutt, E. G., Doyle, A. E., Nigg, J. T., Faraone, S. V., & Pennington, B. F. (2005). Validity of the executive function theory of attention-deficit/hyperactivity disorder: A meta-analytic review. *Biological Psychiatry, 57*(11), 1336–1346.

Yang, L., Cao, Q., Shuai, L., Li, H., Chan, R. C., & Wang, Y. (2011). Comparative study of OROS-MPH and atomoxetine on executive function improvement in ADHD: A randomized controlled trial. *International Journal of Neuropsychopharmacology, 15*(1), 15–26.

Ylvisaker, M., & Feeney, T. (1998). *Collaborative brain injury intervention: Positive everyday routines.* San Diego, CA: Singular Publishing Group.

Ylvisaker, M., & Feeney, T. (2008). Helping children without making them helpless: Facilitating development of executive self-regulation in children and adolescents. In V. Anderson, R. Jacobs, & P. Anderson (Eds.), *Executive functions and the frontal lobes: A lifespan perspective* (pp. 409–438). New York: Taylor & Francis.

Ylvisaker, M., & Feeney, T. (2009). Apprenticeship in self-regulation: Supports and interventions for individuals with self-regulatory impairments. *Developmental Neurorehabilitation, 12*(5), 370–379.

CHAPTER 22

Pediatric Acute-Onset Neuropsychiatric Syndrome

Osman Malik
Davide Martino
Tammy Hedderly

INTRODUCTION

The etiology of mental illness has long been debated and has historically been attributed to myriad causes, from evil spirits to weak-mindedness. Fortunately, we have moved on to scientific exploration of causation. While the idea that mental illness is caused by stress and trauma has been challenged by biological evidence, such as the role of neurotransmitters and genetics, causation remains multifactorial. Among the biological factors that cause mental illness, one proposed etiology involves the immune system causing illness (autoimmune) of the brain and mind. There are well-known models of the immune system turning against the brain causing illness, such as N-methyl-D-aspartate (NMDA) receptor antibody-mediated encephalitis, multiple sclerosis, and Sydenham's chorea. In psychiatric disorders there is evidence that a very small proportion of schizophrenia is due to autoimmune mechanisms (Kayser & Dalmau, 2011). Pediatric autoimmune neuropsychiatric disorder associated with streptococcus (PANDAS; Swedo et al., 1998) and pediatric acute-onset neuropsychiatric syndrome (PANS; Swedo, Leckman, & Rose, 2012) are proposed conditions that explain autoimmunity as the etiology of sudden-onset obsessive-compulsive disorder (OCD) and tics in childhood.

In PANDAS and PANS it has been proposed that, following an infection, antibodies formed against the invading microorganisms cross the blood–brain barrier and attach themselves to certain receptors in the basal ganglia, thus causing OCD/tics. Antibodies are Y-shaped proteins also known as *immunoglobulins* (Ig), produced mainly by a type of white blood cells called *plasma cells*, that neutralize pathogens such as bacteria and viruses by binding to molecules on the surface of these pathogens called *antigens*. Antibodies form an important part of the immune system. Antibodies can sometimes form against our own cells, as the antibodies identify molecules on the surface of human cells as foreign (this is called *autoimmunity*). In PANDAS specifically, it is postulated that following a streptococcal infection, antibodies against streptococcal bacteria (especially group A beta-hemolytic) cross the blood–brain barrier and bind to neuronal surface antigens that appear be similar to streptococcal antigens (Swedo et al., 1998, 2012). It is further postulated that these neurons are likely to be in the basal ganglia, and antibodies tend to bind to dopamine receptors, or the surface of striatal cholinergic interneurons thus modulating their activity (Frick et al., 2018). It is this excitability and release of dopamine, and/or the antibody-mediated dysregulation of striatal cholinergic interneurons, that could then cause tics and other PANDAS symptoms (Cunningham & Cox, 2016). Since the exact antibodies have yet to be detected (both for PANDAS and PANS), the mechanism described here is a postulated hypothesis based on other illness models and clinicians' experience. Thus, due to lack of empirical scientific evidence, there is controversy concerning the PANDAS and PANS models, and questions have been raised about the validity of the proposed disorders.

PANDAS and PANS are defined by some as the features described in Tables 22.1 and 22.2. Some clinicians argue that there is no need for separate terms, as the diagnoses pediatric OCD and Tourette syndrome (TS) encompass the symptoms described in both PANDAS and PANS, and that adding further labels based on possibly different but as yet unproven etiology may confuse clinicians and parents. It is also unclear whether the clinical presentation of PANDAS/PANS can be distinguished from that of an acute behavioral exacerbation in a child with a chronic neurodevelopmental disorder such as chronic tic disorders and autistic spectrum disorder. Some clinicians and parents argue for a need to have PANDAS/PANS as separate, novel disorders to draw a distinction between their treatment course and that of other OCD/tic disorders, advocating the use of antibiotics or immune-modulating treatments in PANDAS/PANS.

HISTORICAL OVERVIEW OF PANDAS AND PANS

The term PANDAS predates PANS by over a decade. PANDAS primarily was intended to describe psychiatric symptoms that arise following a throat infection with group A streptococcus (GAS; as in Table 22.1). The term PANS was proposed in 2012 (Swedo

TABLE 22.1. Proposed PANDAS Diagnostic Criteria (Swedo et al., 1998, 2012)

1. *Presence of OCD and/or a tic disorder.*
2. *Pediatric onset:* Symptoms of the disorder first become evident between 3 years of age and the beginning of puberty.
3. *Episodic course of symptom severity:* Clinical course is characterized by the abrupt onset of symptoms or by dramatic symptom exacerbations. Often, the onset of a specific symptom exacerbation can be assigned to a particular day or week, at which time the symptoms seemed to "explode" in severity. Symptoms usually decrease significantly between episodes and occasionally resolve completely between exacerbations.
4. *Association with group A beta-hemolytic streptococcal (GABHS) infection:* Symptom exacerbations must be temporally related to GABHS infection (i.e., associated with positive throat culture and/or elevated anti-GABHS antibody titers).
5. *Association with neurological abnormalities:* During symptom exacerbations, patients will have abnormal results on neurological examination. Motoric hyperactivity and adventitious movements (including choreiform movements or tics) are particularly common.

TABLE 22.2. PANS Diagnostic Criteria (Swedo et al., 2012; Chang et al., 2015)

1. Abrupt, dramatic onset of OCD or severely restricted food intake.
2. Concurrent presence of additional neuropsychiatric symptoms, with similarly severe and acute onset, from at least two of the following seven categories:
   - anxiety (particularly, separation anxiety)
   - emotional lability (extreme mood swings) and/or depression
   - irritability, aggression and/or severely oppositional behaviors
   - behavioral (developmental) regression (e.g., talking baby talk, throwing temper tantrums)
   - deterioration in school performance
   - sensory or motor abnormalities
   - somatic signs and symptoms, including sleep disturbances, bed-wetting or increased urinary frequency.
3. Symptoms are not better explained by a known neurologic or medical disorder, such as Sydenham's chorea, systemic lupus erythematosus, Tourette syndrome, or others.

et al., 2012), following the proceedings of a workshop held in 2010 to define diagnostic criteria for a broader entity of conditions that lead to acute neuropsychiatric symptoms in childhood, as it was agreed that acute-onset symptoms might occur without a preceding GAS infection. The proceedings of this workshop led to working criteria for a new syndrome (PANS), consisting of dramatic and abrupt onset of OCD or severely restricted food intake, and concurrent sudden onset of at least two of seven categories of additional neuropsychiatric symptoms summarized in Table 22.2. Despite being linked in their conceptualization, PANS and PANDAS are in fact different clinical concepts, in that PANS lacks a unifying etiology or precipitant (unlike the proposed specific streptococcal trigger for PANDAS), and also has additional diagnostic features. For this reason, based on its definition, PANS represents a deliberately broad spectrum proposed by experts with the final goal of subsequently classifying these acute neuropsychiatric presentations according to their multiple causative factors and differing pathogenic mechanisms.

In 2015, a series of articles by clinical researchers from different U.S. institutions (Chang et al., 2015; Frankovich et al., 2017; Murphy et al., 2015b; Toufexis et al., 2015) proposed an initial consensus statement on a detailed diagnostic workup recommended for all patients fulfilling PANS working criteria (Chang et al., 2015), alongside case series addressing treatments, including antibiotics, immune-modifying treatments, and more "traditional" symptomatic treatments for OCD and eating disorders. Since then, PANS experts in the United States have continued to report phenomenological observations indicating the possible coexistence of other symptoms, such as motor disinhibition during rapid eye movement sleep (Gaughan et al., 2016) and psychotic symptoms, particularly complex hallucinations (Silverman et al., 2019). This series of publications has suggested that even with loose etiological boundaries, patients fulfilling PANS criteria could be suffering from an immune-mediated or postinfectious encephalopathic illness. As with PANDAS, the immune-mediated assumption for PANS has, to date, not been corroborated by the discovery of an underlying autoimmune process (Gilbert, Mink, & Singer, 2018). Moreover, the efficacy of an immune-modifying treatment in reducing PANS symptoms still awaits demonstration through high-quality randomized controlled trials (Sigra, Hesselmark, & Bejerot, 2018).

Another milestone in the evolution of the PANS concept is related to the publication of the PANS Research Consortium treatment guidelines (Swedo, Frankovich, & Murphy, 2017; Calaprice, Tona, Parker-Athill, & Murphy, 2017; Calaprice, Tona, & Murphy, 2018; Cooperstock, Swedo, Pasternack, & Murphy, 2017; Jaspers-Fayer et al., 2017). In accordance with the mandate of the PANS multidisciplinary clinic (Brown et al., 2017a, 2017b), these guidelines aim to inform primary care physicians and specialists managing these patients, and suggest psychiatric and behavioral therapies (Thienemann et al., 2017), antibiotic therapy (Murphy et al., 2017), and immune-modifying treatments (Brown et al., 2017a, 2017b; Spartz et al., 2017). Importantly, these guidelines are based on experts' clinical experience but lack a systematic approach to summarize the published evidence with an unbiased methodology and are not corroborated by randomized controlled trials. Another important limitation of the guidelines, which should be addressed in future work, is the lack of a clinical distinction between mild and severe forms that could justify different priorities for trials of potentially harmful antibiotic and immune-modifying therapies. The absence of a biomarker for an immune-mediated mechanism leading to the PANS phenotype is highlighted in Hesselmark and Bejerot's work (2017). These authors subsequently confirmed in a cohort of Swedish patients that the diagnosis of PANS is associated with greater likelihood of treatment with antibiotics or immune-modifying treatment than patients with the OCD and similar symptoms, but not fulfilling the full anecdotal "diagnostic criteria" (Hesselmark & Bejerot, 2019a, 2019b).

Knowledge and evidence gaps notwithstanding, the description of clinical cases characterized by the cardinal features that define PANS highlights an unresolved and controversial clinical challenge (i.e., the diagnostic work-up and appropriate management of this complex population of pediatric patients).

THE DEBATE SURROUNDING PANS/PANDAS

The PANS/PANDAS debate divides clinicians, parents, and scientists, with some doctors refusing to use the term for fear of inducing harm by generating the misconception that the term might imply the presence of "bugs in the brain" (i.e., Streptococcus or "antibodies eating the basal ganglia"). In several clinical cases, anxious concerns of parents have led to the harmful belief that hospital admission, invasive investigations, and heavy immunotherapy are the only ways forward in ensuring their child's health. The repeated use of acute and long-term antibiotics, as recommended by the consensus PANS guidelines (Swedo et al., 2017; Calaprice et al., 2018), comes with a risk of overuse of antibiotics in an era of antibiotic resistance, especially as these guidelines could lead clinicians to consider antibiotic treatment for a number of other chronic, and difficult to treat, psychiatric disorders in children (e.g., OCD and anxiety in the context of autism spectrum disorder [ASD]).

Regardless of the controversies, children do sometimes present very acutely with severe and distressing neuropsychiatric symptoms such as a florid onset of obsessive–compulsive symptoms, associated tics, and behavioral disturbances including rage, aggression, and anxiety. There are a large number and wide range of neurobehavioral, psychological, social, and neurobiological manifestations that lead to the cascade of complex events culminating in the final common endpoint that manifests as an acute behavioral disruption fulfilling criteria for PANS. Diverse examples of the possible etiologies for PANS are genetic copper metabolism abnormalities (e.g., Wilson disease) leading to an OCD, a teenager using recreational drugs and presenting with acutely disturbed behavior, or sudden-onset functional symptoms (i.e., psychogenic or conversion symptoms). In this chapter, we focus our discussion around cases, probably the majority of which fulfill diagnostic criteria for PANS, but in which etiology is undetermined, with negative investigations in terms of cerebrospinal fluid (CSF) analysis, neuroimaging, or electroencephalographic (EEG) findings and therefore not suggestive of encephalitis or known encephalopathies, including autoantibody-mediated forms. Typically, these cases present to the specialist's attention via general pediatric clinics or neurology services or via child and adolescent mental health services. They typically appear otherwise healthy, apart from extreme and often disabling obsessive–compulsive symptoms/tics or eating behavior abnormalities.

The diagnosis and management of PANS is guided *force majeure* by the experience of only a few clinicians and clinical scientists worldwide (Gilbert et al., 2018; Wilbur et al., 2019). Management approaches can also be biased by the clinical discipline of the assessing doctor. Preferring immune-modifying therapies and denying potentially helpful evidence-based psychological therapies such as cognitive-behavioral therapies do not appear to be ethical. The debate regarding administration of antibiotics and immune-modifying medications for managing acute psychiatric symptoms is fueled by the need to consider risks such as side effects and developing resistance to antibiotics, and use of these treatments can also distract the clinician from considering the right treatment. Undoubtedly, despite important initial work (Jaspers-Fayer et al., 2017), a substantial amount of work remains to resolve the debate about this clinical entity and to subtype the PANS spectrum appropriately in order to develop pathogenically driven, reliable diagnostic and therapeutic algorithms. The role of family-related factors (e.g., parental health anxiety, family response to illness, parent–child interaction) also needs further analysis in order to subtype PANS and guide management. Although PANS has a broad definition to include any cause of acute neuropsychiatric symptoms, interest has been mainly focused on possible infectious and immune triggers, though alternative anxiety-driven functional and posttraumatic triggers also occur within this group and are less often considered. The main challenge with formulating a diagnosis of PANS is that it comprises a broad range of sometimes variable and nonspecific symptoms that can also be identified in a range of neurodevelopmental disorders. It is difficult to discriminate PANS, for example, from sudden-onset typical or familial OCD. Differentiating PANDAS from other tic disorders and OCD can be especially difficult, as PANDAS is conceptualized as a fluctuating condition (Swedo et al., 1998, 2012), and hence displays a waxing and waning that is also a very typical pattern in chronic tic disorders.

A recent case–control study compared three groups of patients: those with interview-defined PANS, those "suspected" of having PANS, and those with a psychiatric condition without any suspicion of PANS (Hesselmark & Bejerot, 2019a). Symptoms in patients with interview-confirmed PANS showed an episodic course, with multiple symptoms present at the onset compared with the psychiatric control population. However, individuals with interview-confirmed PANS did not present a more specific symptom profile, despite having more severe symptoms and more frequent exacerbations.

There are no clear biomarkers or investigations that help to differentiate PANS from OCD or chronic tic disorder. Rather, the "diagnosis" (hence, the distinction) is based on a collection of observed symptoms and on the clinician's estimation of whether the onset of symptoms is temporally associated with a possible infection (e.g., a flu or sore throat) or medically definable disorder (e.g., an acquired brain lesion). This temporal association may be proposed by clinicians without specific experience in the diagnosis of neurodevelopmental disorders. The laboratory workup proposed in the PANS consortium guidelines is not based on a traditional evidence basis. Nevertheless, the workup is unlikely to be harmful and when adopted in cases in which a specific etiology is suspected, could lead to the identification of associated treatable disorders, such as Wilson disease. Guidelines are best considered *aides mémoire* to help the experienced clinician make a decision based on their judgment.

Apart from having an acute onset and high symptom severity, there is little clear demarcation between PANS and neuropsychiatric conditions such as OCD and chronic tic disorders from the perspective of neuropsychological assessment. It is therefore extremely important that clinicians assess any potential PANS referral within a psychiatric and neurodevelopmental framework, and ideally within a multidisciplinary team comprising neurology, psychiatry and neuropsychology/psychology expertise (Chang et al., 2015; Gromark et al., 2019). The team should consider preexisting developmental factors, psychosocial issues, and diverse family genetic history, along with any suspected disorder of the immune system. This approach is particularly important in cases in which the family is striving for immune therapy in the hope of "a cure" (Gabbay et al., 2008). Excessive medical investigations and unnecessary immunomodulatory treatments can potentially cause harm to the child. This may be the case in parents who themselves have preexisting anxiety in the form of excessive and obsessional worry about their or their child's health, and focus on minor symptoms and rumination about the presence of a serious medical disorder. In such instances, ill-health anxiety is often fueled or exacerbated by doctors. In cases where there is already a genetic predisposition to have OCD in the family, it is our personal observation that parents can become engaged in compulsively seeking a medical cure for PANS.

In our experience of acute-onset neuropsychiatric symptoms in children, there appears to be a family history of tics, OCD, or other neurodevelopmental disorders, and this again is similar to what is known of the family history of children with typical tic disorders and OCD (Krebs & Heyman, 2014). On careful history taking these children (or one of the parents) often exhibited very minor tics, obsessional behaviors, or compulsive rituals earlier in life (Hedderly & Malik, 2018). Thus, a considerable proportion of new cases that meet the criteria for PANS and/or PANDAS can also fulfil diagnostic criteria for TS, ASD, or familial (genetically based) OCD. A study within an OCD/Tourette clinic found that 31 of 176 (18%) of children referred for tics or OCD had been previously diagnosed with PANDAS (Gabbay et al., 2008); however, only 12 of the 31 (38%) met established PANDAS diagnostic criteria. In another study of PANS multidisciplinary assessment and treatment in Sweden (Gromark et al., 2019), more than 1,500 patients were referred to a specialized OCD clinic and only 47 (about 3%) met criteria for PANS. It is possible that due to the stigma around mental health issues, and perceived incurability of psychiatric disorders, many families (and some providers) tend to prefer "infection and neurological" to "psychiatric" explanations, which could contribute to parents seeking a PANS/PANDAS diagnosis, with a hope for a cure.

CURRENT STATUS: NEUROSCIENCE-BASED EVIDENCE

A brief review of the research exploring the link between GAS putative immune markers, PANS/PANDAS symptomatology, and possible response to treatments is useful in considering the status of these conditions.

Examining the Proposed Link with GAS Infection

To date, research proving a causative role of streptococci in PANDAS is limited, and most children who have PANDAS symptoms will not have an infection with streptococcal bacteria, nor will a majority of young people with a known streptococcal infection/Strep sore throat develop features of PANDAS. Below we summarize research that examines the link between GAS infection and PANDAS.

Mell, Davis, and Owens (2005) identified 144 cases of new-onset OCD, TS, or tic disorder along with 609 matched controls and found that patients with new-onset OCD, TS, or tic disorder were significantly more likely to have had streptococcal infections diagnosed in the year before illness onset. When TS was considered separately, having more than one GAS infection in the 12 months before the tic onset date was 13-fold more common among cases with TS than controls (odds ratio [OR]: 13.6; 95% confidence interval [CI]: 1.93, 51.0).

Two studies have focused on identifying PANDAS in children in community pediatric clinics (Perrin et al., 2004; Murphy et al., 2004). In one, streptococcal infection was present in 411 of 814 (50%) children (4–11 years), presumed viral pharyngitis was present in 207 (25%), and 196 children (24%) had no infections. Parents completed a PANDAS symptoms checklist at the initial study time point, then 2 and 12 weeks thereafter. At 12 weeks, there were no differences across the three groups for obsessive–compulsive behaviors, tics or other neuropsychiatric symptoms (Perrin et al., 2004). In the second study, 693 healthy children (ages 3–12 years) were recruited. Streptococcal infection data (via throat cultures) were collected, as well as clinical examinations and behavioral ratings over an 8-month period. Using a temporal criterion of 3 months from the streptococcal infection to symptoms, the authors reported no increased risk of tics or chorea. They identified significantly more frequent "swaying" and "nontic grimacing" in 37 (19%) children with infection compared to 28 (6%) without infections, and more frequent nonspecific problem behaviors in 68 (35%) children with infections compared to 91 (18%) without. Furthermore, they reported a dose–effect linking more streptococcal infections with more problem behaviors. Despite these associations, the study's causality criteria, which included a strength, timing, and dose–effect, failed to confirm an association between a preceding streptococcal infection and a PANDAS diagnosis (Murphy et al., 2004).

Another study examining the role of strep in chronic tic disorders (CTDs) and TS is the EMTICS (European Multicentre Tics in Children Studies; Martino et al., 2021). This longitudinal, observational multicenter study recruited 715 children with CTD in 16 specialist clinics from nine countries and followed them for 16 months on average. Tic, obsessive–compulsive symptom (OCS), and attention-deficit/hyperactivity disorder (ADHD) severity were assessed during four monthly study visits and telephone interviews. Exposure to GAS was analyzed using measures based on pharyngeal swab and serological testing. The associations between GAS exposures and tic exacerbations or changes of tic,

OCS, and ADHD symptom severity were measured. Exacerbations occurred 455 times in 308 of 715 (43%) participants. The authors did not detect any significant association between GAS exposure and tic exacerbations (OR ranging between 1.006 and 1.235, all *p* values > .3). GAS exposures were associated with longitudinal changes of hyperactivity–impulsivity symptom severity. The authors concluded that the study did not support GAS exposures as contributing factors for tic exacerbations in children with CTD. They recommended that specific workup or active management of GAS infections is unlikely to modify the course of tics in CTD and is therefore not recommended.

Two prospective multicenter studies enrolled children who met PANDAS criteria (Kurlan, Johnson, & Kaplan, 2008; Leckman et al., 2011). The objective was to identify whether a streptococcal infection preceded the exacerbation of OCD or tic symptoms. In the first study (Kurlan et al., 2008), 40 children with stringent criteria for PANDAS were compared to 40 matched children with OCD or tic disorders. All had monthly throat cultures, three monthly antibody tests, and monthly phone or in-clinic evaluations. The PANDAS group had a significantly higher rate of GAS infections, as well as a higher rate of clinical exacerbations. However, no more than 25% of the exacerbations in the PANDAS cases were temporally associated with a GAS infection, this percentage dropped to 6% if exacerbations in the non-PANDAS group were also included. There was no relationship between changes in antistreptococcal antibody titers and occurrence of clinical exacerbations. This suggests that acute onset cases had more exacerbations and severity in the course, but these ongoing symptoms had no correlation with streptococcal infection or ASO (antistreptolysin-O, an antibody against GAS).

In the second study (Leckman et al., 2011), consecutive clinical ratings of tic and OCS severity were obtained for 31 PANDAS subjects and 53 non-PANDAS subjects. Clinical symptoms and laboratory values (throat cultures and streptococcal antibody titers) were evaluated at regular intervals during a 25-month period. Additional testing occurred at the time of any tic or OCS exacerbation. New GAS infections were established by throat swab cultures and/or recent significant rise in streptococcal antibodies. No group differences were observed in the number of clinical exacerbations or the number of newly diagnosed GAS infections. On only 6 of a total of 51 (12%) occasions, a newly diagnosed GAS infection was followed, within 2 months, by an exacerbation of tic and/or OCS. In every instance, this association occurred in the non-PANDAS group. The authors concluded that their study provided no evidence for a temporal association between GAS infections and tic/OCS exacerbations in children who met the PANDAS diagnostic criteria.

Two further longitudinal studies of children meeting PANDAS criteria (without choreiform movements) failed to identify a temporal association between symptom exacerbation and elevations in the purported antibodies (Singer et al., 2015; Morris-Berry, Pollard, Gao, Thompson, & Singer, 2013). The presence of overlapping results in children with Sydenham's chorea and those with "PANDAS plus choreiform movements" has raised the question of whether the latter group actually had Sydenham's chorea.

Examining the Proposed Link with Autoimmune Responses and Potential Antibodies

Patients with TS have some predisposition to autoimmune responses, indicated by the reduced frequency of regulatory T cells, which induce tolerance toward self-antigens, as well as overrepresentation of autoimmune illness in the family (Martino, Zis, & Buttiglione, 2015). Moreover, there are some interesting observed differences in immune response and in allergy tendency in some children with tics and OCD (Chang et al., 2011).

It is also known that autoimmune diseases, such as systemic lupus erythematosus, rheumatoid arthritis, and Hashimoto's thyroiditis, are more prevalent in individuals with OCD/tic disorder and in family members of individuals with OCD (Pérez-Vigil et al., 2016; Mataix-Cols et al., 2018). In the same way association studies show that tic disorders and OCD are over-represented in individuals with autoimmune disorders or those with family history of autoimmune disease (Perez-Vigil et al., 2016; Mataix-Cols et al., 2018), but demonstrating an association is not the same as proving causality. Tic disorders have also been shown to share a genetic/familial link with autoimmune conditions (Mataix-Cols et al., 2018), but despite these links, tic disorders and OCD are not yet considered to be autoimmune conditions themselves—as no specific antibodies or target antigens are known, as in other established autoimmune disorders.

To explore this bidirectional association, common pathological pathways need to be explored, with special emphasis on genetic and environmental factors, in particular psychosocial stress. Clinical observations and studies of tic disorders, early-onset OCD, ADHD, and pediatric depression suggest that these disorders are highly sensitive to psychosocial stress (Lin et al., 2007). Psychosocial stress significantly influences immune and endocrine stress responses, as well as increasing rates of infection—including GAS infections (Luo et al., 2004; Corbett, Mendoza, Baym, Bunge, & Levine, 2008; Lin et al., 2010). Hence, genetics and stress may be shared, common precursors to immune, infectious, and psychological disorders.

Considering research on potential pathological antibodies, a PANDAS hypothesis encourages a search for antistreptococcal antibodies against neurons in the basal ganglia that are purported to bind to dopamine receptors or the surface of striatal cholinergic interneurons (Frick et al., 2018), yet no single antibody marker has been identified so far. Initial studies and ongoing observational investigations (e.g., Lepri et al., 2019) have focused on antibodies commonly produced in response to streptococci (i.e., ASO and anti-DNase B). In the case of PANS, it is proposed that this may include streptococci or any other range of pathogens and antibodies against these pathogens or other immune or postinfectious mechanisms that can influence the brain, such as inflammatory mediators or postsynaptic signaling abnormalities.

The site or nature of neuropathology in PANDAS has not been established, nor has the location at which any putative antibodies could be acting. A volumetric brain magnetic resonance imaging (MRI) study of children with OCD and tics associated with streptococcal infection ($n = 34$) suggested larger central gray matter structures (caudate, putamen, globus pallidus), compared to healthy controls ($n = 82$), but there was no correlation between basal ganglia size and symptom severity, the and authors did not compare findings with those in children with OCD and tics without streptococcal infection (Giedd, Rapoport, Garvey, Perlmutter, & Swedo, 2000). A positron emission tomography study utilizing a marker for activated microglia (neuroinflammation) evaluated 17 children with PANDAS and compared results with 12 children with TS and 15 healthy adults (controls). Compared to adults, both children with TS and those with PANDAS had increased signal in bilateral caudate nuclei, and the PANDAS group showed an increased signal in the lentiform nuclei. However, these findings are difficult to interpret because of the non-age-matched control population (Kumar, Williams, & Chugani, 2015), and overall support the probability of overlapping clinical phenotypes.

Studies attempting to confirm antibody binding in the striatum have been inconsistent. Pavone and coworkers (2004) compared serum antibrain antibodies to human basal ganglia sections assessed by indirect tissue immunofluorescence in two groups: a PANDAS group of 22 patients who met PANDAS criteria and had tics or OCD, or both; and a control group of 22 patients with clinical evidence of active GAS infection confirmed by throat culture and elevated ASO titers, but without history or clinical evidence of tics or OCD. They observed positive antibasal ganglia staining in 14/22 (64%) patients in the PANDAS group, but only 2/22 (9%) in the GAS control group ($p < .001$). These results suggest that in a proportion of children with PANDAS, antibrain antibodies are present but cannot be explained by a history of GAS infection (Pavone et al., 2004). In contrast, another study found no association between PANDAS diagnosis and immunofluorescent positivity in PANDAS, TS, and controls ($n = 30$ in each group) (Morris, Pardo-Villamizar, Gause, & Singer, 2009).

The EMTICS included tic-free younger siblings of patients with tic disorders, as there is a 10-fold chance of a sibling having tics compared to someone from the general population. Recruiting tic-free younger siblings would mean that many would go on to develop tics (new-onset tics) in the duration of the study period (5 years), and this would allow researchers to study immune and other phenomena right at tic onset. One group in the EMTICS consortium (Baglioni et al., 2019) examined serum for antibodies from children with new-onset tic disorders (siblings) and those with CTD. Serum of 30 siblings with new-onset tics before and after the first tic onset (onset group) was examined for antibodies, along with serum of 158 patients in the chronic phase undergoing an acute relapse (exacerbation group) for the same antibodies. Researchers screened for antibodies to anti-*N*-methyl-D-aspartate receptor (NMDAR), contactin-associated protein-like 2 (CASPR2), leucine-rich glioma inactivated 1 (LGI1), AMPA receptors (AMPAR), and gamma-aminobutyric acid (GABA). Only two individuals (one preclinical, one chronic) had antibodies binding the NMDAR, and the binding was only weakly positive. No other specific antibodies were detected. Despite some immunoreactivity toward neuronal antigens on brain tissue, this was not mirrored by antibodies binding to live neurons, suggesting the presence of nonspecific antibodies or those that bind nonpathogenic intracellular epitopes. NMDAR or the other neuronal surface antibodies tested were very infrequent in these patients. The authors concluded that the evidence for pathogenic antibodies being causative of TS is weak.

In a 2019 prospective study (Baumgaertel et al., 2019), 20 adult patients with TS were tested for specific and unspecified autoantibodies against various antigens (NMDA-, CASPR2-, LGI1-, AMPA-, and GABAB1/B). Researchers did not find any specific surface-autoantibodies or unspecified autoantibodies. Immunohistochemistry on tissue-sections also did not show any specific binding patterns.

Animal models have also been used to explore the autoimmune hypothesis in PANDAS (Mora, Martín-González, Flires, & Moreno, 2020). Rats immunized with GAS manifested several features similar to Sydenham's chorea and PANDAS (Yaddanapudi et al., 2010) and antibodies against the dopamine receptors were isolated from these rats. The rats were noted to engage in excessive grooming and displayed motor control impairments.

Transferring serum immunoglobulin G (IgG) obtained from these rats into the striatum of naive rodents caused some similar behavioral and motor symptoms, suggesting that the antibodies in the serum from immunized rates possibly caused the motor disturbance in the naive rodents.

ASO antibodies commonly used in clinical practice to identify possible PANDAS patients are too nonspecific and are often present for 12 months after a GAS infection, and therefore are not meaningful and often are misleading. Given the challenges with ASO and anti-DNase-B as reliable antibodies or disease markers for PANDAS, other sets of antibodies have been explored. These have also been used as recommended tests in PANS cases, and have been organized within the so-called "Cunningham panel" (Cunningham & Cox, 2016), which encompasses antibodies against dopamine D1 receptor (*DRD1*), dopamine D2L receptor (*DRD2L*), lysoganglioside GM1, and tubulin, plus a functional assay involving the calcium-dependent calmodulin protein kinase II (*CaMKII*). One study was conducted to assess the diagnostic accuracy of the Cunningham panel in patients with suspected PANS or PANDAS and compared their antibody profile with healthy controls (Hesselmark & Bejerot, 2017). A majority of the healthy controls had pathological Cunningham panel results and test–retest reliability proved insufficient (Hesselmark & Bejerot, 2017), suggesting that the use of the Cunningham panel of antibodies in the diagnoses of PANDAS/PANS is questionable.

Though there is an ongoing search for the putative antibody, it is not always through antibodies that immune-mediated neuropsychiatric symptoms occur. For instance, there has been research on the role of inflammatory markers such as C-reactive protein, cytokines, interleukins, and tumor necrosis factor- α in psychiatric disorders (Najjar, Pearlman, Alper, Najjar, & Devinsky, 2013; Khandaker et al., 2018a; Khandaker, Zammit, Burgess, Lewis, & Jones, 2018b). Singer, Gause, Morrix, and Lopez (2008) examined the role of cytokines in children with PANDAS in a longitudinal study, although they did not find a correlation between cytokine levels and clinical exacerbations. More research is needed to explore how inflammatory chemicals affect mental state, especially in vulnerable brains, for instance, in those of children with neurodevelopmental disorders. The question of whether this is a direct effect of these inflammatory markers or, rather, that these markers up-regulate or down-regulate certain neurotransmitter receptors in the brain, thus potentially perpetuating behavioral symptoms even when an inflammatory trigger is not present, remains to be answered.

Can Specific Investigations Clarify a Diagnosis of PANS/PANDAS?

Testing for GAS infections should not be considered equivalent to testing for PANDAS. Both throat cultures and serological streptococcal antibody tests indicate exposure to streptococci but do not distinguish between otherwise healthy children with no OCD or tics and those suspected to have PANDAS. Positive throat cultures can indicate active infection or a benign carrier state and do not prove that streptococci are causative for OCD/tic symptoms. Throat cultures can remain positive in nearly 20% of children 12 months after an acquired infection (Johnson, Kurlan, Leckman, & Kaplan, 2010). Similarly, elevated blood titres for streptococcal antibodies (ASO and anti-DNase B) only indicate a prior streptococcal infection, but do not provide reliable information about the time of onset or duration of that infection. These antibodies remain elevated for more than 12 months in over 50% of children (Johnson et al., 2010). Therefore, a single antibody titre elevation does not link a streptococcal infection to tic or OCD onset.

In summary, all published PANDAS data show that streptococcal cultures, antistreptococcal antibodies, and antibrain antibodies have a high potential to mislead both clinicians and parents (Gilbert et al., 2018; Chiarello, Spitoni, Hollander, Matucci Cerinic, & Pallanti, 2017). Moreover, if both antibody levels and behavioral symptoms fluctuate, and these fluctuations are not correlated, then repeated longitudinal testing also becomes problematic. Thus, although protocol-based streptococcal testing remains critical for acute rheumatic fever, there is little evidence to support these tests in children with OCD or tics.

Treatment Studies

In their clinical overview on treatment approaches to PANDAS, Murphy, Lewin, Parker-Athill, Storch, and Mutch (2013) reported that, based on case series and reports, surgically removing tonsils and adenoids does not prevent the onset of PANDAS. Clinical trials of antibiotics have used small sample sizes and detected weak effects. Trials involving penicillin and azithromycin had significant design flaws (e.g., inadequate blinding or control arm, or reliance on use of clinician-rated measures), but despite limited evidence of benefit, antibiotics are being prescribed to children with PANS and PANDAS presentations and antibiotics are suggested in the PANS treatment guidelines (Cooperstock, Swedo, Pasternack, Murphy, & the PANS/PANDAS Consortium, 2017) from the PANS/PANDAS Consortium USA. To demonstrate this challenge, we summarize the antibiotic studies that form part of the basis of these guidelines. In one antibiotic study of PANDAS, a double-blind, randomized controlled trial compared prophylaxis with penicillin versus azithromycin for 12 months, but without a placebo arm (Snider, Lougee, Slattery, Grant, & Swedo, 2005). In this study, the rates of streptococcal infections and neuropsychiatric symptom exacerbations were compared between the study year and the year prior to entry. The authors noted a significant decrease in streptococcal infections during the study year in both the penicillin and the azithromycin groups ($p < .01$). They also noted a significant reduction in neuropsychiatric exacerbations during the study year in both groups ($p < .01$). The absence of a placebo arm limited the conclusions that could be drawn from the study, and the observed improvement might have simply been erroneously attributed to the effect of antibiotics, as it could have reflected the natural course of PANDAS (i.e., less exacerbation with time, whatever medication is used). In a double-blind, randomized, placebo-controlled pilot-study of azithromycin for acute-onset OCD (Murphy et al., 2017), the authors concluded that there was a trend toward benefit produced by antibiotics, hence leading to their statement that antibiotics "may be used" as a treatment approach. These authors found no significant treatment effect of azithromycin based on the Children's Yale–Brown Obsessive–Compulsive Scale (CY-BOCS), but this treatment produced a modest effect as assessed by a clinical global impression scale. Sample size was also rather small. Another randomized pilot study of Cefdinir found that this antibiotic helped OCD and tic symptoms compared to placebo, but these improvements were not statistically or clinically significant (Murphy et al., 2015a).

Antibiotic treatment is common, even in the absence of any laboratory evidence of infection, highlighting the frequent and potentially harmful misuse of the term PANDAS.

This is especially concerning if the PANS/PANDAS label prevented access to psychological therapies that can help manage symptoms of OCD and tics.

A small study of the effects of administration of intravenous human immunoglobulins (IVIG) treatment in children with severe, infection-triggered exacerbations of OCD or tic disorders compared 1-month outcomes for IVIG ($n = 9$), plasma-exchange (plasmapheresis) ($n = 10$), and placebo (sham saline solution) ($n = 10$) (Perlmutter et al., 1999). Symptom severity was rated at baseline, and at 1 month and 12 months after treatment by use of standard assessment scales for OCD, tics, anxiety, depression, and global function. The study showed that the plasma-exchange group had the best outcome, and both the plasmapheresis and IVIG groups had strikingly better outcome than the placebo group in OCD, anxiety and overall function, but only the plasma-exchange group showed improvement in tics. The numbers were very small and findings were not replicated with larger numbers or by another group. Most of the immune-based treatment approaches show weak or conflicting evidence. A recent comprehensive review of PANS/PANDAS treatment by Sigra, Hesselmark and Bejerot (2018) identified 12 treatment studies with published outcome data. Eleven of the 12 studies showed a moderate or high risk of bias, including selection bias, performance bias, detection bias, attrition, reporting bias, or a combination of these issues. The exception was a randomized, controlled clinical trial comparing IVIG with placebo for treatment of PANDAS OCD (moderate to severe) following documented exposure to streptococcal infection or exposure within 6–8 weeks prior to illness onset, in 35 children (ages 4–16 years), which showed no difference between the IVIG and placebo groups in OCD severity scores or proportion of responders (Williams et al., 2016). The follow-up open-label treatment part of this trial reported improvement in all participants regardless of their initial treatment group assignment. In summary, the Williams et al. study showed that IVIG was not superior to placebo for treatment of OCD in patients with a PANDAS phenotype. There was substantial and significant improvement in all groups over time, regardless of treatment modality. It is therefore unclear whether IVIG and immune therapies are useful in the long-term outcome of PANS, and PANDAS/PANS may be self-limiting conditions.

Nadeau and colleagues (2015) conducted a study of effectiveness of cognitive-behavioral therapy (CBT) for OCD in 11 children with PANS, who had incomplete response to antibiotics (i.e., despite antibiotics, they had residual OCD). In these children, all 11 had a minimum eight sessions of CBT with 49% symptom reduction on the CY-BOCS at the end of treatment, and 50 % reduction at 1- and 4-month follow-ups, at which point they also noted reductions in anxiety. Larger-scale trials of CBT are needed in this group of children.

In a systematic review, 65 case reports (individual and series) were included in the PANS treatments review by Sigra et al. (2018). These described treatment with antibiotics, tonsillectomy/adenoidectomy, IVIG, plasma exchange, corticosteroids, nonsteroidal anti-inflammatory drugs, monoclonal antibodies, psychotropic medications, CBT, or a combination. Many of these reports are confounded by the use of combination therapy, ascertainment bias, and the fluctuating course of symptoms within PANS/PANDAS diagnoses. Sigra et al. found that there was not enough evidence to say any of the interventions are effective treatments.

There are currently insufficient data to justify proposal of antibiotic or immune modulating treatment for PANDAS and PANS. There is, however, extensive literature on effective management of typical pediatric OCD and tic disorders through various treatment modalities (for a comprehensive review, see Freeman et al., 2018; Krebs & Heyman, 2015; for a comprehensive review of evidence-based treatment for tics, see Whittington et al., 2016).

EXEMPLARY CASE EPITOMIZING THE PROBLEM OF OVERDIAGNOSIS OF PANS

Sam, age 9 years, had an existing diagnosis of ASD. He had a sore throat about 2 weeks prior to traveling abroad for a vacation. During the vacation, he developed a sudden onset of a severe stutter, some motor neck thrusting and shoulder shrugging tics, and marked anxiety about leaving the hotel room. He was diagnosed with PANS and PANDAS by doctors where he was traveling, who prescribed antibiotics, including azithromycin and co-amoxiclav, and ibuprofen. Extensive investigations included full blood count, copper, caeruloplasmin, thyroid peroxidase antibodies, antigliadin and antitransglutaminase IgG and IgA, antinuclear antibodies, antibasal ganglia antibodies, antistretptolysin O titre (ASOT), anti-DNase B, anti-NMDA-R antibodies, anti-VGKC (voltage-gated potassium channel) antibodies, biotinidase, lactate, amino acids, C-reactive protein, erythrocyte sedimentation rate, thyroid and renal function tests, *Borrelia burgdorferi* serology, urine for organic acids, routine EEG and brain MRI, which were all normal. Physical and neurological examination was normal. A course of steroids, initiated by a pediatric neurologist, also did not improve symptoms. Parents were considering IVIG. Neuropsychiatric assessment led to the observation of previously undiagnosed minor tics reported over the previous 2 years. Current gaps in knowledge about the concept of PANS were explained to parents in a discussion of how pre-existing autism could make Sam more vulnerable to acute-onset neuropsychiatric symptoms. Clonidine was prescribed at night to help him sleep and to decrease vocal tics. Psychoeducation and anxiety work was carried out with the parents over a few sessions around the role of anxiety contagion, focusing on a reduced monitoring of symptoms and a reduction in verbal and nonverbal expression of worry around illness. This resulted in significant recovery. Sam is currently coping well at home and school.

CONCLUSIONS

At present, the concept of PANS represents more a postulated phenomenon than a well circumscribed clinical entity. Pathophysiological mechanisms have so far been proposed but not demonstrated, and treatment guidelines are based on clinical consensus rather than on empirical evidence. In the clinic, the focus should prioritize evidence-based treatments for neuropsychiatric symptoms, as the search for potential, pathogenic biomarkers or the use of experimental treatments could become detrimental.

Regarding treatment with antibiotics, it is interesting to note that antibiotics can have antidepressant effects (Rosenblat & McIntyre, 2018), all medications can have placebo or anxiolytic effects, and, at the same time, some psychotropic medications can have antiviral/antimicrobial effects (Macedo et al., 2017). The sudden onset of illness in children following infections or hospital admissions may also have a functional component, and such symptoms respond well to placebo effects. An overestimation of the clinical effect following initial doses of antibiotics or reports of behavioral improvement within 20–30 minutes of an ibuprofen administration are not uncommon. Therefore, drawing conclusions based on clinical experience of treatment of a postulated condition such as PANS/PANDAS without a clear underlying pathophysiology is fraught with misleading paths and requires rigorous research and empirical evidence to guide clinicians and families.

We need to understand the scale of the problem and therefore need to perform surveillance studies of prevalence and incidence of acute, sudden-onset childhood neuropsychiatric illnesses. In addition to recording child symptoms, we need to explore family factors, documenting the presence of neurodevelopmental difficulties, as well as OCD/tics in siblings, parents, and extended family. The question remains: How do PANS/PANDAS children and families differ, if at all, from those with TS and OCD?

Future research should help to identify any inflammatory or immune biomarkers that will help guide children amenable to immune modulation therapy versus standard psychological/behavioral management and use of selective serotonergic reuptake inhibitors (SSRIs). At the same time, there are likely to be advantages in defining in-depth clinical phenotypes, as well as in including a detailed neuropsychological profile of children and families. This approach is likely to advance our understanding, if and when biomarkers emerge, and will aid the exploration of the neurobiological mechanisms leading to phenotypic heterogeneity.

Finally, all children presenting acutely with severe symptoms of OCD (whatever the cause) deserve assessment and consideration from an expert neurodevelopmental multidisciplinary team including neurology, psychiatry and neuropsychology/psychology. The emergence of symptoms in such an acute presentation is extremely distressing for all involved. There is a clear need to further the understanding of this phenomenon, while recognizing that the acuteness of presentation should not distract from trying to identify the wider contextual factors within a biopsychosocial framework.

REFERENCES

Baglioni, V., Coutinho, E., Menassa, D., Giannoccaro, M., Jacobson, L., Buttiglione, M., . . . EMTICS Collaborative Group. (2019). Antibodies to neuronal surface proteins in Tourette Syndrome: Lack of evidence in a European paediatric cohort. *Brain, Behavior and Immunity, 81*, 665–669.

Baumgaertel, C., Skripuletz, T., Kronenberg, J., Stangel, M., Schwenkenbecher, P., Sinke, C., . . . Sühs, K.-W. (2019). Immunity in Gilles de la Tourette-Syndrome: Results from a cerebrospinal fluid study. *Frontiers In Neurology, 10*, Article 732.

Brown, K., Farmer, C., Farhadian, B., Hernandez, J., Thienemann, M., & Frankovich, J. (2017a). Pediatric acute-onset neuropsychiatric syndrome response to oral corticosteroid bursts: An observational study of patients in an academic community-based PANS clinic. *Journal of Child and Adolescent Psychopharmacology, 27*(7), 629–639.

Brown, K., Farmer, C., Freeman, G., Spartz, E., Farhadian, B., Thienemann, M., & Frankovich, J. (2017b). Effect of early and prophylactic nonsteroidal anti-inflammatory drugs on flare duration in pediatric acute-onset neuropsychiatric syndrome: An observational study of patients followed by an academic community-based pediatric acute-onset neuropsychiatric syndrome clinic. *Journal of Child and Adolescent Psychopharmacology, 27*(7), 619–628.

Calaprice, D., Tona, J., & Murphy, T. (2018). Treatment of pediatric acute-onset neuropsychiatric disorder in a large survey population. *Journal of Child and Adolescent Psychopharmacology, 28*(2), 92–103.

Calaprice, D., Tona, J., Parker-Athill, E., & Murphy, T. (2017). A survey of pediatric acute-onset neuropsychiatric syndrome characteristics and course. *Journal of Child and Adolescent Psychopharmacology, 27*(7), 607–618.

Chang, K., Frankovich, J., Cooperstock, M., Cunningham, M., Latimer, M., & Murphy, T., . . . PANS Collaborative Consortium. (2015). Clinical evaluation of youth with pediatric acute-onset neuropsychiatric syndrome (PANS): Recommendations from the 2013 PANS Consensus Conference. *Journal of Child and Adolescent Psychopharmacology, 25*(1), 3–13.

Chang, Y., Li, Y., Muo, C., Chen, S., Chin, Z., & Kuo, H., . . . Chou, I.-C. (2011). Correlation of Tourette syndrome and allergic disease: Nationwide population-based case–control study. *Journal of Developmental and Behavioral Pediatrics, 32*(2), 98–102.

Chiarello, F., Spitoni, S., Hollander, E., Matucci Cerinic, M., & Pallanti, S. (2017). An expert opinion on PANDAS/PANS: Highlights and controversies. *International Journal of Psychiatry in Clinical Practice, 21*(2), 91–98.

Cooperstock, M., Swedo, S., Pasternack, M., Murphy, T., & the PANS/PANDAS Consortium. (2017). Clinical management of pediatric acute-onset neuropsychiatric syndrome: Part III—Treatment and prevention of infections. *Journal of Child and Adolescent Psychopharmacology, 27*(7), 594–606.

Corbett, B., Mendoza, S., Baym, C., Bunge, S., & Levine, S. (2008). Examining cortisol rhythmicity and responsivity to stress in children with Tourette syndrome. *Psychoneuroendocrinology, 33*(6), 810–820.

Cunningham, M., & Cox, C. (2016). Autoimmunity against dopamine receptors in neuropsychiatric and movement disorders: A review of Sydenham chorea and beyond. *Acta Physiologica, 216*(1), 90–100.

Frankovich, J., Swedo, S., Murphy, T., Dale, R., Agalliu, D., & Williams, K., . . . PANS/PANDAS Consortium. (2017). Clinical management of pediatric acute-onset neuropsychiatric syndrome: Part II-Use of immunomodulatory therapies. *Journal of Child and Adolescent Psychopharmacology, 27*(7), 574–593.

Freeman, J., Benito, K., Herren, J., Kemp, J., Sung, J., & Georgiadis, C., & Edmunds, J. (2018). Evidence base update of psychosocial treatments for pediatric obsessive–compulsive disorder: Evaluating, improving, and transporting what works. *Journal of Clinical Child and Adolescent Psychology, 47*(5), 669–698.

Frick, L., Rapanelli, M., Jindachomthong, K., Grant, P., Leckman, J., & Swedo, S., . . . Pittenger, C. (2018). Differential binding of antibodies in PANDAS patients to cholinergic interneurons in the striatum. *Brain, Behavior, and Immunity, 69*, 304–311.

Gabbay, V., Coffey, B., Babb, J., Meyer, L., Wachtel, C., Anam, S., & Rabinovitz, B. (2008). Pediatric autoimmune neuropsychiatric disorders associated with Streptococcus: Comparison of diagnosis and treatment in the community and at a specialty clinic. *Pediatrics, 122*(2), 273–278.

Gaughan, T., Buckley, A., Hommer, R., Grant, P., Williams, K., Leckman, J., & Swedo, S. (2016). Rapid eye movement sleep abnormalities in children with pediatric acute-onset neuropsychiatric syndrome (PANS). *Journal of Clinical Sleep Medicine, 12*(07), 1027–1032.

Giedd, J., Rapoport, J. L., Garvey, M. A., Perlmutter, S., & Swado, S. E. (2000). MRI Assessment of children with obsessive–compulsive disorder or tics associated with streptococcal infection. *American Journal of Psychiatry, 157*(2), 281–283.

Gilbert, D., Mink, J., & Singer, H. (2018). A pediatric neurology perspective on pediatric autoimmune neuropsychiatric disorder associated with Streptococcal infection and pediatric acute-onset neuropsychiatric syndrome. *Journal Of Pediatrics, 199*, 243–251.

Gromark, C., Harris, R., Wickström, R., Horne, A., Silverberg-Mörse, M., Serlachius, E., & Mataix-Cols, D. (2019). Establishing a pediatric acute-onset neuropsychiatric syndrome clinic: Baseline clinical features of the pediatric acute-onset neuropsychiatric syndrome cohort at Karolinska Institutet. *Journal of Child and Adolescent Psychopharmacology, 29*(8), 625–633.

Hedderly, T., & Malik, O. (2018). Childhood acute neuropsychiatric syndromes . . . furthering the discussion PANS and PANDAS. *European Journal of Paediatric Neurology, 22*(2), 223–224.

Hesselmark, E., & Bejerot, S. (2017). Biomarkers for diagnosis of pediatric acute neuropsychiatric syndrome (PANS)—Sensitivity and specificity of the Cunningham Panel. *Journal of Neuroimmunology, 312*, 31–37.

Hesselmark, E., & Bejerot, S. (2019a). Clinical features of paediatric acute-onset neuropsychiatric syndrome: Findings from a case–control study. *BJPsych Open, 5*(2), Article e25.

Hesselmark, E., & Bejerot, S. (2019b). Patient satisfaction and treatments offered to Swedish patients with suspected pediatric acute-onset neuropsychiatric syndrome and pediatric autoimmune neuropsychiatric disorders associated with Streptococcal infections. *Journal of Child and Adolescent Psychopharmacology, 29*(8), 634–641.

Jaspers-Fayer, F., Han, S., Chan, E., McKenney, K., Simpson, A., & Boyle, A., . . . Stewart, S. E. (2017). Prevalence of acute-onset subtypes in pediatric obsessive–compulsive disorder. *Journal of Child and Adolescent Psychopharmacology, 27*(4), 332–341.

Johnson, D., Kurlan, R., Leckman, J., & Kaplan, E. (2010). The human immune response to streptococcal extracellular antigens: Clinical, diagnostic, and potential pathogenetic implications. *Clinical Infectious Diseases, 50*(4), 481–490.

Kayser, M., & Dalmau, J. (2011). The emerging link between autoimmune disorders and neuropsychiatric disease. *Journal of Neuropsychiatry, 23*(1), 90–97.

Khandaker, G., Stochl, J., Zammit, S., Goodyer, I., Lewis, G., & Jones, P. (2018a). Childhood inflammatory markers and intelligence as predictors of subsequent persistent depressive symptoms: A longitudinal cohort study. *Psychological Medicine, 48*(9), 1514–1522.

Khandaker, G., Zammit, S., Burgess, S., Lewis, G., & Jones, P. (2018b). Association between a functional interleukin 6 receptor genetic variant and risk of depression and psychosis in a population-based birth cohort. *Brain, Behavior, and Immunity, 69*, 264–272.

Krebs, G., & Heyman, I. (2015). Obsessive–compulsive disorder in children and adolescents. *Archives of Disease in Childhood, 100*(5), 495–499.

Kumar, A., Williams, M., & Chugani, H. (2015). Evaluation of basal ganglia and thalamic inflammation in children with pediatric autoimmune neuropsychiatric disorders associated with streptococcal infection and Tourette syndrome. *Journal of Child Neurology, 30*(6), 749–756.

Kurlan, R., Johnson, D., & Kaplan, E. (2008). Streptococcal infection and exacerbations of childhood tics and obsessive–compulsive symptoms: A prospective blinded cohort study. *Pediatrics, 121*(6), 1188–1197.

Leckman, J., King, R., Gilbert, D., Coffey, B., Singer, H., & Dure, L., IV, . . . Kaplan, E. L. (2011). Streptococcal upper respiratory tract infections and exacerbations of tic and obsessive-compulsive symptoms: A prospective longitudinal study. *Journal of the American Academy of Child and Adolescent Psychiatry, 50*(2), 108–118.

Lepri, G., Rigante, D., Bellando Randone, S., Meini, A., Ferrari, A., & Tarantino, G., . . . Falcini, F. (2019). Clinical-serological characterization and treatment outcome of a large cohort of Italian children with pediatric autoimmune neuropsychiatric disorder associated with streptococcal infection and pediatric acute neuropsychiatric syndrome. *Journal of Child and Adolescent Psychopharmacology, 29*(8), 608–614.

Lin, H., Katsovich, L., Ghebremichael, M., Findley, D., Grantz, H., & Lombroso, P., . . . Leckman, J. F. (2007). Psychosocial stress predicts future symptom severities in children and adolescents with Tourette syndrome and/or obsessive-compulsive disorder. *Journal of Child Psychology and Psychiatry, 48*(2), 157–166.

Lin, H., Williams, K., Katsovich, L., Findley, D., Grantz, H., & Lombroso, P., . . . Leckman, J. F. (2010). Streptococcal upper respiratory tract infections and psychosocial stress predict future tic and obsessive–compulsive symptom severity in children and adolescents with Tourette syndrome and obsessive–compulsive disorder. *Biological Psychiatry, 67*(7), 684–691.

Luo, F., Leckman, J. F., Katsovich, L., Findley, D., Grantz, H., Tucker, D. M., . . . Bessen, D. E. (2004). Prospective longitudinal study of children with tic disorders and/or obsessive-compulsive disorder: relationship of symptom exacerbations to newly acquired streptococcal infections. *Pediatrics, 113*(6), e578–e585.

Macedo, D., Filho, A., Soares de Sousa, C. N., Quevedo, J., Barichello, T., Júnior, H., & Freitas de Lucena, D. (2017). Antidepressants, antimicrobials or both?: Gut microbiota dysbiosis in depression and possible implications of the antimicrobial effects of antidepressant drugs for antidepressant effectiveness. *Journal of Affective Disorders, 208*, 22–32.

Martino, D., Schrag, A., Anastasiou, Z., Apter, A., Benaroya-Milstein, N., Buttiglione, M., . . . EMTICS Collaborative Group (2021). Association of Group A *Streptococcus* exposure and exacerbations of chronic tic disorders: A multinational prospective cohort study. *Neurology, 96*(12), e1680–e1693.

Martino, D., Zis, P., & Buttiglione, M. (2015). The role of immune mechanisms in Tourette syndrome. *Brain Research, 1617*, 126–143.

Mataix-Cols, D., Frans, E., Pérez-Vigil, A., Kuja-Halkola, R., Gromark, C., & Isomura, K., . . . Larsson, H. (2018). A total-population multigenerational family clustering study of autoimmune diseases in obsessive–compulsive disorder and Tourette's/chronic tic disorders. *Molecular Psychiatry, 23*(7), 1652–1658.

Mell, L., Davis, R. L., & Owens, D. (2005). Association between streptococcal infection and obsessive–compulsive disorder, Tourette's syndrome, and tic disorder. *Pediatrics, 116*(1), 56–60.

Mora, S., Martín-González, E., Flores, P., & Moreno, M. (2020). Neuropsychiatric consequences of childhood group A streptococcal infection: A systematic review of preclinical models. *Brain, Behavior, and Immunity, 86*, 53–62.

Morris, C., Pardo-Villamizar, C., Gause, C., & Singer, H. (2009). Serum autoantibodies measured by immunofluorescence confirm a failure to differentiate PANDAS and Tourette syndrome from controls. *Journal of the Neurological Sciences, 276*(1–2), 45–48.

Morris-Berry, C., Pollard, M., Gao, S., Thompson, C., & Singer, H. (2013). Anti-streptococcal, tubulin, and dopamine receptor 2 antibodies in children with PANDAS and Tourette syndrome: Single-point and longitudinal assessments. *Journal of Neuroimmunology, 264*(1–2), 106–113.

Murphy, T., Brennan, E., Johnco, C., Parker-Athill, E., Miladinovic, B., Storch, E., & Lewin, A. (2017). A double-blind randomized placebo-controlled pilot study of azithromycin in youth with acute-onset obsessive–compulsive disorder. *Journal of Child and Adolescent Psychopharmacology, 27*(7), 640–651.

Murphy, T., Lewin, A., Parker-Athill, E., Storch, E., & Mutch, P. (2013). Tonsillectomies and adenoidectomies do not prevent the onset of pediatric autoimmune neuropsychiatric disorder associated with Group A Streptococcus. *Pediatric Infectious Disease Journal, 32*(8), 834–838.

Murphy, T., Parker-Athill, E., Lewin, A., Storch, E., & Mutch, P. (2015a). Cefdinir for recent-onset pediatric neuropsychiatric disorders: A pilot randomized trial. *Journal of Child and Adolescent Psychopharmacology, 25*(1), 57–64.

Murphy, T., Patel, P., McGuire, J., Kennel, A., Mutch, P., & Parker-Athill, E., . . . Rodriguez, C. A. (2015b). Characterization of the pediatric acute-onset neuropsychiatric syndrome phenotype. *Journal of Child and Adolescent Psychopharmacology, 25*(1), 14–25.

Murphy, T., Sajid, M., Soto, O., Shapira, N., Edge, P., & Yang, M., . . . Goodman, W. K. (2004). Detecting pediatric autoimmune neuropsychiatric disorders associated with streptococcus in children with obsessive–compulsive disorder and tics. *Biological Psychiatry, 55*(1), 61–68.

Nadeau, J., Jordan, C., Selles, R., Wu, M., King, M., & Patel, P., . . . Storch, E. A. (2015). A pilot trial of cognitive-behavioral therapy augmentation of antibiotic treatment in youth with pediatric acute-onset neuropsychiatric syndrome-related obsessive–compulsive disorder. *Journal of Child and Adolescent Psychopharmacology, 25*(4), 337–343.

Najjar, S., Pearlman, D., Alper, K., Najjar, A., & Devinsky, O. (2013). Neuroinflammation and psychiatric illness. *Journal of Neuroinflammation, 10*(1), Article 816.

Pavone, P., Bianchini, R., Parano, E., Incorpora, G., Rizzo, R., Mazzone, L., & Trifiletti, R. (2004). Anti-brain antibodies in PANDAS versus uncomplicated streptococcal infection. *Pediatric Neurology, 30*(2), 107–110.

Pérez-Vigil, A., Fernández de la Cruz, L., Brander, G., Isomura, K., Gromark, C., & Mataix-Cols, D. (2016). The link between autoimmune diseases and obsessive–compulsive and tic disorders: A systematic review. *Neuroscience and Biobehavioral Reviews, 71*, 542–562.

Perlmutter, S., Leitman, S., Garvey, M., Hamburger, S., Feldman, E., Leonard, H., & Swedo, S. (1999). Therapeutic plasma exchange and intravenous immunoglobulin for obsessive–compulsive disorder and tic disorders in childhood. *Lancet, 354*(9185), 1153–1158.

Perrin, E., Murphy, M., Casey, J., Pichichero, M., Runyan, D., & Miller, W., . . . Swedo, S. (2004). Does Group A β-hemolytic streptococcal infection increase risk for behavioral and neuropsychiatric symptoms in children? *Archives of Pediatrics and Adolescent Medicine, 158*(9), 848–856.

Rosenblat, J., & McIntyre, R. (2018). Efficacy and tolerability of minocycline for depression: A systematic review and meta-analysis of clinical trials. *Journal of Affective Disorders, 227*, 219–225.

Sigra, S., Hesselmark, E., & Bejerot, S. (2018). Treatment of PANDAS and PANS: A systematic review. *Neuroscience and Biobehavioral Reviews, 86*, 51–65.

Silverman, M., Frankovich, J., Nguyen, E., Leibold, C., Yoon, J., & Mark Freeman, G., . . . Thienemann, M. (2019). Psychotic symptoms in youth with pediatric acute-onset neuropsychiatric syndrome (PANS) may reflect syndrome severity and heterogeneity. *Journal of Psychiatric Research, 110*, 93–102.

Singer, H., Gause, C., Morris, C., & Lopez, P. (2008). Serial immune markers do not correlate with clinical exacerbations in pediatric autoimmune neuropsychiatric disorders associated with streptococcal infections. *Pediatrics, 121*(6), 1198–1205.

Singer, H., Mascaro-Blanco, A., Alvarez, K., Morris-Berry, C., Kawikova, I., & Ben-Pazi, H., . . . Cunningham, M. W. (2015). Neuronal antibody biomarkers for Sydenham's chorea identify a new group of children with chronic recurrent episodic acute exacerbations of tic and obsessive compulsive symptoms following a streptococcal infection. *PLoS ONE, 10*(3), e0120499.

Snider, L., Lougee, L., Slattery, M., Grant, P., & Swedo, S. (2005). Antibiotic prophylaxis with azithromycin or penicillin for childhood-onset neuropsychiatric disorders. *Biological Psychiatry, 57*(7), 788–792.

Spartz, E., Freeman, G., Brown, K., Farhadian, B., Thienemann, M., & Frankovich, J. (2017). Course of neuropsychiatric symptoms after introduction and removal of nonsteroidal anti-inflammatory drugs: A pediatric observational study. *Journal of Child and Adolescent Psychopharmacology, 27*(7), 652–659.

Swedo, S., Frankovich, J., & Murphy, T. (2017). Overview of treatment of pediatric acute-onset neuropsychiatric syndrome. *Journal of Child and Adolescent Psychopharmacology, 27*(7), 562–565.

Swedo, S. E., Leckman, J. F., & Rose, N. R. (2012). From research subgroup to clinical syndrome: Modifying the PANDAS criteria to describe PANS (pediatric acute-onset neuropsychiatric syndrome). *Pediatrics and Therapeutics, 2*, 1–8.

Swedo, S. E., Leonard, H. L., Garvey, M., Mittleman, B., Allen, A. J., Perlmutter, S., . . . Dubbert, B. K. (1998). Pediatric autoimmune neuropsychiatric disorders associated with streptococcal infections: clinical description of the first 50 cases. *American Journal of Psychiatry, 155*(2), 264–271.

Thienemann, M., Murphy, T., Leckman, J., Shaw, R., Williams, K., & Kapphahn, C., . . . Swedo, S. (2017). Clinical management of pediatric acute-onset neuropsychiatric syndrome: Part I—Psychiatric and behavioral interventions. *Journal of Child and Adolescent Psychopharmacology, 27*(7), 566–573.

Toufexis, M., Hommer, R., Gerardi, D., Grant, P., Rothschild, L., & D'Souza, P., . . . Murphy, T. K. (2015). Disordered eating and food restrictions in children with PANDAS/PANS. *Journal of Child and Adolescent Psychopharmacology, 25*(1), 48–56.

Whittington, C., Pennant, M., Kendall, T., Glazebrook, C., Trayner, P., & Groom, M., . . . Hollis, C. (2016). Practitioner Review: Treatments for Tourette syndrome in children and young people—A systematic review. *Journal of Child Psychology and Psychiatry, 57*(9), 988–1004.

Wilbur, C., Bitnun, A., Kronenberg, S., Laxer, R., Levy, D., & Logan, W., . . . Yeh, E. A. (2019). PANDAS/PANS in childhood: Controversies and evidence. *Paediatrics and Child Health, 24*(2), 85–91.

Williams, K., Swedo, S., Farmer, C., Grantz, H., Grant, P., & D'Souza, P., . . . Leckman, J. F. (2016). Randomized, controlled trial of intravenous immunoglobulin for pediatric autoimmune neuropsychiatric disorders associated with streptococcal infections. *Journal of the American Academy of Child and Adolescent Psychiatry, 55*(10), 860–867.

Yaddanapudi, K., Hornig, M., Serge, R., De Miranda, J., Baghban, A., Villar, G., & Lipkin, W. (2010). Passive transfer of streptococcus-induced antibodies reproduces behavioral disturbances in a mouse model of pediatric autoimmune neuropsychiatric disorders associated with streptococcal infection. *Molecular Psychiatry, 15*(7), 712–726.

CHAPTER 23

Sluggish Cognitive Tempo

Lisa A. Jacobson

Mary's family has nicknamed her "Miss Molasses." At age 9, she is still having trouble starting and finishing work and needs substantial adult prompting to move along—even though she reportedly is capable of comprehending and completing the work. Mary is slow to perform routine personal tasks such as getting dressed or eating meals. "Hurry up, please!" is a common refrain in the household. Her teacher notes that Mary is often one of the last to turn in classwork and typically runs out of time on tests and timed assignments. He also describes Mary as "unmotivated," as she is very slow to begin tasks even when he believes she knows what to do.

Despite her lack of work completion, Mary is not a "discipline problem" and is typically compliant. She is not aggressive or oppositional and generally gets along with others. She willingly completes tasks that she understands—she just tends to need more time. At times, she appears "spacey" or "in a fog," but is not necessarily overtly distractible in terms of being easily drawn off task, and usually works persistently on tasks for as long as it takes to get them done.

Her parents want to know "Why is Mary so slow?" Does she have attention-deficit/hyperactivity disorder? Is she depressed? Is something else going on? Is there a diagnostic category that captures Mary's presentation of slowness, underactivity, spaciness, and slow initiation?

HISTORICAL OVERVIEW

With the publication of the third edition of the *Diagnostic and Statistical Manual of Mental Disorders* (DSM-III; American Psychiatric Association, 1980) in 1980, the disorder currently known as attention-deficit/hyperactivity disorder (ADHD) was conceptualized to include symptoms of attention deficit disorder (ADD) *with or without* hyperactivity. As a distinct new entity, the criteria for this subtype of ADD without hyperactivity included symptoms of inattention and impulsivity that were not also accompanied by hyperactivity. Subsequent studies examining children who met criteria for the new disorder revealed that these children were likely to present with greater sluggishness, drowsiness, "spaciness," confusion, hypoactivity, and passivity, as well as more anxiety and depressive symptoms, fewer overt externalizing behaviors, and more social withdrawal and difficulty with peers than those who met symptom criteria for ADD with hyperactivity (Lahey & Carlson, 1991; Carlson & Mann, 2000). Apart from a brief period of combining the ADHD subtypes into a single disorder (e.g., DSM-III-R; American Psychiatric Association, 1987), the separate presentations for more inattentive versus more hyperactive/impulsive symptoms of ADHD have been maintained through the present version (i.e., DSM-5; American Psychiatric Association, 2013). Over the intervening period, much work has attempted to clarify the differences between ADHD presentations and identify potentially unique profiles of impairments and comorbidities, resulting in further investigations of attentional differences within or overlapping with the ADHD primarily inattentive presentation.

During the field trials for DSM-IV (Lahey et al., 1994) and in studies examining the factor structure of behavioral symptom ratings associated with DSM-III ADD (Lahey et al., 1988; Lahey & Carlson, 1991), a distinct subset of symptoms was identified that differed from the ADHD subtypes previously described in DSM-III. These included symptoms such as "sluggish," "drowsy," "daydreamy," or "forgetful," or together, "inconsistent alertness" (McBurnett, Pfiffner, & Frick, 2001). Although potentially consistent with the greater sluggishness and internalizing symptoms observed in individuals meeting criteria for DSM-III ADD without hyperactivity, when examined more closely these symptoms were found to load on a separate factor from inattention and impulsive symptoms (Lahey et al., 1988; McBurnett et al., 2001; Milich, Balentine, & Lynam, 2001). The symptom constellation was subsequently described as "sluggish tempo" or "sluggish cognitive tempo" (SCT), and the term has remained in usage despite concerns about the negative nature of the nomenclature (Saxbe & Barkley, 2014).

SCT symptoms were ultimately discarded from inclusion in DSM-IV due to poor negative predictive power (Frick et al., 1994) related to DSM inattention symptoms and interest in consistency of symptomatology across subtypes (Lahey et al., 1994). Specifically, although SCT symptoms were more strongly associated with the predominantly inattentive subtype than the predominantly hyperactive subtype, most inattentive individuals meeting symptom criteria for the inattentive subtype did not exhibit SCT symptoms. Instead of dampening enthusiasm for the construct of SCT as a potentially poor measure of DSM-defined inattention, this finding and related work fueled growing interest in the construct as characteristic of a specific subset of inattentive symptoms. Further work specifically examining DSM inattentive symptoms suggested that sluggish symptoms might differentiate a unique and potentially more homogeneous subgroup of individuals within the ADD without hyperactivity subtype (Carlson & Mann, 2000; McBurnett et al., 2001; Milich et al., 2001). Given the emerging evidence (e.g., Lahey et al., 1988) suggesting a close relationship between DSM inattention and symptoms of sluggishness and related characteristics, this cluster as a whole (without a specific symptom list) was included in DSM-IV-TR (American Psychiatric Association, 2000) as a possible subset of characteristics of ADHD. The example descriptors of ADHD not otherwise specified (314.9) in DSM-IV-TR read, in part, "Individuals with clinically significant impairment who present with inattention and whose symptom pattern does not meet full criteria for the disorder but have a behavioral pattern marked by *sluggishness, daydreaming, and hypoactivity*" (American Psychiatric Association, 2000, p. 93; italics added). Although there has been increasing interest in SCT symptoms and their association with ADHD since then, this symptom constellation was not included in DSM-5 (American Psychiatric Association, 2013). Milich and colleagues (2001) describe the omission of items that purportedly tap SCT from the DSM ADHD symptom criteria as an error impacting both understanding of the inattentive presentation and potential accuracy of diagnostic classifications.

In spite of its omission from DSM-5, there is a growing body of evidence examining the construct of SCT. At the time of writing this chapter, based on specific search terms of *sluggish cognitive tempo* or *sluggish tempo*, there were 168 published manuscripts in PubMed, with a noticeable jump into double-digits beginning in 2014 and a meta-analysis in 2016 (Becker et al., 2016). The evidence base is clearly not yet consistent with that of other recognized developmental disorders, but there is continued progress with regard to defining the core symptoms of SCT, as well as its prevalence, developmental course, and profile of psychological and neuropsychological comorbidities. Note that, for the purposes of this (pediatric) text, this chapter focuses most heavily on work examining SCT and its comorbidities in children and adolescents, which also reflects the state of the literature (although there are a small number of studies exploring the construct in adults).

DEBATE OR CONTROVERSY?

In spite of increasing interest in the construct, it is perhaps not surprising that SCT is not yet recognized as a unique diagnostic condition, nor was included in the most current DSM version. There remain a number of issues and questions to be addressed. These include developing a consensus for core symptoms of SCT, determining how best to define and measure the construct, clarifying prevalence and distinctiveness of the symptom constellation, and determining its developmental course and symptom trajectory.

Development of Rating Scales Specific to SCT, or Have We Adequately Identified the Construct?

The history of SCT and its emergence from work examining DSM-defined inattention has placed the disorder squarely within the construct of ADHD. Early work characterized individuals with SCT symptoms as a subset of the ADHD inattentive subtype (Carlson & Mann, 2000; McBurnett et al., 2001; Milich et al., 2001), raising a question as to whether SCT is a unique set of symptoms at all. However, multiple factor-analytic studies show that SCT symptoms of hypoactivity, sluggishness and drowsiness, forgetfulness, and daydreaminess are related to, but consistently separable from, inattentive symptoms, providing validity for SCT as a construct distinct from DSM-defined inattention.

Early studies took advantage of existing child psychopathology scales containing items such as "seems sluggish or drowsy" or "daydreams," yielding examinations of two (Carlson & Mann, 2002), three (McBurnett et al., 2001, two SCT items plus "forgetful" from the ADHD inattention symptom list) or four items (Lahey et al., 1988) mirroring those included in DSM-III inattention criteria. The next decade's studies tended to rely upon four parent-rated or five teacher-rated items identified by Carlson and Mann (2002) from the Child Behavior Checklist and corresponding Teacher Report Form (CBCL; Achenbach & Rescorla, 2001), or similar items (e.g., Hartman, Wilcutt, Rhee, & Pennington, 2004). While these items proved sufficient to demonstrate the distinctness of an SCT cluster from DSM inattention and hyperactivity, a larger item pool was needed to more comprehensively examine and characterize SCT as a construct.

In the last decade, several scales have been developed to specifically examine SCT, its symptom constellation, and factor structure (see Table 23.1 for examples). Penny, Waschbusch, Klein, Corkum, and Eskes (2009) developed a 14-item SCT scale based on review of the literature to date, expert consensus, and factor-analytic methods, and acquired normative data from parent and teacher ratings of a large sample of schoolchildren in Canada. This scale exhibited a multiple-factor structure, yielding three factors (Slow, Sleepy, and Daydreamer) from parent ratings and two factors (Sleepy, Daydreamer, Slow) from teacher ratings (Penny et al., 2009). Others validating this new measure in referred samples in the United States confirmed a multiple-factor structure to SCT, suggesting three factors (Sleepy/Sluggish, Slow/Daydreamy, Low Initiation/Persistence) in teacher (Jacobson et al., 2012) and parent (Jacobson, Geist, & Mahone, 2018) ratings. Based in part upon this work, Barkley (2013) developed a slightly different 14-item SCT scale, finding that 12 of the items loaded uniquely on a SCT factor rather than the ADHD inattentive factor. McBurnett and colleagues (2014) sought to more comprehensively identify and evaluate potential items for this domain, generating 44 items purporting to measure SCT based on various clinical descriptions and variations of item phrasing. Examining these potential items in a sample of 165 elementary-age children with ADHD inattentive presentation reduced the pool to 15 items retained, as they did not load strongly (e.g., > .30) on the ADHD Inattentive factor, demonstrating their uniqueness as measures of SCT rather than inattention. These items loaded strongly onto three SCT factors for both parent and teacher ratings (Daydreams, Working Memory, Sleepy/Tired; McBurnett et al., 2014). Burns and colleagues subsequently developed a 16-item SCT scale as part of the Child and Adolescent Behavior Inventory (CABI; Burns, Lee, Servera, McBurnett, & Becker, 2018; final version included 15 SCT items), a measure subsequently validated outside of the United States. Taking this foundation into account, a recent meta-analysis examining 73 papers and over 19,000 participants found that 13 items across studies appeared to load consistently on a SCT factor rather than ADHD factors (Becker et al., 2016).

While these and related studies clearly show progress toward identifying symptoms that are associated with SCT and not with ADHD inattention, a question remains regarding how best to understand the nature of the comorbidity between these two symptom clusters and whether statistical control for the other symptom set is adequate, particularly within referred samples. A particular challenge for understanding the core features of SCT is its comorbidity with ADHD; should studies striving to understand the nature of SCT-specific characteristics and comorbidities entirely exclude individuals who also meet criteria for ADHD or not? Further questions include the degree to which variability in the structure of SCT (e.g., subscales or subcomponents of SCT) might be useful in understanding and predicting outcomes, and whether this may vary with the referred nature of the sample. For example, the inclusion of items potentially assessing working memory on the McBurnett scale (see Table 23.1) may reflect use and development of that measure within a sample referred to an ADHD clinic as opposed to a community sample.

Furthermore, SCT also appears correlated with other aspects of developmental psychopathology. A recent meta-analysis found SCT symptoms to be more strongly associated with internalizing (weighted correlations in the .30–.50 range; stronger associations

TABLE 23.1. SCT Scale Items across Measures

	SCT scale items from published work				
CBCL (Achenbach & Rescorla, 2001)	Penny et al. (2009)	Barkley (2013)*	McBurnett et al. (2014)*	Becker et al. (2016) meta-analysis	CABI SCT scale (Burns et al., 2018)*
	Lethargic[A]	Lethargic	Lacks energy[3]/ Gets tired easily[3]	Tired/lethargic	Easily tired
	Drowsy[A]	Drowsy/sleepy Trouble staying alert/awake	Seems drowsy[3]	Sleepy/drowsy	Drowsy or sleepy
Apathetic (teacher only)	Apathetic[A]	Apathetic/ withdrawn		Apathetic/ unmotivated	Lacks motivation/ apathetic
Underactive, slow moving, lacks energy	Underactive[A]	Underactive		Underactive/ slow moving	Low level of activity/ underactive
Sluggish/slow to respond	Sluggish[A]	Slow moving/ sluggish		Sluggish	Behavior is slow
	Yawning[A]		Yawns[3]		
	Unmotivated[B]				Lacks motivation/ apathetic
	Slow/delayed[B]	Doesn't process quickly		Slow thinking/ processing	Thinking is slow
	Needs extra time[B]	Slow/needs more time+			
	Lacks initiative[B]	Lacks initiative/ effort fades quickly+			
	Effort fades[B]				
	Lost in thoughts[C]	Lost in thoughts	Lost in thought[1]	Lost in thoughts	Gets lost in thoughts
Daydreams or gets lost in thoughts	Daydreams[C]	Prone to daydreaming	Daydreams[1]	Daydreams	Daydreams
	In own world[C]		Off in own world[1]		
Stares blankly		Stares a lot	Stares into space[1]	Stares blankly	Stares blankly

(continued)

TABLE 23.1. *(continued)*

CBCL (Achenbach & Rescorla, 2001)	Penny et al. (2009)	Barkley (2013)	McBurnett et al. (2014)	Becker et al. (2016) meta-analysis	CABI SCT scale (Burns et al., 2018)
Confused or seems to be in a fog				In a fog	Lost in a fog
		Mentally foggy/ easily confused	Gets confused[2]	Easily confused	Easily confused
			Loses train of thought[2]	Loses train of thought/ cognitive set	Loses train of thought
		Spacey	Spaces out[1]	Spacey	Spaces or zones out
			Mind drifts off[1]		
			Forgets what was he or she going to say[2]		Forgets what he or she was going to say
			Gets tongue-tied[2]		Difficulty expressing thoughts/tongue-tied
			Gets mixed up[2]		Gets mixed up

Note. Numeric/letter superscripts reflect loadings onto SCT subscales; no superscripts indicates one factor or not reported. CBCL, Child Behavior Checklist; CABI, Child and Adolescent Behavior Inventory; +items ultimately not included due to loading more highly on ADHD Inattentive than SCT factor.

with withdrawn and depressive symptoms than anxiety) than externalizing (.21–.32 range) symptoms (Becker et al., 2016). Notably, the associations between SCT and internalizing symptoms appear to remain even after controlling for inattention, but associations with externalizing symptoms do not (Becker et al., 2016).

Prevalence of SCT

The challenge for ascertaining definitive prevalence estimates for SCT is twofold. First, prevalence estimates in advance of a consensus regarding the construct and its measurement are likely premature and may be inconsistent with those obtained once the field agrees on how best to assess the construct of SCT (see below). Second, there is not yet consensus in the field regarding how many symptoms should be present in order to definitively rule in the condition. Barkley (2013) found that elevated ratings on at least three of 14 SCT symptoms in a nationally representative U.S. sample of just under 2,000 parents of school-age youth (e.g., 6–17 years) approximated the prevalence threshold set by the

DSM diagnostic criterion of six symptoms of inattention or hyperactivity (e.g., 94th percentile). Using this criterion, 5.67% of the sample exhibited significant SCT symptoms, of whom 59% also met criteria for ADHD; conversely, 39% of those with clinically elevated ADHD symptoms also met criteria for SCT. Importantly, these data suggest that a substantial proportion (41%) of those with SCT did not also have ADHD, providing further evidence for the discrimination of SCT from ADHD.

Based on this foundation, more recent work has applied the criterion of top 5% of the sample to identify cut-scores indicative of SCT. For example, Servera, Sáez, Burns, and Becker (2018) sought to replicate Barkley's U.S. study in a sample of parents and teachers of school children (ages 8–13 years) in Spain, using the CABI (Burns et al., 2018; 16 SCT items rated on a scale of 0–5). Examining the top 5% of the sample across SCT items yielded cutoff scores of over 3.0 across raters (e.g., 3.78 for mothers, 3.33 for fathers, and 4.22 for teacher ratings). Burns and Becker (2021) examined a nationally representative U.S. sample of mothers of elementary-age students (e.g., kindergarten through sixth grade) and likewise defined the clinical range as greater than the 95th percentile, or a cutoff point of mean symptom ratings at or above 2.73 (based upon the CABI 15-item version SCT scale).

Given variations in method and scales used, it remains unclear how to harmonize cutoff scores for application to other, potentially smaller and less nationally representative samples. For example, is the cutoff score difference of > 1.0 between maternal ratings in these studies indicative of the change in the measure (e.g., dropping of 1 SCT item from the measure used), cultural—and potentially idiomatic—differences (e.g., "in a fog") in the construct between countries, or simply sample variability that requires further examination? Some earlier work suggests that measurement of SCT may vary by age (Becker et al., 2016; Camprodon-Rosanas et al., 2016; Jacobson et al., 2018), so would cutoff scores therefore also need to be adjusted to be more developmentally sensitive as in most other measures of developmental psychopathology? Although SCT does not appear to show the same greater male prevalence as ADHD, it also remains to be seen whether subcomponents of SCT are more likely to be present in girls versus boys, and whether this also varies with age. On the assumption that SCT may to some degree reflect internalizing psychopathology, and thus may be more likely to be captured by self rather than informant ratings, there has been some work to establish parallel self-report versions for children (Becker, 2015) and adults (e.g., Barkley, 2012b), although as noted earlier, such work may be premature given the variety of informant reports in use.

Other work in more targeted samples has demonstrated that SCT symptoms are also evident, and remain distinct from ADHD, in samples outside the United States (Belmar, Servera, Becker, & Burns, 2015; Burns, Becker, Servera, Bernad, & García-Banda, 2017; Camprodon-Rosanas et al., 2016; Preszler et al., 2019; Khadka, Burns, & Becker, 2016; Lee, Burns, & Becker, 2018). These data provide initial evidence for the cross-cultural validity of the construct, although further work is needed.

Stability of the Construct

Given initial evidence that SCT and/or its associations with other constructs may vary with age, a key question to investigate is that of longitudinal stability. Although test–retest reliability over periods of 4 weeks up to 2 years appears consistently good for both parent and teacher ratings of SCT (Bernad et al., 2014; Burns et al., 2017; Lee, Burns, Snell, & McBurnett, 2014; Penny et al., 2009), evidence remains mixed at this point for stability across longer developmental periods. However, it is worth noting that inconsistencies in SCT scale versions and the ages and characteristics of samples in which SCT is examined add to the complexity of understanding stability of the construct over time.

For example, examining stability of SCT assessed with seven items in a community sample over 10 years (e.g., preschool through ninth grade), Leopold and colleagues (2016) found both ADHD and SCT to be highly stable across development. Furthermore, the trajectory of symptoms of SCT differed from that of ADHD inattentive symptoms in that SCT appeared to increase slightly over time, while inattention remained stable. Likewise, in a community sample recruited from economically disadvantaged areas, SCT assessed with four core items showed adequate stability from age 3 years to fifth grade, and mean levels of SCT tended to increase slightly with age (Dvorsky, Becker, Tamm, & Willoughby, 2021). In contrast, Vu, Thompson, Willcutt, and Petrill (2019) found that while SCT assessed with five items from the CBCL showed some temporal stability over shorter periods of up to 2 years, it did not exhibit similar stability over a 7-year period or a pattern of increase in SCT symptoms over time. Examining state and trait invariance, several studies have found greater trait than occasion-specific variance, suggesting the potential for SCT to be considered trait-like to a similar degree to ADHD inattention and other developmental psychopathologies (Becker et al., 2018; Burns, Becker, Geiser, Leopold, & Willcutt, 2020; Preszler et al., 2019).

Measurement of SCT

With regard to fully characterizing the disorder or understanding its comorbidities, another important question regarding measurement remains to be answered. Most work to date has defined SCT by a constellation of symptoms reported by caregivers and/or teachers and has examined comorbidities and potential domains of impairment in the same fashion. Are informant ratings alone adequate for identifying individuals with SCT or is there a role for performance-based measures? If SCT as a construct is conceptually defined by slowed responding and/or thinking and general sluggishness, then behavioral measures of cognitive processing efficiency, motor speed, or even reaction time may prove valuable to fully characterizing the symptom constellation and understanding the nature of the "sluggishness" feature. Such studies may help clarify whether the slowed processing in SCT reflects slowed motor responding, slowed cognitive processing, or some combination (e.g., Jacobson et al., 2012).

Only a few studies have examined the association between informant ratings of SCT and such performance-based measures, and unsurprisingly—given uncertainty around measurement of the construct—these findings have been inconsistent. Several studies have found SCT severity is not uniquely associated, beyond ADHD inattention, with oral naming, motor/graphomotor processing speed, or reaction time across samples of varying ages (Bauermeister, Barkley, Bauermeister, Martinez, & McBurnett, 2012; Baytunca et al., 2018; Becker et al., 2018; Kofler et al., 2019; Skirbekk, Hansen, Oerbeck, & Kristensen, 2011; Tamm, Brenner, Bamberger, & Becker, 2018; Ünsel-Bolat et al., 2019; Wood, Potts, Lewandownskki, & Lovett, 2017). In contrast, other work has found small associations with reduced processing speed and/or reaction time, even after controlling for ADHD inattention (Becker, Marsh, Holdaway, & Tamm, 2020; Camprodon-Rosanas et al., 2020; Hinshaw, 2002; Jacobson et al., 2018; Willcutt et al., 2014). More work is needed in this area, ideally in large samples, with consistent measures of SCT and a variety of performance-based measures of speed.

CURRENT STATUS WITHIN NEUROPSYCHOLOGY

Although the evidence is clearly still accruing regarding how best to define and measure SCT symptoms, a potential profile is beginning to emerge as researchers examine associations between informant reports of SCT symptoms and domains of developmental psychopathology, impairment, academic skills, and neurocognitive functioning in areas such as attention and executive function. Consistency of findings is likely affected to some degree by use of varying measurement tools, but core SCT symptoms appear to be represented across various rating scales in use (e.g., as shown in Table 23.1). With this in mind, SCT appears to show clear differences from childhood ADHD inattentive or hyperactive profiles in some domains, while further work is needed to clarify less well-studied domains. This distinction from ADHD is important for demonstrating external validity of the SCT construct by differentiating it from other domains of psychopathology.

Externalizing Disorders

In contrast to ADHD, SCT appears to be consistently negatively associated (or not associated at all) with externalizing psychopathology such as disruptive behavior disorders, aggression, or oppositional defiant disorder (Becker et al., 2016; Bernad, Servera, Grases, Collado, & Burns, 2014; Carlson & Mann, 2002; Hartman et al., 2004; Lee et al., 2014; Penny et al., 2009). Consistent with factor analyses that have repeatedly shown SCT symptoms to be separable from ADHD hyperactivity symptoms, the comorbidities commonly associated with this ADHD presentation seem likewise inconsistent with SCT.

Internalizing Disorders and Social Problems

SCT appears to be more strongly and positively associated with internalizing psychopathology such as anxiety, social withdrawal, and depression than is ADHD (Becker et al., 2016; Carlson & Mann, 2002; Garner, Marceaux, Mrug, Patterson, & Hodgens, 2010; Hartman et al., 2004; Jacobson et al., 2012; Penny et al., 2009; Willcutt et al., 2014). This association remains even when symptoms of ADHD inattention are statistically removed (Becker, Luebbe, Fite, Stopplebein, & Greening, 2014; Lee et al., 2014; Vu et al., 2019). SCT symptoms predict poorer concurrent social skills (Bauermeister et al., 2012; McBurnett et al., 2014), and appear to predict peer relationship difficulties over the course of a school year, even when initial peer difficulties and other symptoms are taken into account (Becker, 2014). However, evidence remains somewhat inconsistent for specific internalizing symptoms and may reflect the nature of the samples (e.g., referred or community); in a national community sample, Barkley (2013) found that, relative to controls, children with SCT but not ADHD had higher rates of depression but not anxiety.

Academic Impairment

SCT symptoms have been associated with ratings of academic impairment, with a generally moderate effect size (Bauermeister et al., 2012; Becker et al., 2016; Jacobson et al., 2012; Langberg, Becker, & Dvorsky, 2014; Smith & Langberg, 2017; Tamm et al., 2016; Watabe, Owens, Evans, & Brandt, 2014), although these associations have not been shown to consistently remain after controlling for inattention and/or intellectual ability/IQ (e.g., Becker & Langberg, 2013; Carlson & Mann, 2002; Marshall, Evans, Eiraldi, Becker, & Power, 2014). Some data suggests that in community (e.g., nonreferred) samples, children with SCT but not ADHD may not have higher rates of reading or math disorders than controls (Barkley, 2013). Other work has found that some but not all SCT dimensions show association with reported academic impairment (e.g., Slow SCT factor; Tamm et al., 2016) or grade point average (e.g., the Slow SCT factor was associated with reduced grades, while the Daydreamy factor was associated with higher grades; Smith & Langberg, 2017).

At this point, only a few studies have examined objectively measured academic skills (e.g., standardized test scores) and the initial findings have been inconsistent. Some evidence suggests that SCT is weakly (but significantly) associated with performance on measures of word reading, reading comprehension, math, and written language (Willcutt et al., 2014), even after controlling for ADHD symptoms. Other studies have observed SCT associations with reading but not math (Hartman et al., 2004; Tamm et al., 2016), or with math but not reading (Bauermeister et al., 2012). Still other work has not supported the association between SCT and academic performance beyond effects of ADHD (Bauermeister et al., 2012; Cook et al., 2019; Langberg et al., 2014; Marshall et al., 2014; Vu et al., 2019). Early evidence suggests that children with diagnosed learning disabilities may be more likely to manifest SCT symptoms than those without (Camprodon-Rosanas et al., 2016). Further work is needed to clarify whether SCT might represent a manifestation of the deficit in processing speed shared between ADHD and learning disabilities (McGrath et al., 2011).

Examining timed academic performance while controlling for untimed within-domain skills as well as inattention and motor speed, SCT was found to consistently predict reading and math fluency (Jacobson & Mahone, 2019), although these associations varied slightly by SCT subscale and were stronger in younger participants. In contrast, Wood et al. (2017) found college students with self-reported SCT were not slower on timed reading tasks, potentially suggesting developmental change in the relationship between SCT and academic fluency. Further work examining effects of informant and self-reported SCT on timed and untimed performance-based academic measures will be important for clarifying the SCT profile and any potential developmental changes.

Adaptive/Community Impairment

Functional daily impairment has been one of the most consistently researched domains in youth with SCT. The data consistently show that SCT symptoms convey impairment in global as well as specific domains of social, self-care, and home living skills, beyond contributions of ADHD symptoms (Barkley, 2013; Bauermeister et al., 2012; Becker et al., 2016; Burns et al., 2017; Burns & Becker, 2021; Cook et al., 2019; Jacobson et al., 2012; Sáez, Servera, Becker, & Burns, 2019; Willcutt et al., 2014).

Neurocognitive Function

A few studies have examined whether there are unique associations between SCT and measures of attention and executive function, after controlling for DSM inattentive symptoms. Given the recognized association between ADHD symptoms and executive dysfunction, control for ADHD symptoms is critical to ascertain SCT-specific contributions to functioning within this domain. Taken together, preliminary findings are heterogeneous and not yet strongly supportive of unique neurocognitive deficits in SCT.

With regard to performance-based measures of attention span and sustained attention, some data suggest that SCT is associated with poorer sustained attention, after controlling for ADHD inattentive symptoms (Becker et al., 2018; Wåhlstedt & Bohlin, 2010; Willcutt et al., 2014), although some evidence suggests the opposite (Jacobson, Ryan, & Mahone, 2019). Additionally, some individuals with ADHD and high ratings of SCT have been shown to exhibit better sustained attention than those with ADHD alone (Capdevila-Brophy et al., 2014).

Considering ratings of daily executive behaviors, evidence from a large community sample found ADHD symptoms rather than SCT symptoms to be more strongly associated with parent-rated deficits in application of executive function in day-to-day tasks, although youth with SCT exhibited more difficulty than controls (Barkley, 2013). SCT symptoms were most particularly associated with cognitive regulation difficulty, such as organization and problem-solving weaknesses. This pattern was replicated in college students (Jarrett, Rapport, Rondon, & Becker, 2017). Several studies have examined informant ratings on the Behavior Rating Inventory of Executive Function (BRIEF; Gioia, Isquith, Guy, & Kenworthy, 2000) and the Barkley Deficits in Executive Functioning Scale—Children and Adolescents (BDEFS-CA Short Form; Barkley, 2012a), with studies both finding (Becker & Langberg, 2014; Burns & Becker, 2021; Duncan, Tamm, Birnschein, & Becker, 2019; Koriakin, Noonan, Mahone, & Jacobson, 2015b; Wood et al., 2017) and not finding (Tamm et al., 2018) independent associations between SCT and ratings of executive function. Where positive findings exist, across measures, SCT appears more likely to be associated with problems in cognitive regulation and/or regulation of emotion than behavioral regulation (Burns & Becker, 2021; Duncan et al., 2019; Jarrett et al., 2017; Wood et al., 2017), with some work suggesting associations may be SCT-subscale specific (e.g., Slow SCT, but not Sleepy or Daydreamy SCT; Becker & Langberg, 2014; Sleepy/Sluggish and Low Initiation, but not Daydreamy; Koriakin, Mahone, & Jacobson, 2015a).

With regard to performance-based measures of executive function, the few existing studies suggest that SCT symptoms are not uniquely associated with scores on measures of inhibitory control, attention shifting, cognitive flexibility/set shifting, or problem solving when controlling for ADHD inattention (Bauermeister, 2012; Kofler et al., 2019; Tamm et al., 2018; Willcutt et al., 2014). With regard to working memory, while several studies failed to find independent associations with SCT (Bauermeister et al., 2012; Jacobson et al., 2019; Tamm et al., 2018), a recent clinic-based study found SCT to be associated with working memory and inhibition speed, such that youth with SCT took longer to perform the mental manipulations required for working memory tasks and were more likely to more quickly inhibit responses or initiation of responses, including intended responses, than those without SCT (Kofler et al., 2019). Another study examining a large, referred pediatric sample found SCT did contribute uniquely to inhibitory control and set shifting, after controlling for inattention and verbal ability (Jacobson et al., 2019). Findings were specific to SCT subscales; the Slow/Low Initiation subscale—but not Daydreamy or Sleepy/Sluggish—uniquely contributed to inhibitory control, while both Slow/Low Initiation and the Sleepy/Sluggish scale contributed to set shifting. On the whole, weaknesses in core executive skills appear to be more consistently associated with ADHD than SCT (Bauermeister et al., 2012; Baytunca et al., 2018; Becker et al., 2018; Kofler et al., 2019; Tamm et al., 2018; Wåhlstedt & Bohlin, 2010; Willcutt et al., 2014), though clearly more data are needed in these domains.

Early Evidence for Potential Neurobiology and Etiology

A few initial studies have begun to examine neurobiological and etiological underpinnings of SCT. Examining heritability of SCT in a large sample of school-age twins, Moruzzi, Rijsdijk, and Battaglia (2014) found that SCT symptoms showed moderate heritability but were less heritable than ADHD inattention and hyperactivity. SCT also showed larger nonshared environmental influences than ADHD dimensions. An initial functional magnetic resonance imaging (fMRI) study found that in adolescents with ADHD, greater SCT symptoms were associated with reduced activity in the left superior parietal lobule (Fassbender, Kraft, & Schweitzer, 2015). A more recent structural and functional imaging study suggested that in contrast to the reduced frontal volumes evident in ADHD, children with SCT may have larger frontal cortical regions, particularly in right-sided dorsal prefrontal regions and frontal operculum, and abnormal white matter connectivity involving dorsal prefrontal regions (Camprodon-Rosanas et al., 2019). Associations remained significant after controlling for ADHD symptom scores. Similar to ADHD symptoms, SCT symptoms were associated with altered frontal connectivity within the default mode network, a white matter circuit implicated in attentional control and mind wandering (Posner, Park, & Wang, 2014). Notably, these studies relied on only a few SCT items to characterize the samples; further work using a more comprehensive symptom constellation will be important. However, although clearly much more work is needed, these findings begin to implicate networks critical for executive function and sustained attention.

FUTURE DIRECTIONS

As identified throughout this chapter, more wore work is needed to help clarify the nature of the SCT construct and its comorbidities. First and foremost, consensus on the primary symptoms and their measurement, as well as use of a consistent scale for measurement of both primary and related symptoms, will be critical. It is not yet clear whether the field is ready to agree on a single set of symptoms, or whether additional work examining a broader conceptualization of symptoms still has potential to further our understanding of SCT. Likewise, it will be important to clarify whether the SCT subscale structure has additional value given work suggesting potential for differential prediction from specific subscales. Forward progress and comparability of results across studies and samples will be facilitated by consensus in these areas.

Second, the field needs more work examining the neurobehavioral phenotype of individuals rated as having characteristics of SCT, using the agreed-upon symptom set or definition of SCT across ages and countries. Much of the work to date has relied on informant reports of symptoms, as well as of comorbidities and impairment, rather than objective measurements or behavioral tasks. While one might argue that this practice has been at the core of common diagnostic practice in ADHD (Pritchard, Nigro, Jacobson, & Mahone, 2012), more comprehensive measurement and clarification of the nature of the construct may allow for a clearer understanding of whether SCT should be considered a distinct disorder or not. The field needs further validation of external correlates as well as etiology, treatment options and responsiveness, and neurobiological underpinnings of SCT. All of these rely on consensus of a symptom set, as well as greater consistency of performance-based findings on neuropsychological measures.

Furthermore, given the inconsistent data related to processing speed and reaction time, it will be important to more carefully examine whether such individuals are actually slow or "sluggish," as the name of the disorder implies. If so, what aspects of processing (e.g., Jacobson et al., 2011; Kofler et al., 2019) might be slowed, and how consistently slow are these individuals? In ADHD, the profile of high response variability led to initial characterizations of overall slowed responding (Kofler et al., 2013). Is this profile of inconsistently slowed responding also present in SCT or are individuals with SCT more consistently slow compared to those with ADHD? It may be that this profile depends on whether SCT is comorbid with ADHD or not, but additional work is needed.

More comprehensive and consistent measurement of SCT symptoms will facilitate further examination of neurobiological characteristics and etiologies. It will be important to replicate the initial work examining genetic contributions and neuroimaging differences between SCT and ADHD. Ultimately, a better understanding of the construct and its course will allow for a better definition of the phenotype, which in turn will support these kinds of biological studies. Furthermore, some initial work suggests associations with childhood sleep problems and daytime sleepiness (Becker, Garner, & Byars, 2016; Koriakin et al., 2015a; Smith, Eadeh, Breaux, & Langberg, 2019), suggesting additional examination of these linkages and potential sleep-related interventions may be important for ameliorating SCT symptoms.

Given that impairment has been noted fairly consistently across studies, another question that needs to be addressed is that of effective treatments that might remediate this symptom presentation. Some evidence suggests that aspects of SCT symptomatology (e.g., Sluggish/Sleepy, but not Daydreamy) may be predictive of stimulant nonresponse or placebo response on informant reported inattention in youth with ADHD (Froehlich et al., 2018). There is some limited work examining the potential of nonstimulant medications (McBurnett et al., 2017; Wietecha et al., 2013) as well as behavioral interventions (Smith & Langberg, 2020) on SCT symptoms, but it is not yet clear whether this profile of cognitive inefficiency can be remediated with such strategies. While practice via additional rehearsal with concrete information or motor responses can improve automaticity in other populations, evidence is needed to determine whether this would be productive in SCT.

Ultimately, it is clear that additional work is needed to refine our understanding of SCT, its profile of comorbidities and biological underpinnings, and potential interventions. Further evidence may help to refine our understanding of ADHD as well, given the clear overlap between these conditions and symptomatology. With more information, it may be possible to determine whether SCT reflects a distinct and unique disorder or a dimensional, cross-diagnostic process or set of processes that might be useful in predicting risks and outcomes, and guiding treatment decisions, across a range of developmental psychopathologies, consistent with the National Institutes of Mental Health's Research Domain Criteria (RDoC) initiative. While Saxbe and Barkley (2014) have proposed the former, Becker and Willcutt (2019) recently proposed the possibility that the profile of SCT symptoms and comorbidities might be best investigated within the dimensional framework of the RDoC constructs of attention, arousal, and negative valence systems. Only with further work examining most or all of these possibilities will we more fully understand the nature of SCT and be able to potentially rename it appropriately to ameliorate the "disrespectful semantic baggage" (Saxbe & Barkley, 2014) of the terminology.

REFERENCES

Achenbach, T. M., & Rescorla, L. A. (2001). *Manual for the ASEBA School-Age Forms and Profiles.* Burlington: University of Vermont, Research Center for Children, Youth, and Families.

American Psychiatric Association. (1980). *Diagnostic and statistical manual of mental disorders* (3rd ed.). Washington, DC: Author.

American Psychiatric Association. (1987). *Diagnostic and statistical manual of mental disorders* (3rd ed., text rev.). Washington, DC: Author.

American Psychiatric Association. (2000). *Diagnostic and statistical manual of mental disorders* (4th ed.). Washington, DC: Author.

American Psychiatric Association. (2013). *Diagnostic and statistical manual of mental disorders* (5th ed.). Arlington, VA: Author.

Barkley, R. A. (2012a). *Barkley Deficits in Executive Functioning Scale–Children and Adolescents (BDEFS-CA).* New York: Guilford Press.

Barkley, R. A. (2012b). Distinguishing sluggish cognitive tempo from attention-deficit/hyperactivity disorder in adults. *Journal of Abnormal Psychology, 121*(4), 978–990.

Barkley, R. A. (2013). Distinguishing sluggish cognitive tempo from ADHD in children and adolescents: Executive functioning, impairment, and comorbidity. *Journal of Clinical Child and Adolescent Psychology, 42*(2),161–173.

Bauermeister, J. J., Barkley, R. A., Bauermeister, J. A., Martinez, J. V., & McBurnett, K. (2012). Validity of the sluggish cognitive tempo, inattention, and hyperactivity symptom dimensions: Neuropsychological and psychosocial correlates. *Journal of Abnormal Child Psychopathology, 40,* 683–697.

Baytunca, M. B., Inci, S. B., Ipci, M., Kardas, B., Unsel Bolat, G., & Ercan, E. S. (2018). The neurocognitive nature of children with ADHD comorbid sluggish cognitive tempo: Might SCT be a disorder of vigilance? *Psychiatry Research, 270,* 967–973.

Becker, S. P. (2014). Sluggish cognitive tempo and peer functioning in school-aged children: A six-month longitudinal study. *Psychiatry Research, 217*(1–2), 72–78.

Becker, S. P. (2015). *Child Concentration Inventory, Second Edition (CCI-2).* Cincinnati, OH: Author.

Becker, S. P., Burns, G. L., Leopold, D. R., Olson, R. K., & Willcutt, E. G. (2018). Differential impact of trait sluggish cognitive tempo and ADHD inattention in early childhood on adolescent functioning. *Journal of Child Psychology and Psychiatry, 59*(10), 1094–1104.

Becker, S. P., Garner, A. A., & Byars, K. C. (2016). Sluggish cognitive tempo in children referred to a pediatric Sleep Disorders Center: Examining possible overlap with sleep problems and associations with impairment. *Journal of Psychiatric Research, 77,* 116–124.

Becker, S. P., & Langberg, J. M. (2013). Sluggish cognitive tempo among young adolescents with ADHD: Relations to mental health, academic, and social functioning. *Journal of Attention Disorders, 17*(8), 681–689.

Becker, S. P., & Langberg, J. M. (2014). Attention-deficit/hyperactivity disorder and sluggish cognitive tempo dimensions in relation to executive functioning in adolescents with ADHD. *Child Psychiatry Human Development, 45,* 1–11.

Becker, S. P., Leopold, D. R., Burns, L., Jarrett, M. A., Langberg, J. M., Marshall, S. A., . . . Willcutt, E. G. (2016). The internal, external, and diagnostic validity of sluggish cognitive tempo: A meta-analysis and critical review. *Journal of the American Academy of Child and Adolescent Psychiatry, 55*(3), 163–178.

Becker, S. P., Luebbe, A. M., Fite, P. J., Stopplebein, L., & Greening, L. (2014). Sluggish cognitive tempo in psychiatrically hospitalized children: Factor structure and relations to internalizing symptoms, social problems, and observed behavioral dysregulation. *Journal of Abnormal Child Psychology, 42*(1), 49–62.

Becker, S. P., Marsh, N. P., Holdaway, A. S., & Tamm, L. (2020). Sluggish cognitive tempo and processing speed in adolescents with ADHD: Do findings vary based on informant and task? *European Journal of Child and Adolescent Psychiatry, 29,* 1371–1384.

Becker, S. P., & Willcutt, E. G. (2019). Advancing the study of sluggish cognitive tempo via DSM, RDoC, and hierarchical models of psychopathology. *European Journal Child and Adolescent Psychiatry, 28*(5), 603–613.

Belmar, M., Servera, M., Becker, S. P., & Burns, G. L. (2015). Validity of sluggish cognitive tempo in South America: An initial examination using mother and teacher ratings of Chilean children. *Journal of Attention Disorders, 21*(8), 667–672.

Bernad, M. M., Servera, M., Grases, G., Collado, S., & Burns, G. L. (2014). A cross-sectional and longitudinal investigation of the external correlates of sluggish cognitive tempo and ADHD-inattention symptoms dimensions. *Journal of Abnormal Child Psychology, 42,* 1225–1236.

Burns, G. L., & Becker, S. P. (2021). Sluggish cognitive tempo and ADHD symptoms in a nationally representative sample of U.S. children: Differentiation using categorical and dimensional approaches. *Journal of Clinical Child and Adolescent Psychology, 50,* 267–280.

Burns, G. L., Becker, S. P., Geiser, C., Leopold, D. R., & Willcutt, E. G. (2020, July 1). Are sluggish cognitive tempo, ADHD, and oppositional defiant disorder trait- or state-like constructs from prekindergarten to fourth grade? *Journal of Clinical Child and Adolescent Psychology.*

Burns, G. L., Becker, S. P., Servera, M., Bernad, M. M., & García-Banda, G. (2017). Sluggish cognitive tempo and ADHD inattention in the home and school contexts: Parent and teacher invariance and cross-setting validity. *Psychological Assessment, 29*(2), 209–220.

Burns, G. L., Lee, S., Servera, M., McBurnett, K., & Becker, S. P. (2018). *Child and Adolescent Behavior Inventory–Parent Version 1.1.* Pullman, WA: Author.

Camprodon-Rosanas, E., Batlle, S., Estrada-Prat, X., Aceña-Díaz, M., Petrizan-Aleman, A., Pujals, E., . . . Ribas-Fitó, N. (2016). Sluggish cognitive tempo in a child and adolescent clinical outpatient setting. *Journal of Psychiatric Practice, 22*(5), 355–362.

Camprodon-Rosanas, E., Pujol, E., Martınez-Vilavella, G., Blanco-Hinojo, L., Medrano-Martorell, S., . . . Sunyer, J. (2019). Brain structure and function in school-aged children with sluggish cognitive tempo symptoms. *Journal of the American Academy of Child and Adolescent Psychiatry, 58*(2), 256–266.

Camprodon-Rosanas, E., Ribas-Fitó, N., Batlle, S., Persavento, C., Alvarez-Pedrerol, M., Sunyer, J., & Forns, J. (2020). Association between sluggish cognitive tempo symptoms and attentional network and working memory in primary schoolchildren. *Journal of Attention Disorders, 24,* 1787–1795.

Capdevila-Brophy, C., Artigas-Pallarés, J., Navarro-Pastor, J. B., García-Nonell, K., Rigau-Ratera, E., & Obiols, J. E. (2014). ADHD predominantly inattentive subtype with high sluggish cognitive tempo: A new clinical entity? *Journal of Attention Disorders, 18*(7), 607–616.

Carlson, C. L., & Mann, M. (2000). Attention-deficit/hyperactivity disorder, predominantly inattentive subtype. *Child and Adolescent Psychiatric Clinics of North America, 9*(3), 499–510.

Carlson, C. L., & Mann, M. (2002). Sluggish cognitive tempo predicts a different pattern of impairment in the attention deficit hyperactivity disorder, predominantly inattentive type. *Journal of Clinical Child and Adolescent Psychiatry, 31*(1), 123–129.

Cook, N. E., Braaten, E. B., Vuijk, P. J., Lee, A., Samkavitz, A. R., Doyle, A. E., & Surman, C. B. H. (2019). Slow processing speed and sluggish cognitive tempo in pediatric attention-deficit/hyperactivity disorder: Evidence for differentiation of functional correlates. *Child Psychiatry and Human Development, 50,* 1049–1057.

Duncan, A., Tamm, L., Birnschein, A. M., & Becker, S. P. (2019). Clinical correlates of sluggish cognitive tempo in adolescents with autism spectrum disorder. *Autism, 23*(6), 1354–1362.

Dvorsky, M. R., Becker, S. P., Tamm, L., & Willoughby, M. T. (2021). Testing the longitudinal structure and change in sluggish cognitive tempo and inattentive behaviors from early through middle childhood. *Assessment, 28,* 380–394.

Fassbender, C., Kraft, C. E., & Schweitzer, J. B. (2015). Differentiating SCT and inattentive symptoms in ADHD using fMRI measures of cognitive control. *NeuroImage: Clinical, 8,* 390–397.

Frick, P. J., Lahey, B. B., Applegate, B., Kerdyck, L., Ollendick, T., Hynd, G. W., . . . Waldman, I. (1994). DSM-IV field trials for the disruptive behavior disorders: Symptom utility estimates. *Journal of the American Academy of Child and Adolescent Psychiatry, 33*(4), 529–539.

Froehlich, T. E., Becker, S. P., Nick, T. G., Brinkman, W. B., Stein, M. A., Peugh, J., & Epstein, J. N. (2018). Sluggish cognitive tempo as a possible predictor of methylphenidate response in children with ADHD: A randomized controlled trial. *Journal of Clinical Psychiatry, 79*(2), Article 17m11553.

Garner, A. A., Marceaux, J. C., Mrug, S., Patterson, C., & Hodgens, B. (2010). Dimensions and correlates of attention deficit/hyperactivity disorder and sluggish cognitive tempo. *Journal of Abnormal Child Psychology, 38*, 1097–1107.

Gioia, G. A., Isquith, P. K., Guy, S. C., & Kenworthy, L. (2000). *BRIEF: Behavior Rating Inventory of Executive Function.* Lutz, FL: Psychological Assessment Resources.

Hartman, C. A., Willcutt, E. G., Rhee, S. H., & Pennington, B. F. (2004). The relation between sluggish cognitive tempo and DSM-IV ADHD. *Journal of Abnormal Child Psychology, 32*(5), 491–503.

Hinshaw, S. P. (2002). Preadolescent girls with attention-deficit/hyperactivity disorder: I. Background characteristics, comorbidity, cognitive and social functioning, and parenting practices. *Journal of Consulting and Clinical Psychology, 70*(5), 1086–1098.

Jacobson, L. A., Geist, M., & Mahone, E. M. (2018). Sluggish cognitive tempo, processing speed, and internalizing symptoms: the moderating effect of age. *Journal of Abnormal Child Psychology, 46*, 127–135.

Jacobson, L. A., & Mahone, E. M. (2019). Sluggish cognitive tempo predicts academic fluency, beyond contributions of core academic skills, attention, and motor speed. *Journal of Attention Disorders, 23*(14), 1703–1710.

Jacobson, L. A., Murphy-Bowman, S. C., Pritchard, A. E., Tart-Zelvin, A., Zabel, T. A., & Mahone, E. M. (2012). Factor structure of a sluggish cognitive tempo scale in clinically-referred children. *Journal of Abnormal Child Psychology, 40*(8), 1327–1337.

Jacobson, L. A., Ryan, M., & Mahone, E. M. (2019, March). *Sluggish cognitive tempo, but not inattention, consistently predicts cognitive control.* Poster presented at the annual meeting of the Society for Research in Child Development, Baltimore, MD.

Jacobson, L. A., Ryan, M., Martin, R. B., Ewen, J., Mostofsky, S. H., Denckla, M. B., & Mahone, E. M. (2011). Working memory influences processing speed and reading fluency in ADHD. *Child Neuropsychology, 17*(3), 209–224.

Jarrett, M. A., Rapport, H. F., Rondon, A. T., & Becker, S. P. (2017). ADHD dimensions and sluggish cognitive tempo symptoms in relation to self-report and laboratory measures of neuropsychological functioning in college students. *Journal of Attention Disorders, 21*(8), 673–683.

Khadka, G., Burns, G. L., & Becker, S. P. (2016). Internal and external validity of sluggish cognitive tempo and ADHD inattention dimensions with teacher ratings of Nepali children. *Journal of Psychopathology and Behavior Assessment, 38*(3), 433–442.

Kofler, M. J., Irwin, L., Sarver, D. E., Fosco, W. D., Miller, C. E., Spiegel, J. A., & Becker, S. P. (2019). What cognitive processes are "sluggish" in sluggish cognitive tempo? *Journal of Consulting and Clinical Psychology, 87*(11), 1030–1042.

Kofler, M. J., Rapport, M. D., Sarver, D. E., Raiker, J. S., Orban, S. A., Friedman, L. M., & Kolomeyer, E. G. (2013). Reaction time variability in ADHD: A meta-analytic review of 319 studies. *Clinical Psychology Review, 33*(6), 795–811.

Koriakin, T. A., Mahone, E. M., & Jacobson, L. A. (2015a). Sleep difficulties are associated with parent report of sluggish cognitive tempo. *Journal of Developmental Behavioral Pediatrics, 36*(9), 717–723.

Koriakin, T. A., Noonan, N., Mahone, E. M., & Jacobson, L. A. (2015b). The contribution of sluggish cognitive tempo to executive and adaptive functioning [Abstract]. *Journal of the International Neuropsychological Society, 21*(S1), 285.

Lahey, B. B., Applegate, B., McBurnett, K., Biederman, J., Greenhill, L., Hynd, G. W., . . . Shaffer, D. (1994). DSM-IV field trials for attention deficit hyperactivity disorder in children and adolescents. *American Journal of Psychiatry, 151*, 1673–1685.

Lahey, B. B., & Carlson, C. L. (1991). Validity of the diagnostic category of attention deficit disorder without hyperactivity: A review of the literature. *Journal of Learning Disabilities, 24*(2), 110–120.

Lahey, B. B., Pelham, W. E., Schaughency, E. A., Atkins, M. S., Murphy, H. A., Hynd, G., . . . Lorys-Vernon, A. (1988). Dimensions and types of attention deficit disorder. *Journal of the Ameri-*

can Academy of Child and Adolescent Psychiatry, 27(3), 330–335.

Langberg, J. M., Becker, S. P., & Dvorsky, M. R. (2014). The association between sluggish cognitive tempo and academic functioning in youth with attention-deficit/hyperactivity disorder (ADHD). *Journal of Abnormal Child Psychology, 42*(1), 91–103.

Lee, S., Burns, G. L., & Becker, S. P. (2018). towards establishing the transcultural validity of sluggish cognitive tempo: Evidence from a sample of South Korean children. *Journal of Clinical Child and Adolescent Psychology, 47*(1), 61–68.

Lee, S., Burns, G. L., Snell, J., & McBurnett, K. (2014). Validity of the sluggish cognitive tempo symptom dimension in children: Sluggish cognitive tempo and ADHD-inattention as distinct symptom dimensions. *Journal of Abnormal Child Psychology, 42*(1), 7–19.

Leopold, D. R., Christopher, M. E., Burns, G. L., Becker, S. P., Olson, R. K., & Willcutt, E. G. (2016). Attention-deficit/hyperactivity disorder and sluggish cognitive tempo throughout childhood: Temporal invariance and stability from preschool through ninth grade. *Journal of Child Psychology and Psychiatry, 57*(9), 1066–1074.

Marshall, S. A., Evans, S. W., Eiraldi, R. B., Becker, S. P., & Power, T. J. (2014). Social and academic impairment in youth with ADHD, predominately inattentive type and sluggish cognitive tempo. *Journal of Abnormal Child Psychology, 42*(1), 77–90.

McBurnett, K., Clernow, D., Williams, D., Villodas, M., Wietecha, L., & Barkley, R. (2017). Atomoxetine-related change in sluggish cognitive tempo is partially independent of change in attention-deficit/hyperactivity disorder inattentive symptoms. *Journal of Child and Adolescent Psychopharmacology, 27*(1), 38–42.

McBurnett, K., Pfiffner, L. J., & Frick. P. J. (2001). Symptom properties as a function of ADHD type: An argument for continued study of sluggish cognitive tempo. *Journal of Abnormal Child Psychology, 29*(3), 207–213.

McBurnett, K., Villodas, M., Burns, G. L., Hinshaw, S. P., Beaulieu, A., & Pfiffner, L. J. (2014). Structure and validity of sluggish cognitive tempo using an expanded item pool in children with attention-deficit/hyperactivity disorder. *Journal of Abnormal Child Psychology, 42*, 37–48.

McGrath, L. M., Pennington, B. F., Shanahan, M. A., Santerre-Lemmon, L. E., Barnard, H. D., Willcutt, E. G., . . . Olson, R. K. (2011). A multiple deficit model of reading disability and attention-deficit/hyperactivity disorder: Searching for shared cognitive deficits. *Journal of Child Psychology and Psychiatry, and Allied Disciplines, 52*(5), 547–557.

Milich, R., Balentine, A. C., & Lynam, D. R. (2001). ADHD combined type and ADHD predominantly inattentive type are distinct and unrelated disorders. *Clinical Psychology Science and Practice, 8*, 463–488.

Moruzzi, S., Rijsdijk, F., & Battaglia, M. (2014). A twin study of the relationships among inattention, hyperactivity/impulsivity and sluggish cognitive tempo problems. *Journal of Abnormal Child Psychology, 42*, 63–75.

Penny, A. M., Waschbusch, D. A., Klein, R. M., Corkum, P., & Eskes, G. (2009). Developing a measure of sluggish cognitive tempo for children: Content validity, factor structure, and reliability. *Psychological Assessment, 21*(3), 380–389.

Posner, J., Park, C., & Wang, Z. (2014). Connecting the dots: A review of resting connectivity MRI studies in attention-deficit/hyperactivity disorder. *Neuropsychology Review, 24*(1), 3–15.

Preszler, J., Burns, G. L., Litson, K., Geiser, C., Servera, M., & Becker, S. P. (2019). How consistent is sluggish cognitive tempo across occasions, sources, and settings?: Evidence from latent state–trait modeling. *Assessment, 26*(1), 99–110.

Pritchard, A. E., Nigro, C. A., Jacobson, L. A., & Mahone, E. M. (2012). The role of neuropsychological assessment in the functional outcomes of children with ADHD. *Neuropsychology Review, 22*(1), 54–68.

Sáez, B., Servera, M., Becker, S. P., & Burns, G. L. (2019). Optimal items for assessing sluggish cognitive tempo in children across mother, father, and teacher ratings. *Journal of Clinical Child and Adolescent Psychology, 48*(6), 825–839.

Saxbe, C., & Barkley, R. A. (2014). The second attention disorder?: Sluggish cognitive tempo vs. attention-deficit/hyperactivity disorder: Update for clinicians. *Journal of Psychiatric Practice, 20*, 38–49.

Servera, M., Sáez, B., Burns, G. L., & Becker, S. P. (2018). Clinical differentiation of sluggish cognitive tempo and attention-deficit/hyperactivity disorder in children. *Journal of Abnormal Psychology, 127*(8), 818–829.

Skirbekk, B., Hansen, B. H., Oerbeck, B., & Kristensen, H. (2011). The relationship between sluggish cognitive tempo, subtypes of attention-deficit/hyperactivity disorder, and anxiety disorders. *Journal of Abnormal Child Psychology, 39*(4), 513–525.

Smith, Z. R., Eadeh, H. M., Breaux, R. P., & Langberg, J. M. (2019). Sleepy, sluggish, worried, or down?: The distinction between self-reported sluggish cognitive tempo, daytime sleepiness, and internalizing symptoms in youth with attention-deficit/hyperactivity disorder. *Psychological Assessment, 31*(3), 365–375.

Smith, Z. R., & Langberg, J. M. (2017). Predicting academic impairment and internalizing psychopathology using a multidimensional framework of sluggish cognitive tempo with parent- and adolescent reports. *European Journal Child and Adolescent Psychiatry, 26*(9), 1141–1150.

Smith, Z. R., & Langberg, J. M. (2020). Do sluggish cognitive tempo symptoms improve with school-based ADHD interventions?: Outcomes and predictors of change. *Journal of Child Psychology and Psychiatry, 61,* 575–583.

Tamm, L., Brenner, S. B., Bamberger, M. E., & Becker, S. P. (2018). Are sluggish cognitive tempo symptoms associated with executive functioning in preschoolers? *Child Neuropsychology, 24*(1), 82–105.

Tamm, L., Garner, A. A., Loren, R. E. A., Epstein, J. N., Vaughn, A. J., Ciesielski, H. A., & Becker, S. P. (2016). Slow sluggish cognitive tempo symptoms are associated with poorer academic performance in children with ADHD. *Psychiatry Research, 242,* 251–259.

Ünsel-Bolat, G., Ercan, E. S., Bolat, H., Süren, S., Bacanlı, A., Yazıcı, K. U., & Rohde, L. A. (2019). Comparisons between sluggish cognitive tempo and ADHD-restrictive inattentive presentation phenotypes in a clinical ADHD sample. *ADHD Attention Deficit and Hyperactivity Disorders, 11,* 363–372.

Vu, A., Thompson, L., Willcutt, E., & Petrill, S. (2019). Sluggish cognitive tempo: longitudinal stability and validity. *Attention Deficit and Hyperactivity Disorders, 11,* 463–471.

Wåhlstedt, C., & Bohlin, G. (2010). DSM-IV-defined inattention and sluggish cognitive tempo: Independent and interactive relations to neuropsychological factors and comorbidity. *Child Neuropsychology, 16*(4), 350–365.

Watabe, Y., Owens, J. S., Evans, S. W., & Brandt, N. E. (2014). The relationship between sluggish cognitive tempo and impairment in children with and without ADHD. *Journal of Abnormal Child Psychology, 42*(1), 105–115.

Wietecha, L., Williams, D., Shaywitz, S., Shaywitz, B., Hooper, S. R., Wigal, S. B., & McBurnett, K. (2013). Atomoxetine improved attention in children and adolescents with attention-deficit/hyperactivity disorder and dyslexia in a 16 week, acute, randomized, double-blind trial. *Journal of Child and Adolescent Psychopharmacology, 23*(9), 605–613.

Willcutt, E. G., Chhabildas, N., Kinnear, M., DeFries, J. C., Olson, R. K., Leopold, D. R., . . . Pennington, C. F. (2014). The internal and external validity of sluggish cognitive tempo and its relation with DSM-IV ADHD. *Journal of Abnormal Child Psychology, 42*(1), 21–35.

Wood, W. L. M., Potts, H. E., Lewandowski, L. J., & Lovett, B. J. (2017). Sluggish cognitive tempo and speed of performance. *Journal of Attention Disorders, 21*(8), 684–690.

PART VI
CONCLUSIONS

CHAPTER 24

From Knowledge Base to Clinical Case

Jane Holmes Bernstein
Adam R. Cassidy

In the 350+ years since the first peer-reviewed scientific paper was published, the recorded base of human knowledge has grown to well over 50 million published entries (Jinha, 2010). In the past 5 years, more than 350,000 articles have been added to the psychology literature alone, not to mention the 500 or so pages contained within this volume. The sheer amount of information represented by these estimates is truly awesome, as is the challenge it presents to the pediatric neuropsychologist seeking to access and apply relevant knowledge in the service of the individual child. This challenge—which we call the "knowledge base to clinical case (or KB→CC) problem"—is one that we as pediatric neuropsychologists strive to manage on a day-to-day basis, yet it is anything but ordinary. Indeed, going from knowledge base (KB) to clinical case (CC) is actually quite difficult and not at all straightforward.

THE "KB→CC PROBLEM"

The Extent of the Knowledge Base

The breadth of the knowledge base underlying clinical neuropsychological assessment is immense and not always fully appreciated. First, it is not monolithic. Multiple knowledge bases can be brought to bear on clinical case conceptualization. In the instructions for this book, for example, authors were asked to provide a discussion of the history, epidemiology, etiology/neuropathology/neural substrates, neuropsychological consequences, developmental considerations, predictors and moderators, and treatment/intervention for each of their respective disorders. Each of these topics has its own knowledge base! Add to this the knowledge bases pertaining to the nature of the organism to which the condition is happening (here, the child), the processes underlying behavioral measurement and diagnostic decision making, and the functional capacities of the organism doing the decision making (the clinician)—at a minimum. Then add the fact that all of these knowledge bases are not just learned once and for all but are continually being added to and refined—and that cogent disagreements occur among well-meaning practitioners of both the science and the clinical work about what findings mean and how they should be interpreted. The challenge is enormous.

Different Methodological Value Systems

The methodological value systems of research and practice are not aligned (McCall, 2009). The knowledge (i.e., evidence) base is typically derived from research investigations involving multiple individuals (N = many). In contrast, clinical practice is conducted as an "experiment with an N of 1" (Bernstein, 2000). Whereas *research*, in its adherence to the Kantian nomothetic tendency, prioritizes universals, is variable-centered, and worries about internal validity (i.e., investigative control/precision), *practice* espouses a more idiographic/humanistic tendency that prizes individuals, is person-centered, and is concerned about external validity (relevance/utility in real life). Historically, in neuropsychology, the overt focus on brain and biology effectively created an imbalance in which "neuro" was granted privileged status over "psycho." Although much of the knowledge base for actual clinical practice is found within the psychology literature, the integration of psychological principles and practice (derived from fields such as cognitive psychology on the one hand and from skills such as interviewing, creating rapport/therapeutic alliances, and managing transference on the other) as these apply in the context of neuropsychological assessment has not been fully articulated.

Defining Outcomes

A primary and shared goal of both clinical research and practice is the optimization of outcomes following adverse experiences, medical/biological and otherwise. The field of neuropsychology has at times been accused of being better at identifying problems than fixing them. There is truth to this. Neuropsychologists have done a masterful job of describing the impact of neurological breakdown and identifying how this can affect behavior. The rapid establishment and reach of the field attests to this. The challenge, though, is that we do not have a comparable evidence base that proves that our clinical services add value (in the modern financial parlance) in terms of improving the well-being of the patients we see. We need more research on outcomes arising from clinical practice. But this is not easy, largely because delineation of practice outcomes does not lend itself to a controlled research investigation strategy. The first challenge is one of definition: What are you going to consider a desired outcome and when? Is the desired outcome better control of a specific nonoptimal behavior across, say, 6 months? Or is it successful completion of grade 3, or 6, or high school? Or is a successful outcome a 25-year-old with a job and friends? Or a 30-year-old with a partner and children? The second challenge may be that of the clinician's philosophy vis-à-vis the responsibility of the clinician to the client. Is the desired outcome an endpoint that the clinician can more or less specify, or is the clinician's role one of partnership in the ongoing construction of the family's narrative?

A third problem arises, however. As renowned cognitive psychologist, Amos Tversky, once said, "It is sometimes easier to make the world a better place than to prove you have made the world a better place" (Lewis, 2016, p. 230). Indeed, evaluating outcomes against rigorous research criteria is hard, perhaps impossible, when what a clinician does for one child and family at, say, 8 years of age is credited by them for the success of the young adult at 22! How do you know? How could you prove it? Yet every clinician who has been in practice for any length of time can tell you such stories. Even harder is proving at the individual level that you *prevented* something adverse from happening by your intervention, be it co-constructing a new narrative with child and family, recommending a specific therapy, or designing an alternative education program—yet this is what many clinicians, particularly those working in a public health or prevention model, including ourselves, believe they do. Clinicians also run the very real risk that when they do their work well, they effectively render themselves invisible: Their interventions are not remembered as discrete events but become part of the ongoing child and family narrative, which is much harder to capture empirically.

Evidence-Based Practice: The Challenge of "Expertise"

How does a clinician use all or even some of the knowledge available? This question invokes the construct of clinical expertise. But we do not have a firm grasp of what clinical expertise is, how it can be fostered, and how it can be effectively evaluated. We do not understand how aspiring clinicians acquire the expertise to use the knowledge base in the first place, nor how established practitioners adapt, develop, and enrich their repertoires over time in the face of new knowledge.

In clinical neuropsychology, mobilizing the knowledge base in the service of the individual child is done via the "complex clinical activity" (Vanderploeg, 1994, p. 38) that is the clinical assessment. This process is undertaken in the context of evidence-based practice defined by the Institute of Medicine (IOM; 2001, p. 147) as "the integration of best research evidence with clinical expertise and patient values." The relevant evidence is recognized to come from a wide range of possible sources (Greenberg & Newman, 1996)—from randomized controlled trials to large observational studies to process analyses, meta-analyses, and single-case designs, as well as from "practice-based evidence" methodologies (Barkham & Mellor-Clark, 2003; Grodzinsky, Forbes, & Bernstein, 2010). Central to evidence-based practice approaches is the goal of improving outcomes—important both to the individual patient and to the health care system in general. A framework for evidence-based practice in neuropsychology, with a focus on outcomes, has been laid out by Chelune (2010).

The recommendations of the IOM report have been important and widely influential—although there have been many critiques that have been incisive and pertinent (Greenhalgh et al., 2014). Our critique is with the repeated alignment of "expertise" with "research evidence" and "client values." We believe that this alignment is misleading. It obscures the fact that evidence and values provide relevant data for clinical decision making, whereas expertise *is* the clinical decision making; that is, the application of expertise is what yields the diagnostic formulation and guides case management. Expertise is thus a superordinate process whereby the relevant data are rendered coherent and useful to the child and family (Figure 24.1). We also take issue with the discussion of "clinical expertise" in the APA Presidential Task Force on Evidence-Based Practice in Psychology (American Psychological Association, 2006). In our opinion the analysis of clinical expertise in terms of "components" actually invokes additional knowledge bases and fails to

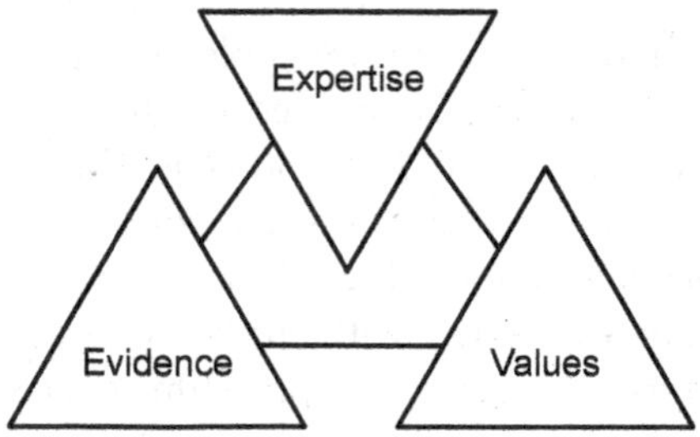

FIGURE 24.1. Expertise as superordinate.

clarify the nature of expertise itself, diluting the meaning of this critical competence at the core of a clinical discipline.

Expertise—the ability to *choose* relevant evidence and *use* it effectively—is key, yet is not well understood. Expertise cannot be acquired via "book learning" alone but is derived from intensive supervision by more experienced clinicians who are responsible for directing and guiding the training needed to provide this level of professional development. The acquisition of expertise takes place in the context of delivering clinical services. In psychological disciplines, this experience is typically—in the U.S. setting—introduced during clinical practica in graduate school, continues during internship, and is consolidated throughout postdoctoral fellowship training. In the transition to fellowship training, a general assumption seems to be that when students complete their doctoral work, they have mastered a core set of disciplinary knowledge bases, and then proceed to fellowship to extend and refine their knowledge in a specialty area by providing services under supervision. This assumption is true but partial. Fellowship does not simply expose a student to more and more specialized knowledge; it provides a critical element in professional development by making the clinician aware of, and then nurturing and refining, clinical expertise. This is perhaps the most important responsibility of the fellowship supervisor.

To do justice to the centrality of clinical expertise, evidence-based practice requires that the clinician activate a *thinking process* that integrates the data relevant to diagnostic decision making and case management. Thus, expertise is not achieved by accruing more data; rather, it is the thinking activity that enables any and all relevant evidence to be used effectively—essentially, "evidence-based thinking." This process encompasses not only knowledge of the biological factors associated with disorders/conditions and, in neuropsychology, the brain–behavior relationships that these elucidate, but must also entail knowledge of *principles* underlying human behavior and learning, social integration, functional adaptation, and plausible interventions—as well as *principles* underlying the measurement of human behavior (not human behavior in the laboratory, but human behavior "in the field" of real life). The knowledge (evidence) base informs the clinician about what is expected neuropsychologically; expertise enables the clinician to make that information meaningful to a particular child/family. Vanderploeg's "complex clinical activity" thus encompasses all the potentially relevant knowledge bases that inform our understanding of how the individual child builds a brain from conception to adulthood.

How does such thinking take place? What do clinicians bring to bear? Part of the answer is that the knowledge base is not accessed directly. The knowledge base yields a variety of theoretical models that guide the organization of behavioral data. Such models are tools for thinking: In both the research lab and the clinical office, thinking (i.e., the organization of data into theoretically coherent constructs) is based on an ongoing interaction between models and evidence. In practice, such models, which are debated and constantly refined, yield the theoretical framework of the discipline (Bernstein, 2010). The development of appropriate models is thus the critical mediating variable between the knowledge base and the clinical case; the challenge we face would be better captured as a KB→M^n→CC problem—where the relevant M (model) could be derived from one or many knowledge bases (Table 24.1).

The Lens of Development

To a significant extent, the knowledge base of neuropsychology comprises studies aiming to characterize the conditions that change brain–behavior relationships, further elucidating these wherever possible. When these disorders affect a developing child, both theories and the models they generate must be grounded in the dynamics of development wherein, as Maureen Dennis so eloquently described, "neural and behavioral outcome is constructed through transactions between plastic and homeostatic processes and the

TABLE 24.1. Major Knowledge Bases at Play in Neuropsychological Assessment of the Developing Child

Knowledge bases	Representative principles
Medical condition	Nature, timing, location, duration of condition; etiology; pathophysiology
Brain–behavior relationships	Localization and lateralization by lesion/imaging/cognitive paradigms; cortical and subcortical processing loops
Developmental science	Continuity and change; interactive specialization; canalization; role of experience (positive, adverse, lacking); cascades; expected/alternative trajectories; responsive relationships/attachment; risk and resilience
Neurobiology	Genetics/genomics; epigenetics; neural plasticity; stress responsivity; homeostasis/allostasis
Evolution/adaptation	Evolutionary/ontogenetic change/conservation; survival needs; brain–context–development transactional model; brain as both dependent and independent variable
Assessment	Collection/organization of behavioral data (integrated Q^2 model; diagnostic behavioral clustering); principles of measurement, psychometrics, statistics
Psychology	Information processing (cognitive, affective, social); behavior regulation; sociality/interpersonal dynamics; personality
Society	Systems analysis—family, community, culture; school design, curriculum, special education; vocational pathways

environment" (Dennis et al., 2014, p. 390). Developmental dynamics are thus crucial to an understanding of both outcomes and the trajectories by which they are achieved (Karmiloff-Smith, 1998).

The goal of this book is to make a contribution to the knowledge base by updating available knowledge vis-à-vis the *nature* of the disorders under discussion (i.e., their pathophysiology and developmental dynamics). As clinicians working with the individual child, however, we are equally invested in the *fact* of a disorder; that is, the presence of disorder (any disorder) in a developing child necessarily perturbs the dynamics underlying the developmental course in its entirety.

Thus, for the clinician working with children, the fundamental model in the KB→M^n→CC equation is that of *development*. Thinking developmentally in neuropsychology, however, does not simply mean scrutinizing changes in scores on tasks tapping specific domains as children get older. This is a test-centered approach. What it does require is the integration of principles of development—developmental expression, brain–world interaction, developmental change—to gain a more complete understanding of how this child's brain was sculpted over time from conception to the time of evaluation. This is a whole-child, child-centered approach. Seeing behavior through a developmental lens thus entails incorporating a set of fundamental principles that structure our thinking, requiring us to frame our task around a coherent theory of the developing person rather than limiting it to a cross-sectional analysis of a child's current behavior. To this end, the developmental lens requires that we revisit some of the ways we think. For example, outcomes are not just something in the future that we aim to influence by our actions; the evaluation itself documents an outcome—of the child's developmental course to date. Similarly, chronological age is not only a metric of time passing, but it also serves as an index of "developmental time" during which a child has been acquiring (or failing to acquire) the experiences that build brain and behavioral competencies. Furthermore, through the developmental lens, adverse experiences of all kinds are potential threats to development itself.

All neurodevelopmental disorders change the interactions between the organism and the environment; they all change the experience on which subsequent development depends. Such "brain changers" can threaten behavioral development from the beginning by establishing alternative developmental trajectories (e.g., genetic disorders, congenital heart disease) or they can derail a developmental trajectory that was proceeding in an expectable fashion prior to the given insult (e.g., acquired insults). Development of the brain—and thus behavior—is also seriously threatened by any sustained lack of the expectable experiences upon which brain health depends, including emotional nurturance, sensitive and responsive caregiving, adequate nutrition, physical safety (self, caretakers), and opportunities to learn (both socially created and secondary to treatment). All can be manifest as a failure to acquire expectable skills at the right time and in the right order (Dennis, 1988). The expected skills can be typically "caught" or acquired from interaction with the environment ("biologically primary"), or they can depend heavily on direct instruction, that is, "taught" directly ("biologically secondary"; Geary, 2008).

Adverse events can, of course, occur independently of a known medical disorder; they can also complicate the outcome of one. Their effects can be both buffered and exacerbated by variables associated with family style, expectations, and coping strategies, as well as cultural values and beliefs (e.g., Yeates et al., 2007; Yeates, Taylor, Walz, Stancin,

& Wade, 2010). Moreover, adverse events may be experienced as a relatively discrete event (exposure to a single violent event; successful surgical treatment of brain tumor) or may extend over time (chronic abuse/neglect, extended medical treatment/hospitalization). Under no circumstance, however, is the resulting perturbation a one-off experience. The change itself is incorporated into the ongoing developmental course, becomes an integral part of the organism's neurobehavioral repertoire, and shapes the individual's adaptation from then on. Indeed, "the effects of early injury cascade through the developing neurobehavioral system . . . inducing not one instance of reorganization, but rather altering the entire trajectory of development" (Stiles, Reilly, Levine, Trauner, & Nass, 2012, p. 339).

The clinician's work is anchored in outcomes at every stage of development. When a clinician sees a child for an assessment, he or she is seeing the outcome of that child's developmental course to date, that is, what they have been able to learn (or not) as a function of optimal and nonoptimal experiences. The outcome of the assessment is the understanding that will allow the clinician to act to promote optimal outcomes for the child into the future. Thus, the clinician also functions as a potential "brain changer"—or, at least, developmental trajectory rerouter—in developing a management plan and interventions, with the goal of nudging the child's ongoing trajectory in the direction that will most closely approximate age-expected adaptive capacities in the future. For some individuals, this will be mastery of activities of daily living, while for others, it will be strategies for managing high-level abstract materials. Both the trajectories and the endpoints of recovery are legion (Dennis et al., 2014; Krueger & Bear, 2010). The goal is to help a child and family to match now-changed capacities to the real demands of everyday life—to optimize their *lived experience*. For the clinician, the knowledge required thus ranges far beyond the biological parameters of the medical condition. The clinical analysis must be centered on the child and his or her developmental trajectory: How has this child developed? When did the derailment occur? How has the child developed from the time of insult? What are the child's future goals? What constraints on future development are in place? Can these constraints be mitigated and how?

Assessing the Developing Child

For us, the entire assessment process is guided by the systemic neurodevelopmental model (Bernstein, 2000; Holmes-Bernstein & Waber, 1990; Bernstein & Weiler, 2000). Central to our thinking is that CONTEXT-based and DEVELOPMENT-based experiences shape BRAIN directly—and are not, at least not initially, to be viewed as moderator variables. For BRAIN, the primary questions are *what* (the pathophysiology of the condition), *where* (the location of the insult), and *how* (the conditions under which the insult was sustained; the mechanics of injury). For DEVELOPMENT, four questions are critical for all relevant behavioral domains. First, has the child had the relevant experience to promote the acquisition of this domain? Second, has there been any lack of expectable input? Third, have there been any specific adverse experiences ('brain changers') operating at different times? Adverse experiences can include the medical condition and also its treatment (e.g., hospitalization, procedures, toxic exposures), as well as psychosocial stressors at the level of the child, the family, the community, and the culture. Fourth, when (during which developmental epoch) did these adverse experiences occur? For CONTEXT, the questions involve not only the nature and timing of adverse events, but also the opportunities and resources (e.g., social, educational) available to the child and family at different times, and the beliefs, values, and goals of the child and family in the community/(ies) to which they belong. These can both facilitate and constrain a child's progress over time.

The assessment is bipartite, consisting of evaluation on the one hand and management on the other. In conducting the evaluation, the clinician specifies *products*, analyzes *processes*, and understands the impact of *systems*. *Products*, both biologically primary and biologically secondary, are the outcome of the developmental course to date (i.e., what has been learned in the interactions between child and world over time). The success of their acquisition is defined by society via the education system (grades, academic placement) and measurement tools (educational and psychological measures; behavioral rating scales). They lead to societally defined services where necessary. The analysis of *processes* tells us how the brain might support or mediate the behavior in question, informs our understanding of how development might unfold, provides critical clues as to how and why it can go wrong, and is central to rehabilitation efforts. Knowledge of relevant *systems* tells us who this child is—the whole lived experience of this child in his or her actual circumstances. The systems are the context in which the clinician works to promote optimal outcomes for each child and family. Understanding the products, the processes, and the systems operative at the time of the assessment is critical. The clinician has to situate the impact of brain function and its derailment in the context of the life experiences of a particular child in his or her family, community, and culture. The same quantitative profile may be realized in very different lived experiences in different individuals; it may play out very differently over time given important differences in family values, beliefs, and goals.

The evaluation strategy involves a systematic review of the major neurobehavioral systems, from arousal to higher-order abstract thinking, that have been identified and parsed in the research investigations of the neuropsychological evidence base (i.e., brain–behavior relationships). This review always takes place against the background of developmental dynamics, that is, evaluation of the integrity of any behavior is always age- and developmental-stage referenced. The diagnostic model is based on the *integration* of quantitative and qualitative data (the Q2 model) obtained from each of the primary neurobehavioral domains. In our setting, the review of systems is facilitated by a *Review of Neurobehavioral Systems* (RNbS) tool that structures the capture of behavior from standardized tests and rating scales in addition to the observed or described behavior that is otherwise "invisible" to standardized measures, behavior that deviates from expectation in both positive (too much) and negative (too little) directions, and behavior that emerges from the transactions inherent in relationships (clinician and child—directly observed, child- and others-reported). The clinician provides information about the relationship dynamics by monitoring his or her own behavior and behavior change in transactions with the child or parent as a diagnostic tool in and of itself. Our position is that such diagnostically important behaviors must be incorporated explicitly into clinical decision-making strategies and that we should develop and refine the tools for so doing. We will then be in a position to be equally explicit in our teaching of rigorous Q2 models.

In an integrated Q2 model, both quantitative and qualitative information relating to each of the major neurobehavioral domains are derived from the history, from observations of the child by the clinician and others, and from test scores and performances. The data are then scrutinized to determine their membership in a diagnostic behavioral cluster. This comprises both converging and discriminating findings or observations whose co-occurrence is determined by the theoretical model derived from the larger evidence base. The approach allows the full range of relevant knowledge bases to be accessed in a systematic fashion. The review of systems strategy is fundamental to the approach, keeping the window through which diagnostically relevant behaviors are observed as wide open as possible in order to reduce the potential for bias secondary to premature diagnostic closure. It directly counters any potential for choosing a diagnosis first, then essentially "cherry-picking" the data to make the case for that diagnosis.

The assessment itself is not a unidirectional collection of data but an iterative process, with the clinician circling back to reevaluate the diagnostic import of data collected so far as new data are obtained (Figure 24.2). This means that the clinician is always open to the possibility that relevant data may be obtained throughout the entirety of the assessment, from record and referral review to the feedback session. Reframing of the child's overall presentation during feedback often prompts parents to provide information that they had not reported before. This can elicit a very different perspective on the current

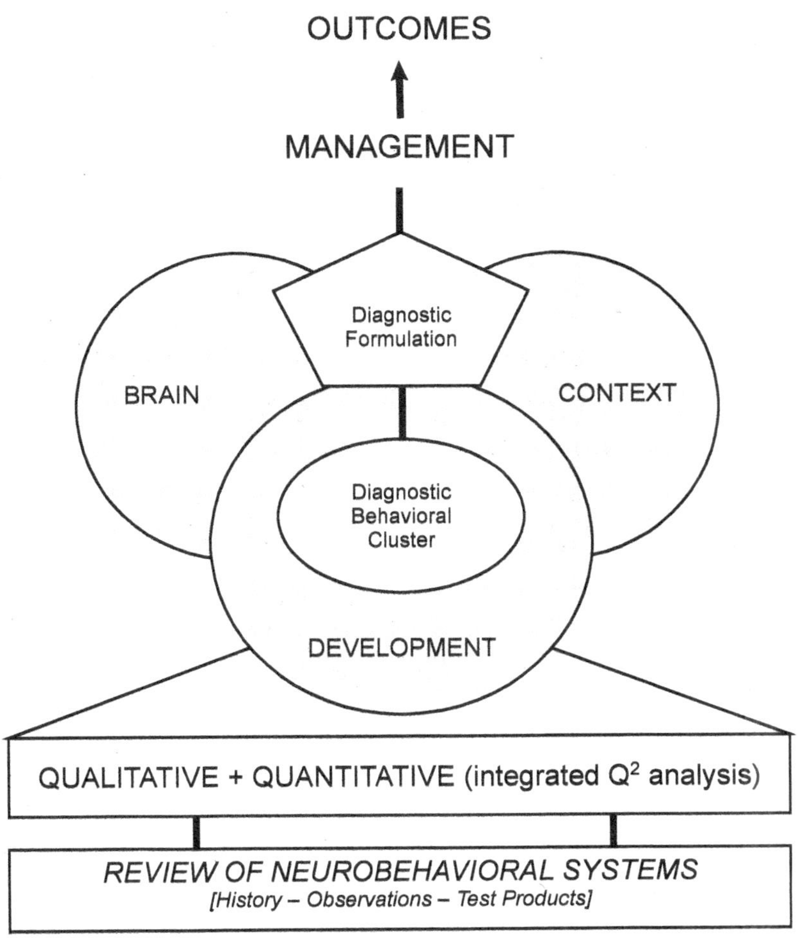

FIGURE 24.2. Systemic neurodevelopmental model.

formulation. Drafting a report for the feedback session but not providing the final copy at that time is an important procedural step that allows such new diagnostic information to be incorporated into the final written document.

Quantifying Quality

The use of qualitative data is not a casual undertaking. It requires a high degree of rigor both in observing and collecting the relevant behavioral data and in integrating this with quantitative data in a coherent diagnostic model. Emphasizing the importance of qualitative data in the diagnostic model does not mean, however, that we should treat the numbers casually, or that we should fail to incorporate advances in psychometric theory and in diagnostic decision-making algorithms. What it does mean is that we should always appreciate that the clinical job cannot depend on the numbers alone.

A significant limitation of quantified (or actuarial) diagnostic strategies alone lies in the fact that many diagnostically relevant behaviors are effectively "invisible" to psychometric measures. Such behaviors do not lend themselves to the static requirements of standardized measures that are well suited to the evaluation of a child's cognitive skills (e.g., acquired knowledge, information processing). The target behaviors typically reflect a child's mastery of self-regulatory capacities (e.g., behavioral modulation, problem solving) and their match with the situation at hand; these are experienced in an online and dynamic fashion and are elicited in specific contexts and relationships. At the "micro" level, examples of the latter include problem-solving strategies en route to task solution, inability to maintain age-expected inhibitory control (of movement or verbal output) while simultaneously processing information, manifestations of anxiety or distress in the context of testing, and so forth. At the "macro" level, examples involve failure to match behavior to the expectations or constraints of the context, as seen in atypical patterns of motor activity level, verbal activity level, or emotional expression, or failure to appreciate culturally expected interpersonal distances or individual interpersonal boundaries.

Failing to capture diagnostically important but "invisible" behaviors is not the only constraint. Even with the best of current algorithms—ones that can, say, correctly assign 85% of presenting patients to a given diagnostic category—the clinician is still tasked with the decision as to whether the individual in front of him or her is in the 85% or the 15%. Moreover, just because a given patient sample is identified through rigorous empirical methods as having, on average, a distinctive neurobehavioral profile does not mean that most (or even any) of the individuals within that sample have a profile matching that average. Formal analytic methods for improving clinical decision making using quantitative data are available (e.g., receiver operating characteristic analysis; Youngstrom, 2014) and have promise for neuropsychological assessment (Ransom et al., 2016). As these and other advances in automation and technology (e.g., computer-aided test administration) are incorporated into everyday neuropsychological practice, the need for a better understanding of the nature of clinical expertise will only increase (Miller & Barr, 2017).

We acknowledge that, in principle, all clinical observations could be operationalized and thus quantified. The rise of "Big Data" and Artificial Intelligence (AI), especially integrated with neurosymbolic models (e.g., Smolensky, 2019), means that it will presumably be possible one day to create algorithms with sufficiently fine-grained analyses of moment-to-moment behavior changes between clinician and child to render highly individualized diagnostic formulations to guide equally individualized management plans. The application of such developing technologies to neuropsychology and their value in making the evidence base for the discipline more meaningful has been discussed by Bilder (2011). Without a doubt, advances in any field come from advances in technology (Bernstein, 2010). However, the ability to choose and use the knowledge so gained in the service of an individual is not inherent in the technology; the challenge of understanding how we do this remains. In the meantime, more rigorous analysis of what clinicians actually do to achieve positive clinical outcomes is needed, for clinicians and AI algorithm developers, as well as our patients and their families.

IN CONCLUSION

In this chapter we have raised several themes that we believe to be important for the field of pediatric neuropsychology as it moves from research to practice, and back again. First, what skilled clinicians learn to do on behalf of children and families is quite remarkable. We need to understand it better. The clinician's role has at various times been viewed as one of "formulator," "interpreter," "conceptualizer," or "translator." Yet, from our perspective, none of these metaphors truly captures the essence of the clinician's thinking process; they all seem too static and unidirectional. Metaphors are, however, powerful tools for thinking (Lakoff & Johnson, 1980; Thibodeau, Matlock, & Flusberg, 2019) and creativity in both scientific and artistic domains (Ox & Van Der Elst, 2011), and can be particularly valuable when the goal is to communicate complex and dynamic processes of thinking that cannot be captured by linear narratives. We find two complementary metaphors useful in trying to capture the dynamic creativity that we believe is at the core of expertise: one, an attractor in a dynamical system; the other, the spreading activation of nodes within a dynamic network. Both try to capture the actively changing nature of the clinician's thinking process. An attractor network in a dynamical system (Kenrick, 2001; van Geert, 2009) is a set of values toward which a system tends to evolve from a wide variety of starting conditions. As the clinician obtains each new piece of information on a moment-to-moment basis, the continually evolving (often latent) knowledge bases available through training and experience are activated—and relevant attractors (possible diagnoses, formulations, etc.) form and reform until equilibrium around a diagnostic formulation is achieved. In contrast to the spiraling shape of an attractor as typically represented, the dynamic network metaphor (e.g., Stam, 2014) highlights more of a starburst pattern in which, over time, nodes link, relink, and link again according to changing probabilities, creating new structures of relationships between behaviors and behavioral domains that shape the eventual diagnosis (see Plate 24.1 in the color insert).

Second, we need to pay more systematic attention to the development of clinical expertise and the teaching of evidence-based thinking. How is it learned? How do we teach it? As a rough approximation, formal training programs provide exposure to the evidence, the knowledge bases of the discipline; advanced clinical training (fellowship, professional certification programs) fosters the expertise that is at the core of clinical work through application, feedback, practice, and refinement (Mehta & Fine, 2019). The latter can only be developed through experience with actual patients and in real time with the help of supervisors whose role it is to prompt the trainee's attention to one knowledge base or another, facilitating access to relevant data for the ongoing analysis, and nudging the trainee toward the equilibrium/structure at the core of the clinical thinking process.

Third, the clinical neuropsychologist is in a strange, almost contradictory, space. On the one hand, he or she is tasked with assessing an individual with a given condition and needs to understand the nature and impact of the condition. Here, the primary unit of analysis is the condition. On the other hand, the goal of the clinical work itself is the optimization of the child's lived experience over time. Here, the child is the primary unit of analysis. On the one hand, developmental variables can be considered almost as moderator variables acting on the trajectory of a specific disorder. On the other hand, development itself is the core underlying process. From this perspective, the specific disorders function as moderator variables to derail or divert an optimal developmental trajectory for each child. Central to the KB→CC problem is the need to negotiate this apparent contradiction.

And finally, given that we deal in "broken brains," clinical neuropsychologists need to remember that these cannot be fixed like broken bones. Central to our professional identity is the fact that we are also psychologists and, as such, deal in adaptation and coping, resilience and wellness. Our goal is to help a child and family to match available capacities to the real demands of everyday life, that is, to optimize their *lived experience.* Success in life is highly personal; it depends on one's own conception of success within one's own sociocultural environment (Sternberg, 1999). Subsequent to neuropsychological disorder, success in life may be achieved because some derailed capacities can be rendered functionally adaptive through rehearsal and practice. Other successes will require realistic matching of available capacities, environmental demands, and personal values to achieve individual goals. Still others will only follow from a reenvisioning of the child's future. In most instances, a combination of these approaches contributes to positive outcomes.

Increasing the knowledge base does not in and of itself address the clinician's primary responsibility: to make a meaningful difference to the lived experience of a child developing along a nontypical or new trajectory. Efforts to expand the knowledge base are necessary but are by no means sufficient to do the job. Only by means of evidence-based thinking by the clinician, drawing on both the knowledge base and models that are informed by the transactions between brain and context throughout development, can we hope to achieve the outcomes we desire for our patients. Without the mediation of the skilled clinician, the knowledge base is just that—knowledge. It is the clinician who conceptualizes that knowledge clinically; it is the clinician who makes it relevant not to a "case" but to a child.

CASE EXAMPLE

Referral: 11-year-old girl, high-risk acute lymphoblastic leukemia (ALL) diagnosed at age 7, treated with cranial irradiation and high-dose methotrexate; now presenting with academic and socioemotional difficulties.

Method-Clinician: Consults knowledge base for ALL+treatment; reviews medical variables, neurobehavioral profile, and outcomes of disorder; recognizes that ALL is not a local lesion; appreciates developmental dynamics associated with extended treatment with toxic agents in the developing child and potential dynamics as child continues to develop. Presents case to supervisor: 11-year-old girl–history: family, developmental, medical, psychological, academic–neurobehavioral profile: age-expected knowledge and skills overall; domains implicated: language, executive skills, verbal and visual recall (poor input processing limits recall of information); psychological adjustment of concern. In discussion, provides excellent analysis of what was actively developing over the time frame of treatment and how this might be reflected in the neurobehavioral profile at the time of evaluation.

Method-Supervisor: Notes age at time of insult/age at time of testing; prompts consideration of a longer developmental perspective by querying details of the child's lived experience from the very beginning; obtains history of significant adverse events in the child's first year of life, raising questions as to the integrity of the developmental trajectory prior to birth and immediately thereafter.

Result: Activation of another (critical) knowledge base for the clinician, that of the nature and impact (both immediate and long term) of specific types of adverse events. In this particular situation, the clinician needs to take into account the experience of medicalization/hospitalization for a child whose system may already be upregulated with respect to managing allostasis (Danese & McEwen, 2012); this can be expected to amplify the stressors of the medical condition and its treatment.

Impact: What difference does this make? Not much perhaps with respect to the diagnostic statement (in terms of numbers, domains of behavior affected) at the time of testing, but potentially a great deal to the overall *formulation*—in terms of an understanding of the child, their development and their adjustment—that can be expected to have specific implications for the overall management plan, now and in the future. In fact, the new information changes the landscape significantly. The ALL-and-its-treatment is not a new perturber of the system that changes the developmental dynamics thereafter. The perturbation secondary to the ALL+treatment is taking place in a system that was already perturbed by an earlier event. The knowledge base relevant to the medical condition needs to be added to the knowledge base relevant to the impact of major psychosocial stressors in early life on brain (and thus behavior) development thereafter. This "double whammy" is all too likely to shape the child's coping strategies throughout her lifetime. Delineation of the neuropsychological profile at age 11, however expert and detailed, does not access all the relevant knowledge bases needed to do justice to the child's experience, nor does it provide the level of understanding on the basis of which the clinician can make a meaningful difference to the child's future adjustment.

REFERENCES

American Psychological Association, Presidential Task Force on Evidence-Based Practice. (2006). Evidence-based practice in psychology. *American Psychologist, 61*(4), 271–285.

Barkham, M., & Mellor-Clark, J. (2003). Bridging evidence-based practice and practice-based evidence: Developing a rigorous and relevant knowledge for the psychological therapies. *Clinical Psychology and Psychotherapy, 10,* 319–327.

Bernstein, J. H. (2000). Developmental neuropsychological assessment. In K. O. Yeates, M. D. Ris, & H. G. Taylor (Eds.), *Pediatric neuropsychol-*

ogy: Research, theory, and practice (pp. 405–438). New York: Guilford Press.

Bernstein, J. H. (2010). Developmental models in pediatric neuropsychology. In J. Donders & S. J. Hunter (Eds.), *Principles and practice of lifespan developmental neuropsychology* (pp. 17–40). Cambridge, UK: Cambridge University Press.

Bernstein, J. H., & Weiler, M. D. (2000). Pediatric neuropsychological assessment examined. In G. Goldstein & M. Hersen (Eds.), *Handbook of psychological assessment* (3rd ed., pp. 263–300). New York: Pergamon.

Bilder, R. M. (2011). Neuropsychology 3.0. *Journal of the International Neuropsychological Society, 17*(1), 7–13.

Chelune, G. J. (2010). Evidence-based research and practice in clinical neuropsychology. *Clinical Neuropsychologist, 24,* 454–467.

Danese, A., & McEwen, B. S. (2012). Adverse childhood experiences, allostasis, allostatic load, and age-related disease. *Physiology and Behavior, 106,* 29–39.

Dennis, M. (1988). Language and the young damaged brain. In T. Boll & B. K. Bryant (Eds.), *Clinical neuropsychology and brain function* (pp. 85–123). Washington, DC: American Psychological Association.

Dennis, M., Spiegler, B. J., Simic, N., Sinopoli, K. J., Wilkinson, A., Yeates, K. O., . . . Fletcher, J. M. (2014). Functional plasticity in childhood brain disorders: When, what, how, and whom to assess. *Neuropsychology Review, 24*(4), 389–408.

Geary, D. C. (2008). An evolutionarily informed education science. *Educational Psychologist, 43,* 179–195.

Greenberg, L. S., & Newman, F. L. (1996). An approach to psychotherapy change process research: Introduction to the special section. *Journal of Consulting and Clinical Psychology, 64,* 435–438.

Greenhalgh, T., Howick, J., Maskrey, N., Brassey, J., Burch, D., Burton, M., . . . Spence, D. (2014). Evidence based medicine: A movement in crisis? *BMJ (Online), 348,* 1–7.

Grodzinsky, G. M., Forbes, P. W., & Bernstein, J. H. (2010). A practice-based approach to group identification in nonverbal learning disorders. *Child Neuropsychology, 16*(5), 433–460.

Holmes-Bernstein, J. H., & Waber, D. P. (1990). Developmental neuropsychological assessment: The systemic approach. In A. A. Boulton, G. B. Baker, & M. Hiscock (Eds.), *Neuromethods: Neuropsychology* (pp. 17–40). Clifton, NJ: Humana Press.

Institute of Medicine. (2001). *Crossing the quality chasm: A new health system for the 21st century.* Washington, DC: National Academies Press.

Jinha, A. (2010). Article 50 million: An estimate of the number of scholarly articles in existence. *Learned Publishing, 23*(3), 258–263.

Karmiloff-Smith, A. (1998). Development itself is the key to understanding developmental disorders. *Trends in Cognitive Sciences, 2*(10), 389–398.

Kenrick, D. T. (2001). Evolutionary psychology, cognitive science, and dynamical systems: Building an integrative paradigm. *Current Directions in Psychological Science, 10*(1), 13–17.

Krueger, D. D., & Bear, M. F. (2010). Toward fulfilling the promise of molecular medicine in fragile X syndrome. *Annual Review of Medicine, 62,* 411–429.

Lakoff, G., & Johnson, M. (1980). *Metaphors we live by.* Chicago: University of Chicago Press.

Lewis, M. (2016). *The Undoing Project: A friendship that changed our minds.* New York: Norton.

McCall, R. B. (2009). Evidence-based programming in the context of practice and policy and commentaries. *Social Policy Report, 23*(3), 1–20.

Mehta, J., & Fine, S. (2019). *In search of deeper learning: The quest to remake the American high school.* Cambridge, MA: Harvard University Press.

Miller, J. B., & Barr, W. B. (2017). The technology crisis in neuropsychology. *Archives of Clinical Neuropsychology, 32*(5), 541–554.

Ox, J., & Van Der Elst, J. (2011). How metaphor functions as a vehicle of thought: Creativity as a necessity for knowledge building and communication. *Journal of Visual Art Practice, 10*(1), 83–102.

Ransom, D. M., Burns, A. R., Youngstrom, E. A., Vaughan, C. G., Sady, M. D., & Gioia, G. A. (2016). Applying an evidence-based assessment model to identify students at risk for perceived academic problems following concussion. *Journal of the International Neuropsychological Society, 22*(10), 1038–1049.

Smolensky, P. (2019). Next-generation architectures bridge gap between neural and symbolic representations with neural symbols. Retrieved from *www.microsoft.com/en-us/research/blog/next-generation-architectures-bridge-gap-between-neural-and-symbolic-representations-with-neural-symbols.*

Stam, C. J. (2014). Modern network science of neurological disorders. *Nature Reviews Neuroscience, 15*(10), 683–695.

Sternberg, R. J. (1999). The theory of successful intelligence. *Review of General Psychology, 3*(4), 292–316.

Stiles, J., Reilly, J. S., Levine, S. C., Trauner, D. A., & Nass, R. (2012). *Neural plasticity and cognitive development: Insights from children with perinatal brain injury*. New York: Oxford University Press.

Thibodeau, P. H., Matlock, T., & Flusberg, S. J. (2019). The role of metaphor in communication and thought. *Linguistics and Language Compass, 13*(5), e12327.

van Geert, P. (2009). Nonlinear complex dynamical systems in developmental psychology. In S. J. Guastello, M. Koopmans, & D. Pincus (Eds.), *Chaos and complexity in psychology: The theory of nonlinear dynamical systems* (pp. 242–281). New York: Cambridge University Press.

Vanderploeg, R. D. (1994). Interview and testing: The data collection phase of neuropsychological evaluations. In *Clinician's guide to neuropsychological assessment* (pp. 1–41). Cambridge, MA: Erlbaum.

Yeates, K. O., Bigler, E. D., Dennis, M., Gerhardt, C. a, Rubin, K. H., Stancin, T., . . . Vannatta, K. (2007). Social outcomes in childhood brain disorder: a heuristic integration of social neuroscience and developmental psychology. *Psychological Bulletin, 133*(3), 535–556.

Yeates, K. O., Taylor, H. G., Walz, N. C., Stancin, T., & Wade, S. L. (2010). The family environment as a moderator of psychosocial outcomes following traumatic brain injury in young children. *Neuropsychology, 24*(3), 345–356.

Youngstrom, E. A. (2014). A primer on receiver operating characteristic analysis and diagnostic efficiency statistics for pediatric psychology: We are ready to ROC. *Journal of Pediatric Psychology, 39*(2), 204–221.

Index

Note. t, f, or *n* after a page number indicates a table, a figure, or a note.

B

C

E

F

G

N

O

P

T

U

V

W

X